ST. ALBANS CITY HOSPITAL
LIBRARY

KU-346-620

THE SPLEEN

To Madeleine

THE SPLEEN
Structure, function and clinical significance

Edited by
Anthony J. Bowdler

Professor of Medicine
Marshall University School of Medicine
Huntington, West Virginia

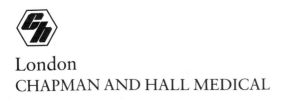

London
CHAPMAN AND HALL MEDICAL

First published in 1990 by
Chapman and Hall Ltd
11 New Fetter Lane, London EC4P 4EE

Published in the USA by
Van Nostrand Reinhold
115 Fifth Avenue, New York, NY 10003

© 1990 Chapman and Hall

Typeset in 10/12 Sabon by
Acorn Bookwork, Salisbury
Printed in Great Britain at the
University Press, Cambridge

ISBN 0 412 29120 7
(USA) 0 442 31209 1

All rights reserved. No part of this book may be
reprinted or reproduced, or utilized in any form or
by any electronic, mechanical or other means,
now known or hereafter invented, including photo-
copying and recording, or in any information storage
and retrieval system, without permission in writing
from the publisher.

British Library Cataloguing in Publication Data

The Spleen.
  1. Man. Spleen
  I. Bowdler, Anthony J.
  612'.41

ISBN 0 412 29120 7

Library of Congress Cataloguing in
Publication Data available

CONTENTS

CONTRIBUTORS

DAVID R. ANDERSON MD
Research Fellow
Department of Medicine,
McMaster University Medical Centre,
Hamilton, Ontario, Canada.

PETER S. AMENTA I PhD
Professor and Chairman,
Department of Anatomy,
Hahnemann University School of Medicine,
Philadelphia, Pennsylvania, United States.

PETER S. AMENTA II MD, PhD
Assistant Professor of Pathology and
   Laboratory Medicine,
Hahnemann University School of Medicine,
Philadelphia, Pennsylvania, United States.

ANTHONY J. BOWDLER MD, PhD, BSc,
   FRCP Lond, FRC Path, FACP
Professor of Medicine,
Marshall University School of Medicine,
Huntington, West Virginia, United States.

JACK K. CHAMBERLAIN MD, FACP
Associate Professor of Medicine,
East Carolina University School of Medicine,
Greenville, North Carolina, United States.

T. K. CHAN MD, FRCP, FRCPE
Professor of Medicine and Head,
Department of Medicine,
University of Hong Kong,
Queen Mary Hospital,
Hong Kong.

STEBBINS B. CHANDOR MD
Professor and Chairman,
Department of Pathology,
Marshall University School of Medicine,
Huntington, West Virginia, United States.

ABRAHAM H. DACHMAN MD
Associate Professor of Radiology,
Uniformed Services University of the Health
   Sciences,
Bethesda, Maryland and
Chief, Section of Gastrointestinal Radiology,
Walter Reed Army Medical Center,
Washington, DC, United States.

W. JEAN DODDS DVM
Chief, Laboratory of Hematology,
Wadsworth Center for Laboratories and
   Research,
State of New York Department of Health,
Albany, New York, United States.

PETER N. FOSTER BA, BM, BCh, MRCP
Senior Registrar,
Yorkshire Regional Health Authority,
Yorkshire, England.

GEOFFREY J. GORSE MD, FACP
Associate Professor of Medicine,
Division of Infectious Diseases,
Department of Internal Medicine,
St Louis University School of Medicine,
St Louis, Missouri, United States.

ALAN C. GROOM PhD
Professor and Immediate Past-Chairman,
Department of Medical Biophysics,
University of Western Ontario,
London, Ontario, Canada.

JOHN G. KELTON MD
Professor of Medicine and Pathology,
McMaster University Medical Centre and
Deputy Director, Canadian Red Cross Blood
   Transfusion Service,
Hamilton Centre, Ontario, Canada.

WILLIAM C. KOPP PhD
Assistant Professor,
Department of Microbiology,
Marshall University School of Medicine,
Huntington, West Virginia, United States.

M. S. LOSOWSKY MD, FRCP
Professor of Medicine and Head, Department
    of Medicine,
University of Leeds,
St James' Hospital,
Leeds, England.

PETER C. RAICH MD, FACP
American Cancer Society Professor of Clinical
    Oncology,
and Chief, Section of Hematology/Oncology,
West Virginia University Health Sciences
    Center,
Department of Medicine,
Morgantown, West Virginia, United States.

RICHARD J. ROLFES MD
Associate Chief Resident, Department of
    Radiology,
University of Florida College of Medicine,
Gainesville, Florida, United States.

PABLO R. ROS MD
Associate Professor and Director,
Division of Abdominal Imaging, Department
    of Radiology,
University of Florida College of Medicine,
Gainesville, Florida, United States.

CAROL E. H. SCOTT-CONNER MD, PhD,
    FACS
Associate Professor of Surgery,
University of Mississippi Medical Center,
Jackson, Mississippi, United States.

ERIC E. SCHMIDT BSc, MCS
Research Technologist,
Department of Medical Biophysics,
University of Western Ontario,
London, Ontario, Canada.

G. R. SERJEANT CMG, MD, FRCP
Director, Medical Research Council
    Laboratories,
University of the West Indies,
Kingston, Jamaica, WI.

MICHAEL T. SHAW MD, FRCP, FACP, DCH
Clinical Professor of Medicine, Department of
    Medicine,
Mariopa Medical Center,
Phoenix, Arizona, United States.

DAVID TODD MD, FRCP, FRCPE, FRCP,
    Glasg, FRACP
Professor and former Head, Department of
    Medicine,
University of Hong Kong,
Queen Mary Hospital,
Hong Kong.

P. J. TOGHILL MD, FRCP
Consultant Physician, Department of Medicine,
University Hospital,
Nottingham, England.

AAGE VIDEBAEK MD
Professor of Internal Medicine,
Gentofte University Hospital,
Copenhagen, Denmark.

LEON WEISS MD
Grace Lansing Lambert Professor of Cell
    Biology,
The Laboratory of Experimental Hematology
    and Cell Biology,
School of Veterinary Medicine,
Professor of Cell Biology (Division of
    Hematology) Medical School,
University of Pennsylvania,
Philadelphia, Pennsylvania, United States.

ACKNOWLEDGEMENTS

Dr Leon Weiss acknowledges the permission of Baillière Tindall Ltd to use Figure 3.1 which is modified from Figure 2 of L. Weiss (1983) *Clinics in Haematology*, **12**, 381.

Dr Jack Chamberlain wishes to thank M. Kashimura and T. Fujita for the use of Figure 2.1; T. Fujita, M. Kashimura and K. Adachi for Figure 2.2; T. Fujita, M. Kashimura and K. Adachi for Figure 2.3; T. Fujita for Figures 2.5, 2.6 and 2.8; L. T. Chen and L. Weiss for Figure 2.9; S. Sasou for Figure 2.10 and their respective publishers as cited in the figure captions.

Dr Alan Groom and E. E. Schmidt acknowledge with thanks the permission to use the following figures in Chapter 4: W. B. Saunders of Philadelphia for Figure 4.1; the Oxford University Press of New York for Figure 4.23; the American Physiological Society for Figures 4.29 and 4.33. In addition permission was given by the publishers of the *American Journal of Physiology* for Figures 4.2, 4.4, 4.5 and 4.6; by *Microvascular Research* for Figures 4.3, 4.25 and 4.26; by the *Archivum Histologicum Japonicum* for Figures 4.7 and 4.8; by the *Journal of Morphology* for Figures 4.10, 4.14, 4.15, 4.16, 4.20, 4.30, 4.31, 4.34 and 4.39; by the *American Journal of Anatomy* for Figures 4.13, 4.17, 4.18, 4.21, 4.22, 4.35, 4.40 and 4.41; by the *Journal of Electron Microscopy* for Figures 4.11 and 4.36; by the *Anatomical Record* for Figure 12; by *Blood Cells* for Figure 24; and by *Cell and Tissue Research* for Figures 4.27, 4.37a, 4.37b and 4.38. These authors also acknowledge the support of research funding from the Medical Research Council of Canada.

Dr W. Jean Dodds acknowledges the support of the National Heart, Lung and Blood Institute (USA) provided by NIH Research Grant HL 09902 for her work described in Chapter 6.

Drs A. J. Bowdler and A. Videbaek acknowledge the permission to publish granted by Baillière Tindall Ltd for Figure 8.3, and the American College of Physicians for Figure 8.1. Likewise they wish to thank Blackwell Scientific Publications Ltd for permission to reproduce Figures 8.4, 8.6, 8.9 and 8.10 from the *British Journal of Haematology*, and to acknowledge the use of Figures 8.7 and 8.8 from the *Scandinavian Journal of Haematology*.

Drs P. N. Foster and M. S. Losowsky acknowledge the permission granted by *Pediatrics* to reproduce Figure 11.3, originally published in *Pediatrics*, **76**, 392 (1985).

Drs David R. Anderson and John Kelton acknowledge with thanks the permission of Grune and Stratton, Inc. to use Figure 13.2 in Chapter 13. These authors also acknowledge the grant made to them by the Medical Research Council of Canada which supported part of the work described in Chapter 13.

Dr Michael Shaw acknowledges the permission of Blackwell Scientific Publications Ltd, publishers of the *British Journal of Haematology*, **43**, 69–77 (1979) to reproduce Figure 14.1.

Dr Peter C. Raich acknowledges support from The American Cancer Society and the assistance of Annorah Cale and Margo Neal in preparing the manuscript for Chapter 15.

Dr G. R. Serjeant acknowledges the permission of the publishers to reproduce the following figures: Baillière Tindall Ltd for Figure 16.2; Blackwell Scientific Publications for Figure 16.3; the *New England Journal of Medicine* for Figure 16.4; the *Archives of Diseases of Child-*

hood for Figures 16.5 and 16.8; the *Journal of Pediatrics* for Figure 16.7; the Oxford University Press for 16.9; and the *British Medical Journal* for 16.11.

Drs R. J. Rolfes, P. R. Ros and A. H. Dachman wish to thank Williams and Wilkins for permission to reproduce Figure 17.22 from the *American Journal of Radiology*, and the publishers of *Radiology* for the use of Figures 17.40 and 17.41.

Dr C. E. H. Scott-Conner acknowledges the skilled assistance of Michael P. Schenk who was responsible for the illustrations of Chapter 18.

PREFACE

INTRODUCTION

The last several years have seen a remarkable improvement in our understanding of the spleen, especially with respect to structure, and how this is related functionally to the many formed elements which perfuse the spleen from the general circulation. To this must be added the very considerable body of knowledge which has evolved from clinical experience. This book is the work of many authors of diverse expertise; each has provided an overview of his own area of interest, sometimes as a summary of the present state of the field, and sometimes with new information which has yet to be integrated into a more global understanding of the organ.

The spleen as yet belongs to no single discipline, and interest is shared among anatomists, basic circulatory physiologists, hematologists, immunologists, infectious disease physicians, surgeons and many others. It is our intent that this book will present an overview of current understanding of the spleen, and provide a stimulus to continuing interest in the organ across many specialties. Several areas of considerable interest have had to be addressed in the context of other primary subjects, in order to keep the book within a moderate compass. However, individual authors have not been prevented from discussing some aspects of subjects which are given in greater detail in other chapters, when these have been relevant to their principal theme. In an expanding field of interest it is to be expected that specific concepts and data will be perceived differently from various specialized viewpoints. Consequently I have not rigorously excluded some overlap in the subject matter, where this has been important to the development of the themes of more than one contributor.

THE STUDY OF THE SPLEEN

CLASSICAL STUDIES OF SPLEEN STRUCTURE AND FUNCTION

Of all the formed organs studied in the fields of medicine and mammalian biology, the spleen has until recently been the most difficult to place within the economy of the organism. Speculation concerning the spleen in the classical period commonly ascribed a digestive function to the organ: Hippocrates, Aristotle and subsequently Galen supported the concept of an interchange of humors between the spleen and the stomach, probably through the short gastric vessels. However, there was later considerable doubt as to the mechanism of such a process, and for centuries the spleen remained Galen's 'organ of mystery'. It was for Vesalius (1514–1564 AD) to demonstrate that the postulated transfer was untenable on anatomical grounds. Nevertheless, the concept of a secretory function for the spleen died slowly, and even Malpighi inclined to the view that the lymphoid follicles of the spleen were minute secretory glands.

An insight into the special relationship between circulating blood and the spleen was evident in the suggestion by van Leeuwenhoeck (1632–1723 AD) that the spleen plays a role in the elaboration and 'purification' of the blood. Stukely, in his Goulstonian lecture of 1722, showed remarkable prescience when, relying essentially on macroscopic structure, he rejected a secretory function for the organ, and proposed that it was a 'diverticulum of the systemic circulation, filling and emptying with blood and acting as a controller of blood volume'. This idea, with modifications, was supported by investigators such as Cooper, Winslow, Heister, and Hodgkin. In 1854 Gray, of Gray's *Textbook of Anatomy*, described his extensive researches into the comparative anatomy of the spleen, and concluded that its function 'is to regulate the quantity and quality of the blood'. He was especially impressed by the variable size of the equine spleen, and was also aware of the reservoir function of the spleen in diving mammals. Subsequently the control of the quantity of circulating red cells by the spleen received much more attention than the control of quality, and researches by Barcroft and his colleagues in the period between 1923 and 1932 clarified many of the factors influencing this control in small mammals. Other studies relevant to this function were performed by Scheunert, Cannon and Cruickshank. Unfortunately it was many years before it was recognized that the physiological storage of blood cells is not a significant feature of the human spleen: indeed, with an average red cell content of 30–50 ml, there is no potential for augmenting the circulating red cell mass by the human spleen.

CLINICAL CONCEPTS: AN INTERMEDIATE PERIOD

One of the principal barriers to developing an understanding of the physiology of the human spleen has been the considerable interspecies variability of both function and structure. Among these are the variable degree of smooth muscle development in the capsule and trabeculae, the structural differences between sinusal and non-sinusal spleens, and the relative development of arteriolar sheaths. These all suggest variations in function, which has made more complex the interpretation of animal studies and their relevance to human pathophysiology.

Uncertainty with respect to the validity of available animal models led clinicians to organize their clinical experiences conceptually in terms of postulated or apparently necessary splenic functions. Once the operation of splenectomy had been shown to be a reasonably safe procedure, and experience had been gained in the context of trauma to the organ, it was applied to the treatment of various disorders showing cell deficits in the blood. Conditions now identified as hereditary spherocytosis and idiopathic thrombocytopenic purpura were treated successfully by removal of the spleen, and later the procedure was applied to a heterogeneous group of disorders showing blood cell deficits under the rubric of 'hypersplenism'.

The original concept of 'hypersplenism' was that of a pathogenic process whereby the spleen affected the hemopoietic activity of the bone marrow by a process analogous to the excessive endocrine activity of hyperthyroidism. This concept, first put forward by Chauffard in relation to hereditary spherocytosis in 1907, later culminated in a prolonged debate in the literature, between Dameshek as the proponent of a humoral influence on the bone marrow, and those such as Doan, who proposed that cell deficits such as thrombocytopenia are due to cell destruction mediated by the spleen.

The concept of 'hypersplenism' has proved useful in a strictly clinical context, in that it describes a situation commonly found with one or more cell deficits in the peripheral blood, usually associated with enlargement of the spleen, and with a normal or excessive representation of the relevant cell precursors in the bone marrow. The term also carries the implication that the deficit will be corrected by splenectomy. It is important, however, to recognize that this is purely a syndromatic connotation, and does not imply a specific mechanism for the deficit. Indeed, the cause of a cytopenia is often multifactorial, and it is of interest that the early debates on mechanism did not recognize the possibility of a dilutional form of anemia, which is probably the commonest factor in these circumstances. Nor did they recognize the 'maldistribution thrombocytopenia' resulting from increased platelet pooling in the enlarged spleen.

Following this period, further clinical studies were made of hereditary spherocytosis, in which splenectomy corrects anemia without affecting the underlying membrane disorder of the spherocytes. The work of Lawrence Young, T. A. J. Prankerd, Robert Weed and others showed that the spleen responds to the abnormal shape of red cells by impeding their flow through the organ, conditioning them to hemolysis both in the spleen and elsewhere, and disposing of a proportion of the damaged red cells in the organ itself.

Study of the mechanisms affecting the survival of red cells in conditions such as hereditary spherocytosis, in which the spleen plays so predominant a part, led to recognition of the importance of physical factors in the relationship of the spleen to blood cells. These gave pathophysiological meaning to concepts such as cell deformability, membrane rigidity, cell fragmentation, conditioning and cell pooling. In one sense, such physical concepts have been a counterpoise to the assumptions made with respect to the special biological processes ascribed to the spleen, such as sequestration and hypersplenism, and have introduced a rigor into the investigation of the spleen which has been highly productive.

In a more general context, Crosby introduced the idea of the complete removal ('culling') and partial removal ('pitting') of red cells from the circulation. Such clinicopathological concepts were instrumental in leading to a search for the basic structures whereby the spleen could interact with red cells in this fashion.

CHANGING CONCEPTS OF THE SIGNIFICANCE OF THE SPLEEN

It is still within the professional memory of many physicians still practising, that removal of the spleen by splenectomy was believed to carry no subsequent functional penalty, and indeed that there was no indispensable function of the spleen which could not be undertaken by organs and tissues elsewhere. Likewise it was commonly believed that the clinically enlarged spleen was invariably abnormal, and conversely that the abnormal spleen necessarily showed enlargement. Even though these clinical expectations have now been critically modified, it is of interest to look at the seminal concepts of the last 30 years, to identify those observations which have markedly changed the clinician's view of the significance of splenic disorders.

Studies with labeled red cells

The advent of radionuclide labeling for red cells, and later with more difficulty for platelets, radically changed the level of understanding of the relationship between the spleen and blood cells. In view of the red cell debris and liberated iron which remained in the spleen following the phagocytosis of red cells, it was anticipated that hemolysis would result in the accumulation of the labeling nuclide, usually chromium-51, in the organ responsible for destruction. Nuclide accumulation was detectable at the body surface, and patterns of increase in surface radioactivity were described; these were initially held to reflect a process of 'sequestration'. Sequestration was at first regarded as equivalent to destruction, but more careful analysis showed that radioactivity detectable at the body surface had several components, each of which varied individually with time. These consisted of the background radioactivity from red cells in the general circulation, that from a pool of red cells very slowly exchanging with the circulating red cells, and the subsequently slowly accumulated nuclide from cells destroyed in the organ. The processes of conditioning and spleen-dependent destruction at other sites were identified largely but not exclusively by inference.

The evidence of an exchanging red cell pool was especially important, as it implied that in pathological circumstances the circulation through the spleen might depart critically from normal. No other organ has been shown to have a comparable pooling component, and in some circumstances it appears to have an important effect on red cell life span. With respect to the red cell, pooling in man is essentially pathological; however, it was subsequently shown that platelets also pool in the spleen, and in this case the pool is present in normal circumstances, and expands when the spleen enlarges.

The postsplenectomy state

The recognition that splenectomy in infancy and early childhood could result in exceptional susceptibility to infection abruptly increased the clinical significance of the loss of splenic function. This has resulted in practical changes in clinical management, such as the deferring of elective splenectomy in young children, and has directed attention to the detailed consequences of impaired function of the spleen. The study of the hyposplenic state has, in fact, contributed extensively to the present understanding of the functions of the spleen, and indeed has proved to be much more informative than the investigation of 'hypersplenism'. It has also stimulated detailed investigation of the immune functions of the spleen, and has led to new surgical approaches to disorders involving the spleen, such as subtotal splenectomy, in order to reduce the disadvantages of the completely hyposplenic state.

The list of disorders which can contribute to the hyposplenic state continues to lengthen, and emphasizes the fact that the spleen has functions which are not readily matched by the compensatory activity of the immune system elsewhere. Recognition that the spleen has a very special role in defense against infection has given a special cogency to recent studies of the function of the red pulp, which are proceeding in both the ultrastructural and clinical fields. Dr Weiss in Chapter 3 describes his recent observations of the red pulp in experimental malaria, which demonstrate the mechanism by which the spleen can exclude intraerythrocytic parasites from infecting healthy red cells.

These observations illustrate well the import-

ance of the spleen to human survival, and perhaps primate evolution. It has been estimated that more than half the deaths which have occurred since the emergence of the human species have been due to malaria, which emphasizes the very significant role which the organ must have played in protecting the survival and evolution of the species.

The significance of the lymphocyte

If the spleen was at one time the classical 'organ of mystery', it is equally true that until recently one of the most enigmatic of cells has been the lymphocyte. The extensive body of knowledge now available on the functions and identity of the lymphocyte has obscured how recent has been the elucidation of its functions, its complex taxonomy, and the subset interactions. It now appears that the spleen has a unique role in the immune system, and houses perhaps one-third of all the circulating lymphocytes. Of special interest to the hematologist is the significance of the spleen to the pathways of spread of the pathological cells in lymphomata, and the relationship of the surface characteristics of lymphocytes to the distribution of disease in these disorders.

Dilution and cell-distribution as mechanisms for blood cell deficits

One mechanism contributing to anemia and other cell deficits which has been recognized since the earlier discussions on 'hypersplenism', has been the dilutional effect caused by the presence of an excess plasma volume in relation to the mass of circulating red cells. Frequently in the anemia accompanying splenomegaly the red cell mass is little changed from that which would be expected from the subject's height and weight. Anemia is then the result of an expansion of plasma volume, in circumstances in which a proportionate expansion of the red cell mass has not occurred despite an increase in total blood volume. This does not seem to be the consequence of control of plasma volume by the spleen, but to result from an expanded total blood volume without a proportionate increase in the number of red cells. It is of interest that such a phenomenon is unrelated to the principal functions of the spleen as presently understood; it appears to be the consequence of the additional vascularity of the organ, and its specific locus in the splanchnic pattern of blood vessels. An additional contributor to the blood cell deficits commonly present with splenomegaly is a maldistribution phenomenon: this is especially evident in the thrombocytopenia associated with the enlarged spleen, since the splenic pool of platelets enlarges in proportion to spleen volume. It is not yet clear why this does not produce a compensatory output of cells from the bone marrow, but a similar phenomenon also contributes in some cases to the anemia of splenomegaly.

Prospects for the clinical management of disorders of the spleen

The study of the spleen has been passing through a particularly productive period, and this is reflected in changes in the surgical approach to the organ. These have yet to be proved effective empirically, but there has evolved a more flexible approach, and a willingness to review long-standing concepts of management in this field. One may reasonably hope that as the properties of the lymphoid system and pulp vasculature become increasingly well defined, there will be a basis for developing a new pharmacology for splenic disorders.

ACKNOWLEDGEMENTS

This appears to be an especially appropriate time to summarize recent and current work, which has proceeded so far in many different fields. I am most grateful to many former colleagues and collaborators for their generous contributions to this work, and also to the publishers for encouraging this restatement of the clinical significance of the spleen, and of the basic biology which makes its understanding possible. I wish to thank the many contributors for their cooperation and high expertise, and to make clear that if there are deficiencies in this work then the responsibility is entirely mine. To any of the workers in this field who may have felt that their efforts have remained unrecognized, I offer my apologies and express the sincere hope that they will not be discouraged from continuing their efforts to unravel the enigmas of this fascinating organ.

Finally, I must acknowledge the influence of John Z. Young, FRS, Emeritus Professor of Anatomy at University College, London, who many years ago introduced me to the task of identifying the functional basis of perceived structure; and also to recall the late Robert I. Weed, MD, who personified the matching of intellectual insight by ingenuity in experiment. I also wish to thank Carolyn Endicott, Jennifer Long and Patsy Dallas of the Word Processing Unit of the Marshall University School of Medicine, for their unfailing patience and expertise. I am also grateful to my wife, Madeleine, who has contributed more than she knows to the completion of this work.

Anthony J. Bowdler
Huntington, West Virginia

A BIBLIOGRAPHY OF THE SPLEEN

Gray, H. (1854) *On the Structure and Use of the Spleen*. Astley Cooper Prize Essay. J. W. Parker, London.

Lewis, S. M. (1983) The spleen – mysteries solved and unresolved. *Clin. Haematol.*, **12**, 363–73.

McCuskey, R. S. (1985) New trends in spleen research. *Experientia*, **41**, 143–284.

Macpherson, A. I. S., Richmond, J. and Stuart, A. E. (1973) *The Spleen*. American Lecture Series, No. 893. Charles C. Thomas, Springfield, Ill.

Moynihan, B. (1921) *The Spleen and Some of its Diseases*. W.B. Saunders, Philadelphia.

Prankerd, T. A. J. (1963) The spleen and anemia. *Br. Med. J.*, **2**, 517–24.

Rosse, W. F. (1987) The spleen as a filter. *N. Engl. J. Med.*, **317**, 704–5.

Videbaek, Aa., Christensen, B. E. and Jonsson, V. (1982) *The Spleen in Health and Disease*. Yearbook Medical Publishers, Copenhagen and Chicago.

Weiss, L., Geduldig, U. and Weidanz, W. (1986) Mechanisms of splenic control of murine malaria: reticular cell activation and the development of a blood-spleen barrier. *Am. J. Anat.*, **176**, 251–85.

Wolf, B. C. and Neiman, R. S. (1988) *Disorders of the Spleen*. W.B. Saunders, Philadelphia and London.

PART ONE

THE STRUCTURE AND FUNCTIONS OF THE SPLEEN

THE ANATOMY OF THE SPLEEN 1

Peter S. Amenta I and Peter S. Amenta II

1.1 INTRODUCTION

The spleen (Gr: splen, L: lien), is a large, soft, vascular lymphatic organ about the size of a clenched fist, possessing the greatest aggregation of lymphoid tissue in the body. Unlike the lymph nodes, which are interposed in chains of lymphatic vessels to filter lymph, the spleen is situated in the course of the blood vascular system to filter blood.

1.2 DEVELOPMENT OF THE SPLEEN

The development of the spleen begins in the fifth week of intrauterine life. Mesenchymal cells, between the two mesothelial layers of the mesogastrium, aggregate and differentiate as the anlage of the spleen. Primitive vessels, during the second month of gestation, vascularize these cellular aggregates to form a lobulated embryonic spleen. Continued growth and formation occurs during fusion of the splenic lobules. By the third fetal month the spleen assumes a recognizable form. From the fourth to the eighth month, the spleen participates with the liver in hemocytopoiesis. After the eighth month and throughout postnatal life, the spleen resumes hemocytopoiesis only when bone marrow is incapable of meeting the demands of the body (extramedullary hemocytopoiesis), or in pathological circumstances. This is discussed further in Chapter 14.

1.3 DIMENSIONS

The measurements of the spleen vary from 12 to 15 cm in length, 4 to 8 cm in width and 3 to 4 cm in thickness. At birth, the difference in average organ weight between males (10.5 g) and females (10.4 g) is insignificant. However, the average weight of the spleen in adult males (180 g) surpasses that of the adult female by 40 g. In later adult life a gradual weight loss occurs, until in the seventh and eighth decades the total weight lost is about 60 g. In disease states the spleen may achieve weights of 2000 g or more. In 1854, a spleen weight of 9 kg was recorded in a patient with malaria (Clemente, 1985).

Size differences may reflect the physiological condition of the subject; for example, an increase in blood pressure is usually accompanied by enlargement, and an increase occurs during and after meals. Starvation and death are characterized by substantial decrease in size. During enlargement or in disease, the spleen protrudes anteriorly and inferiorly so that it may be palpated below the left costal margin. In this position its relationship to the stomach may be appreciated when patients complain of early satiety. Variations in mass and overall dimensions in one individual, and from one individual to another reflect physical condition, time of day, age and sex (see also Chapter 10).

1.4 GENERAL ANATOMY

1.4.1 RELATIONSHIPS

Located superiorly and posteriorly to the cardia of the stomach at the level of the 9th, 10th and

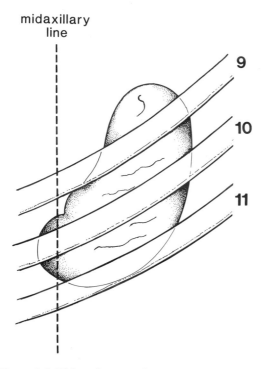

Figure 1.1 This figure demonstrates the diaphragmatic surface of the spleen and its relationship to the 9th, 10th and 11th ribs. Note the fissures on the convex surface.

11th ribs, the spleen nestles between the fundus of the stomach and the diaphragm. Its longest axis parallels the 10th rib (Figure 1.1), with the posterior border extending medially toward the epigastric region. In anatomically embalmed cadavers, the soft, friable spleen is shaped by adjacent, firmer viscera. Against the concavity of the diaphragm, the superior (diaphragmatic) surface assumes a convex shape. Three concavities are impressed into the inferior (visceral) surface: (1) a gastric surface facing anteromedially and superiorly, produced by the greater curvature of the stomach, (2) a renal surface, directed inferomedially, produced by the superior pole of the kidney, and (3) a flat triangular colic surface, produced by the left flexure of the colon (Figure 1.2). The latter is commonly in contact with the tail of the pancreas, which may leave a fourth or pancreatic impression.

1.4.2 ANATOMICAL VARIATION

The variations observed in living subjects in a variety of normal and pathological conditions, should be expected, recognized and appreciated. Resembling a large coffee bean, the spleen is indented on its anterior border by one or more notches, resulting from the fusion of several splenules during histogenesis. Below the notches, where the three concavities of the inferior surface meet, is the hilum, which provides an entrance and an exit for components of the neurovascular bundle (Figure 1.2). Similar notches may appear on the posterior and inferior borders. Fissures on the diaphragmatic surface do not appear to reflect embryonic or primitive lobulation. Occasional isolated spherical nodules of splenic tissue (accessory or supplemental spleens) may reside in the vicinity of the spleen. Commonly called splenculi* (liencu-

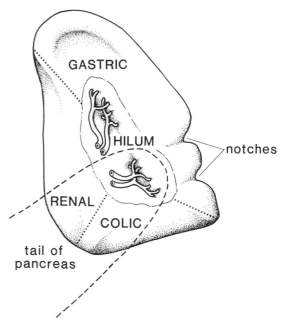

Figure 1.2 This figure reveals the concave surface of the spleen with its three major impressions, notches, hilum and the relationship to the tail of the pancreas. Splenic vessels are also placed in the hilum.

*Commonly known to clinicians as accessory spleens or 'splenunculi'. (ed.)

li), these miniature spleens vary in number from one to 25, and may occur in a condition known as polysplenia. These splenculi range from the size of a garden pea to a meatball. Usually found in connective tissue surrounding the hilum, they also occur in the greater omentum, gastrosplenic ligament, transverse mesocolon and the connective tissue surrounding the splenic vessels. The proximity of the spleen, during development, to the developing testis and ovaries accounts for splenogonadal fusion. Agenesis (asplenia) associated with developmental anomalies of the heart also occurs.

1.4.3 PERITONEAL RELATIONS

Investment by visceral mesothelium forms strong suspensory peritoneal folds which connect the spleen to: (1) the stomach (the gastrosplenic (gastrolienal) ligament), (2) the diaphragm (the phrenicosplenic (phrenicolienal) ligament), and (3) the kidney (the splenorenal (lienorenal) ligament). Branches of the splenic (lienal) artery course in the gastrosplenic ligament. The inferior pole of the spleen is cradled in the gastrocolic ligament (a portion of the greater omentum).

1.4.4 STROMA AND PARENCHYMA

The stroma of the spleen is composed of a thick, fibrous capsule from which collagenous trabeculae emerge to converge upon the hilum. Interconnecting thinner trabecular collagenous bundles subdivide the areas between major trabeculae into small compartments several millimeters in diameter. Delicate reticular fibers radiate from the outer capsule and trabeculae, forming a spongy network which confines and supports the free parenchymal cells and the specialized vasculature.

The parenchyma in fresh surgical specimens appears as grayish-white areas, the white pulp, scattered in a spongy deep-reddish-purple substance, the red pulp. The white pulp consists of 0.2—0.8 mm masses of diffuse and nodular lymphatic tissue surrounding small arteries called central arteries. Like most lymphoid tissue, the white pulp undergoes involution between the ages of 10 and 14. After age 60, the spleen as a whole undergoes involution. The red pulp possesses unique *venous sinuses* supported in a spongy reticular stroma containing free erythrocytes, macrophages, reticular cells and other cells.

1.4.5 BLOOD SUPPLY

The blood supply to the spleen is provided by the *splenic* (lienal) artery, the largest of the three branches of the celiac artery. This tortuous vessel travels horizontally along the body of the pancreas for about 8—32 cm until it reaches the hilum of the spleen. During its course, it sends branches to (1) the stomach (*via* the left gastroepiploic artery and the short gastric artery), (2) the pancreas (*via* the pancreatic artery) and (3) the spleen (*via* the end of the splenic [lienal] artery). About 3.5 cm from the spleen, the splenic artery divides into superior and inferior terminal branches, each of which further subdivides into several smaller branches prior to penetrating the hilum of the spleen. It is not unusual to find several smaller intermediate branches which supply the poles of the spleen. Ramifications of the splenic artery occur internally as the branches pass into the trabeculae. When smaller arterial branches leave trabeculae to enter the small compartments, and acquire coats of diffuse and nodular lymphatic tissue, they are termed central arteries. When an artery decreases to a diameter of 50 μm, it emerges from the coat of lymphatic tissue and ramifies in the red pulp as penicillar arteries composed of endothelium while lacking muscle or adventitial coats. However, when macrophages and reticular cells ensheath some of the penicillar arteries they are named sheathed capillaries, which are more common in lower species. These peculiar capillaries run relatively short distances prior to dividing into terminal, naked (unsheathed), non-fenestrated capillaries. The precise mechanism by which blood is delivered to the spleen's unique venous sinuses is incompletely understood (see Chapters 2, 3 and 4). Some authors postulate that terminal capillaries insert directly into venous sinuses ('closed' theory of circulation). Others maintain that the capillaries pour blood into the red pulp and that erythrocytes enter the venous sinuses from the periphery, by insinuating themselves between elongate endothelial cells arranged along the longitudinal axis of the venous sinus ('open' theory of circulation). (The latest *Nomina Histologica* designates each component cell as endotheliocytus fusiformis, or spindle-shaped endothelial cell.) A compromise suggests that both theories are possible according to physiological demands.

The venous drainage commences in the venous sinuses, located in the red pulp. These flaccid vessels are capable of confining large quantities of blood under low pressure, and may exceed 40 μm in diameter. The fusiform endothelial cells are compared to the staves of a barrel, where reticular fibers (the hoops of the barrel) spiral around the periphery to bind and provide external support. Veins of the red pulp, receiving blood from the venous sinuses, drain into trabecular veins which accompany the trabecular arteries. The trabecular veins terminate in nine branches which unite to form the splenic veins at the hilum. The large diameter splenic vein coursing along the dorsal and superior portion of the pancreas, ultimately joins the portal vein to provide blood to the liver. The splenic vein, with its large caliber, is not as large as the splenic artery under normal conditions. However, in patients with increased portal pressures (such as occurs in cirrhosis) the lumen may achieve a large diameter and the vein can become tortuous. The proximity of the splenic vein to the renal vein has been used to the advantage of patients for anastomoses to bypass a cirrhotic liver and decompress the hypertensive portal venous system.

Lymphatic vessels in the red or white pulp of the human spleen are few. Lymphatic capillaries originating in the capsule and trabeculae converge on lymph nodes of the hilum and pancreatico-duodenal lymph nodes. Efferent vessels from these nodes drain into the celiac preaortic lymph nodes along with the lymphatics from the stomach and pancreas. Nodes in the splenic hilum are often involved in disease processes such as lymphoma, when the spleen is involved. Accessory spleens may be confused with these lymph nodes on gross examination.

1.4.6 NERVE SUPPLY

Nerves (vasomotor postganglionic sympathetic) leave the celiac plexus and follow the splenic artery to the hilum of the spleen, to supply the musculature of the branching vessels. Preganglionic parasympathetic fibers of the right vagus nerve also accompany the splenic artery into the spleen.

TERMINOLOGY

NB Terminology (including spelling) employed in this chapter is recommended by: *Nomina Anatomica* 6th edn, Churchill Livingstone, Edinburgh/London, 1989. (This is a revision by the International Anatomical Nomenclature Committee approved by the 11th International Congress of Anatomists in Mexico City, 1980. *Nomina Histologica* is included in this edition.)

RECOMMENDED BIBLIOGRPAHY

Each of the following has sections or other material devoted to the gross anatomy of the spleen:

Amenta, P. S. (1983) *Histology*, 3rd edn. Medical Examination Publishing Company, Inc., New Hyde Park, New York.
Amenta, P. S. (1987) Elias-Pauly's *Histology and Human Microanatomy*, 5th edn. John Wiley, New York and Toronto.
Bloom, W. and Fawcett, D. W. (1986) *Histology*, 11th edn. W. B. Saunders, Philadelphia, London and Toronto.
Clemente, C. D. (ed.) (1985) Gray's *Anatomy of the Human Body*, 30th American edn, Lea and Febiger, Philadelphia.
Ellis, H. (1974) *Clinical Anatomy*, 5th edn. Blackwell Scientific Publications, Oxford and London.

Grant, J. C. B. (1980) *Method of Anatomy*, 10th edn. (ed. J. V. Basmajian), Williams and Wilkins, Baltimore and London.

Hall-Craggs, E. C. B. (1985) *Anatomy as a Basis for Clinical Medicine*. Urban and Schwarzenberg, Baltimore and Munich.

Hollinshead, W. H. and Rosse, C. (1985) *Textbook of Anatomy*, 4th edn. Harper and Row, Philadelphia.

Moore, K. L. (1985) *Clinically Oriented Anatomy*, 2nd edn. Williams and Wilkins, Baltimore and London.

Nomina Anatomica (1983) 5th edn. Williams and Wilkins, Baltimore and London.

Poirier, J. and Dumas, J.-L. R. (1977) *Review of Medical Histology*. (edited and adapted by P. S. Amenta), W.B. Saunders, Philadelphia, London and Toronto.

Weiss, L. (1983) *Histology, Cell and Tissue Biology*, 5th edn. Elsevier Biomedical, New York, Baltimore and Oxford.

THE MICROANATOMY OF THE SPLEEN IN MAN

Jack K. Chamberlain

2.1 INTRODUCTION

The spleen is a uniquely adapted lymphatic organ which is specialized for the processing of the components of the blood, predominantly in relation to its immunoprotective function (Groom, 1987; McCuskey, 1985; Weiss, 1983). The general structural characteristics of the mammalian spleen are reviewed in Chapter 3, with emphasis on the anatomical basis of the mechanisms whereby particulate elements are removed from the circulation, and by which normal cells passing through the spleen are protected from parasitization from trapped affected cells (Weiss, Geduldig and Weidanz, 1986). Details of the fine structure of the mammalian spleen are further developed in Chapter 4, with emphasis on those concepts which have been accessible to experimentation. The present chapter reviews the ultrastructure of the human spleen and the inferences which can be made with respect to its function and pathophysiology.

In man the organ is highly vascular and distensible, and it receives up to 10% of the cardiac output at rest (Groom, 1987). It is a 'defense' spleen in Weiss's term, rather than a 'storage' spleen, and does not normally contain sufficient red cells in the red pulp to support the function of physiological augmentation of the circulating red cell mass (Wadenvik and Kutti, 1988; Weiss, 1983; see also section 3.2.1).

2.2 THE FUNCTIONS OF THE SPLEEN

The structure of the spleen is largely oriented in relation to its blood vessels, and the microvasculature reflects the principal functions of the organ in both organization and structure (see *inter alia* section 4.3.13). Experimentally these functions have been shown to include the trapping and processing of blood cells (such as reticulocytes and morphologically abnormal cells), the filtration of abnormal particles, the separation of plasma from red cells ('skimming'), and the presentation of particulate materials and their derivatives to cells of the immune system (Groom, 1987; Kashimura and Fujita, 1987; McCuskey, 1985; Weiss, 1983, 1985). In man many of these functions have not been systematically observed in the normal state, but the response of the spleen to abnormal circumstances has provided evidence that such processes occur. For example, radionuclide studies have shown that pathological red cell pooling in the spleen is accompanied by an increase in the concentration of the red cells (Bowdler, 1969; Wadenvik and Kutti, 1988; see also section 8.2.3), suggesting that a plasma skimming mechanism is operative. Reticulocyte counts rise in the peripheral blood following splenectomy, which is consonant with delay (and perhaps maturation) of the cells during passage through the spleen. Pathological red cell pooling may be inhibited by administering epinephrine, which suggests blood flow regulation at the vascular level, since the human spleen shows little capsular muscle (Faller, 1985; Groom, 1987; Reilly, 1985). Furthermore, abnormal particles, such as red cells modified chemically or by antibody, may be shown to be trapped readily by the spleen in man (section 11.2.3). Consequently the principal normal functions of the mammalian spleen, with the exception of storage pooling of red cells, can be inferred to have their counterparts in the spleen in man, although their demonstration has been limited in detail.

Additional functions of the spleen related to normal blood cells include:

1. Trapping of monocytes produced by the bone marrow, and facilitating their transformation to macrophages, many of which develop specialized functions such as antigen presentation (Weiss, 1983; see also sections 5.2.3 and 5.2.4).
2. Recruitment of both T and B lymphocytes and their accessory cells from the circulation, and their conduction into specialized zones of the splenic lymphoid structure where immune responses are mediated (Eikelenboom *et al.*, 1985; McCuskey, 1985; van Ewijk and Nieuwenhuis, 1985; Weiss, 1983, 1985; see also section 5.2.1).
3. Pooling of granulocytes, possibly by means of the exaggeration of the margination of cells, as in small blood vessels elsewhere (McCuskey, 1985; Wadenvik and Kutti, 1988; Weiss, 1983; see also section 8.4).
4. Pooling of platelets, which even in normal circumstances may amount to as many as 30% of the total platelet mass (Groom, 1987; McCuskey, 1985; Wadenvik and Kutti, 1988; Weiss, 1983; see also sections 8.1 and 8.3).

2.3   THE STRUCTURE OF THE HUMAN SPLEEN

2.3.1   THE CAPSULE AND TRABECULAE

The human spleen weighs approximately 150 g in adults. It is enclosed by a capsule composed of dense white connective tissue which contains little smooth muscle (Faller, 1985; Weiss, 1983, 1985). This reflects the minimal role played by active contraction of the capsule and trabeculae in modifying the volume of the human spleen in normal circumstances. The capsule measures 1.1–1.5 mm in thickness, and is covered by serosa except at the hilus where blood vessels, lymphatics and nerves enter the spleen. The capsule consists of two layers of connective tissue distinguished by the orientation of their fibers (Faller, 1985). The fibers themselves are relatively uniform and of medium thickness, consisting principally of collagen: these become finer in the deeper regions where transition to pulp fibers occurs. Elastic fibers are also present in the capsule: these are fine in form in the superficial connective tissue layer, and coarser in the deeper layer of the capsule.

The inner surface of the capsule gives rise to a rich branching network of trabeculae, which subdivides the spleen into a series of communicating compartments, each several millimeters across. The blood and lymphatic vessels are carried into the splenic pulp in the trabeculae.

2.3.2   THE SPLENIC PULP

The splenic pulp consists of the white pulp, an intermediate marginal zone, and the red pulp (Figure 2.1) (Kashimura and Fujita, 1987; Sasou *et al.*, 1986; van Krieken and te Velde, 1988; see also sections 5.2.3 and 5.2.4).

The white pulp (WP)

The white pulp consists predominantly of lymphocytes, together with macrophages and other free cells, lying in a specialized reticular meshwork composed of concentric layers of stromal cells (Fujita, Kashimura and Adachi, 1982, 1985). Its organization is closely related to the arteries of the splenic vasculature, for which it provides a cellular adventitia: tapering cylinders of white pulp surround the central arteries and constitute the periarterial lymphatic sheaths (PALS). The free cells in the sheaths are

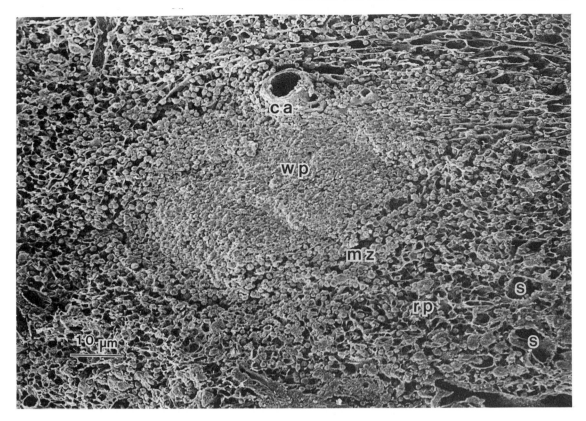

Figure 2.1 Scanning electron micrograph of the human spleen at low power. Central artery (ca), white pulp (wp), marginal zone (mz), red pulp (rp) and sinuses (s) in a freeze-cracked surface of the splenic pulp. (Reproduced with permission from Kashimura, M. and Fujita, T. (1987) *Scanning Microscopy*, **I**, 843, Figure 1.)

predominantly T cells, while B cells are concentrated in the lymphatic nodules, which are often situated more peripherally or at sites of arterial branching. The central artery supplies radial branches to the white pulp, the marginal zone and the red pulp, and terminates in an attenuated vessel of variable structure supplying the red pulp (Figure 2.2). The distal portion of the vessel may be surrounded by Weiss's periarterial macrophage sheath (PAMS), which is usually not highly developed in man (Figure 2.3) (Buyssens, Paulus and Burgeois, 1984; Weiss, 1983; Weiss, Powell and Schiffman, 1985). It is however more prominent in younger subjects. Deep efferent lymphatic vessels are also present in relation to central arteries; they arise distally in the white pulp and run towards and through the trabeculae to leave the spleen at the hilus.

The red pulp (RP)

Three-quarters of the volume of the human spleen consists of the red pulp, which comprises four vascular structures in sequence: slender non–anastomosing arterial vessels (penicilli), the splenic cords of Billroth, the venous sinuses and the pulp veins. The walled vessels are suspended within a reticular meshwork, and the splenic cords are formed from spaces within the network (Figures 2.4–2.6). The human spleen is of the sinusal type and the splenic sinuses comprise approximately one-third of the volume of the red pulp (van Krieken and te

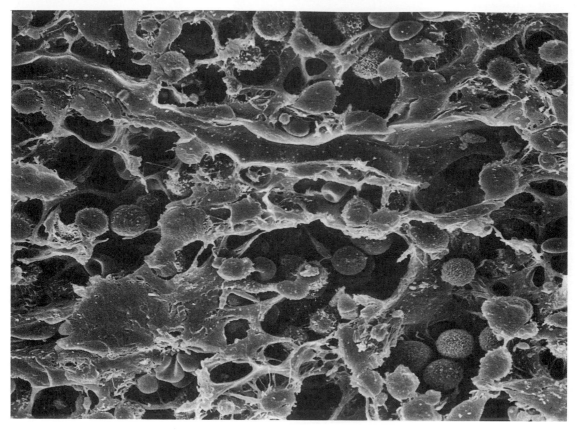

Figure 2.2 Scanning electron micrograph of the human spleen. A longitudinally fractured arterial capillary terminates in the cordal spaces of the red pulp. The arterial capillary fans out to the right-hand side, where fenestrations provide openings to the cordal spaces. (×1350). (Adapted by permission of the authors and publisher, Birkhauser Verlag of Basel, from Fujita, T., Kashimura, M. and Adachi, K. (1985) *Experientia*, **41**, 174, Figure 15.)

Velde, 1988); they consist of long anastomosing vascular channels, which ultimately drain into the pulp veins. The sinuses have a unique endothelium with cells arranged longitudinally like the staves of a barrel; these run parallel to the long axis of the sinus and show tight junctional complexes at regular intervals along their lateral surfaces. Potential slit-like spaces, which can be penetrated by cells flowing from the pulp cords, separate the endothelial cells (Figures 2.5–2.9). A fenestrated basement membrane is applied to the external (pulp) surface of the

---

Figure 2.3 Scanning electron micrograph of the human spleen to show a sheathed artery enveloped by macrophages and reticular cells. The specimen is taken from the spleen of a patient with immune thrombocytopenia: the honeycombing of the cytoplasm of the macrophages is due to the phagocytosis of platelets. (×4000). (Reproduced with permission from Fujita, T., Kashimura, M. and Adachi, K. (1985) *Experientia*, **41**, 174, Figure 14.)

Figure 2.4 Scanning electron micrograph of the red pulp of the human spleen. The meshwork is formed by reticular cells (R), their processes and reticular fibers. Critical point drying has produced cell retraction, so that the cells shrink against the reticular fibers which they surround. (×1500).

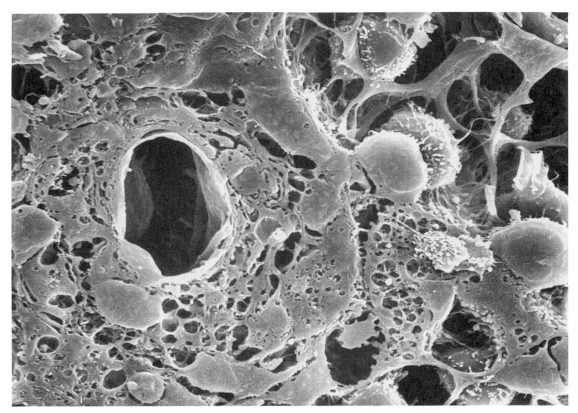

Figure 2.3

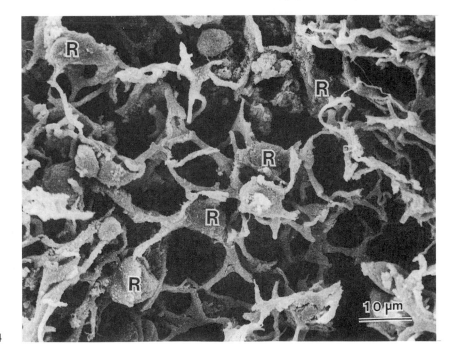

Figure 2.4

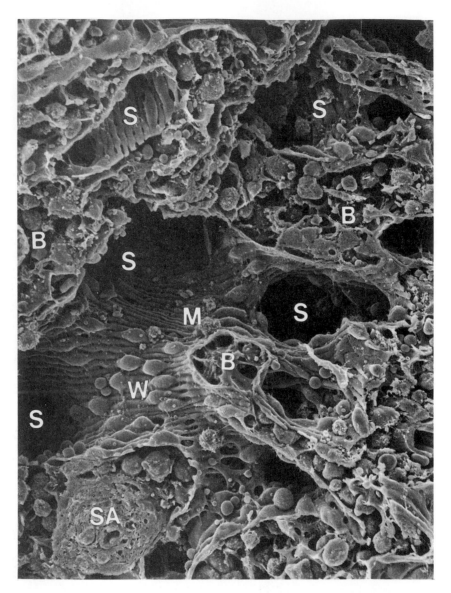

Figure 2.5 Scanning electron micrograph of the red pulp of the human spleen at low power. The splenic cords (B) are fractured, and the sinuses (S) are seen mainly from the surface. The endothelial cells (or 'rod cells of Weidenreich', W) are arranged in parallel and show enlarged nuclear portions which project into the lumen of the sinus. Red cells can be seen protruding into the sinuses through the junctions of the endothelial cells. M, macrophages. SA, sheathed artery. (×875). (Reproduced with modification from Fujita, T. (1974) *Archivum Histologicum Japonicum*, 37, 190, Figure 2 with the permission of the author and publisher.)

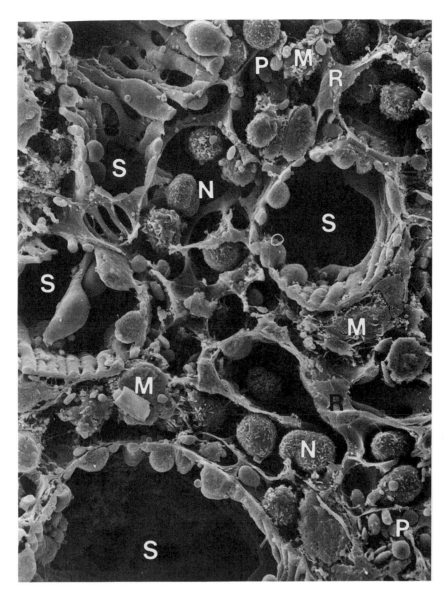

Figure 2.6 Scanning electron micrograph of the red pulp of the human spleen, at higher power than Figure 2.5. The splenic cords are seen to be supported by reticulum cells (R), and the cord meshwork contains macrophages (M), leukocytes, mainly neutrophils (N) and blood platelets (P). The endothelial pattern of the sinuses (S) is demonstrated; the sinuses in the upper part of the micrograph suggest a perforated structure. (×1800). (Reproduced by permission of the author and publisher from Fujita, T. (1974) *Archivum Histologicum Japonicum*, **37**, 191, Figure 3.)

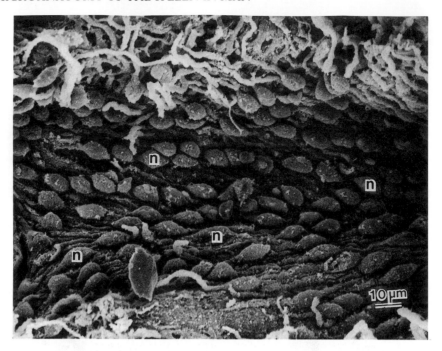

Figure 2.7 Scanning electron micrograph of the human spleen, showing the luminal surface of a vascular sinus. The endothelial cells are arranged in parallel rows. The portions of the cells containing nuclei (n) bulge into the lumen; there are no visible gaps between the endothelial cells. (×3000).

endothelial cells; its transverse ring-like component reinforces the sinusal structure like the hoops of a barrel (Figure 2.8) (Groom, 1987; Weiss, 1983).

The endothelial cells have two sets of cytoplasmic filaments: one set, the tonofilaments, is loosely arranged, while the other is tightly organized into dense bands in the basal cytoplasm (Drenckhahn and Wagner, 1986). These bands arch between attachments to circumferential components of the basement membrane; they have been shown to contain actin and myosin, and can probably contract to vary the tension in the endothelial cell and the dimensions of the interendothelial slits (IES). Since the interendothelial slits are a critical point in the flow pathway of particulates through the spleen, this may constitute an important regulator of selective particulate flow (Figure 2.9; see also sections 4.3.4, 4.3.5 and 4.3.10 and Figures 4.25 and 4.26).

In the human spleen the basement membrane of the venous sinuses has a well-marked circumferential component and a lesser longitudinal component. It is continuous with the reticular fibres of the surrounding cords and is overlaid with reticular cells. The junction of the venous sinuses with the pulp veins requires a transition from rod-like endothelial cells with a fenestrated basement membrane to the flattened endothelium of the veins and a basement membrane without apertures: this transition can be quite abrupt and without an intermediate structural organization (Weiss, 1983).

The marginal zone (MZ)

The marginal zone, as its name implies, lies at the periphery of the white pulp and its outer surface blends with the structure of the red pulp. In the human spleen the reticular meshwork is fine, and the zone is the site of termina-

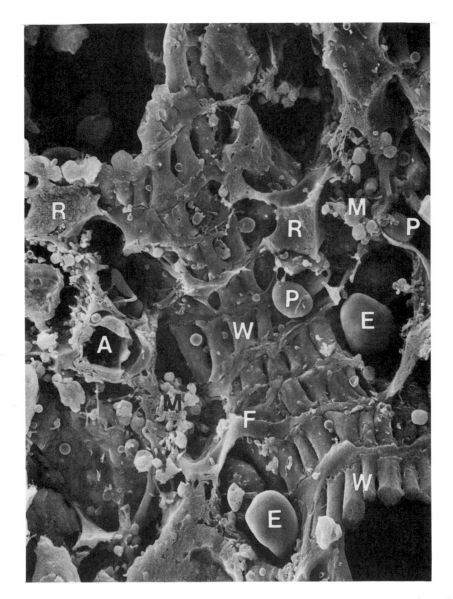

Figure 2.8 Scanning electron micrograph of the human spleen, showing the abluminal surface of a vascular sinus. The rod-like endothelial cells are crossed by the encircling hoops of basement membrane. Sinus endothelial cells (W). Reticular cell foot processes (F). Artery (A). Erythrocytes (E). Macrophage (M). Platelets (P). Reticulum cells (R). (×3700). (Reproduced by permission of the author and publisher from Fujita, T. (1974) *Archivum Histologicum Japonicum*, 37, 199, Figure 12.)

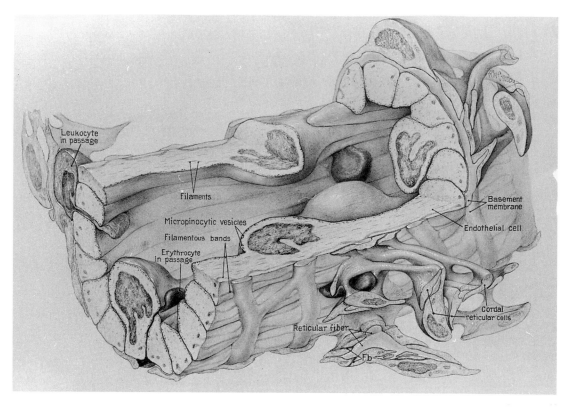

Figure 2.9 A schematic diagram of a red pulp sinus. The parallel orientation of the sinus endothelial cells is shown, with endothelial nuclei causing protrusion into the sinus lumen. On the abluminal surface of the sinus is the fenestrated basement membrane, to which the cordal macrophages are attached. A blood cell, in this case a leukocyte, is passing between adjacent endothelial cells to enter the lumen from the pulp cord. (Reproduced with permission from Chen, L. T. and Weiss, L. (1972) *American Journal of Anatomy*, **134**, 457, plate 13, with acknowledgement to the Wistar Institute Press.)

tion of many arterioles, which frequently bifurcate just before their termination (Figure 2.10). On the efferent side, many venous sinuses are within or close to the marginal zone. This appears to be an area of heavy blood traffic and filtration, and a zone of considerable importance to the distribution of blood components to other parts of the spleen. However, the detailed vascular structures of the human spleen in the marginal zone have been the subject of some controversy: the marginal sinus evident in many species appears to be poorly developed. There is however a structure apparently unique to the human spleen, known as the perimarginal cavernous sinus, which drains into the venous sinuses (Groom, 1987; Sasou *et al.*, 1986; Schmidt, MacDonald and Groom, 1988; see also section 4.3.9).

2.4 THE PATHWAYS OF BLOOD FLOW

The afferent arterial vessels course through the WP as central arteries, and their radial branches supply the MZ or RP, or return from the red pulp to terminate in the MZ or the lymphatic nodules. The attenuated mainstem of a central artery drains in most instances into the reticular meshwork of the RP. In man, the majority of the arterial terminations have no endothelial continuity with venous structures, and the cir-

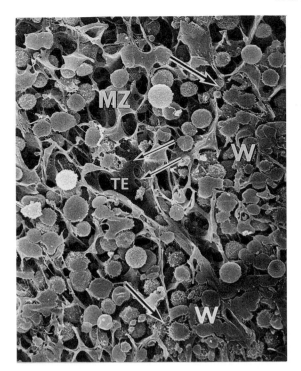

Figure 2.10 Scanning electron micrograph of the human spleen, showing the terminal end (TE) of a follicular artery in the marginal zone (MZ). The thin arrows show openings in the flat reticular cells which demarcate the marginal zone (MZ) from the white pulp (W). (Reproduced with permission of Dr Shunichi Sasou and the publishers of *Scanning Electron Microscopy*, **III**, 1986, 1065–69, Figure 3).

Groom and his colleagues have demonstrated vascular pathways in the marginal zone which have the potential for by-passing the red pulp: these are discussed in more detail in Chapter 4. Open-ended venous sinuses have not been identified unequivocally by electron microscopy of the human spleen, although Sasou found small venous sinuses in the MZ, close to the RP, which are continuous with larger sinuses. The walls of these sinuses consist of broader endothelial cells than are seen elsewhere, and they may in fact be flattened reticular cells and represent open-ended pathways (Sasou *et al.*, 1986).

2.5   THE REGULATION OF SPLENIC BLOOD FLOW

The regulation of volume and distribution of blood flow is critical to the effective functioning of the spleen. A high proportion of a bolus of abnormal red cells entering the spleen is retained on initial passage through the organ, indicating that the filtration process is dependent on structures 'in place', mainly on the afferent aspect of the circulation, and does not require adaptive changes and prolonged flow (Groom, 1987). The arterial structures appear to direct plasma to the MZ, marginated cells to WP and MZ, and the axial flow (especially red cells) to the RP.

The arteries of the human spleen appear to have sympathetic innervation but parasympathetic innervation has not been convincingly demonstrated (Reilly, 1985). Plasma skimming appears to require an intact nerve supply, while pooling and the concentration of red cells are inhibited by sympathomimetic drugs (sections 4.5.3 and 8.3).

The MZ receives a disproportionately large number of terminal arterial vessels. Blood entering the MZ is directed selectively to other arterial beds: lymphocytes and their accessory cells pass to the WP and are preferentially sorted into the B and T zones (van Ewijk and Nieuwenhuis, 1985). Should there be no functional reaction, the lymphocytes leave the spleen through the deep efferent lymphatics.

culation is predominantly 'open' in form, with the pathway of blood flow crossing a connective tissue space. This does not mean that in normal circumstances there is a random process of flow in the intermediate circulation, since the orientation of the arterial terminations to the splenic sinus walls effectively produces an unimpeded pathway. As a consequence the greater part of the blood *flow* through the human spleen passes through a functional 'fast pathway', in contrast to the very small fraction of flow which traverses the slow pathway (Groom, 1987). However, the *volume* of blood is greater in the 'slow pathway' due to its slow turnover: this occupies part of the pulp cords where they are both physiologically and structurally 'open'.

The reticular stroma of the MZ and the PALS contains numerous cells with smooth muscle actin and myosin (Toccanier-Pelte et al., 1987): these are not present in the red pulp. Transmission electron microscopy shows these myoid cells to have slender cytoplasmic processes containing bundles of microfilaments associated with reticular fibers. Their location in areas of high blood flow suggests that they have a role in controlling blood flow and directing cell traffic. Likewise some of the arterioles in the red pulp bear a small PAMS prior to termination, and the smooth muscle represented in these structures suggests that this is another site where blood flow is regulated (Buyssens, Paulus and Burgeois, 1984; Sasou et al., 1986).

Buckley et al. (1987) have studied the macrophages of the spleen by means of immunohistochemical techniques using monoclonal antibodies; they have demonstrated phenotypically different subpopulations in discrete locations, and have suggested that they are subsets with functional specialization. Distinctive antigenic markers were shared by macrophages forming clusters about the blood vessels and macrophages located in the marginal zones: it is suggested that this reflects a common function in the trapping and processing of circulating antigens.

Blood which enters the red pulp is in an 'open' anatomical system in which significant filtration can occur. The formation of efficient, sometimes functionally closed, channels is described in Chapter 3, and the dynamics of flow at the sinus wall in Chapter 4. Structural studies suggest the presence of comparable processes in the human spleen.

Blood which enters the red pulp is in an continues through the pulp veins, trabecular veins and subsequently the splenic veins at the hilus. Since the splenic vein enters the portal vein, any increase in portal pressure increases the blood contained in the spleen and consequently the volume of the spleen: when of long-standing this may result in 'congestive splenomegaly'. The myoelastic structure of the splenic vein suggests that the diameter of the vein can be actively varied to modify both intrasplenic pressure and venous flow (Reis and Ferraz de Carvalho, 1988). Secondary splenic distention could in turn modify the relationship of the arterial terminations to the sinus walls, increasing the length and duration of the flow pathway and improving the filtration efficiency of the red pulp.

It is thus possible to infer significant regulation of blood flow at several sites in the spleen, notably:

1. in the central arteries and their radial branches, where plasma separation will be an important effect;
2. in the marginal zone, where flow can be directed to the filtration beds of the white pulp or the red pulp, or to a bypass pathway;
3. in the PAMS, where clearance of blood-borne particles is a major function;
4. in the red pulp, where flow can be modified by contractile reticular cells, and by the formation of reticular cell syncytia;
5. at the venous sinus wall, where contractile elements in the endothelial cells can vary the resistance to flow of the interendothelial spaces (MacDonald et al., 1987); and
6. in the splenic vein, which can retard venous outflow and modify the functional state of the red pulp.

2.6   THE FUNCTIONAL SIGNIFICANCE OF SPLEEN STRUCTURE

The unique vascular structure of the spleen principally subserves mechanisms for the separation of plasma from the particles suspended in the blood, and the sorting of the particles (principally cells) into functional zones where appropriately sequenced phagocytosis and lymphocyte activity, such as antigen recognition, occurs. These defensive processes are outlined in greater detail in Chapter 5.

The regulation of blood flow is clearly a significant factor in the separation and sorting of particles from the circulation. The experimental aspects of the related processes are discussed in Chapter 4, but the overall consequence of controlled flow is to reduce the flow rate of particles, so that their contact with macrophages and other reactive cells is prolonged and the distractive forces separating interactive cells are minimized. The factors influencing cell contact in the slowly flowing pathways of the spleen are principally physicochemical and are related to surface properties such as loss of surface charge, the inhibition of membrane sulfhydryl groups, surface adhesiveness and the presence of antibody. Loss of cell deformability and increased sphericity in red cells leads to impaired flow at the sinus endothelial wall (Groom, 1987; MacDonald *et al.*, 1987).

A further consequence of impaired flow is a change in the properties of the splenic environment, which may show sufficient reduction in pH, oxygen tension and glucose concentration to impair the viability of entrapped cells, especially red cells. More needs to be known of the physiological significance of modified splenic blood flow, but the part played by modified flow in the pathological pooling of blood cells is critical in some red cell disorders (Chapter 8).

REFERENCES

Bowdler, A. J. (1969) Regional variations in the proportion of red cells in the blood in man. *Br. J. Haematol.*, **16**, 557–71.

Buckley, P. J. *et al.* (1987) Human spleen contains phenotypic subsets of macrophage and dendritic cells that occupy discrete microanatomic locations. *Am. J. Pathol.*, **128**, 505–20.

Buyssens, N., Paulus, G. and Burgeois, N. (1984) Ellipsoids in the human spleen. *Virchows Arch. (Path. Anat.)*, **403**, 27–40.

Drenckhahn, D. and Wagner, J. (1986) Stress fibers in the splenic sinus endothelium in situ: molecular structure, relationship to the extracellular matrix and contractility. *J. Cell Biol.*, **102**, 1738–47.

Eikelenboom, P. *et al.* (1985) Characterization of lymphoid and nonlymphoid cells in the white pulp of the spleen using immunohistoperoxidase techniques and enzyme histochemistry. *Experientia*, **41**, 209–15.

Faller, A. (1985) Splenic architecture as reflected in the connective tissue structure of the human spleen. *Experientia*, **41**, 164–7

Fujita, T., Kashimura, M. and Adachi, K. (1982) Scanning electron microscopy studies of the spleen – normal and pathological. *Scanning Electron Microscopy*, **I**, 435–44.

Fujita, T., Kashimura, M. and Adachi, K. (1985) Scanning electron microscopy and terminal circulation. *Experientia*, **41**, 167–79.

Groom, A. C. (1987) Microcirculation of the spleen: new concepts, new challenges. *Microvasc. Res.*, **34**, 269–89.

Kashimura, M. and Fujita, T. (1987) A scanning electron microscope study of human spleen: relationship between the microcirculation and functions. *Scanning Microscopy*, **I**, 841–51.

MacDonald, I. C. *et al.* (1987) Kinetics of red cell passage through interendothelial slits into venous sinuses in rat spleen, analysed by *in vivo* microscopy. *Microvasc. Res.*, **33**, 118–34.

McCuskey, R. S. (1985) New trends in spleen research: Introduction. *Experientia*, **41**, 144.

Reilly, F. D. (1985) Innervation and vascular pharmacodynamics of the mammalian spleen. *Experientia*, **41**, 187–92.

Reis, F. P. and Ferraz de Carvalho, C. A. (1988) Functional architecture of the splenic vein in the adult human. *Acta Anat.*, **132**, 109–13.

Sasou, S. *et al.* (1986) Scanning electron microscopic features of the spleen in the rat and human: a comparative study. *Scanning Electron Microscopy*, **III**, 1063–9

Schmidt, E. E., MacDonald, I. C. and Groom, A. C. (1988) Microcirculatory pathways in normal human spleen demonstrated by scanning electron microscopy of corrosion casts. *Am. J. Anat.*, **181**, 253–66.

Toccanier-Pelte, M. F. *et al.* (1987) Characterization of stromal cells with myoid features in lymph nodes and spleen in normal and pathologic conditions. *Am. J. Pathol.*, **129**, 109–18.

van Ewijk, W. and Nieuwenhuis, P. (1985) Compartments, domains, and migration pathways of lymphoid cells in the splenic pulp. *Experientia*, **41**, 199–208.

van Krieken, J. H. J. M. and te Velde, J. (1988) Normal histology of the human spleen. *Am. J. Surg. Path.*, **12**, 777–85.

Wadenvik, H. and Kutti, J. (1988) The spleen and pooling of blood cells. *Eur. J. Haematol.*, **41**, 1–5.

Weiss, L. (1983) The spleen, in *Histology, Cell and Tissue Biology*, 5th edn, Ch 16. (ed. L. Weiss). Elsevier Biomedical, New York, Amsterdam and Oxford.

Weiss, L. (1985) New trends in spleen research: Conclusion. *Experientia*, **41**, 243–8.

Weiss, L., Powell, R. and Schiffman, F. J. (1985) Terminating arterial vessels in red pulp of human spleen: a transmission electron microscopic study. *Experientia*, **41**, 233–42.

Weiss, L., Geduldig, U. and Weidanz, W. (1986) Mechanisms of splenic control of murine malaria: reticular cell activation and the development of a blood spleen barrier. *Am. J. Anat.*, **176**, 251–85.

MECHANISMS OF SPLENIC CLEARANCE OF THE BLOOD; A STRUCTURAL OVERVIEW OF THE MAMMALIAN SPLEEN

Leon Weiss

3.1 INTRODUCTION

The spleen is dedicated to the clearance of blood cells, microorganisms and other particles from the blood. This chapter deals with cell and tissue biological matters related to the mechanisms of splenic clearance, which include the vascular organization of the spleen and the character of the intermediate circulation, the mechanisms and regulation of clearance, the representation of the reticuloendothelial system in the spleen, and the development of barriers by a newly-recognized fibroblastic lineage of barrier cells. From experimental morphological studies in my laboratory, I believe that these topics have common roots. I shall set out the vascular context of the spleen, including its comparative aspects, and discuss each of the above topics in turn. Then I shall attempt to establish how they are related, and present a working model of the structure and function of the spleen.

3.2 THE ANATOMICAL ORGANIZATION OF THE SPLEEN

The mammalian spleen consists of an encapsulated, trabeculated pulp made up of stroma and vasculature supporting a large population of circulating, migrating, and differentiating blood and hematopoietic cells (Figures 3.1–3.6). The vascular layout of the spleen is as follows: arteries enter the pulp and terminate there, opening up into filtration beds. A system of venous vessels in the marginal zones (MZ) and red pulp (RP) drain blood from the filtration beds. MZ are shells of pulp surrounding the white pulp (WP), interposed between WP centrally and RP peripherally. They are heavily trafficked by blood, receiving blood from many arterial terminals, and selectively distributing its components to other parts of the spleen. The MZ also store erythrocytes, platelets, monocyte-macrophages, and initiate their processing. The red pulp is that large part of the pulp that extends outward from the MZ. It too receives arterial terminals, clears, tests and stores erythrocytes, and is primed for erythroclasia and erythropoiesis. The WP lies centrally, ensheathing the arterial vessels as they enter and run through the pulp: it clears lymphocytes and their accessory cells selectively from the blood and prepares them for immunological reactions. The WP is drained by a specialized set of deep lymphatic vessels.

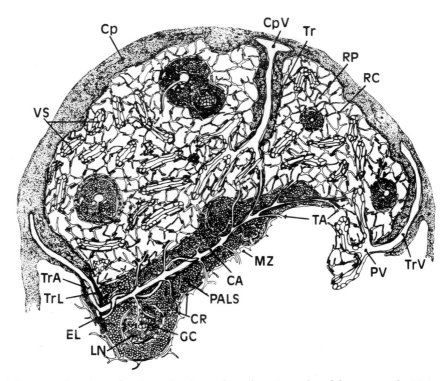

Figure 3.1 Schematic drawing of a sinusal spleen: the spleen is enclosed by a capsule (Cp) and from its internal surface trabeculae (Tr) branch to compartmentalize the pulp. The splenic artery pierces the capsule and branches into trabecular arteries (TrA). The trabecular artery enters the pulp as an artery, the central artery (CA), which runs in the central axis of the periarteriolar lymphatic sheath (PALS). This is the component of the white pulp (WP) in which T-cells are concentrated. The second major component of the white pulp consists of the lymphatic nodules (LN), which occur as nodules within the PALS, where their presence forces the central artery into an eccentric position. LN are sites of concentration of B-cells and may contain germinal centres (GC) when there is a high level of antibody formation. Branches of the central artery supply LN and pass laterally through the white pulp to terminate in the marginal zone (MZ) which closely surrounds the WP. In addition to its arterial vessels, efferent lymphatic vessels (EL) drain the white pulp, entering the trabeculae as trabecular lymphatics (TrL).

In this schema the lymphocytes of the WP are shown and, with the vasculature, dominate the picture. Note, however, that there is a circumferential reticulum (CR) limiting the periphery of WP. The MZ and red pulp (RP) which occupy the bulk of the spleen are schematized and show no free cells. The red pulp consists of terminating arterial vessels (TA), a meshwork, or filtration bed, consisting of reticular cells (RC) and associated reticular fibers, and a system of venous vessels. The proximal venous vessel which receives blood from the filtration beds is the venous sinus (VS). These distinctive vessels end blindly, anastomosing richly, deeply penetrating the filtration beds of RP, supported by the reticular meshwork. VS receive blood through their interendothelial slits, which then drains into pulp veins (PV), trabecular veins (TrV), and capsular veins (CpV).

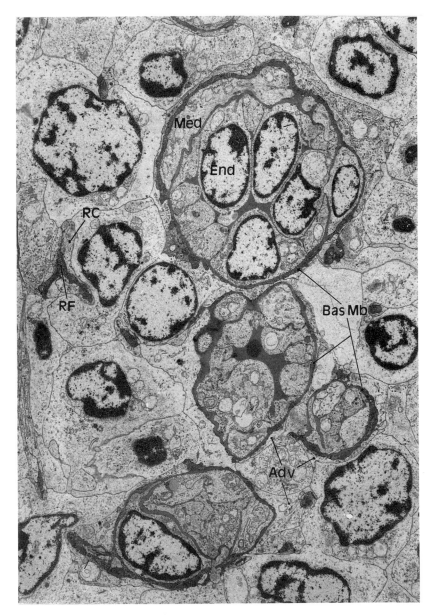

Figure 3.2 White pulp, human spleen: four cross-sections of an arteriole and its smaller branches lie in white pulp. Each of the vessels may possess an endothelium (End), basement membrane (Bas Mb), media (Med) and adventitia (Adv). Especially in the smaller vessels the media and adventitial layers are rather incomplete. Lymphocytes occupy much of the rest of this field, held in a meshwork of reticular cells (RC) and reticular fibers (RF). (×6250).

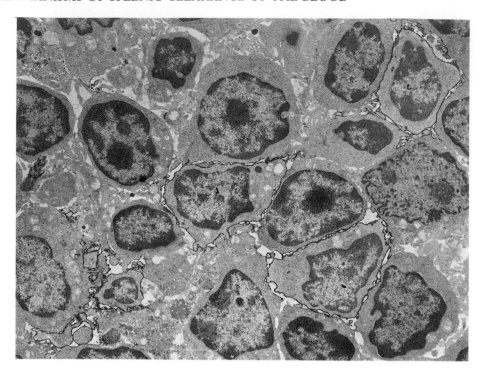

Figure 3.3 Normal murine white pulp stained for T-cells: the field consists largely of T-cells, the surfaces of some of which are stained by immunocytochemistry for the T-cell marker, Thy 1.2. Note the short cell processes of many of the lymphocytes, establishing transient junctional complexes with vicinal cells. (×2500).

3.2.1 CAPSULE AND TRABECULAE

The splenic capsule is a sympathetically innervated, species-dependent blend of smooth muscle and collagenous tissue. The capsule is continuous on its inner surface with a richly ramified system of trabeculae which penetrates and supports the pulp. In certain species the capsule and trabeculae are quite rich in smooth muscle. These spleens, of which the equine and feline are examples, are termed storage spleens. Contraction of the capsule and trabeculae by the mediation of the sympathetic nerves, causes delivery of large reserves of blood to the circulation. The horse has a huge spleen and its outstanding athletic prowess appears to depend upon the spleen's capacity to boost the oxygen-carrying capacity of the circulation by 'internal transfusion'. In fact, splenic reserves of mature erythrocytes are so large and so readily mobil-ized that the horse seldom shows circulating reticulocytes, although the marrow produces reticulocytes, holds them in reserve and can release them; it uses the splenic store of mature erythrocytes to compensate for all but persistent, long-term blood loss. In contrast, the spleen of the human being, rabbit and mouse, and its erythrocyte reserves, are quite small. These spleens do retain some significant storage capacity, however, holding large numbers of platelets in ready reserve. Because such small spleens have been thought to have great immunological and other antimicrobial capacity they been termed defense spleens.

3.2.2 ARTERIAL VESSELS

Arteries pierce the capsule at the hilus and ramify through the trabeculae which carry them

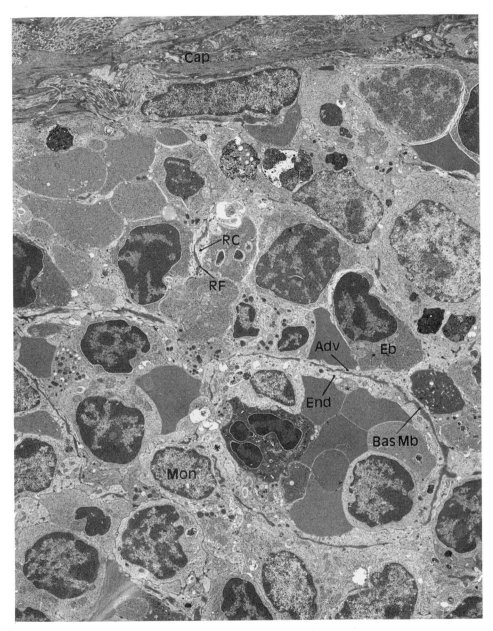

Figure 3.4 Subcapsular red pulp mouse spleen: the capsule is rich in muscle and collagen. The subjacent red pulp contains a bifurcating pulp vein. The right limb has endothelium (End), basement membrane (Bas Mb) and adventitia (Adv) labelled. A mononuclear cell (Mon) sends delicate cytoplasmic processes into the vascular wall, penetrating adventitia and basement membrane[*]. The perivascular red pulp is pervaded by a reticular meshwork consisting of reticular cells (RC), which branch from the adventitial layer of pulp veins, and reticular fibers (RF). The reticular meshwork of mouse red pulp is, however, typically quite scanty. The red pulp contains many reticulocytes and some erythroblasts (Eb). (×5000).

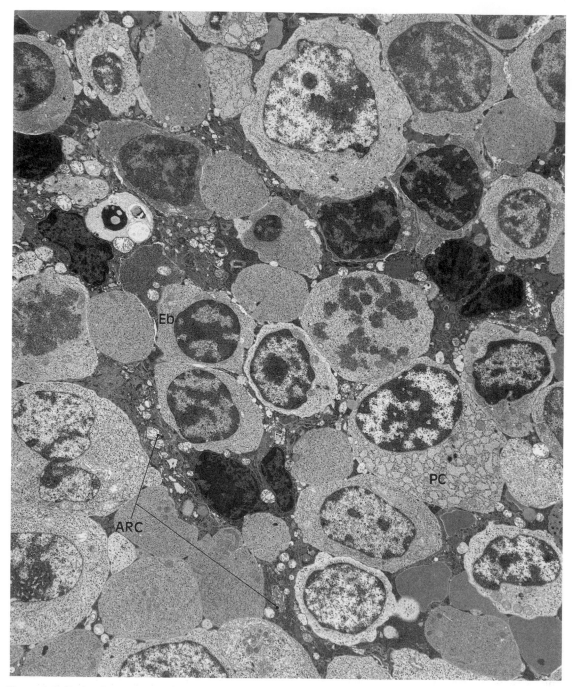

Figure 3.5 Red pulp, murine spleen in malaria: this field of red pulp in precrisis *Plasmodium yoelii* malaria consists of many erythroblasts (Eb), some in mitosis, and a few plasma cells (PC). Note the dark, syncytially fused stromal cells forming a complex, extensive membrane which constitutes a barrier, surrounding many free cells. These stromal cells are barrier cells (ARC). (×5000).

in prominent numbers through the pulp. Arteries then leave the trabeculae, and enter the pulp, tunneling through the WP, to branch a number of times and emerge from the WP. When they reach the MZ or RP they terminate, having devolved to the structural level of metarteriole or capillary. The termination may be rather abrupt and unadorned, almost as if the vessel were simply transected, and the blood it carries empties into the pulp. There are a number of variations in the configuration of arterial terminals: an ending may be flared or ampullary. Just before termination, moreover, the endothelial cells typically lose junctional complexes on their lateral surfaces. Blood cells, therefore, may leave an arterial vessel not only at its termination, but through interendothelial slits just prior to this point.

Macrophages are always present around arterial terminations: these may be rather loosely arranged, as in the human, mouse and rabbit, or organized into a rather large, tight cluster or nodule. This is seen in the canine, feline, herbivore and avian spleen, where the macrophages surround the terminal arterial vessel as a tight cuff or sheath. This cuff has been termed the ellipsoid, but it has been suggested that the term periarterial macrophage sheath (PAMS) be used instead; this term is informative and homologous with the periarterial lymphatic sheath (see below), whereas the term ellipsoid is often inaccurate, and suggests inappropriately a unique mechanical form.

3.2.3   VENOUS AND LYMPHATIC VESSELS

While arteries alone bring blood into the spleen, both veins and lymphatics drain it. Veins and lymphatics originate as anastomosing, blindly ending, large-lumened, thin-walled vessels. In sinusal spleens (see below) the most fully developed of the initial veins are the venous sinuses whose endothelium, basement membrane, and adventitia are each distinctive. The endothelium consists of cells shaped as tapered rods arranged longitudinally, close together, side-by-side, and connected to one another by

adherent junctions. Sinusal endothelial cells possess bundles of longitudinal basal intermediate filaments identified as myosin. To enter the lumen of these sinuses and leave the spleen, blood cells must pass through narrow interendothelial slits, which may offer resistance to the passage of rigid cells.

In the heyday of monophyletic–polyphyletic hematopoietic stem cell dialectics, these endothelial cells were recognized as distinctive from other endothelial cells and termed littoral (*syn.* shore) cells. They were regarded as phagocytic and as multipotent hematopoietic stem cells, capable of rounding off the endothelium and differentiating into any line of blood cells. We recognize these cells, by electron microscopy, as reluctant phagocytes, phagocytic only with heavy, sustained phagocytic loads, as in congenital hemolytic anemias. There is no competent evidence that they are, or become, multipotent hematopoietic stem cells. The basement membrane is, as are other basement membranes, a thin acellular sheet of carbohydrate–protein complexes, rich in collagens. The sinusal basement membrane is distinctive, however, in being broadly and regularly fenestrated, giving the appearance of being made of transverse and longitudinal fibers. In general, as shown by the human spleen, the transverse or annular component is stout, the longitudinal slender. This membrane may be deeply stained by the periodic acid–Schiff (PAS) method for carbohydrate–protein complexes, and by silver salts (argyrophilia).

Reticular cells (RC) lie on the outer surface of the basement membrane, forming the adventitial layer, and branch into the surrounding perivascular tissue. They ensheathe argyrophilic fibers, continuous with the sinusal basement membrane, and presumably synthesize them: they are, therefore, fibroblastic. Cytochemically they can be shown to contain actin and myosin and are therefore contractile. Like the capsule and trabeculae, they are innervated by sympathetic fibers, which have been shown in the horse and the dog by electron microscopy. RC, capsule and trabeculae thereby possess a vaso-

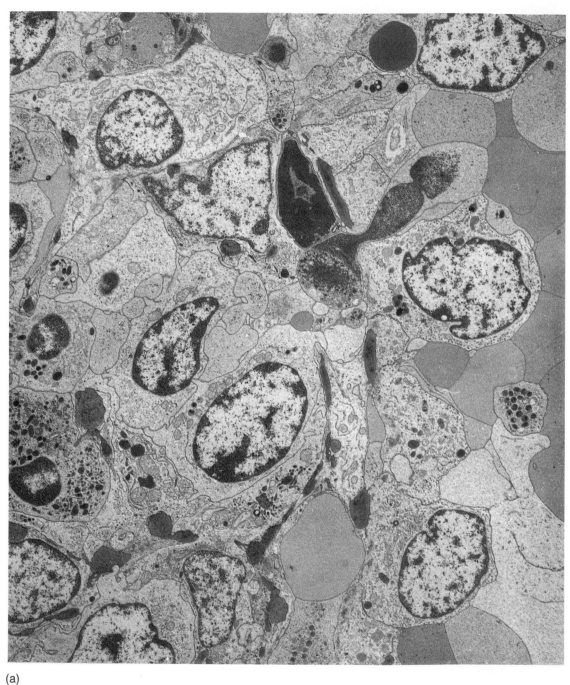

(a)

Figure 3.6 (a) Transmission micrograph; (b) key to part (a). Red pulp, human spleen, thalassemia: human spleen is a sinusal spleen, and this field contains a venous sinus. Its wall runs vertically, its luminal surface to

motor character, which underscores their essentially vascular nature. RC have been regarded, as had the sinusal endothelium, as phagocytic and hematopoietically multipotential. However, as in the case of the endothelium, RC are slightly to moderately phagocytic only with heavy, sustained phagocytic loads. There is no evidence that they are hematopoietic stem cells.

Non-sinusal spleens lack venous sinuses, and efferent blood is received initially by pulp veins.

These vessels often lie against trabeculae and enter them, becoming trabecular veins. In mouse, dog and horse, pulp veins are thin-walled, large-lumened vessels with squamous endothelium. Their wall, unlike that of the venous sinuses, offers little impedance to the passage of blood cells because they bear large transmural apertures.

In contrast to the superficial lymphatics that relate mainly to the capsule, the deep efferent

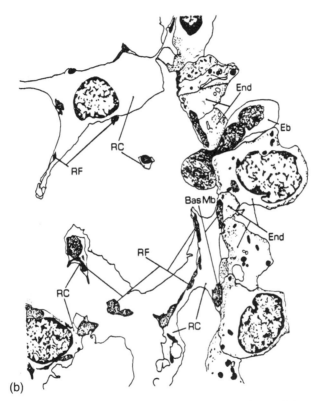

the right lined by cross-sections of the rod-shaped endothelial cells (End). Nuclei are present in three of these endothelial cells. The basal portion of the endothelial cell is rich in longitudinally running filaments which stipple the cell, and when interwoven, present as dense plaques. The fenestrated basement membrane appears in short segments (Bas Mb) at the base of the endothelium. Red cells in thalassemia vary considerably in appearance and are 'floppy', tending to fold flexibly on one another. Many reticulocytes are present, and erythroblasts circulate. An erythroblast (Eb), with its nucleus deeply constricted in two places, is passing through the endothelium in an interendothelial slit. (The erythroblast itself is deeply constricted in the interendothelial slit at the lower nuclear constriction.) The cord on the left is rather fully packed with leukocytes and reticular cells (RC). The latter serve as the fibroblastic stroma of the cord, and ensheathe reticular fibers (RF). (×8000).

splenic lymphatic vessels are well developed but inconspicuous because, running in lymphocyte-crowded beds and possessing a lymphocyte-crowded lumen surrounded by the thinnest of vascular walls, they stand out poorly from their background. In fact, for a long time the existence of deep splenic lymphatics was denied. They originate deep in the WP and, entwining the arterial vessels, run from the WP into the trabeculae and then leave the spleen at the hilus. Thus they carry lymph countercurrent to the flow of blood in the arterial vessels they encumber. They provide splenic lymphocytes with a major efferent pathway, which constitutes an intrasplenic limb for the migrations of the immunologically competent lymphocytes of the recirculating lymphocyte pool.

3.3 FILTRATION BEDS

The tissue interposed between the terminal arterial vessels and the initial venous vessels is a reticulum or reticular meshwork, composed of reticular cells and their ensheathed reticular fibers. In the human spleen, and indeed in sinusal spleens in general, the pulp consists of a reticular meshwork in which arterial and venous vessels are suspended by adventitial reticular cells which branch out perivascularly and contribute to the reticular meshwork. If the meshwork is big enough it will contain reticular cells that are entirely confined to the reticulum, without an adventitial relationship to blood vessels. In the human spleen and other sinusal spleens, the reticular meshwork is well developed. Reticular cell branches are sheet-like in character. The reticular cells thus form a system of thin-walled locules reinforced by reticular fibers. The locules communicate with one another and, as a system, are open, directly or indirectly, to the blood that enters the spleen. Variations in locular location, arrangement and development result in a variety of types of reticular meshwork. These meshworks are the fundamental elements that filter or clear the blood. Hence, I term them filtration beds.

Two types of filtration bed make up the WP.

Periarterial lymphatic sheaths (PALS) are long, conical sleeves coaxially surrounding the larger arterial vessels as they emerge from the trabeculae and proceed through the pulp. PALS are thick around the larger arteries and taper until they finally disappear as the vessels become finer, permitting the main stem of the arterial vessel (now a small arteriole) to run beyond them as fine, free, arteries of the MZ and RP. PALS are limited peripherally by the reticulum arranged in two or more concentric, circumferential layers. The outermost layer faces out onto the MZ, constituting its innermost boundary. PALS constitute a filtration bed specialized for the clearance of T-cells, and provide an immunologically reactive microenvironment for T-cells. Should T-cells fail to react, they provide migration pathways, including deep efferent lymphatics, for their exit from the spleen.

The second type of filtration bed of the WP is the lymphatic nodule (LN). LN are ovoid structures bounded by circumferential reticulum: they lie within PALS, and appear to distend them. Like their counterparts in the cortex of lymph nodes, splenic LN clear and hold B-lymphocytes and permit them to react immunologically or, should they fail to do so, provide them with a route of exit from the spleen *via* the lymphatics. Primary LN are solidly packed with small, migratory B-cells. When a nodule engages in high-level antibody formation, a germinal center occupies its center and the nodule forms a larger, secondary nodule. Many B-lymphocytes which had filled the primary nodule are now compressed into a peripheral mantle layer.

In sinusal spleens, including the human spleen, the filtration beds comprising the MZ are unusually fine-meshed, and MZ receive a disproportionately large number of terminal arterial vessels. MZ are among the most highly trafficked parts of the spleen, receiving and processing large volumes of blood. Blood cells entering the MZ may migrate selectively to other filtration beds. Lymphocytes, for example, may go to the WP, there to be sorted into T-

and B-cell zones. In addition, blood cells may be held in the MZ and processed there. Imperfect erythrocytes are pooled and phagocytized; monocytes are sequestered and differentiate to macrophages there; platelets in large numbers may be stored in the MZ in ready reserve, for quick release to the circulation.

A lobule of red pulp consists of a terminating arterial vessel emptying into a reticular meshwork, or filtration bed, drained by venous vessels. RP filtration beds, identified as pulp spaces, are quite extensive in non-sinusal spleens, because the terminal arterial vessels take little space (except, in some spleens, for PAMS) and the veins are set back against the trabeculae. In sinusal spleens, on the other hand, an extensive anastomosing system of venous sinuses penetrates deeply into the RP and leaves the filtration beds restricted to cords between branches of the venous sinuses. Macrophages, always present in the RP, may quickly increase in number due to trapping and differentiation of circulating monocytes. Some human and rodent arterial terminals bear small periarterial macrophage sheaths (PAMS), while others do not. Rabbit spleen lacks PAMS. PAMS in dog and cat spleen are quite large. RP filtration beds process erythrocytes, permitting the final maturation of reticulocytes before their release to the circulation, and, at the other end of their life span, phagocytizing them. Filtration beds of murine RP regularly hold erythroid stem cells (CFU-E and BFU-E), and, especially in paratrabecular beds, support erythropoiesis. They also support antibody production, holding sheets of plasma cells, often mixed with erythroblasts.

3.3.1 THE INTERMEDIATE CIRCULATION OF THE SPLEEN

The intermediate circulation of the spleen comprises that part of the vascular bed that includes terminal arterial vessels at one end and veins at the other. There has been controversy about whether this circulation is 'open' or 'closed'. Such controversy, reported through many editions of many textbooks, has been sustained, perhaps unnecessarily, by failing to distinguish between the anatomical layout of blood vessels and the physiology of flow.

By anatomical definition, open circulation means that there is no endothelial continuity from artery to vein, and closed circulation means that there is endothelial continuity from artery to vein. By analysis of light or electron microscopic sections of mammalian spleen there is virtually unanimous agreement that the splenic circulation is anatomically open. Arterial vessels end in different sites in the filtration beds, and some endings are quite close to the walls of veins, even sharing a basement membrane over a short distance, but there is no evidence by light or electron transmission microscopy that endothelial continuity occurs between arterial and venous vessels.

By physiological definition, the intermediate circulation of the spleen is, for the most part, closed: this means that over 90% of the blood circulating through the spleen flows through in seconds, which is as rapidly as through tissues with conventional, anatomically closed vasculatures. The spleen also offers minor delayed circulations, moderately delayed (taking minutes) or greatly delayed (taking an hour). In the human spleen it has been determined, using the Fick principle and erythrocytes labeled with ^{51}Cr, that 98% of the blood entering the spleen flows through in about 30 s. By kinetic analysis of red cell washout of perfused isolated cat spleen, Groom and his colleagues have identified three compartments (see also Chapter 4). The first provides a 30-second transit to 90% of the splenic red cells. The second provides 9% of the splenic circulation, with a transit time of 8 minutes. The third handles about 1% of blood flow with a transit time of 1 hour. The first compartment behaves as if the circulation were closed. The second represents stored or marginated blood cells: if the spleen is induced to contract (a process known to eject stored blood cells) this compartment is greatly reduced. The third compartment probably includes cells, such as reticulocytes just received from bone marrow, and offers them terminal maturation before release to the general circulation.

There are other methods of determination of the patterns of blood flow. One can study blood flow by light microscopy in transilluminated living spleen, an approach initiated by Knisely in the 1930s. The resolution and contrast offers a picture of blood flow, but not a satisfactory picture of the structure of blood vessels. Knisely and others concluded that the circulation is closed; other students of the living splenic circulation concluded that it is open. This approach was brought to its apogee by McCuskey and McCuskey (1985) who recorded observations of the living transilluminated circulation by light microscopy, by a method refined by the use of intense, cold xenon light and high-resolution cinematography. They then fixed the living light-microscopic field under observation and sectioned it for electron microscopy. It was concluded that the circulation is anatomically open and physiologically closed. Another valuable method, also morphological, involves intravascular injection of a fluid substance, such as liquid latex or monomeric plastic, and then, when the vessels are filled, hardening the injectate and thereby obtaining a cast of the lumen of the blood vessels. A cast, as it were, is obtained by this means of the pathway of blood flow. The tissue may then be dissolved away, leaving the cast which can be studied by stereomicroscopy and/or scanning electron microscopy. This material does not give direct information on the structure of the vasculature, although a delicate cast of the luminal surface of endothelial cells and their intercellular junctions may be obtained. Using this method, one can, of course, attempt to extrapolate to the anatomy of the blood vessels. But the presence of a cylindrical segment of plastic does not necessarily mean that the cylinder was contained in a blood vessel: it represents simply the shape of the stream of blood and might, as discussed below, result from the blood being contained in a cylindrical segment, or shunt, of the reticular cell filtration bed. Studies from Groom's laboratory have shown tubular or cylindrical paths of blood flow in contracted spleens, and diffuse, less-confined blood flow in relaxed spleens.

I believe that the following conclusions on the intermediate circulation of the mammalian spleen are warranted. The intermediate vasculature in the MZ and RP of both sinusal and non-sinusal spleen is anatomically open. Arteries and veins are suspended in a reticular meshwork which functions as a filtration bed. This meshwork is interposed between the arterial termination and the vein, although in some instances the arterial vessel may end so close to the vein there is scarcely any interposed meshwork. When the spleen contracts, the capsule, trabeculae and the filtration beds appear to contract, causing many cells held in the filtration beds to be expressed into the circulation, and arterial endings and venous walls to come closer together. When the orifice of an arterial termination is brought close to an interendothelial slit of a venous sinus, conditions are set for blood flow to be as efficient and effective as through an anatomically closed pathway. The combination of an anatomically open vasculature and a physiologically closed circulation is quite nicely expressed in non-sinusal spleens because the separation of arterial ending and vein in a relaxed spleen is quite great, and the veins bear large mural apertures; these spleens develop massive splenic congestion after administration of such relaxants as the barbital anesthetics. However, when these spleens contract, bringing the orifices of arterial terminals upon the venous mural apertures, very efficient, direct blood flow should result.

Even with minimal contraction the spleen is set for some physiologically closed circulation in that there are arterial vessels positioned so close to the venous wall that, despite the endothelial disjunction, blood may well flow efficiently through the filtration bed. Moreover, when one visualizes by scanning electron microscopy the broad sheet-like processes of reticular cells making up the filtration bed, it appears that tubules fashioned from these processes may connect arterial and venous vessels across the filtration beds, as efficiently as bona-fide vessels. Furthermore, such tubules may come and go in a manner more transient than is the case with blood vessels. By diverse means the filtration beds of the spleen may actively admit the flow of blood and thereby clear it, with this segment of the circulation now being delayed. Conversely, the filtration beds may be closed off from the circulation by contraction and tubular formation of the filtration beds, and (as shown below) by the activity of barrier cells. Such a segment of the circulation is now rapid. Thus the nature of the intermediate circulation is dynamic and changeable, involving at different times the passage into, or the by-passing of, the filtration beds. The nature of the circulation is thus tied to the function of clearance of the blood, and clearance of the blood is at the root of virtually all functions of the spleen.

3.3.2 THE CLEARANCE OF BLOOD BY THE SPLEEN

The spleen possesses an extraordinary capacity for clearing the blood of blood cells, infectious organisms, particles and macromolecules. This clearance is effected by the splenic filtration beds. The spleen then acts on the cleared material, the filtration beds providing the appropriate micro-environments for phagocytosis, cell differentiation, proliferation, and so on. Under normal conditions, aged erythrocytes are cleared from the blood by the filtration beds of the MZ and RP, and inclusion-containing erythrocytes, such as those containing Heinz bodies, may be pitted of their inclusions and returned to the circulation. Lymphocytes, both T- and B-cells, and their accessory cells (including monocytes-macrophages and veiled cells-interdigitating cells) are sequestered in the filtration beds of the WP, and are organized there to engage in immune responses, or to emigrate from the spleen *via* the deep lymphatics. Monocytes are cleared from the circulation in all beds of the spleen and readily differentiate into macrophages. Bacteria and other infectious particles such as the plasmodial-parasitized erythrocytes of malaria, are cleared from the circulation by the spleen. Slightly to moderately damaged erythrocytes, such as occur in such congenital hemolytic diseases as hereditary spherocytosis and other spectrin deficiencies, and erythrocytes damaged by such extrinsic factors as autoantibodies, parasites, and heat, are cleared by the spleen and phagocytized or repaired. Inert particles such as carbon are cleared from the blood by the spleen; this has proved to be of great experimental value, nicely displayed in the many clearance studies in the 1950s, and even today in experimental determinations of splenic clearance. The repertoire of particles and molecules used for such experimental or clinical assays of the reticuloendothelial system has increased to include radionuclide-labeled erythrocytes damaged by heat, phenylhydrazine or sulfhydryl-blocking agents, and many other materials, some of which are discussed later (see Chapter 13).

In most classical, and even in contemporary, studies the mechanisms of splenic clearance have been assumed to center on the macrophage. While the macrophage is essential to clearance, I believe other elements of the reticuloendothelial system are as important, if less obviously so. I shall now consider the reticuloendothelial components of the spleen.

3.4 THE RETICULOENDOTHELIAL SYSTEM (RES) IN THE SPLEEN

As formulation of the RES has evolved, the conception of the system has become more complex both with respect to its cellular make-up and to the functions ascribed to it. By the 1930s three major stromal-vascular cells were identified: macrophages, endothelial cells of vascular sinuses, and reticular cells. More recently, interdigitating cells, and other cells of the Langerhans' system of antigen-presenting cells, have been included because they have been thought to be related to or derived from macrophages.

The reticuloendothelial nature of the spleen has been inferred from its capacity to clear particles from the blood, this capacity, as indicated above, being largely ascribed to macrophages. The spleen is of course, a major locus of macrophages, the number and degree of activation of which may be swiftly raised. The spleen acquires its macrophages by the immigration of marrow-produced monocytes, and perhaps of circulating macrophages, by differentiation of splenic-based monocyte–macrophage stem cells (CFU-GM), and by some division of differentiated splenic macrophages. Macrophages are clearly not simply phagocytic cells, and knowledge of their functional repertoire has undergone a steady expansion. They are secretory, producing components of complement, interferon, hematopoietic colony-stimulating factors, and fibroblastic stimulating factors; they enhance the immunogenicity of antigens, present antigens, and assume other roles in immune reactions; they are key players in many phases of inflammation; and they regulate hematopoiesis. They possess many capacities ascribed to the RES and many of the properties of the RES are ascribed to them. As the complexity and coherence of macrophages and their cognate cells were increasingly appreciated, it appeared useful to investigators who studied them to abstract them from the RES and recognize them as a system, namely, the Mononuclear Phagocytic System (MPS).

In studies in the 1930s, the endothelial cells of the vascular sinuses were considered to be different from common endothelium in being both phagocytic and hematopoietically multipotent, and consequently they were thought to be deserving of a special name, i.e. lining cells or littoral (syn. shore) cells. Electron microscopic studies have shown that sinusal endothelium in human spleen may, in fact, become phagocytic when presented with long-term, large-scale phagocytic loads, such as the imperfect erythrocytes of hemolytic anemias. But the notion that these endothelial cells round up from the vascular wall and become hematopoietic stem cells has no contemporary support. Splenic sinusal endothelium is quite specialized, with such features as interendothelial slits, in-

termediate filaments aligned in basal bundles, luminal surface vesicles, and so on. But a distinctive name may not be necessary because it is increasingly appreciated that no endothelium is merely a mechanical lining; rather it is a complex biologically active tissue, secreting factors, controlling such major functions of the blood as coagulation and inflammation, and offering variations from place to place in respect to such morphological characteristics as the development of basement membrane, endothelial configuration, and the presence of endothelial cell fenestrations. The term 'endothelium', therefore, should be sufficient to encompass specializations and complexities, including those of the splenic sinuses.

Reticular cells, which are dendritic, fibroblastic, contractile, innervated stromal cells, form the scaffolding or meshwork which springs from the inner surface of the capsule and from the surface of trabeculae, and occupies the pulp, where it supports the vasculature and holds free cells in its interstices. RC, like the endothelium of venous sinuses, become phagocytic only when presented with long-term and large-scale phagocytic loads. Earlier notions that reticular cells may round up off the reticulum to become multipotent hemotopoietic stem cells have also not been supported by modern studies. RC are associated with argyrophilic reticular fibers and ensheathe them in their cytoplasmic processes. RC look like fibroblasts and it would appear they produce the reticular fibers, containing collagen type III, with which they remain associated. So closely do reticular cells and reticular fibers coincide that one may recognize as coincident, a cellular reticulum consisting of reticular cells, and a fibrous reticulum of reticular fibers, together constituting a reticulum; this is the salient, most consistent stromal arrangement of the spleen. I have recognized the reticulum as constituting the filtration beds, receiving blood, directly or indirectly from terminal arterial vessels and draining into veins or lymphatics. The curved, sheet-like cytoplasmic processes of reticular cells, reinforced by reticular fibers, form the locules of these filtration beds.

These locules can be open to one another and to the circulation, or can be closed off, so that the blood is shunted past them. The regulation of these filtration beds is central and critical to an understanding of the actions of the spleen, and its cellular basis is discussed in the following section.

Simple conceptions of these complex cells will not suffice. Just as monocyte-macrophages are not merely phagocytic, and endothelial cells of the vascular sinuses do not merely line vascular sinuses, reticular cells are not merely fibroblastic. Indeed, fibroblastic cells have been accorded important roles in the induction of differentiation of many tissues, including the hematopoietic system. As studies in my laboratory have emphasized, reticular cells enjoy great morphological range and even additional regulatory functions. It may be appropriate at this time to recognize RC and barrier cells (vide infra), as was done for the MPS, as sufficiently distinctive, coherent and important, to constitute an hegemony of the RES. Indeed, such a system, dependent upon the activation of fibroblastic cells, is proposed in the following section.

3.4.1 BARRIER-FORMING SYSTEMS

Reticular cells constitute a substantive, rather stable component of the filtration beds of hematopoietic tissues. Splenic filtration beds do not normally show a high level of filtration since more than 90% of the blood circulates through the spleen as rapidly as through tissues with a conventional vasculature. Yet splenic behavior may change rapidly in stress, and the organ become hypersplenic. I recognize a lineage of fibroblastic cells which appears to superimpose a dynamic, responsive character on the relatively stable reticulum, and permits one to rationalize the extraordinary clearance capacities of the stressed, and even of the normal spleen. The cells of this lineage appear fibroblastic and contractile, and fuse with one another in the filtration beds of the spleen to form complex, branched syncytial cellular sheets which form a variety of barriers. These cells had been termed activated reticular cells (Weiss, Geduldig, and Weidanz, 1986) but on the basis of continued study, I now term them barrier cells, because I think it appropriate to recognize them as an entity. I believe, moreover, that they warrant inclusion in the Reticuloendothelial System. Barrier cells are present in large numbers in murine and human spleen under conditions in which splenic clearance appears heightened pathologically (including sickle cell disease, spectrin deficiency, congenital spherocytic anemia, thalassemia, malaria and Hodgkin's disease). They occur in small numbers in the normal spleen. Barrier cells proliferate and show morphologic signs related to intense protein synthesis: large nucleoli, dense hyaloplasm, and a widened perinuclear cisterna continuous with endoplasmic reticulum, so branched and expanded that it imparts a lacy appearance to the cytoplasm.

Barrier cells originate by activation of fibroblasts on the surface of trabeculae and the adventitial aspect of blood vessels; activation is signalled by densification of the cytoplasm, with many lamellated packets of rough endoplasmic reticulum, and dilated mitochondria. Barrier cells also originate from circulating stem cells: circulating blood contains fibroblast stem cells (CFU-F), as determined in tissue culture assay, some of which must constitute barrier cell stem cells. Barrier cells initially accumulate in the spleen perivascularly, as dense, round cells with relatively short cell processes. Fusing with one another, they then move out from the initial perivascular location and in many instances apply themselves upon the existing reticulum, insinuating themselves along the reticular fibers, and associating themselves with established reticular cells. They thereby augment the functions and structure of the basic reticular cell filtration beds.

Barrier cells enclose blood vessels, providing an adventitial layer. They tightly surround single blood cells and multicellular hematopoietic colonies. They infiltrate the existing circumferential reticulum and layer upon its outside (marginal zone) surface, transforming the circumferential reticulum into a more effective barrier surrounding and protecting the white pulp. In the MZ and cords of RP of human (sinusal) spleens, where filtration locules are well developed, barrier cells insinuate into locules, often leaving a free portion which serves as a flap or valve which may open and close them. In contrast, in murine (nonsinusal) spleen, the reticulum composing the filtration locules in RP and MZ is scanty and poorly developed. Yet in these spleens, as in the sinusal spleens, barrier cells are present as extensive, branched, syncytial membranes. But with scant reticulum to infiltrate, barrier cells largely float free in the blood of the pulp, tethered only to the adventitial surface of blood vessels by adventitial RC. These nonsinusal spleens may well depend upon barrier cells to provide normal basal filtration to RP and MZ. In the sinusal spleen, I believe that barrier cells augment the basal filtration activity of the locules of the filtration beds, serving to regulate them, by opening and closing the beds, and to extend them.

Barrier cells provide dynamic, diverse blood–spleen barriers which, acting in co-ordination with macrophages and other stromal cells, regulate splenic filtration and its intrasplenic consequences, including blood flow, cell homing and migration, hematopoietic and immune responses, and the clearance of infectious organisms. They trap circulating infectious organisms and monocytes on their adherent surfaces, clearing them from the blood and positioning them so that the monocyte, differentiating into a macrophage, phagocytizes the microorganisms. Barrier cells enclosing hematopoietic colonies are positioned to confine factors controlling colony growth and differentiation. They may protect colonies from parasitization, as, for example, erythroblastic colonies in malaria. Activated circumferential reticulum may close off WP rather effectively. An initial antigenic stimulus is thereby met by a complete response, which confines the lymphokines, cytokines, and other regulatory substances to the WP, and prevents epiphenomenal antigen from dissipating immunologic resources. Closing off the white pulp in the presence of contiguous tissue damage would reduce autoimmune responses. As barrier cells close off locules of the filtration beds, they constitute a shunt, permitting an efficient closed circulation between arterial terminals and veins. The spleen, unlike bone marrow, lacks a cellular barrier between hematopoietic tissues and the blood. Barrier cells provide such barriers, thereby conferring upon the spleen certain attributes of the marrow. Barrier cells may be evoked by administration of interleukin-1a.

3.5   CONCLUSION

In a normal spleen the level of filtration activity may well be regulated by (1) the degree of contraction of the filtration beds, the capsule and trabeculae, (2) the placement of the terminating arterial vessels, and (3) the capacity of the sheet-like processes of the reticular cells to configure tubular connections between arterial and venous vessels. The normal spleen does not appear to depend heavily upon its barrier cells. These are of fibroblastic lineage, and fuse with one another, providing systems of dynamic membranous barriers which, in concert with the more stable reticulum, provide a dynamic character to the filtration beds. This accounts for much of the pattern of behavior of stressed spleens. Even in the normal spleen, however, barrier cells may appear, insinuated into the circumferential reticulum bounding white pulp, and, especially in non-sinusal spleens, as floating membranes in the MZ and RP. In pathological spleens in which the locules of the filtration bed become tightly crowded as a result of heightened filtration, the spleen becomes quite firm and enlarged; consequently, the mechanisms regulating blood flow under normal circumstances cannot function since the spleen is distended and becomes incapable of contraction. The syncytial membrane and meshworks produced by fusion of barrier cells now become the means by which the character of blood flow is determined. The character of blood flow, in turn, determines whether or not the filtration beds are perfused, whether the circulation is open or closed, and whether or not the blood is cleared.

BIBLIOGRAPHY

This list contains a series of references of significance to an understanding of spleen structure, and does not refer only to papers quoted in the text.

Butcher, E. C. and Weissman, I. L. (1984) Lymphoid tissues and organs, in *Fundamental Immunology* (ed. W. Paul), Raven Press, New York, p. 109.

Fujita, T., Kashimura, M. and Adachi, K. (1985) Scanning electron microscopy and terminal circulation. *Experientia*, **40**, 167–78.

Gowans, J. L. (1959) The recirculation of lymphocytes from blood to lymph in the rat. *J. Physiol.*, **146**, 54.

Groom, A. C. and Song, S.H. (1971) Effects of norepinephrine on washout of red cells from the spleen. *Am. J. Physiol.*, **22**, 255–8.

Knisely, M. H. (1936) Spleen studies, I. Microscopic observations of the circulatory system of living unstimulated mammalian spleen. *Anat. Rec.* **65**, 23.

McCuskey R. S. and McCuskey R. P. (1985) *In vivo* and electron microscopy studies of the splenic microvasculature in mice. *Experientia*, **40**, 179–87.

Pellas, T. C. and Weiss, L. (1989a) Migration pathways of recirculating Murine B cells, CD4[+] and CD8[+] T lymphocytes. *Am. J. Anat.* (in press).

Pellas, T. C. and Weiss, L. (1989b) Deep splenic lymphatic vessels in the mouse: A route of splenic exit for recirculating lymphocytes. *Am. J. Anat.* (in press).

Physiology of the Reticulendothelial System. A Symposium. (1957) The Council for International Organizations of Medical Sciences. Unesco and WHO, Paris, France, (eds B. N. Halpern, B. Benacerraf and J. F. Delafresnaye), Blackwell, Oxford.

Reilly F. D. (1985) Innervation and vascular pharmacodynamics of the mammalian spleen. *Experientia*, **40**, 187–92.

Reticuloendothelial Structure and Function (1958) Third International Symposium. The International Society for Research of the Reticuloendothelial System. Rapallo, Italy. (ed. J. H. Heller), Ronald Press, New York.

Schiffman, F. J., Weiss, L. and Cadman, E. C. (1988) Erythrophagocytosis by venous sinus endothelial cells of the spleen in autoimmune hemolytic anemia. *Hemat. Reviews*, **2**, 327–43.

Seifert, M. F. and Marks, Jr, S. C. (1985) The regulation of hemopoiesis in the spleen. *Experientia*, **40**, 192–8.

Tischendorf, F. (1985) On the evolution of the spleen. *Experientia*. **40**, 145–52.

van Ewijk, W. and Nieuwenhius, P. (1985) Compartments, domains and migration pathways of lymphoid cells in the splenic pulp. *Experientia*, **40**, 199–208.

Weiss, L. (ed.) (1988a) *Cell and Tissue Biology*, 6th edn, Urban and Schwarzenberg, Baltimore and Munich, Chs 12–17.

Weiss, L. (1988b) Interleukin 1-induced fibroblastic barrier forming systems in infectious disease. ASCB/ASBMB Meeting 1/29/89–2/2/89, San Francisco. *J. Cell Biol.*, Abstr. 3955, p. 699a.

Weiss, L. (1988c) Hegemonies of the reticuloendothelial system: Barrier forming systems of activated reticular cells. RES Soc. Meeting Oct. 27–30, 1988, Washington, D.C. *J. Leuk. Biol.*, Abstr. 100, p. 283.

Weiss, L. (1989a) Barrier-forming systems of activated reticular cells regulating clearance, blood flow, cell migration and hematopoiesis in the spleen. Am. Assoc. Anat. Meeting, April 24–28, 1988, Cincinnati, Ohio. *Am. J. Anat.* (in press).

Weiss, L. (1989b) Barrier cells: A newly defined, interleukin 1a evoked, lineage of fibroblastic cells which fuse to form barriers in spleen, bone marrow and reticuloendothelial system. *Science* (submitted).

Weiss, L. (1989c) Mechanisms of splenic control of murine malaria: Cellular reactions of the spleen in lethal (strain 17XL) plasmodium yoelii malaria in BALB/c mice, and the consequences of preinfective splenectomy. *Am. J. Trop. Med. Hyg.* (in press).

Weiss, L., Powell, R. and Schiffman, F. J. (1985) Terminating arterial vessels in red pulp of the spleen. *Experientia*, **40**, 233–42.

Weiss, L., Geduldig, U. and Weidanz, W. (1986) Mechanisms of splenic control of murine malaria: Reticular cell activation and the development of a blood–spleen barrier. *Am. J. Anat.*, **176**, 251–85.

GLOSSARY

A list of definitions of structural terms may be useful for those who work with the spleen but infrequently deal with its structure. The term, its acronym, and its definition are provided. This glossary is drawn from Weiss (1988a).

Barrier cells. Reticular cells (RC) are the dendritic, fibroblastic, contractile, innervated stromal cells which make up the splenic filtration beds and constitute the outermost (adventitial) layer of blood vessels. See Reticular cells. Normally the locules and enclosures formed by RC are communicating and rather incomplete, with the result that only imperfect barriers result. But to some degree normally, and in certain cases of splenomegaly to a pronounced degree, a newly recognized lineage of fibroblastic cells, termed 'barrier cells' appears. Barrier cells are 'turned on' to intense protein synthesis and secretion, which can be inferred from such cytological changes as a dilated perinuclear space extending, as endoplasmic reticulum, deep into the cytoplasm. Nucleoli become prominent and mitosis, rare among non-activated reticular cells, is common. Barrier cells may develop from existing splenic fibroblasts and may also differentiate from circulating fibroblastic progenitors in the spleen. Barrier cells then fuse with one another to form complex, extensive, syncytial cellular sheets which form a variety of barriers. They may enwrap blood vessels, insinuate into existing reticulum, and form sacs. Tethered to the outside surface of blood vessels or trabeculae, they may float in the blood circulating in the pulp spaces (as in mouse spleen) serving as adherent membranes, clearing microbes and other particles from the blood. They may reinforce the circumferential reticulum of white pulp, for example, sealing it off rather effectively from encroachment by antigens. They may form sacs holding hematopoietic colonies (brood-sacs as it were), isolating these colonies from the blood, and therefore from parasites of the blood, and concentrating hematopoietic regulatory factors. They may also form vascular shunts. They contain microfilaments and are presumably contractile.

Blood–spleen barriers. Although the spleen is the quintessential filter of the blood, its filtration beds may be closed off from the blood, usually in a dynamic, reversible manner. Under normal circumstances to a limited degree, and in some pathological spleens to considerably augmented degrees, cellular sheets or barriers of fused barrier cells, are formed. These syncytial cellular sheets close off filtration beds, envelop blood vessels, and divert the circulation: in short, they constitute blood–spleen barriers. See Barrier cells.

Capsule and trabeculae. The capsule, and the trabeculae which spring from its internal surface, consist of connective tissue and smooth muscle, the proportions and amount being species-dependent. In storage spleens, such as that of the horse, the capsule and trabeculae are thick and rich in smooth muscle, while in defense spleens (as in rabbits) they are thin and rich in collagen. Trabeculae subdivide the pulp, carry blood vessels and nerves into the interior, and are a source of fibroblastic stromal cells both normally and during activation of reticular cells.

Circumferential reticulum. The reticulum of the PALS tends to be arranged circumferentially about the central artery rather than in the non-oriented, rather symmetrically branched conformation it assumes in many sites. About the periphery of the PALS the circumferential disposition is often both well developed and stout, providing a peripheral boundary to the white pulp, a central boundary to the surrounding marginal zone, and a barrier to the penetration of materials into the white pulp from the marginal zone. Lymphatic nodules may be enclosed by a slighter circumferential reticulum.

Filtration beds. This term was coined to apply to the reticular meshworks of the spleen, recognizing their physiological capacity for clearing blood cells, antigens and other particles from the blood. Filtration beds are distinctive in different parts of the spleen. Those in the periarterial lymphatic sheaths selectively filter out T-cells; lymphatic nodules accumulate B-cells. Monocyte-macrophages are filtered out of the blood by virtually all the filtration beds. The beds of the marginal zone and red pulp hold and process erythroid cells, platelets and granulocytes. Filtration beds may be opened or closed responsively (see Barrier cells) providing delayed (physiologically open) and direct (physiologically closed) circulations.

Germinal center. See Lymphatic nodules.

Interendothelial Slit (IES) of proximal veins. These are the slits between the endothelial cells of venous sinuses, and in the pulp veins of many non-sinusal spleens (such as that of the mouse), through which blood cells, and other elements of the blood, must flow in order to enter the venous system and leave the spleen. These slits, like Millipore filters, may provide considerable impedance to flow and therefore be a site where rigid cells are held up or 'culled'. It is generally believed that this is the site at which erythrocytes containing rigid inclusions, such as Heinz bodies or malarial plasmodia, may be 'pitted' of their inclusions. In animals such as the cat and horse with a non-sinusal spleen, whose proximal pulp veins display large mural defects or apertures, pitting may not occur. Thus Heinz bodies may remain in the circulation in the cat, both because of the propensity of feline hemoglobin to form them, and to the presence of large mural venous apertures.

Intermediate circulation. This is the level of the circulation that occurs between terminal arterial vessels and the proximal venous vessels (*viz:* the venous sinuses in sinusal spleens). There has been controversy over whether this circulation is open or closed, or a mixture of the two.

Lymphatic nodules (LN). These are present in that part of the filtration beds of white pulp lying in the proximal, thicker parts of the periarterial lymphatic sheaths; they appear as ovoid nodules comprising a specialized reticular meshwork consisting preponderantly of B-cells and their accessory cells. When composed of closely packed small lymphocytes, the nodule is recognized as a primary nodule. In a sustained or secondary antibody response the central zone of the LN may be occupied by large lymphocytes (both T- and B-cells), together with macrophages and other accessory cells. These cells form a pale-staining central zone, the germinal center (GC). The periphery of the LN, consisting of a shell of small B-lymphocytes surrounding the GC, has been termed 'mantle'. LN containing GC are termed secondary nodules. In their proliferative early and middle stages germinal centers are high-level monoclonal antibody producers. GC will wane after weeks or months and macrophages may become the predominant cells, 'mopping up' the debris of the structure. Such terminal germinal centers have been termed reaction centers.

Mantle. See Lymphatic nodules.

Marginal Zone (MZ). The filtration bed interposed between the white pulp (on its central surface) and the red pulp (on its peripheral surface). MZ is the major traffic zone of the spleen, receiving a disproportionately great number of arterial endings and possessing, in many species, a fine-meshed reticulum (*syn.* filtration bed). The MZ is thus the great vestibule or reception center of the spleen, receiving many blood cells and despatching them to different parts of the spleen for further processing.

Mononuclear Phagocytic System (MPS). Finding the concept of the RES inadequate, one group of investigators abstracted the macrophage and its associated cells, and proposed the term Mononuclear Phagocytic System (MPS). I believe that the term is awkward, unsophisticated and imprecise. Mononuclear, like round cells, has long been used as informal scientific shorthand or argot, in setting lymphocytes and monocytes aside from polymorphonuclear cells. It means, of course, having one nucleus, which is scarcely defining since it characterizes almost every cell. The word phagocytic hardly sets these cells apart, and characterizes only their salient characteristic, but not their secretory factor producing, and immunological functions, which may be more significant. Such cavil notwithstanding, the term seems to have gained acceptance to some degree. As tends to happen to encompassing terms, the term MPS is creeping into use with respect to other cells and functions, blurring its boundaries. It has been extended to interdigitating cells, for example, whose relationship to macrophages is still unclear.

Non-sinusal spleen. This refers to the type of spleen in which proximal venous vessels, the pulp veins, possess 'common' flat endothelium, a conventional basement membrane, and adventitial reticular cells. Circulating blood cells enter the lumen of pulp veins by passing through interendothelial slits (or mural apertures) which, depending upon the species, can be quite large, offering little impedance to flow (e.g. cat, horse).

Open vs closed circulation. Unless the distinction is made between anatomically open or closed and physiologically open or closed, confusion is sure to result. An anatomically open circulation or, better, vasculature, is one in which there is no endothelial continuity between terminal arterial vessels and proximal veins. An anatomically closed circulation, or vasculature, which is typical of virtually all the tissues of the body, is one in which there is endothelial continuity between terminal arterial vessels and proximal veins. A physiologically closed circulation is one in which blood flow is as rapid, and even as confined, as that through kidney, muscle or liver, but in which there need be no complete continuity of endothelium. A physiologically open circulation is one in which the circulation is delayed and, possibly not as confined, as that through tissues which possess an anatomically closed vasculature. A major problem that must be reconciled in the spleen is the existence of physiologically closed circulations through anatomically open vasculatures.

Periarterial Lymphatic Sheath (PALS). This is the part of the filtration beds of white pulp that surrounds the central artery as a coaxial sheath, concentrating T-cells and their accessory cells. That part of the PALS that first surrounds the artery as it emerges from a trabecula and enters the pulp is relatively thick. As the artery runs in the pulp, branching and growing finer in caliber, the PALS ensheathing it branches with it, and later tapers down and disappears. After it emerges from the attenuated PALS the artery continues on to terminate in the marginal zone or red pulp.

Periarterial Macrophage Sheath (PAMS) or Ellipsoid. Terminal arterial vessels in the spleen always open into a filtration bed, surrounded by many macrophages. These macrophages may lie rather loosely and diffusely in the neighborhood of the arterial ending or be rather tightly organized into a nodular cuff through which the arteriole runs just before ending. In fact the macrophages in this cuff may be supported by reticular cells and joined by other cell types, such as interdigitating cells (Figure 2.3).

Reticular Cell (RC). A dendritic, fibroblastic, contractile, innervated stromal cell which, with other RC, forms the meshworks or reticula or filtration beds of the spleen. RC contain microfilaments and appear to synthesize, and remain associated with, argyrophilic fibers. At least in some species, they are innervated by sympathetic autonomic nerves. The conformation of reticular cells is dependent on species and intrasplenic location. Steady-state reticular cells seldom divide.

Reticular Fibers (RF). Slender argyrophilic fibers are produced and associated with reticular cells, and form the fibrous reticulum. The conformation and development of RF is dependent on species and intrasplenic location. The substance of RF is sometimes termed reticulin. Modern methods reveal it as a mixture of collagen types. RF share many staining characteristics, such as argyrophilia, with basement membranes. RF are by no means restricted to the spleen or even to hematopoietic tissues, but occur in diverse tissues, such as the liver and endocrine tissues, where they may be synthesized by cells other than RC.

Reticuloendothelial System (RES). This is a pervasive system of cells and vessels whose salient characteristic is pronounced phagocytic capacity. By extension the RES has been accorded roles in such diverse functions as the immune process, inflammation, the control of infectious disease, lipid and carbohydrate metabolism, pigmentation, and hematopoiesis. Major cell types of the RES are reticular cells, endothelial cells of the vascular sinuses of hematopoietic, endocrine and other tissues, and macrophages, all of which were accorded phagocytic and pluripotent differentiative capacity at the time the RES was being defined. The spleen, which is a quintessential filter of the blood and unusually rich in the above cells is the pre-eminent reticuloendothelial organ. The apogee of the spleen's prominence and clear delineation as a RE organ was, perhaps, in the clearance studies where the removal of injected particles was attributed to splenic macrophage beds. Since then, the picture has become more complicated, and more interesting. The RES is difficult to characterize simply scientifically because it has been the subject of much speculation, especially in relation to postulated roles in hematopoiesis, carcinogenesis, etc.

Reticulum. This is a meshwork fashioned of reticular cells and reticular fibers, constituting filtration beds. The reticulum consists of a cellular reticulum (reticular cells) and a fibrous reticulum (reticular fibers). Because the reticular fibers are ensheathed by the reticular cells which produce them, fibrous and cellular reticula are coincident.

Sinusal spleen. This is the form of spleen characterized by distinctive proximal venous vessels, known as venous sinuses and characterized by longitudinally aligned endothelial cells, a fenestrated basement membrane, and adventitial reticular cells. Circulating blood enters the lumen of venous sinuses through interendothelial slits (q.v.).

Splenic pulp. This is the tissue enclosed by capsule and trabeculae. It consists of the reticular meshworks (constituting filtration beds), free cells (cells filtered from the blood and hematopoietic cells produced in the spleen) held in the meshworks, and a vasculature. The splenic pulp is divisible into three major divisions: white pulp, marginal zone and red pulp.

Terminating arterial vessels. Terminating arterial vessels which empty into the filtration beds of mammalian spleen in anatomically open arrangements, terminate in different ways in different places in different species. They end at marginal zone and in red pulp. They end as small arterioles, as metarterioles or as capillaries. They terminate abruptly, as if cleanly transected, or they flare. Their interendothelial slits open just before termination. They may be surrounded by a cuff of macrophages, the periarterial macrophage sheath or ellipsoid. They may end some distance away from the wall of a vein, or at or near the wall of a vein, but there is no endothelial continuity between arterial terminal and vein.

White pulp (WP). This is the splenic filtration bed which selectively filters and sorts out lymphocytes and accessory cells, setting them up to carry out immune responses or, failing that, to recirculate. WP consists of periarterial lymphatic sheaths and lymphatic nodules.

MICROCIRCULATORY BLOOD FLOW THROUGH THE SPLEEN

4

Alan C. Groom and Eric E. Schmidt

4.1 INTRODUCTION

The microcirculation of the spleen is perhaps the most complex of any organ in the body; splenic arterioles lead to capillaries, most of which do not lead to venules but discharge blood into a labyrinthine reticular meshwork. The spleen contains blood with a packed cell volume twice that of arterial blood: it is not yet known why this high hematocrit is necessary, or how it is achieved. Red cell (RBC) transit times through some microcirculatory routes are as short as through skeletal muscle, whereas transit times for other routes can be up to one thousand times longer. The distribution of the total flow among these various routes can change dramatically under neural or hormonal stimulation, and as a result of increased portal venous pressure. Unlike most other organs and tissues studied from a microcirculatory viewpoint, the spleen is not concerned with transcapillary exchange in relation to metabolism but constitutes the only lymphoid organ specialized for the filtration of blood. The unique structure of the microvascular pathways in the spleen must be understood as a reflection of this function.

For humans and a group of common laboratory animals, splenic weight, expressed as a proportion of body weight, is quite variable (Davies and Withrington, 1973). Approximate values are given as 1% (cat, dog), 0.7% (mouse), 0.25% (human, rat), 0.15% (monkey,

guinea pig), and 0.05% (rabbit). The highest values are found in species with an abundance of smooth muscle in the splenic capsule and trabeculae, and in which the organ is known to be contractile. Conversely the intermediate and low values occur in species with little capsular and trabecular smooth muscle and in which active contraction probably does not occur: the spleens with lower weights are probably those which lack the reservoir function. Resting splenic blood flow in all species studied lies in the range of 40–100 ml/min per 100 g of tissue; this corresponds to 1–10% of the cardiac output depending on the species (Davies and Withrington, 1973).

The blood-filled space in the spleen is a large fraction of the total volume of the organ; in the relaxed spleen of the cat this amounts to 50%. When the high hematocrit is taken into consideration, this means that stored red cells represent about 40% of the total volume of the organ. In species with contractile spleens a large proportion of these stored cells can be released promptly into the general circulation when needed. It is possible that this happens to a lesser extent in species such as man, in which the spleen is non-contractile. Because the compliance of the spleen is so great, elevated portal venous pressure can cause a considerable increase in the splenic blood volume, and in the overall size of the organ. When perfused with blood *in vivo* against an outflow pressure of 25 cmH$_2$O, the spleen of cat takes up and stores one-half of the animal's total RBC mass (Levesque and Groom, 1980b). Large numbers of all the cellular elements of the blood are stored in the spleen by a process which is not yet understood, and in normal human subjects the spleen contains about 30% of the total platelet mass of the body. (See also Chapter 8.)

The filtration of blood by the spleen with the removal of blood cells unsuitable for continued circulation, has been studied principally with respect to red cells. Reticulocytes released from bone marrow are retained in the organ (Dornfest, Handler and Handler, 1971; Wade, 1973), perhaps for destruction (Sorbie and Valberg, 1970), maturation (Pictet *et al.*, 1969; Song and Groom, 1971c, 1972), or remodeling (Ganzoni, Hillman and Finch, 1969; Crosby, 1977). Inclusion bodies such as Heinz bodies are removed from RBCs in the spleen ('pitting' function: Koyama, Aoki and Deguchi, 1964; Chen and Weiss, 1973; Klausner *et al.*, 1975; Matsumoto *et al.*, 1977). The selective retention ('culling') of abnormal red cells has been demonstrated for pathological red cells (Weiss and Tavassoli, 1970; Schnitzer *et al.*, 1973) and for normal RBCs altered by thermal stress (Dornfest, Handler and Handler, 1970; Levesque and Groom, 1977; Peters, 1983), by treatment with *N*-ethylmaleimide (Klausner *et al.*, 1975; Levesque and Groom, 1980a), phenylhydrazine (Chen and Weiss, 1973; Klausner *et al.*, 1975), or neuraminidase (Janicik *et al.* 1978; Levesque and Groom, 1980a). Whether or not the spleen culls normally senescent red cells has not yet been demonstrated conclusively. It is thought that culled red cells are subsequently destroyed in the spleen, a process which has been attributed to osmotic hemolysis (Prankerd, 1963; Benbassat, 1969) or to phagocytosis (Rifkind, 1966; Simon and Burke, 1970; Klausner *et al.*, 1975).

Little is known of the mechanism underlying the sequestration and subsequent processing of red cells in the spleen, in terms of the properties of the cells themselves or the morphology of the splenic red pulp. Red cell trapping in sinusal spleens has been described in terms of an intrasplenic filter based on geometrical restrictions (Chen and Weiss, 1973; Boisfleury and Mohandas, 1977). However, it has been proposed that sequestration of immature red cells may be due to an increased tendency for cell-to-cell adhesion (Berendes, 1959; Jandl, 1960; Song and Groom, 1971b, c, 1972, 1974) and that phagocytosis of senescent red cells may occur because of a reduction in the density of electrical charge on the cell surface (Pictet *et al.*, 1969; Skutelsky and Danon, 1970a, b) which unmasks immunoglobulins and leads to recognition and degradation by macrophages (Janicik *et al.*, 1978; Kay *et al.*, 1982). The hypothesis has been widely held that the splenic red pulp provides a hostile metabolic environment for red cells, leading to a selective weakening ('conditioning': Griggs, Weisman and Harris, 1960) of abnormal or senescent red cells in preparation for destruction in the circulation. What configurations of circulatory pathways within the organ subserve these various functions?

Blood vessels enter the spleen along the hilus of its concave surface and are conveyed within trabeculae into the interior of the organ (Figure 4.1). Suspended within the trabecular network is an open three-dimensional web of reticular tissue housing white pulp and red pulp. The white pulp forms a sheath of lymphatic tissue surrounding the arteries after they leave the trabeculae (periarterial lymphatic sheath), and it is thickened in places to form lymphatic nodules. The red pulp, in which the filtration function of the spleen is carried out, occupies most of the parenchyma and amounts to 75% of the normal human spleen (Van Krieken *et al.*, 1985a). Its basic structure, a meshwork of reticular cells and fibers ('reticular meshwork'), appears honeycombed by an anastomosing system of venous sinuses in about 50% of mammalian species examined (Snook, 1950); in other species the venous system begins, instead, as small, fenestrated pulp venules. We refer to 'sinusal' and 'non-sinusal' spleens, the human spleen being of the sinusal type. (See also Chapter 3.)

The red pulp occupies all the space not taken

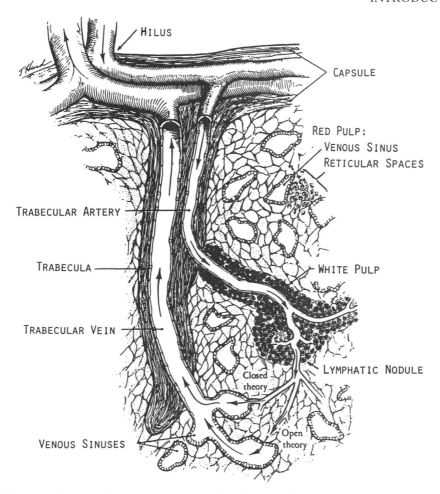

Figure 4.1 Schematic diagram showing structure of sinusal spleen. (Reproduced with permission from J. A. Bellanti (1979) *Immunology: Basic Processes*, W. B. Saunders, Philadelphia.)

up by trabeculae and white pulp, and its interstices are lined with both fixed and free phagocytes which remove abnormal particulate material from the blood passing through. Because cellular components of the blood are concentrated within the spleen, the reticular meshwork is filled with blood of very high hematocrit. It may be seen (Figure 4.1) that blood flows through the white pulp and then the red pulp in series. The white pulp is intimately associated with the arterial tree, whereas the red pulp is similarly associated with the venous system draining the spleen. Most capillaries empty into the reticular meshwork ('open' circulation) to drain into the venous system. Thus, the reticular meshwork constitutes an 'intermediate circulation' between the capillaries and venous channels. Whether direct vascular connections also exist ('closed' circulation), bypassing the intermediate circulation, has been controversial.

How can one study microcirculatory pathways and their perfusion with blood in such a complicated circulatory system? It is necessary to employ several different methods in order to answer key questions about the splenic microcirculation. (See section 4.2; for further discussion see Goresky and Groom (1984) and Groom (1987)).

4.2   METHODS FOR THE STUDY OF SPLENIC MICROCIRCULATORY PATHWAYS AND BLOOD FLOW

4.2.1   THE 'BLACK BOX' APPROACH

One can learn a great deal about intrasplenic blood flow under different conditions, and about splenic retention of abnormal red cells, by considering the organ as a 'black box' and studying input/output relationships. For example, total splenic blood flow has been measured by washout of radioactive gas (^{133}Xe, ^{85}Kr); the presence of both fast and slow pathways for flow was shown by the fact that the washout curves were biexponential (Sandberg, 1972; Zetterstrom, 1973; Braunbeck, Hutten and Vaupel, 1973; Vaupel, Ruppert and Hutten, 1977). Because the spleen is a filter for blood, red cells may be treated differently from plasma during passage through this organ; therefore, there is the need for washout studies of red cells and plasma to be performed separately. Three 'black box' approaches to the study of microcirculatory blood flow through the spleen will now be described.

(a)   RBC and plasma washout during Ringer perfusion

One simple way to study the storage and transit of red cells in the spleen is to isolate the organ and perfuse it with cell-free Ringer's solution, sampling the outflow as a function of time (Song and Groom, 1971a). This system has the advantage that the red cells are not processed first, as with radiolabelling; the red cells collected at the outflow are those which were contained in the spleen *in vivo* at the time of cannulation and are now simply being 'washed out' by Ringer perfusion. Moreover, since this is a non-recirculating system and the perfusate

entering the organ is cell-free, slow as well as fast clearance of red cells from the spleen may be quantitated. Cell concentrations in successive samples of the outflow can be measured very precisely, over several orders of magnitude, by means of an electronic particle counter. If a small quantity of radioiodinated (^{125}I) serum albumin is injected into the general circulation and allowed to equilibrate intravascularly prior to isolating the spleen, then the washout of both red cells and plasma from the organ may be studied simultaneously (Levesque and Groom, 1976a). Red cell and plasma concentrations are plotted semilogarithmically against the sequential volumes of perfusing fluid per gram splenic weight.

An example is given in Figure 4.2. The red cell washout from relaxed spleen of cat shows an initial rapid decrease of red cell concentration by an order of magnitude, followed by a slower rate of decline over the next 1.5 orders of magnitude; there follows an exceedingly slow but consistent rate of decline of concentration thereafter. Although a number of different mathematical models might be fitted to such a washout curve, only in the case of a series of exponentials can the equations be derived as the outcome of a set of rational assumptions. A single exponential component represents washout of a single compartment. If a washout curve contains two exponential components, then the final part of the graph will be a straight line, whereas the earlier part will be curved continuously. By standard mathematical procedures the red cell washout curve of Figure 4.2 may be analyzed into three exponential components, shown as solid lines, each being characterized by a very different volume of perfusate per gram splenic weight needed to reduce the concentration of red cells by one-half. These $V_{1/2}$ values proved to be 0.067, 4.7 and 97 ml/g, respectively, and on that basis the components have been designated as fast, intermediate, and slow, respectively.

The fact that the sum of three exponential terms can describe completely the RBC washout curve indicates that a simple model consist-

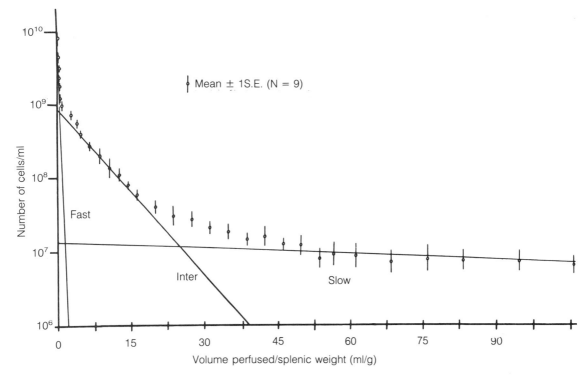

Figure 4.2 Mean red cell washout curve from cat spleens during constant-flow perfusion with Ringer's solution. Cell concentration in outflow is plotted semilogarithmically against cumulative volume of fluid perfused. Washout curve may be expressed as the sum of three exponential components, labeled FAST, INTER, and SLOW. (Reproduced with permission from Levesque and Groom (1976a) *American Journal of Physiology*, **231**, 1665–71.)

ing of three compartments in parallel is sufficient to approximate the red cell washout processes from the spleen. The respective sizes (red cells/g) and perfusion (% of total) of these compartments can then be computed.

(b) Splenic drainage with inflow occluded

This procedure consists of anaerobic collection of blood drained from the organ, during contraction with inflow occluded, as successive discrete samples (Levesque and Groom, 1976b). It provides a means of selectively sampling blood from the reticular meshwork, because expulsion of blood from the fast transit pathways is completed ahead of expulsion of blood from the slower transit pathways of the reticular meshwork. The increase in hematocrit of the

venous outflow during this procedure, from an initial value comparable to that of arterial blood to a final value of almost 80%, suggests that the last samples are indeed representative of blood from the reticular meshwork. This conclusion is also reinforced by the progressive changes in gas tensions and glucose concentrations that are found during drainage.

(c) Bolus injections of abnormal RBCs into Ringer-perfused spleens

The isolated perfused spleen preparation offers a number of advantages over the use of intact animals for studying the sequestration of 'abnormal' red cells. The results do not depend on the ratio of splenic blood flow to cardiac output. They are not complicated by the simultaneous activities of other organs of the mono-nuclear-phagocyte system, such as bone marrow or liver, which in the intact animal can make the interpretation of splenic function difficult. The technique allows for the accurate quantitative assessment of the efficiency of trapping abnormal red cells during a single passage through the spleen. The use of two or three serial injections of red cells offers the means of assessing whether it is possible to saturate the splenic trapping mechanism.

The spleen is isolated and perfused at constant pressure with oxygenated ($5\% CO_2$ in O_2) buffered Ringer's solution to wash out most of the contained red cells. Samples of the outflow are then collected for measurement of the 'background' or preinjection red cell concentration. A small bolus of a red cell suspension containing a known number of cells (approximately 2×10^6 red cells for a 30g spleen of cat) is then injected quickly into the arterial cannula close to the spleen itself. At the same time, rapid sequential sampling of the venous outflow is begun, and is continued until the red cell concentration has returned to its preinjection level. Red cell concentrations are determined by an electronic cell counter, and the cumulative outflows of red cells (expressed as percentages of the number injected) are then used to derive plots of percentage red cell recovery *versus* outflowing volume of perfusate (Levesque and Groom, 1980a).

4.2.2 FIXED SECTIONS OF SPLENIC TISSUE, INCLUDING HISTOLOGICAL STUDIES DURING RED CELL WASHOUT

Much has been learned about microcirculatory pathways from examination of sections of splenic tissue, using either the light microscope or transmission electron microscopy (TEM). For example, the classic study by Snook (1950) used serial histological sections to provide schematic diagrams of microcirculatory routes in spleens of several mammalian species. Greater detail is shown in TEM photographs, especially concerning the cells lining venous sinuses

and blood cells in transit through interendothelial slits (e.g. Blue and Weiss, 1981d). The study of fixed sections by means of light microscopy or TEM is limited by the very small depth of focus, leading to problems in tracing vascular pathways over long distances. The greater depth of focus of the scanning electron microscope (SEM) has allowed three-dimensional views of such pathways to be obtained (e.g. Fujita, 1974).

Information regarding flow has been obtained by preparing histological sections at serial intervals from the start of splenic perfusion with Ringer solution (Song and Groom, 1971b). Perfusion by 1–2 ml of solution per gram spleen weight is sufficient to eliminate virtually all red cells comprising the fast compartment. Perfusion by a larger volume (up to 15 ml/g) will reduce by a factor of ten the red cells of the intermediate compartment. If the volume of solution perfused is increased to 50–150 ml/g, the red cells comprising the intermediate compartment are reduced to zero, while the red cells of the slow compartment remain at roughly one-half the value of the normal blood-perfused spleen. This technique has helped to identify the morphological counterparts of the fast, intermediate and slow compartments identified by the study of red cell washout kinetics.

4.2.3 MICROCORROSION CASTING STUDIES

In this technique a methyl-methacrylate resin of low viscosity (Nopanitaya, Aghajanian and Gray, 1979) is injected into the splenic artery or vein. After polymerization of the resin, the tissue is corroded away using concentrated KOH at 60°C. This leaves a rigid cast which faithfully reproduces the morphology of the blood pathways, including fine details of vascular luminal surfaces. Examination of vascular corrosion casts by SEM offers a way of studying circulatory pathways and their interconnections over a considerable length with the view unobstructed by surrounding tissue. The 'black box' studies of red cell washout showed that in the relaxed spleen 90% of the inflow travels to the splenic vein *via* the fast pathways that occupy only 18% of the total blood space. This suggested that microcorrosion casting could offer a unique opportunity to study the morphology of the fast arteriovenous pathways, provided that very small quantities of material were injected. Under these conditions, extensive filling of slower routes through the reticular meshwork would be avoided. By varying the volume of material injected in successive experiments, other red cell compartments of the splenic microcirculation were studied.

Red cell washout studies also showed that in dilated spleens the customary fast component of flow appears to be absent, whereas in contracted spleens the fast pathways carry almost the entire blood flow. Therefore, in order to demonstrate the morphology of the fast pathways preferentially, one injects minimal amounts of casting material into spleens contracted by norepinephrine. In order to view the slow pathways, minimal injections are used in spleens dilated by perfusion against a high venous pressure. In all cases, clearer views of pathways in the interior of the organ can be obtained by making use of the 'natural dissection' occurring at a boundary between a perfused segment of the spleen and adjacent unperfused tissue. This can be achieved by injection of casting material into an arterial branch supplying only a limited segment of the organ. Fragmentation of the cast, which occurs inevitably at cut faces, may thereby be avoided.

4.2.4 VIDEOMICROSCOPIC STUDIES OF TRANSILLUMINATED SPLEENS *IN VIVO*

In vivo microscopy of the spleen was attempted more than 50 years ago, but the quality of recorded images was not adequate for quantitative analysis of RBC flow within the organ. In addition, the interpretation of *in vivo* observations has been difficult due to lack of a 3-dimensional 'map' of the diverse pathways available for flow, and this has led to contradictory conclusions (Knisely, 1936; MacKenzie, Whipple and Wintersteiner, 1941). Successful *in vivo* microscopy of the spleen requires a method whereby the position of the organ can be completely stabilized for long periods with minimal application of pressure to the capsule. A standard upright microscope requires constant adjustment as the organ moves with respiration and varies in volume spontaneously; in addition, the surface being viewed is often at an angle to the plane of focus. However, if an inverted microscope is used the viewed tissue rests on a stationary coverslip, and problems associated with respiratory movement are minimized. A transparent Saran film can be used to hold the spleen gently against the coverslip, restricting lateral and vertical motion at the plane of focus. Objective lenses of high magnification and short working distance can then be used over a large working area.

Image contrast can be enhanced considerably by using oblique lighting rather than conventional illumination. If a fiberoptic source is positioned at about 45° to the optical axis of the microscope, more light is reflected from one side of each structure than the other. This results in shadowing which imparts a 3-dimensional quality to the image. The extended red sensitivity of the Newvicon videocamera (Panasonic WV-1550) and the ability to adjust the picture brightness and contrast on the videomonitor results in image contrast far superior to that obtained by eye, viewing through the eyepieces of the microscope. Objective lenses from 10 to 100× (oil immersion) may be used, giving magnification of 500 to 5000× on a 21×27 cm monitor and a maximum resolution of $<0.5\,\mu m$. By combining the use of an inverted microscope and oblique lighting with slow-motion video playback, we have obtained the first sequential images of individual red cells flowing within the spleen which are of sufficient quality for still-frame viewing and quantitative analysis (MacDonald *et al.*, 1987).

Use of *in vivo* microscopy is restricted to animal spleens that are sufficiently thin to be transilluminated (e.g. rat, mouse). With the aid of microcorrosion casts of spleens from these same species (Schmidt, MacDonald and Groom, 1985a,b), positive identification can be made of the channels through which the red cells are seen to flow. *In vivo* microscopy permits the direction and kinetics of blood flow to be determined so that one can visualize and describe quantitatively the movement of blood through the various pathways elucidated by other techniques. In addition, *in vivo* microscopy of Ringer-perfused spleens injected with a bolus of abnormal or senescent red cells promises to give valuable information on the sites and mechanisms of RBC trapping during a single passage through the spleen.

4.3 KEY ISSUES CONCERNING SPLENIC MICROCIRCULATORY BLOOD FLOW

4.3.1 FAST VERSUS SLOW PATHWAYS FOR RED CELL FLOW

Studies of red cell washout from cat spleen during Ringer perfusion (section 4.2.1(a)) have shown that the red cells leaving the organ do so as three distinct groups traveling with very different mean velocities (Song and Groom, 1971a; Levesque and Groom, 1976a). These groups are designated fast, intermediate, and slow, based on the volumes of the perfusate required to reduce their concentrations by one-half ($V_{1/2}$:0.067, 4.7, and 97 ml/g splenic weight, respectively). By histological examination of spleens in which Ringer perfusion was terminated after different volumes of perfusate had passed through (section 4.2.2), the locations of red cells have been compared before perfusion and after cells comprising the fast and intermediate components, respectively, have been almost completely washed out. These experiments (Song and Groom, 1971b) showed that the fast component corresponded to red cells in splenic vessels, the intermediate component to free red cells in the interstices of the reticular meshwork, and the slow component to red cells adhering to fine structures of the reticular meshwork ('bound' red cells).

Because the sum of the three exponential terms can completely describe the red cell washout curve, a simple model consisting of three compartments in parallel is sufficient to approximate the washout processes from the spleen. However, histological evidence showed that the bound red cells (slow compartment) are accumulated from blood flowing through the reticular meshwork (Song, 1972; Song and Groom, 1971b); when released from their bound state, they must rejoin the free red cells flowing through. These findings suggest that there are only two vascular compartments within the spleen; namely the vessels constituting the fast pathway, and the reticular spaces of the red pulp. The distinction between the intermediate and slow compartments is entirely the result of a cellular factor. For this reason, the compartment model (Levesque and Groom, 1976a) presented in Figure 4.3 shows the slow and intermediate red cell compartments in a mammillary arrangement rather than in parallel. Because of the great differences in $V_{1/2}$ values, it is

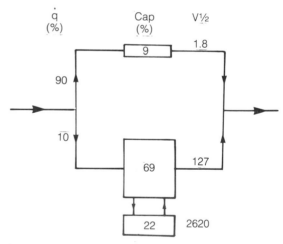

Figure 4.3 Three-compartment model, derived from cell washout kinetics and morphological studies, for distribution of red cells in cat spleen. Cap, capacity of compartment (% of total); q̇, flow to compartment (% of total flow); $V_{1/2}$, desaturation half-volume of compartment (ml perfusate). (Reproduced with permission from Groom (1987) *Microvascular Research*, 34, 269–89).

not possible to distinguish between these two arrangements on the basis of washout kinetics alone.

The model shows that 90% of the flow passes through a small (fast) compartment containing only 9% of the total RBCs, the remaining flow passing to the other two compartments (Figure 4.3). The intermediate compartment is perfused by 9.6% of the total inflow and contains 69% of all splenic RBCs, whereas the slow compartment is perfused by only 0.15% of the inflow and represents 22% of the total RBCs. Results qualitatively similar to the above have also been obtained from RBC washout studies in rats (Cilento *et al.*, 1980; Stock *et al.*, 1983). From microcorrosion casts prepared by the minimal-injection technique, the microcirculatory pathways corresponding to the two vascular compartments, fast and slow, have been identified. Photomicrographs of these pathways will be presented later (sections 4.3.8–4.3.13), but a brief summary of the conclusions is given here.

The *fast* pathways in sinusal spleens (such as human, dog, rat; see Schmidt, MacDonald and Groom, 1982, 1983a, 1985a, 1988) include:

1. Venous sinuses originating as open-ended tubes continuous with the marginal sinus or the marginal zone surrounding the white pulp (this pathway carries a large proportion of the flow).
2. Direct connections of arterial capillaries to venous sinuses (which are more plentiful in some species than in others).
3. Flow from arterial capillaries radially outward through ellipsoid sheaths and into closely adjacent venous sinuses, *via* interendothelial slits in sinus walls. (In some species, such as the rat, ellipsoids are absent.)
4. In human spleen, an additional fast route is provided by the perimarginal cavernous sinus (PMCS) bordering the lymphatic nodules. Flow into the PMCS occurs *via* direct connections with arterial capillaries, *via* connections with ellipsoid sheaths, and *via* connections with the marginal zone.

Drainage from the PMCS occurs directly into venous sinuses.

The fast pathways in non-sinusal spleens (such as the cat, mouse; Schmidt, MacDonald and Groom, 1983b, 1985b) include:

1. Short routes through the reticular meshwork of the red pulp, from arterial capillary terminations to nearby pulp venules. (For details regarding the distinction between pulp venules and venous sinuses, see section 4.3.8.) We have found no direct arteriovenous connections in non-sinusal spleens.
2. Short routes through the reticular meshwork from marginal sinus or marginal zone to pulp venules.
3. Short routes through the reticular meshwork from ellipsoid sheaths (when present as in the cat) to pulp venules.

The *slow* pathways, in both sinusal and non-sinusal spleens, all involve longer distances through the labyrinthine reticular meshwork of the red pulp, where filtration of abnormal red cells takes place. Blood flows into the reticular meshwork from arterial capillary terminations, from the marginal zone, and from ellipsoid sheaths. From the reticular meshwork, blood enters the venous system by passing through interendothelial slits in walls of venous sinuses or, in the case of non-sinusal spleens, by passing into pulp venules *via* their open ends or fenestrated walls.

4.3.2   RED CELL CONCENTRATION IN THE SPLEEN

It has been known for many years that in dogs the hemoglobin concentration of splenic blood is much higher than that of peripheral blood (Barcroft and Poole, 1927; Kramer and Luft, 1951). More recently, measurements on blood drained from excised dog spleens, contracting under electrical stimulation, have shown the hematocrit to be as high as 90% (Opdyke and Apostolico, 1966). These observations confirm the impression gained from histological sections, that the red pulp is packed with red cells in all species studied.

Black box studies of the washout of both red cells and plasma simultaneously have provided the first measurements of the total volume and hematocrit of blood in the fast and slow pathways respectively (cat spleen: Levesque and Groom, 1976a). The plasma washout curve consisted of only two exponential components, the $V_{1/2}$ values corresponding closely to those of the fast and intermediate components of red cell washout (Figure 4.2). There existed no counterpart to the slow component of red cell washout, indicating that the latter must have been caused by a process peculiar to the red cells. By combining the data of both plasma and red cell washout, a single model for the morphological distribution of blood within the spleen was derived (Figure 4.4). This is a two-compartment model, in which the red cells of the intermediate and slow compartments are combined. From the volumes of red cells and plasma in each vascular compartment, the hematocrits were calculated to be 37% (fast pathways) and 75% (slow pathways). The total blood volume was 0.51 ml/g splenic weight, of which more then 80% was located in the slow pathways of the red pulp. Confirmation of the hematocrit values determined by the washout method was obtained by means of the splenic drainage procedure (section 4.2.1(b)). Figure 4.5 shows that the initial hematocrit (representing blood from the fast pathways) was 33.5% comparable to that of peripheral blood, whereas the final hematocrit, reflecting the blood from the slow pathways, was 78.5%.

What is the mechanism of red cell concentration that gives rise to such a high hematocrit in the red pulp? From *in vivo* studies of the transilluminated spleens of mouse, rat and cat, Knisely (1936) suggested that hemoconcentration was a function of venous sinuses. He claimed that the actions of afferent and efferent sinus sphincters caused the sinuses to fill with blood, and then allowed plasma to drain out through fenestrations in their walls; this resulted in

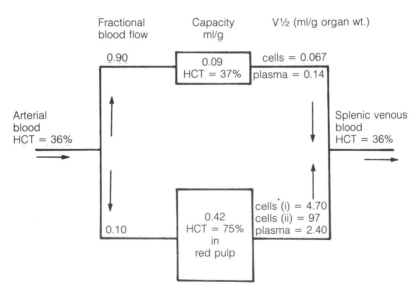

Figure 4.4 Compartmental model for distribution of whole blood in cat spleen (see text). Nine-tenths of splenic arterial blood passes through the smaller compartment that contains blood of similar hematocrit (37%). One-tenth of total blood flow passes through red pulp (the major compartment) that contains blood of hematocrit 75%. (Reproduced with permission from Levesque and Groom (1976a) *American Journal of Physiology*, **231**, 1665–71.)

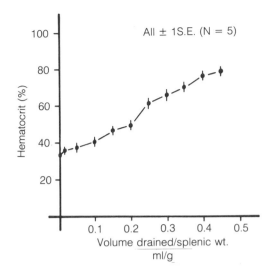

Figure 4.5 Results from splenic drainage (cat) with inflow occluded: see section 4.2.1(b). Mean value (± SE) of hematocrit (%) of successive venous samples is plotted against cumulative volume of blood drained per gram of splenic weight. Initial hematocrit represents that of blood from the fast pathways through the spleen, whereas final hematocrit represents that of blood in the slow pathways through the reticular meshwork. (Reproduced with permission from Levesque and Groom (1976a) *American Journal of Physiology*, **231**, 1665–71.)

sinuses filled with packed red cells, which could be discharged into the venous outflow. However, other investigators were unable to confirm this mechanism (MacKenzie, Whipple and Wintersteiner, 1941; McCuskey and McCuskey, 1977). Furthermore, the spleens of cat and mouse are non-sinusal (Snook, 1950): their 'pulp venules' are quite different from venous sinuses (see section 4.3.8). Yet in spite of the absence of venous sinuses, such spleens as those of cat, mouse, and many other mammalian species also develop hematocrits of twice the arterial value. Consequently, the primary mechanism of red cell concentration must be independent of the presence of venous sinuses.

Other suggestions have been offered to explain red cell concentration in the spleen. (1) The plasma is carried away by lymphatic vessels (Barcroft and Florey, 1928) and the separation

requires splenic innervation (Barcroft and Poole, 1927). (2) Because of the presence of a high endothelium, the terminal arterioles and arterial capillaries may constrict, so that only plasma is passed on and red cell concentration occurs in the proximal segment (Weiss, 1962). However, the total volume of the splenic arterial circulation is undoubtedly too small to accommodate the volume of red cells known to be sequestered. (3) The branching angles in the arterial circulation may promote plasma skimming (Weed, 1970). However, neither histological studies nor *in vivo* microscopy have led to any explanation that has found general acceptance.

More recently Greenway (1979) has developed a method by which the spleen of cat was weighed *in situ* continuously to determine its total blood content; its red cell content was determined simultaneously by the use of ^{51}Cr-labelled red cells and continuous recording of splenic radioactivity by external scintillation counting. After contraction of the organ, the curves for recovery of weight and radioactivity were found to be remarkably similar. This showed that the spleen does not first fill with blood and then concentrate red cells by removal of plasma, but that refilling and red cell concentration proceed simultaneously. Moreover, splenic innervation was not required for red cell concentration to occur, and plasma separated from red cells was not removed by lymphatic vessels because these had been ligated. Furthermore, the removal of 30 ml of lymph in the first 2 minutes of the experiment would have been required. Using the splenic drainage procedure (section 4.2.1(b)), Greenway found that the hematocrit of the outflow reached 80%, whereas after infusion of isoproterenol it reached only 46%. This showed that beta-receptor mediated activity affects the mechanism of red cell concentration, the exact nature of which awaits further elucidation. We propose (section 4.5.3) that the development of a high hematocrit is a side-effect of the low shear conditions necessary in the reticular meshwork for filtration of abnormal red cells to occur.

4.3.3 IMMATURE RED CELLS AND THE SPLEEN

Histological studies at different stages of red cell washout indicated that the slow component consisted of red cells adhering to the reticular meshwork (Song and Groom, 1971b; Song, 1972). What was different about these red cells that became trapped in the reticular meshwork? At different stages of the washout fairly pure (>85%) samples of red cells from each compartment could be collected at the outflow. The specific gravity and cell volume of red cells from the three compartments showed that the cells from the slow compartment differed significantly from those of arterial blood, being larger and lighter (Groom et al., 1971) and suggesting that these were younger cells (Piomelli, Lurinsky and Wasserman, 1967). Supravital staining of blood smears confirmed that they were indeed reticulocytes (Song and Groom, 1972), and measurements showed that the reticulocyte washout curve was almost identical to that of RBCs from the slow compartment. These reticulocytes amounted to 8% of all splenic RBCs and were equal to 1.5 times the total daily production.

Counts of red cell precursors in histological sections (Song and Groom, 1972) showed that the reticulocytes could not have arisen by splenic erythropoiesis, for proerythroblasts were never found, and the ratio of reticulocytes to rubricytes was 75 times the number which would have been expected if they had been derived from red cell precursors in the spleen. These results suggest that reticulocytes released from bone marrow are retained in the spleen for a 1- to 2-day period of maturation, and then returned to the circulation (Song and Groom, 1971c, 1972). It is hardly conceivable that such large numbers of reticulocytes would undergo destruction simultaneously in normal animals. Instead the spleen appears to function as a 'finishing school' with maturation of reticulocytes proceeding within the organ (Song, 1972). Moreover, there is evidence that splenic macrophages serve as 'nurse' cells, assisting in the maturation of immature red cells (Pictet et al., 1969).

4.3.4 NON-SPECIFICITY OF SPLENIC 'FILTRATION' OF ABNORMAL RED CELLS

The role of the spleen in removing abnormal red cells from the circulation has long been recognized (Weisman et al., 1955; Wennberg and Weiss, 1969; Schnitzer et al., 1973). Red cells containing inclusion bodies are 'remodelled' at the interendothelial slits, and probably also by contact with macrophages in the reticular meshwork. Those with impaired deformability, such as the sickle cell, may be subjected to mechanical trauma and lysis before phagocytosis of the cellular fragments. Other abnormal red cells that adhere to the reticular meshwork and macrophages in the red pulp may be phagocytosed. The factors which determine whether there is maturation of young red cells or destruction of old red cells, when these cells adhere to macrophages, are apparently the characteristics of the cells themselves rather than of the macrophages (Pictet et al., 1969). Grossly damaged red cells are taken up in vivo primarily by the liver, which has a much higher mass and blood flow than the spleen (Jacob and Jandl, 1962; Wagner et al., 1962; Kimber and Lander, 1964; Ultmann and Gordon, 1965). However, the spleen has a remarkable ability to remove selectively from the blood those red cells that are so slightly damaged that they would escape retention elsewhere.

What are the key cellular or membrane properties that, when modified, determine whether the initial trapping event will occur? The percentage of altered red cells retained during a single transit through the isolated, Ringer-perfused spleen of the cat has been measured (Levesque and Groom, 1980a). A variety of altered red cells (autologous red cells damaged with glutaraldehyde, heat, neuraminidase, or N-ethylmaleimide; autologous 'bound' red cells drained previously from the spleen; and foreign red cells from a human donor) was used to explore the effects of changes in bulk properties (deformability, shape, and size) and surface properties (adhesiveness) on trapping in the spleen. In every case extensive sequestration occurred. The results showed that no single cellular property uniquely determines whether red cells will be retained in the spleen; the degree of injury is more important than type. Thus red cells are retained because of loss of deformability, increased sphericity, loss of surface charge, inhibition of membrane sulfhydryl groups, immaturity or incompatibility, respectively.

Although the most obvious effect of treating red cells with heat or glutaraldehyde is a reduction in cellular deformability, concomitant changes in membrane properties also occur. Thus, all types of abnormal red cells used in this study would have had membrane properties differing in various ways from those of mature autologous cells; it is significant that splenic sequestration occurred in every case. What happens to red cells after initial trapping will depend on the precise way in which their properties differ from those of normal mature cells. Immature red cells are retained for maturation; most other abnormal cells will ultimately be phagocytosed.

By observing the spleen filtering abnormal red cells from the blood, it should be possible to determine which cellular properties are important for them to function appropriately in the general circulation (Groom, 1980). The unequivocal answer from such experiments seems to be that deformability and suitable surface properties are both important. Therefore, it was surprising to find that cellular deformability alone seems to matter when red cells are in transit through skeletal muscle. In an isolated perfused cat gastrocnemius muscle, recovery of glutaraldehyde-treated RBCs from the venous outflow after intra-arterial injection was only 21%, whereas that of every other type of abnormal red cell studied was not significantly different from 100% (Bowden, 1978). This may indicate that the surface properties of red cells are not as important for safe transit in the general microcirculation; however, it has been shown that reticulocytes are cleared from skeletal muscle much more slowly than mature red cells, and this was attributed to cell adherence to vessel walls (Groom, Song and Campling, 1973). Why then should the spleen sequester autologous red cells with altered surface properties? It is probable that the basic mechanism of filtration of pathological red cells in the reticular meshwork *in vivo* is not mechanical but physicochemical. Alteration of red cell surface properties may 'deceive' the spleen so that it treats functionally adequate red cells as abnormal and filters them out of the circulating blood.

4.3.5 SITES OF TRAPPING OF ABNORMAL RED CELLS

Where and how is red cell 'filtration' carried out? The traditional view is that this occurs solely at interendothelial slits (IES) in walls of venous sinuses. It is known that the IES impede or prevent the movement of abnormal red cells from the reticular meshwork into venous sinuses; a well-studied example is that of red cells containing Heinz bodies induced by phenylhydrazine (Koyama, Aoki and Deguchi, 1964; Chen and Weiss, 1973; Leblond, 1973; Chen, 1980). Although such retention occurs at the IES, for remodeling ('pitting') or subsequent phagocytosis, it is a fact that the spleens of many mammalian species lack venous sinuses (see section 4.3.8). Moreover, our research has shown that retention of immature or abnormal red cells takes place on a large scale within the reticular meshwork itself. Since the interstices of the reticular meshwork are larger than the red cells and do not constitute a test of cell deformability (as do the IES), factors other than bulk properties of the red cells must necessarily be involved. It appears that immature or abnormal cells develop altered surface properties in addition to whatever internal changes may have occurred. Histological evidence demonstrates that these red cells adhere to fine structures of the reticular meshwork (Song, 1972; Song and Groom, 1971b, 1974).

Thus, there are two distinct mechanisms which can form the basis for trapping abnormal red cells: (1) altered surface properties of the red cell membrane, giving rise to adhesion at low shear rates to structures and macrophages within the marginal zone and reticular meshwork; (2) changes in the bulk properties of the cell, such as reduced cellular deformability, which can cause cell retention at the IES. It appears that sinusal spleens have an advantage over non-sinusal spleens in that IES provide a second means of filtering out abnormal red cells from the blood.

In conclusion, it is probable that selective retention of abnormal or immature red cells occurs wherever circulatory paths have an 'open' configuration. Such sites include the reticular meshwork of the marginal zone and red pulp, and possibly the ellipsoid sheaths (Blue and Weiss, 1981a) which are present in many species, including man. This means that red cell filtration is primarily a function of the slow pathways in the spleen. It should be noted that there are other pathways for blood flow (fast pathways) that bypass these sites of trapping of abnormal cells in the reticular meshwork of the red pulp, as well as the IES in sinusal spleens (see section 4.3.l0).

4.3.6   SATURATION OF THE SPLENIC RBC TRAPPING MECHANISM

Under conditions of constant pressure perfusion more than one-third of injected heat-treated red cells become entrapped in the cat spleen during a single transit (Levesque and Groom, 1977). This raises a series of important questions about splenic sequestration of abnormal red cells *in vivo*. Do such cells reduce the total splenic blood flow *in vivo* and change intrasplenic flow distribution? Are normal red cells immobilized behind the sequestered red cells? To what extent does saturation of the splenic trapping mechanism occur?

A study of these questions was carried out in cat spleen (Levesque and Groom, 1977). Heat-treated red cells were injected into the splenic artery *in vivo*, followed 1 hour later by red cell washout during Ringer perfusion. The number of red cells injected (1.6×10^9 cells) was equivalent to only 0.8% of the splenic red cell volume, yet this caused immobilization of 50% of the red cells in the red pulp. Such spleens remained deep red throughout the perfusion, whereas control spleens became very pale. Adhesion of abnormal red cells to the reticular meshwork would retard flow, promoting further sequestration (Holzbach *et al.*, 1964). This could explain extensive 'clogging' of the red pulp as a result of the trapping of only a small volume of heat-treated red cells. Nevertheless, all the plasma remained free to circulate, albeit much of it did so slowly. In sinusal spleens, blocking of interendothelial slits in the walls of venous sinuses by heat-treated red cells (Vaupel, Ruppert and Hutten, 1977) or red cells containing Heinz bodies (Chen, 1980) further contributes to 'clogging' of red pulp.

It has long been recognized that saturation of the sequestration mechanism can occur, even leading to functional asplenia in the case of trapped sickle cells (Pearson, Spencer and Cornelius, 1969), although some authors have thought this to be a consequence of the limited capacity of splenic phagocytes for phagocytosis (Miescher, 1957; Mollison, 1962). Our own results suggest that this explanation may not be correct, since for both neuraminidase- and NEM-treated red cells, the percentage of cells trapped in the spleen decreased significantly with each repeated bolus injection into Ringer-perfused spleens (Levesque and Groom, 1980a). By the third injection of NEM-treated red cells, all the injected cells reached the venous outflow. This suggests that all the slow pathways through the red pulp had been blocked, but a sufficient number of the fast pathways remained open. Thus, the reduced removal of non-viable red cells by the spleen when larger quantities are injected is primarily due to reduced red cell flow through the red pulp. In clinical investigations, therefore, the dose of heat-treated red cells employed is an important consideration when clearance half-times from the blood are to be measured.

4.3.7 'HOSTILE' METABOLIC ENVIRONMENT FOR RED CELLS?

Red cells in the reticular meshwork are exposed to the local splenic environment for long periods, because of their slow transit. It is known that splenic red cells exhibit increased mechanical and osmotic fragility (Emerson *et al.*, 1956) and have a lower sodium–potassium ratio (Prankerd, 1960). It has been hypothesized that the metabolic environment for cells in the red pulp may be similar to that which develops in blood incubated at 37°C *in vitro*, including low pH, O_2 tension and glucose concentration. The red cell membrane loses its deformability at O_2 tensions below 30 Torr (LaCelle, 1970). At a pH of less than 6.8, red cells show increased mean cellular volume, rigidity, blood viscosity at low shear rate, and osmotic fragility (Dintenfass and Burnard, 1966; Murphy, 1967, 1969; LaCelle, 1970). Such physical changes might predispose red cells, especially when abnormal, to destruction in the circulation. The term 'conditioning' has been used to describe the modification of red cells which makes them more susceptible to further challenge within spleen or peripheral circulation (Griggs, Weisman and Harris, 1960).

The hypothesis of low intrasplenic pH, O_2 tension and glucose concentration has been difficult to test, because blood samples from the splenic pulp (either from the cut surface of the spleen or withdrawn by tissue aspiration) are always contaminated with blood from the fast circulation. Use of the splenic drainage procedure permitted selective sampling of blood from the reticular meshwork of the red pulp, as described earlier (section 4.2.1(b)). The measurements showed that the pH in the reticular meshwork is normally 7.20 (Figure 4.6, group A; Levesque and Groom, 1976b). Further experiments showed that intrasplenic pH results from the interplay of two separate factors: pH-determining elements of the splenic tissue that buffer at 6.8 and buffering provided by red cells passing through the reticular mesh-

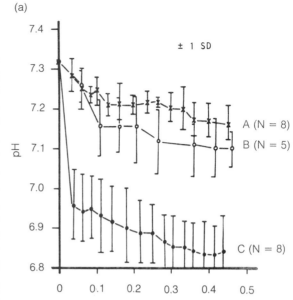

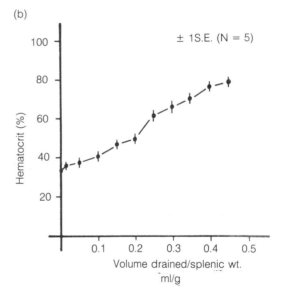

Figure 4.6 The pH and hematocrit of successive samples of venous blood drained from cat spleen after clamping arterial inflow. (a) With no stasis pH fell to 7.16 (group A); with stasis during cannulation procedures (8–10 min) pH fell to 7.10 (group B); and after stasis for 60 min the pH fell to 6.83 (group C). (b) High hematocrit values at end show that blood came from red pulp. (Reproduced with permission from Levesque and Groom (1976b) *American Journal of Physiology*, **231**, 1672–8.)

work. Stasis for 10 minutes (Figure 4.6, group B) or 60 minutes (Figure 4.6, group C) reduced the pH to 7.16 and 6.83 respectively. Measurements of O_2 tension (approximately 54 Torr) and glucose concentration (60% of that in venous blood) in the reticular meshwork showed them to be well above critical values, unless arterial inflow was occluded completely for 20 minutes or more (Groom, Levesque and Bruckschweiger, 1977). Thus, the notion of a hostile environment for red cells in the reticular meshwork simply due to very low values of pH, O_2 tension, and glucose concentration is incorrect. Other explanations must be sought for deleterious changes observed in red cells sequestered in the spleen.

The fact that unfavorable metabolic conditions develop rapidly within the spleen when blood flow is occluded, the principal stress being substrate deprivation, raises the question: Do such unfavorable conditions also develop when red cell stasis occurs following trapping of abnormal cells? (see section 4.3.6). If so, these conditions would promote further deterioration and destruction of trapped cells. When this hypothesis was tested by injecting heat-treated red cells, and then repeating the splenic drainage experiments (Groom *et al.*, 1985), the results showed unequivocally that hostile metabolic conditions did not develop in the red pulp. Inasmuch as red cell stasis was known to be present, there must presumably have been sufficient residual flow of plasma through the reticular meshwork to prevent serious deterioration of the environment.

There is no question that red cells incubated within the splenic pulp show deleterious changes, and these changes may indeed represent direct damage by the spleen in preparation for their eventual destruction (Motulsky *et al.*, 1958). However, it is now clear that the levels of pH, O_2 tension, and glucose concentration in the splenic red pulp are not as low as had been thought previously and that additional explanations must be sought for the deleterious changes observed in red cells sequestered within the spleen.

4.3.8   SINUSAL VERSUS NON-SINUSAL SPLEENS

Although the main features of the arterial circulation are similar in all mammalian spleens (with the exception of the ellipsoid sheaths, which are well developed in some species and absent in others), two quite different types of venous circulation are found, namely those with and those without venous sinuses in the red pulp. In about 50% of mammalian species examined by Snook (1950), venous sinuses were absent (non-sinusal type). Instead, the venous origins in the reticular meshwork consisted of 'primordial veins' (or 'pulp venules': Blue and Weiss, 1981b). The sinusal group includes man, dog and rat, while cat and mouse belong to the non-sinusal group.

Venous sinuses can be distinguished from pulp venules by their larger size, greater abundance, arrangement into a richly anastomosing plexus, and the characteristic structure of their walls, which are encircled by rings of argyrophilic fibers (Snook, 1950). By means of transmission and scanning electron microscopy (TEM, SEM), a more detailed description of the contrasting arrangements of elements in the walls of venous sinuses and pulp venules has been obtained (Blue and Weiss, 1981b,c; Fujita, 1974; Hataba, Kirino and Suzuki, 1981). The walls of venous sinuses consist of long spindle-shaped endothelial cells aligned parallel to the axis of the vessel (Figure 4.7). These cells are held in position by the processes of reticular cells, which fit into transverse grooves in the endothelial cells and thus form 'hoops' around the abluminal surface of the sinus (Figure 4.8). Slit-like gaps exist between the endothelial cells (interendothelial slits: IES); *in vivo* the IES may be very narrow (Weiss, 1974) or exist only as potential spaces (Cho and DeBruyn, 1975), but in many SEM micrographs, the IES appear widened into oval or rounded apertures, probably as a result of drying artefacts. Blood cells from the reticular meshwork penetrate the IES into the lumens of venous sinuses (see section 4.3.10). A clear view of venous sinuses and

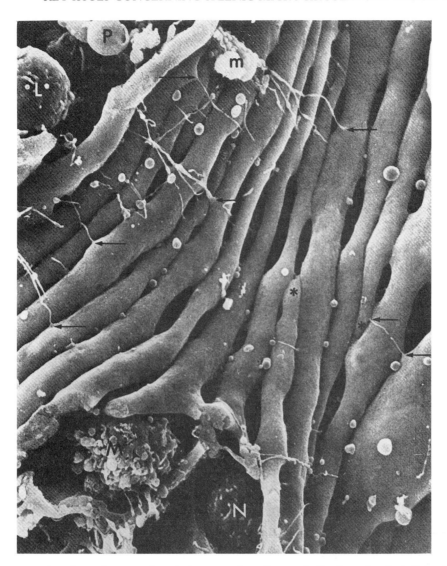

Figure 4.7 Luminal surface of venous sinus in human spleen. Long spindle-shaped endothelial cells lie side by side with slit-like gaps between them; a few cells terminated in tapered end (*). Threadlike processes (→) extend from endothelial cells. Some threads may belong to macrophage (M) processes (m). L, lymphocyte; N, neutrophil; P, platelet. (×3100). (Reproduced with permission from Fujita (1974) *Archivum Histologicum Japonicum*, 37, 187–216.)

their 3-dimensional relationships is obtained by microcorrosion casts (Figure 4.9), if only small amounts of material are injected. It is generally believed that venous sinuses originate in the red pulp or marginal zone as blind-ended sacs, and that inward passage of blood occurs exclusively through the IES; this view has now been shown to be incorrect (section 4.3.10).

The pulp venules in non-sinusal spleens appear, in microcorrosion casts, either as short lateral 'twigs' branching individually from a collecting vein, or as a 'root system' with many

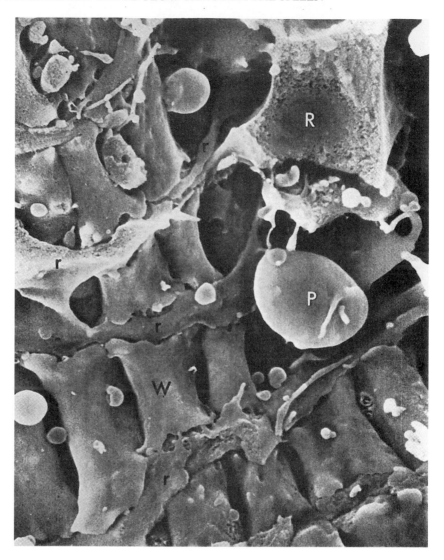

Figure 4.8 Abluminal surface of venous sinus in human spleen. Footlike processes (r) of reticulum cells (R) fit into transverse grooves in endothelial cells (W) and thus form 'hoops' around abluminal surface of sinus. P, platelet. (×7640). (Reproduced with permission from Fujita (1974), *Archivum Histologicum Japonicum*, **37**, 187–216.)

fine rootlets merging into one trunk (Figure 4.10). In contrast to the extensive system of interconnected venous sinuses in sinusal spleens, pulp venules are non-anastomosing, shorter and smaller in caliber, and all receive blood cells which flow freely from the reticular meshwork through the open ends and fenestrations in their walls. SEM of tissue (Hataba, Kirino and Suzuki, 1981) shows that the walls of pulp venules lack the characteristic 'rod cells' aligned parallel to the long axis of the vessel; instead, they are lined with smooth, flattened, irregularly shaped

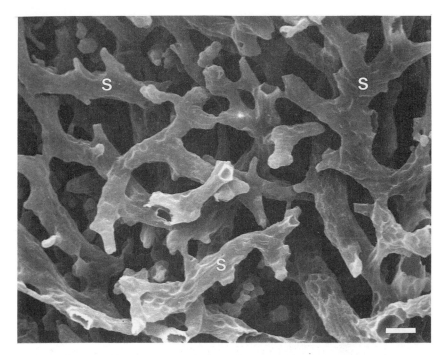

Figure 4.9 Microcorrosion cast of interconnected, three-dimensional network of venous sinuses (S) in normal human spleen. Since only a small amount of casting material was injected (see section 4.2.3) some sinuses are incompletely filled, and reticular meshwork is unfilled. Bar = 20 μm.

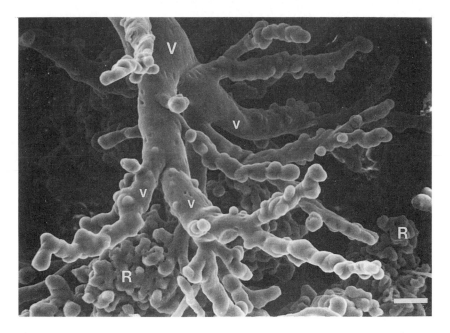

Figure 4.10 Microcorrosion cast from cat spleen (non-sinusal). Rootlike system of non-anastomosing pulp venules (v) drains into collecting vein (V); knobbly appearance results from emergence of material into reticular meshwork (R) *via* fenestrations in venular walls and *via* open ends. Bar = 50 μm. (Reproduced with permission from Schmidt, MacDonald and Groom (1983b) *Journal of Morphology*, **178**, 125–38.)

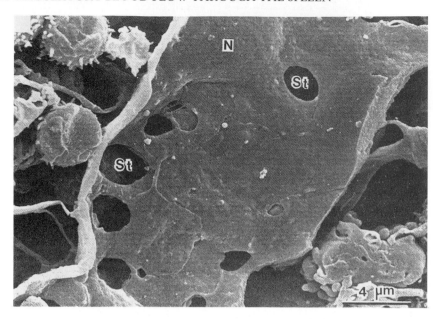

Figure 4.11 Luminal aspect of pulp venule from mouse spleen, showing flattened, irregularly shaped endothelial cells and relatively few, irregularly distributed fenestrations: St, stomata; N, nuclear region of endothelial cell which bulges slightly into lumen. (Reproduced with permission from Hataba, Kirino and Suzuki (1981) *Journal of Electron Microscopy*, 30, 46–56.)

endothelial cells and have relatively few and irregularly distributed fenestrations in their walls (Figure 4.11).

The distinction between venous sinuses and pulp venules has important functional implications. The narrow IES in the walls of venous sinuses serve to impede, or even prevent, entry of red cells into the sinus lumen (section 4.3.10). Pulp venules lack such IES but receive flow freely through the open ends and rounded fenestrations in their walls; the sizes of the fenestrations are mostly large enough to allow unimpeded entry of RBCs into the venule (Blue and Weiss, 1981b). Thus, in non-sinusal spleens trapping of immature and abnormal red cells occurs by adhesion to the fine structures of the reticular meshwork; in sinusal spleens, the reticular meshwork must, presumably, serve a similar function but the IES provide an important second mechanism for trapping red cells.

4.3.9   FLOW PATHWAYS BORDERING THE WHITE PULP

Circulatory routes within, and out of, the region bordering the white pulp constitute a major area of uncertainty: this is especially true in the case of the human spleen. It has been claimed that the human spleen lacks the marginal sinus (MS) found in many other species (Van Krieken *et al.*, 1985b). Barnhart and Lusher (1979) referred to the MS as a 'poorly delimited' component of the marginal zone (MZ) and stated that additional work is necessary to identify the precise vascular routes through this region. The existence of the MS as a distinct vascular space was first described in rat spleen (Andrew, 1946; Snook 1950); it consists of a series of anastomosing vascular spaces lying between the white pulp and the MZ. Serial sections revealed that the MS is not a vessel but a cleft-like space

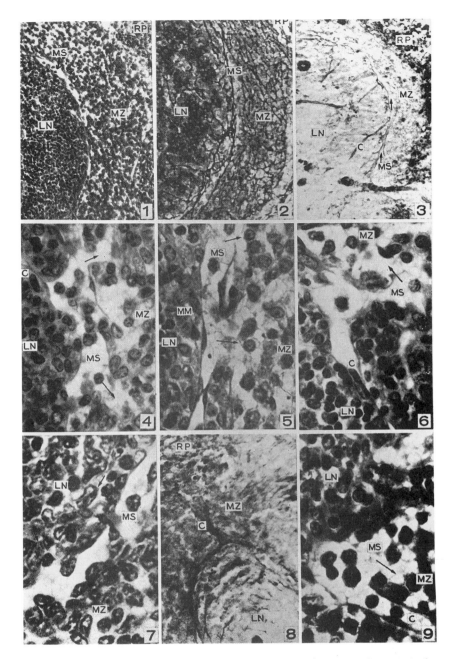

Figure 4.12 Relationship between lymphatic nodule (LN), marginal sinus (MS), marginal zone (MZ), and red pulp (RP) in rat spleen. 1: Overview; hematoxylin and eosin stain (×140). 2: Reticular fiber network of marginal zone/sinus; Snook's reticular stain (×210). 3: White pulp capillaries (C) emptying into marginal sinus (arrows); periodic acid–Schiff stain (×140). 4: Marginal sinus showing pores (arrows) through which red cells pass into marginal zone; pyronin–methyl green stain (×570). 5: Marginal sinus showing endothelial cells and pores (arrows); pyronin–methyl green stain (×570). 6: Ampullary ending of white pulp capillary. Pore (arrow) connects marginal sinus with interstices of marginal zone; pyronin–methyl green stain (×570). 7: Diapedesis of cell through inner lining of marginal sinus; arrows, nuclei of marginal metalophils; Giemsa stain (×620). 8: Capillary from white pulp traversing marginal zone; periodic acid–Schiff stain (×150). 9: Capillary from red pulp opening into marginal sinus; arrow, marginal sinus pore; hematoxylin and eosin stain (×570). (Reproduced with permission from Snook (1964), *Anatomical Record*, **148**, 149–59.)

surrounding the white pulp (Figure 4.12). Many follicular capillaries terminate in the MS, their endothelial walls being in continuity with the cells lining the MS. Red cells have direct access to the MZ through discontinuities in the outer wall of the MS (Figure 4.12). Blood leaving the MS moves outward through the MZ, a well-defined region of reticular meshwork surrounding the white pulp, which contains a large population of medium-sized lymphocytes and other blood cells. Blood then moves on into the red pulp, and joins blood which has entered the red pulp directly from arterial capillaries.

A 3-dimensional view of the interrelationship in the human spleen, between lymphatic nodules, MS, MZ, and venous sinus network in the red pulp may be obtained from microcorrosion casts (Figure 4.13). In this figure, the nodule appears hollow because the white pulp has been corroded away, and an opening in the

MS represents the site where the central artery entered the nodule. (The casts of the artery and follicular capillaries were broken off during processing.) The reticular meshwork of the red pulp is unfilled (due to the small amount of material injected), although the network of venous sinuses and part of a collecting vein can be seen; the thickness of the MZ is not uniform around each nodule, but varies from 200 μm down to a narrow band in the region where two nodules are in close approximation.

The schematic diagram in Figure 4.1 shows clearly that before reaching lymphatic nodules the central artery travels down the axis of a cylindrical sheath of lymphoid tissue, the periarterial lymphatic sheath (PALS). The microcorrosion cast in Figure 4.14 gives a 3-dimensional view of the relationship between the PALS, the central artery, and the surrounding marginal zone and venous sinuses which are

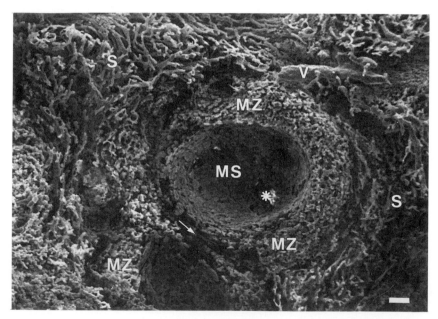

Figure 4.13 Microcorrosion cast of normal human spleen showing relationship between lymphatic nodules (white pulp corroded away), marginal sinus (MS), marginal zone (MZ), and venous sinus network (S) in red pulp. Opening in MS (*) is site where central artery (cast accidentally broken off) entered nodule. In region where two nodules are close together, MZ is narrow (→). A collecting vein (V) has begun to fill. Bar = 100 μm. (Reproduced with permission from Schmidt, MacDonald and Groom (1988) *American Journal of Anatomy*, **181**, 253–66.)

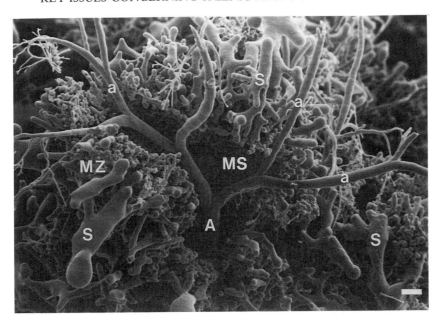

Figure 4.14 Microcorrosion cast of dog spleen showing central artery (A) passing down the axis of periarterial lymphatic sheath (with white pulp corroded away). Many arteriolar branches (a) extend through marginal sinus (MS) and marginal zone (MZ) into red pulp (incompletely filled). Many venous sinuses (S) originating in MS/MZ have begun to fill. Bar = 100 μm. (Reproduced with permission from Schmidt, MacDonald and Groom (1983a) *Journal of Morphology*, **178**, 111–23.)

incompletely filled (dog spleen). The artery bifurcates several times, giving rise to arterioles which extend laterally beyond the PALS and branch repeatedly before ending as capillaries, either in the MS/MZ or further on within the red pulp itself. Many of the casts of the smallest vessels end blindly (Figure 4.14, top left), indicating incomplete filling.

A cast of a lymphatic nodule with intact central artery and follicular capillaries is shown in Figure 4.15 (dog spleen). These follicular capillaries terminate in ampullary dilatations that are continuous with the MS. The major arterioles arising from the central artery pass intact through both the MS and MZ into the red pulp. Many of these arterioles then curve back toward the nodule and branch to form an array of smaller arterioles (penicilli), which terminate as capillaries in the MS or MZ; other arterioles terminate some distance away in the red pulp. (Again, many arterial and venous

vessels are incompletely filled in Figure 4.15.) There is strong evidence that the whole MS is filled by circumferential spreading of the injected material, before radial spreading occurs outwardly into the MZ through fenestrations in the outer surface of the MS. This is shown particularly well in casts from spleens of dog (Figure 4.15) and cat (Figure 4.16); it is also seen in rat, mouse and, to a lesser extent, in humans (Schmidt, MacDonald and Groom, 1985a,b, 1988). When a suitably small volume of casting material is injected, each nodule is surrounded by a thin spherical annulus of material (<10 μm) sharply delineating the outer limits of the nodule but not enclosing it completely (Figure 4.16). In human spleen, the inner aspect of the MS casts adjoining the white pulp appears as a flattened, almost continuous, system of anastomosing spaces (Figure 4.17). We have found consistently that the MS is present in normal human spleens obtained from organ

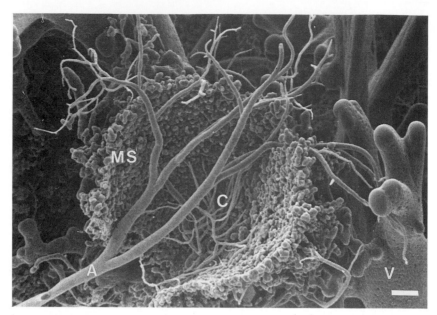

Figure 4.15 Microcorrosion cast of dog spleen. Central artery (A) bifurcates repeatedly within a lymphatic nodule, giving rise to follicular capillaries (C), ending in marginal sinus (MS), and to capillaries in red pulp (casts with 'blind' ends, due to incomplete filling). Collecting veins (V) partially filled. Bar = 100 μm. (Reproduced with permission from Schmidt, MacDonald and Groom (1983a) *Journal of Morphology*, **178**, 111–23.)

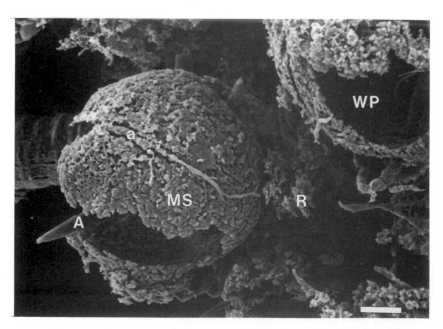

Figure 4.16 Microcorrosion cast of cat spleen showing marginal sinus (MS) surrounding lymphatic nodule (white pulp, WP, corroded away). Marginal sinus appears as a thin spherical annulus, due to circumferential spreading of injectate before outward radial spreading into marginal zone occurred. Arteriole (a) ramifies over convex surface of MS, before terminating there *via* capillaries. Branch of central artery (A) leaves the nodule. Reticular meshwork (R) has just begun to fill between the two nodules. Bar = 100 μm. (Reproduced with permission from Schmidt, MacDonald and Groom (1983b) *Journal of Morphology*, **178**, 125–38.)

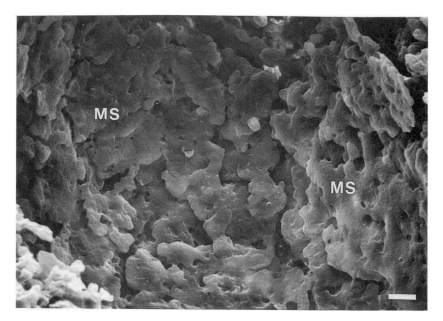

Figure 4.17 Microcorrosion cast of normal human spleen. Marginal sinus (MS) consists of flattened, anastomosing vascular spaces between white pulp (corroded away) and marginal zone. Contrast the sheet-like appearance of MS with the knobbly configuration of marginal zone in Figure 4.22. Bar = 25 μm. (Reproduced with permission from Schmidt, MacDonald and Groom (1988) *American Journal of Anatomy*, **181**, 253–66.)

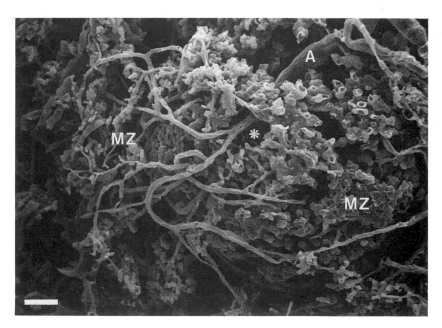

Figure 4.18 Microcorrosion cast of normal human spleen. Central artery (A) passes to marginal zone (MZ) and, at this point (*), gives rise to numerous circumferentially directed arterioles and capillaries, most of which terminate there. Bar = 50 μm. (Reproduced with permission from Schmidt, MacDonald and Groom (1988) *American Journal of Anatomy*, **181**, 253–66.)

transplant donors, whereas it is absent in certain diseases (see section 4.3.13). Relatively few follicular capillaries terminate on the inner aspect of the MS, perfusion occurring mainly through capillaries which terminate on the outer aspect facing the MZ.

Within some lymphatic nodules the arteries are seen to branch many times over a very short distance, the branches remaining together as arteriolar–capillary bundles; after running in parallel for some distance, these vessels fan out 'and terminate in the MZ (Snook, 1975; Schmidt, MacDonald and Groom, 1988). In many instances, however, the central artery continues to the margin of the nodule as a single vessel and, at this point, branches repeatedly in the MZ, thereby giving rise to numerous circumferentially directed arterioles and capillaries which terminate there (Figure 4.18). From the MZ blood enters the venous system through two routes: (1) open-ended venous sinuses in continuity with the outer aspect of the MZ (see section 4.3.10), and (2) a pathway of flow outward into the reticular meshwork of the red pulp, from where it enters venous sinuses through the interendothelial slits in sinus walls (see section 4.3.10).

An additional flow pathway bordering the white pulp, which appears to be unique to the human spleen, is the perimarginal cavernous sinus (PMCS). The PMCS receives flow from the MZ, ellipsoid sheaths, or directly from arterial capillaries, and drains into venous sinuses (see section 4.3.13).

4.3.10   ENTRY OF BLOOD INTO VENOUS SINUSES

It is widely believed that venous sinuses originate in the red pulp or MZ as blind-ended sacs, and that entry of blood into sinuses occurs exclusively through the interendothelial slits (IES) in their walls (Chen and Weiss, 1973; Leblond, 1973; Cho and DeBruyn, 1975; Barnhart and Lusher, 1976; Weiss, Powell and Schiffman, 1985; Fujita, Kashimura and Adachi, 1985). This is represented schematical-

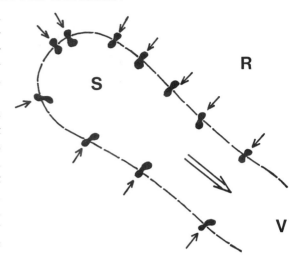

Figure 4.19 Schematic diagram representing traditional view that all venous sinuses originate in the marginal zone or red pulp as blind-ended sacs, and that entry of blood into sinuses occurs exclusively *via* interendothelial slits in their walls. R, reticular meshwork; S, venous sinus lumen; V, collecting vein; arrows indicate direction of flow.

ly in Figure 4.19. However, microcorrosion casts have revealed that there are two additional routes for blood flow into venous sinuses. First, many venous sinuses begin as open-ended tubules continuous with the marginal sinus (MS) or marginal zone (MZ), allowing free entry of blood into the venous system and bypassing the reticular meshwork of the red pulp. Such open-ended sinuses are abundant in all the sinusal spleens we have examined (dog, rat and human spleens; Schmidt, MacDonald and Groom, 1983a, 1985a, 1988). Second, direct connections of arterial capillaries to venous sinuses exist (see section 4.3.11). Thus, blood enters the system of interconnected venous sinuses by three different routes: (1) open-ended sinuses; (2) direct arteriovenous connections, and (3) IES in sinus walls.

Many venous sinuses drain the region bordering the white pulp. In Figure 4.20, open-ended venous sinuses originating in the MS bordering the PALS are shown (dog spleen). The diameters of the regions of continuity are

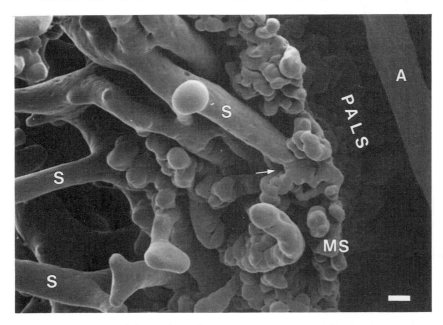

Figure 4.20 Microcorrosion cast of dog spleen showing interconnecting venous sinuses (S) originating in marginal sinus (MS) bordering periarterial lymphatic sheath (PALS). Note continuity (→) between MS and lumen of venous sinus, i.e. the sinus begins as an open-ended tube which has filled before any filling of the reticular meshwork occurred. A, central artery. Bar = 25 μm. (Reproduced with permission from Schmidt, MacDonald and Groom (1983a) *Journal of Morphology*, 178, 111–23.)

20 to 25 μm, the same caliber as venous sinuses, and much larger than would be expected if flow into the sinuses were limited to channels the size of IES. In casts prepared by injection of only very small amounts of material, there is no filling of reticular meshwork around most venous sinuses; the surfaces of the sinuses are quite bare and exposed. These sinuses could not have filled through the IES in their walls. These same features in human spleen are shown in Figure 4.21, where an open-ended venous sinus received its flow freely from the MZ surrounding a lymphatic nodule; this is demonstrated by the continuity that exists between the cast of the sinus (a cylinder at least 10 μm in diameter at its interface with the MZ) and the clusters of casting material representing the MZ. The abundance of such open-ended origins of venous sinuses is shown in Figure 4.22 (human spleen). This particular cast demonstrates well the whole route for blood

flow from the MS, through the meshwork of the MZ, into the interconnected system of venous sinuses by their open-ended origins and from there into collecting veins. The quantity of material which has passed into the venous system indicates that the route provided by open-ended venous sinuses must be one of very low resistance to flow, and represents a major part of the fast pathway through the spleen.

Demonstration of open-ended venous sinuses has been possible for the first time, because the modified microcorrosion casting technique reveals selectively the fast channels for flow, and allows them to be visualized three-dimensionally in the absence of surrounding tissue. Based on SEM of tissue, Fujita and Kashimura (1983) showed the presence of a large 'window' (approximately 10 μm diameter) at the tapered end of a venous sinus in human spleen. This may correspond to the open-ended sinuses we have found. Microcorrosion casts also reveal

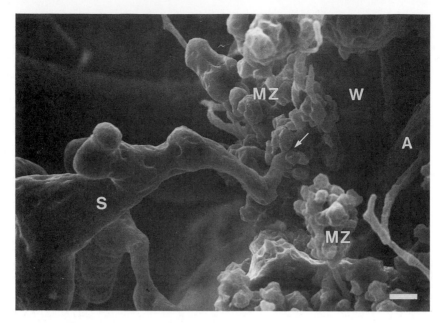

Figure 4.21 Microcorrosion cast from human spleen (patient with lymphocytic leukemia) showing open-ended origin (→) of venous sinus (S) in marginal zone (MZ). Note lack of filling of reticular meshwork surrounding the sinus. A, central artery; W, white pulp corroded away. Bar = 20 μm. (Reproduced with permission from Schmidt, MacDonald and Groom (1988) *American Journal of Anatomy*, **181**, 253–66.)

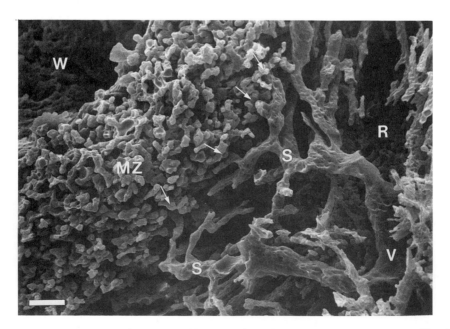

Figure 4.22 Microcorrosion cast from normal human spleen showing many venous sinuses (S) originating *via* open ends (→) in marginal zone (MZ). Note interconnected nature of venous sinus network, draining into collecting vein (V). W, white pulp corroded away; R, reticular meshwork of red pulp mostly unfilled. Bar = 50 μm. (Reproduced with permission from Schmidt, MacDonald and Groom (1988) *American Journal of Anatomy*, **181**, 253–66.)

that some venous sinuses do indeed originate as blind-ended sacs; casts made by venous retrograde injection of material show some well-filled sinuses with genuine blind ends completely covered with endothelial nuclear impressions, in contrast to the artifactual 'blind ends' caused by incomplete filling with casting material (Figure 4.20). The presence of open-ended venous sinuses explains how spleens injected with minimal quantities of casting material fill the venous system without filling the reticular meshwork about the venous sinuses.

That blood can enter venous sinuses by passing through the IES was demonstrated by earlier investigators using transmission and scanning electron microscopy: Figure 4.23 is a TEM micrograph showing red cells caught in passage. It is clear from this figure that the red cells are severely deformed in passing through the narrow IES. A comparable picture is presented in the SEM micrograph in Figure 4.24, where a 3-dimensional view is obtained. It has been noted that the 'heads' of the RBCs are always on the luminal side of the sinus walls, and the 'tails' on the side facing the reticular meshwork; this suggests that the direction of flow is into, not out of, the sinus. However, there has been no universal agreement about this (Chen and Weiss, 1973; Leblond, 1973; Cho and DeBruyn, 1975; Blue and Weiss, 1981a; Weiss, Powell and Schiffman, 1985; Fujita, Kashimura and Adachi, 1985). Compare also Pictet *et al.*, 1969; Tischendorf, 1985. Studies of fixed splenic tissue cannot answer this question directly nor can they address questions regarding the kinetics of red cell flow through the IES: for this, microscopy *in vivo* is necessary.

Videomicroscopy of transilluminated rat spleens *in vivo* (section 4.2.4) has recently analyzed the kinetics of red cell passage through IES (MacDonald *et al.*, 1987). The direction of red cell flow was invariably from reticular meshwork into venous sinuses in normal spleens. Sequential photomicrographs of a red cell squeezing through an IES are shown in Figure 4.25. The time course can be seen from the stopwatch characters at the bottom left of each picture. The venous sinus (diameter 17 μm) runs vertically at the left of each micrograph and is only partially shown (see schematic: Figure 4.25c). Rapid flow of red cells within the lumen is seen only as a blur; to the right of the sinus wall are the reticular spaces of the red pulp, where numerous red cells are visible. Although the IES itself cannot be seen, the position and conformation of the RBC within it reveal its location. In Figure 4.25(a), one red cell has begun to emerge into the lumen of the venous sinus. Figure 4.25(b) shows it at the half-way point in its passage through the IES, whereas in Figure 4.25(f) the red cell has passed into the lumen but remains tethered by a long 'tail' which remains momentarily trapped by the IES, before the cell escapes completely and is swept away by rapid flow in the lumen of the sinus.

The striking feature of the flow of red cells through the IES is that it occurs as a series of brief, discontinuous bursts separated by periods of zero, or near zero, flow (Figure 4.26). Three factors could contribute to this pattern of flow: (1) changes in pressure difference across the sinus wall; (2) changes in supply of red cells to the reticular meshwork in the region of the IES; and (3) changes in flow resistance at the IES itself. Factors (1) and (2) would give rise to synchronous bursts of red cells through closely adjacent IES, whereas (3) would lead, in general, to asynchronous bursts of red cells. Analysis of red cell flow through two such IES simultaneously, for 30 minutes, showed that most of the bursts were asynchronous (Figure 4.26). Thus, changes in flow resistance of the IES itself were primarily responsible for the observed pattern of flow.

Examination of the videorecordings showed that temporary obstruction of IES by white cells or platelet aggregates was not a major cause of the changes in flow resistance although such obstruction did occur occasionally. Therefore, the red cell bursts must have been caused by changes in caliber of IES themselves. Drenckhahn and Wagner (1986) demonstrated the contractility of microfilamentous bundles run-

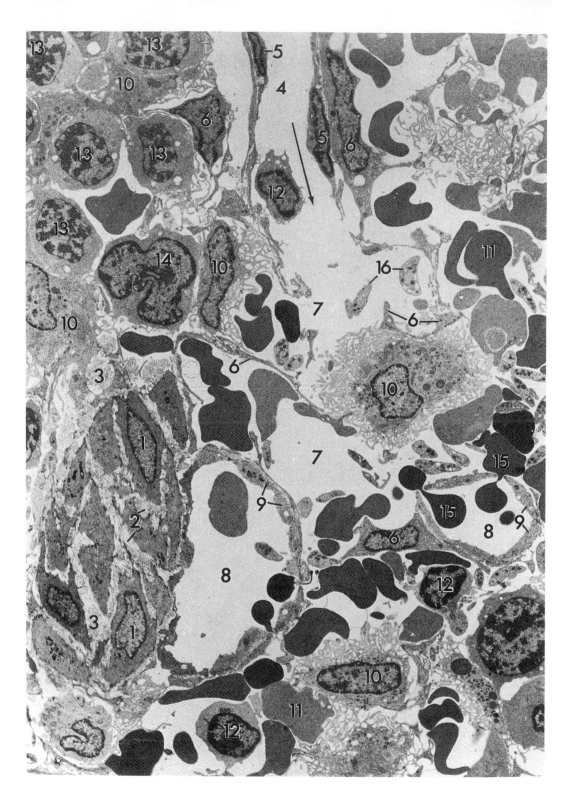

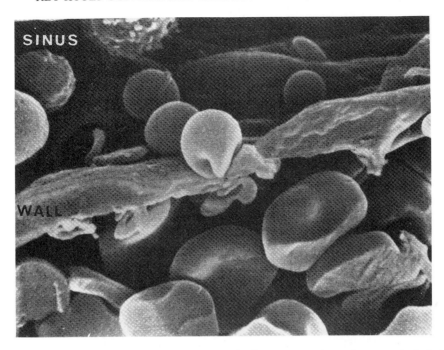

Figure 4.24 SEM micrograph from rat spleen showing red cells squeezing through interendothelial slits in the wall of a venous sinus. (Reproduced with permission from Boisfleury and Mohandas (1977) *Blood Cells*, **3**, 197–208.)

ning along either side of the IES, within the endothelial cells of the sinus wall, and suggested that such contractile activity might control the width of the IES. Our *in vivo* studies support this view: IES can be held closed for considerable periods of time, and only 20% (approximately) of the total number of IES present anatomically allow passage of red cells during any 5 minute period. The mean red cell flow rate per IES was 15 red cells/minute for the six active IES analysed, whereas the maximum instantaneous red cell flow rate was 10 red cells/s. The time required for a red cell to pass through an IES varied greatly; even for a single IES it

ranged from 0.02 to 60 s (MacDonald *et al.*, 1987).

In summary, the view that all venous sinuses originate in the red pulp as blind sacs, into which blood enters solely through the IES in the sinus walls, is incorrect. Two additional routes for blood flow into venous sinuses exist, besides that involving IES: (1) open-ended venous sinuses originating in the marginal sinus or marginal zone, which represent a major component of the fast pathway through the spleen; (2) direct connections of arterial capillaries to venous sinuses, a route that is also part of the fast pathway (see section 4.3.11). The route for

Figure 4.23 Rat spleen. 1, Smooth muscle cells of trabecula; 2, elastic fibers; 3, bundles of collagenous fibrils; 4, open termination of arterial capillary (→, direction of flow); 5, endothelial cells; 6, reticular cells; 7, interstitial space; 8, venous sinuses; 9, endothelial cells lining sinuses; 10, macrophages; 11, red cells; 12, small lymphocytes; 13, proerythroblasts; 14, lymphocyte; 15, red cell squeezing through interendothelial slits in sinus wall; 16, platelets (×1400). (Reproduced with permission from Rhodin (1974) *Histology: A Text and Atlas*, Oxford University Press, New York.)

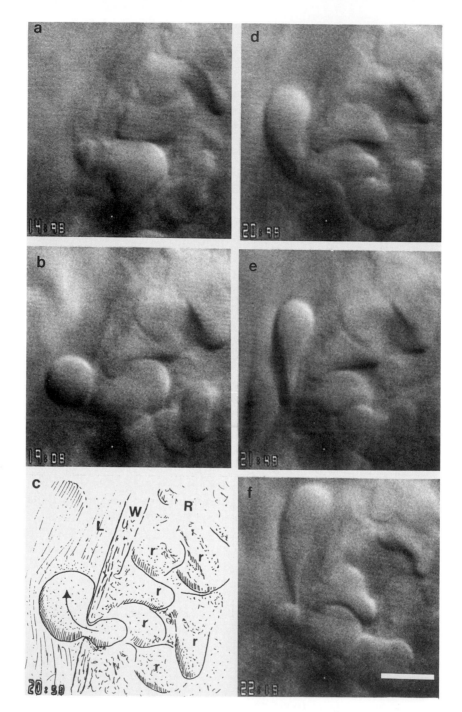

Figure 4.25 Photomicrographs from videomicroscopy of transilluminated rat spleen *in vivo*. Sequential images of a red cell squeezing through an interendothelial slit in the wall of a venous sinus. Numbers in lower left corners give time in seconds and hundredths of a second. The venous sinus (diameter 17 μm) runs vertically at left of photos and is only partially shown. The schematic (Figure 4.25c) shows the locations of the sinus lumen (L), sinus wall (W), and numerous red cells (r) within the reticular spaces of the red pulp (R). Bar = 5 μm. (Reproduced with permission from MacDonald *et al.* (1987) *Microvascular Research*, 33, 118–34.)

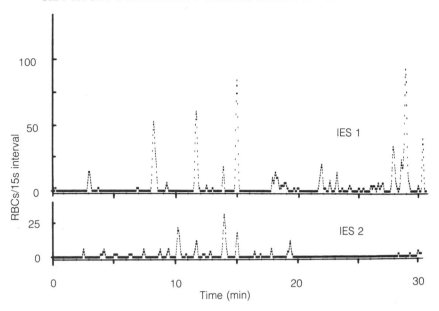

Figure 4.26 Rate of red cell flow (red cells/15 s) through two closely adjacent interendothelial slits (IES) in a venous sinus in rat spleen, measured simultaneously over a 30-minute period by *in vivo* microscopy (see Figure 4.25). Flow consisted of a series of brief, discontinuous bursts of red cells, separated by periods of zero, or near zero, flow (see text). (Reproduced with permission from MacDonald, I.C. *et al.* (1987) *Microvascular Research*, **33**, 118–34.)

flow from the reticular meshwork into venous sinuses through interendothelial slits in sinus walls forms part of the slow pathway through the spleen.

4.3.11   SPLENIC MICROCIRCULATION: 'OPEN', OR BOTH 'OPEN' AND 'CLOSED'?

The question of whether all blood passing through the spleen must flow through the reticular meshwork of the red pulp or marginal zone in order to reach the venous system ('open' circulation), or whether some of the blood flows through direct connections of arterial capillaries to venous vessels, has been the subject of much controversy since the turn of this century (Weidenreich, 1901; Helly, 1902). The controversy came into sharp focus with the radically divergent results of Knisely (1936) and MacKenzie, Whipple and Wintersteiner (1941), both obtained by the same transillumination procedure. Similarly, studies of fixed splenic tissue or corrosion casts examined by light or electron microscopy have produced conflicting results. Most investigators, having failed to find evidence of direct arteriovenous pathways, have concluded that a closed circulation does not exist (Human spleen: Irino, Murakami and Fujita, 1977; Suzuki *et al.*, 1978; Weiss, Powell and Schiffman, 1985; Van Krieken *et al.*, 1985a; Fujita, Kashimura and Adachi, 1985. Sinusal spleens of dog, rat, rabbit: Snook, 1950; Lewis, 1957; Suzuki *et al.*, 1977; Blue and Weiss, 1981d. Non-sinusal spleens of cat, mouse: Snook, 1950; Lewis, 1957; Blue and Weiss, 1981b; Hataba, Kirino and Suzuki, 1981). In contrast, Barnhart, Baechler and Lusher (1976) found evidence of both open and closed pathways in human spleen, while others have maintained that the circulation is entirely closed (Human and other sinusal spleens: Tischendorf, 1969; Pictet *et al.*, 1969; Miyamoto, Seguchi and Ogawa, 1980).

Why is there still controversy? The beautiful

SEM micrographs of arterial capillary endings in the reticular meshwork produced by Suzuki *et al.* (1977: dog) and Irino, Murakami and Fujita (1977: human) demonstrate clearly the existence of an open circulation. Such clear evidence has been lacking for the closed circulation. Although many investigators have not found evidence for a closed circulation, one should not use the 'argument from silence' to conclude that a closed circulation does not exist. Much of the evidence for a closed circulation has been unconvincing, often due to the rarity with which direct arteriovenous connections have been found. Recently, clear evidence of abundant connections of arterial capillaries to venous sinuses (as well as capillary endings in the reticular meshwork) was obtained in dog spleen by means of the microcorrosion casting procedure described in section 4.2.3 (Schmidt, MacDonald and Groom, 1982). Thus, in this species both open and closed circulations exist. This is also the case in rat and human spleens (Schmidt, MacDonald and Groom, 1985a, 1988), although direct connections are less

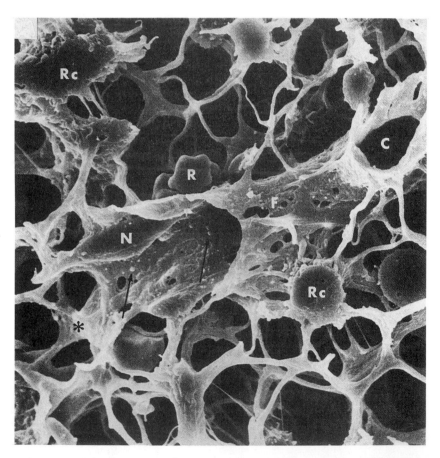

Figure 4.27 Reticular meshwork in red pulp of dog spleen. Loose irregular 3-dimensional network of reticulum cells (Rc) and their fibrous processes. Arterial capillary terminates rather abruptly in red pulp. Processes from reticulum cells are fixed on outer capillary surface supporting vessel. Note transition from endothelial sheet to reticular meshwork (*). Arrows, microvilli of endothelial cells; C, capillary lumen; F, fenestration in capillary wall; N, nuclear elevation of endothelial cell; R, red blood cell. (×2650). (Reproduced with permission from Suzuki, T. *et al.* (1977) *Cell and Tissue Research*, **182**, 441–53.)

abundant than in the dog. In non-sinusal spleens, however, no direct connections of arterial capillaries to pulp venules were found (Schmidt, MacDonald and Groom, 1983b: cat; 1985b: mouse).

Evidence for the open circulation is presented in Figures 4.23 and 4.27–4.32. In TEM micrographs arterial capillaries may sometimes be seen terminating in the reticular meshwork (Figure 4.23), and 3-dimensional views of such open terminations may be obtained by SEM. In Figure 4.27 an arterial capillary terminates rather abruptly in the loose irregular meshwork of reticulum cells and their fibrous processes; such processes are fixed on the outer surface of the capillary, supporting the vessel. The transition from endothelial sheet to reticular meshwork is shown clearly in this figure. In microcorrosion casts, continuity of flow from capillary lumen to reticular meshwork may be seen.

In the example from human spleen (Figure 4.28), only a few of the interstices of the reticular meshwork have begun to fill, whereas in Figure 4.29 (cat spleen) entire pathways from arterial capillary through the reticular meshwork to a pulp venule are shown. The most direct route that we have found in a non-sinusal spleen, from arterial capillary to pulp venule, is shown in Figure. 4.30 (cat spleen); the distance through the reticular meshwork between the two vessels is merely 15–25 μm. Another part of the open circulation consists of flow through fenestrations in the capillary wall radially outward into ellipsoid sheaths (the 'periarterial macrophage sheaths' of Blue and Weiss, 1981a) and on into the reticular meshwork. The interstices of ellipsoid sheaths are considerably smaller than those of the reticular meshwork, as may be seen from Figures 4.31 and 4.32. Ellipsoid sheaths are usually found just before the

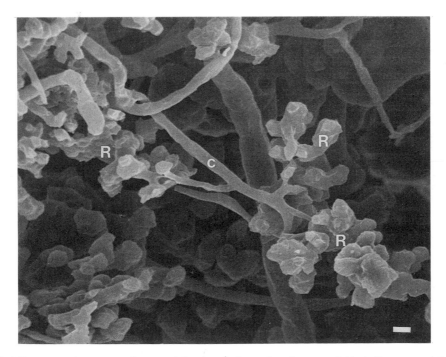

Figure 4.28 Microcorrosion cast of normal human spleen showing arterial capillary (c) endings in the reticular meshwork of the red pulp (R). Due to injection of only a small amount of material the interstices of the reticular meshwork have barely begun to fill. Bar = 10 μm.

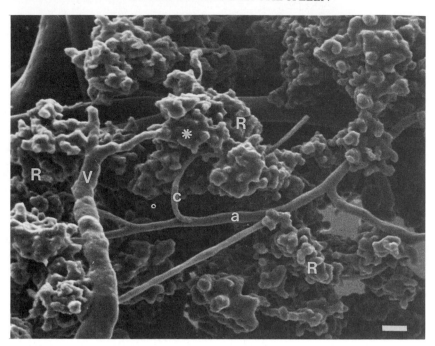

Figure 4.29 Microcorrosion cast of cat spleen (non-sinusal). Large slender arterial vessels (a) branch, forming capillaries (c) which end in reticular meshwork of the red pulp (R). Short pathway (*) through reticular meshwork connects capillary with pulp venule (V). Longer routes through reticular meshwork are unfilled (due to small amount of injectate). Bar = 50 μm. (Reproduced with permission from Goresky and Groom (1984) *Handbook of Physiology*, Section 2, *The Cardiovascular System*, Vol. IV, Microcirculation, Part 2, pp. 689–780. American Physiological Society, Washington, DC.)

termination of arterial capillaries (Figure 4.32), and they are thought to represent sites of filtration of particulate matter from the blood.

Evidence for a closed circulation is presented in Figures 4.33 to 4.36. Abundant direct connections of arterial capillaries to venous sinuses have been demonstrated in dog spleen, by means of the minimal-injection microcorrosion casting technique (section 4.2.3). Typically the terminal arteriole bifurcates repeatedly to give rise to many short capillaries, each of which leads to one end of a venous sinus. This is shown in Figure 4.33 in which at least 10 venous sinuses are fed from the same terminal arteriole.

Figure 4.30 Microcorrosion cast of cat spleen (non-sinusal). (a) Arterial capillary (c) terminates in reticular meshwork (R), closely adjacent to pulp venule (v) which drains into collecting vein (V). Because of retrograde flow, material is beginning to emerge from fenestrations in pulp venule into reticular meshwork. Bar = 25 μm. (b) Close-up of area from (a) shows shortest route found between capillary ending and pulp venule. The forward (capillary, c) and retrograde (venular, v) flows have reached adjacent reticular spaces (R) but have not quite merged. Bar = 10 μm. (Reproduced with permission from Schmidt, MacDonald and Groom (1983b) *Journal of Morphology*, **178**, 125–38.)

Figure 4.31 Microcorrosion cast of dog spleen. Capillary branch (c) from arteriole (a) shows leakage pattern of casting material into ellipsoid sheath (E) and thence into surrounding reticular meshwork (R). Note that interstices of the ellipsoid sheath are considerably smaller than those of the reticular meshwork. Bar = 10 μm. (Reproduced with permission from Schmidt, MacDonald and Groom (1983a) *Journal of Morphology*, **178**, 111–23.)

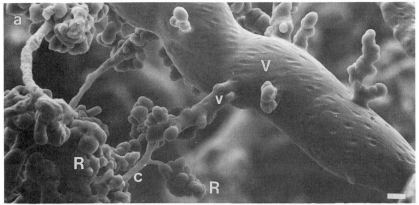

Figure 4.30(a)

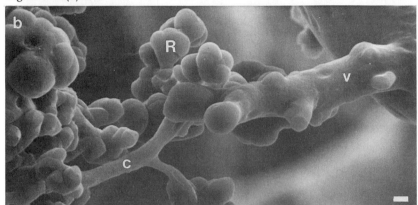

Figure 4.30(b)

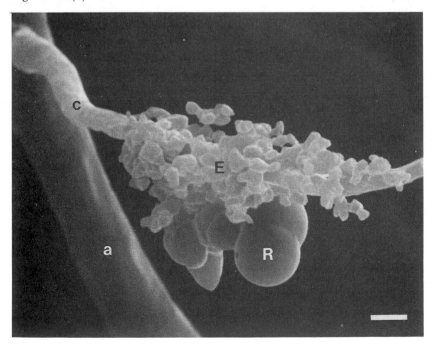

Figure 4.31

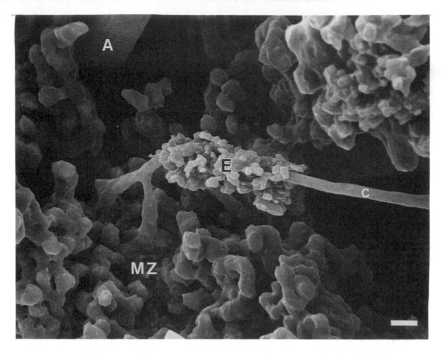

Figure 4.32 Microcorrosion cast of dog spleen showing location of ellipsoid sheath (E) just before the termination of the arterial capillary (c) in the marginal zone (MZ). A, central artery of lymphatic nodule. Bar = 20 μm.

In this particular example the venous sinuses have just begun to fill, whereas in Figure 4.34 more extensive filling of some venous sinuses has occurred. In human spleen, direct connections of arterial capillaries to venous sinuses are fewer than in dog spleen (Schmidt, MacDonald and Groom, 1988). The overview in Figure 4.35(a) shows several long capillaries, one giving off two short branches that terminate in adjacent venous sinuses, after approaching them from a radial direction. At higher magnification it may be seen that the two short branches are indeed continuous with the sinuses (Figure 4.35b,c). Direct connections also occur to the perimarginal cavernous sinus (see section 4.3.13). Although microcorrosion casts cannot demonstrate endothelial continuity between capillary and sinus, these results provide convincing evidence of direct connections. Furthermore, endothelial continuity has been demonstrated in chicken spleen by Miyamoto, Seguchi and Ogawa (1980) and by Olah and Glick (1982). In Figure 4.36 a sheathed artery gives rise to an arterial capillary which is directly connected with venous sinuses: continuity of internal elastic laminae and endothelial cells may be seen.

In summary, the circulation in sinusal spleens appears to be primarily 'open', but a 'closed' circulation also exists; the frequency of 'closed' pathways differs among species. In non-sinusal spleens 'closed' pathways have not yet been demonstrated, and the circulation appears to be exclusively 'open'.

4.3.12 'SWITCHING' OF MICROCIRCULATORY FLOW PATHS

Studies of RBC washout from the spleen during Ringer perfusion (section 4.2.1(a)) have shown that in the relaxed spleen 90% of the inflowing blood travels to the splenic vein by fast path-

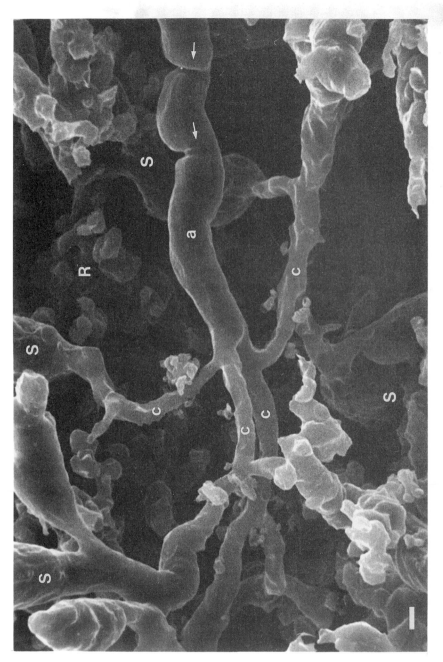

Figure 4.33 Microcorrosion cast of dog spleen showing direct connections of arterial capillaries (c) to venous sinuses (S) i.e. 'closed' circulation. Arteriole (a) entering from right is constricted in two places (arrows); note endothelial nuclear impressions on this vessel. Vessel bifurcates repeatedly in quick succession giving rise to many very short capillaries, each of which leads to one end of a venous sinus. Sinuses are only partially filled because of very small amount of casting material injected; nevertheless 10 venous sinuses are fed from this one terminal arteriole. Between sinuses, areas show start of reticular meshwork filling (R). Bar = 10 μm. (Reproduced with permission from Goresky and Groom (1984) *Handbook of Physiology*, Section 2, *The Cardiovascular System*, Vol. IV, Microcirculation, Part 2, pp. 689–780. American Physiological Society, Washington, DC.)

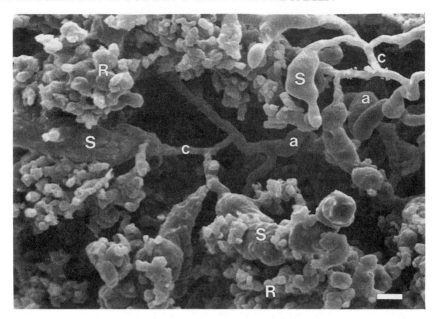

Figure 4.34 Microcorrosion cast of dog spleen. More extensive filling of some venous sinuses has occurred in this cast than that shown in Figure 4.33. Arterioles (a) connect *via* short capillary segments (c) directly to several venous sinuses (S). Little filling of the reticular meshwork of the red pulp (R) has occurred. Bar = 25 μm. (Reproduced with permission from Schmidt, MacDonald and Groom (1983a) *Journal of Morphology*, **178**, 111–23.)

ways (Song and Groom, 1971a: cat), whereas in the norepinephrine-contracted spleen the proportion of the flow carried by fast pathways rises to 98.7% (Groom and Song, 1971). By contrast, when the spleen is dilated by perfusion against an elevated venous outflow pressure of 25 cmH$_2$O, the flow fraction carried by the fast pathways falls to zero (Levesque and Groom, 1980b). These results suggest that 'switching' of flow between alternate paths can occur. Application of the microcorrosion casting technique under each of these conditions has allowed the morphology of the different pathways to be studied selectively (section 4.2.3).

In the contracted spleen of cat, the casts showed that flow occurred through short routes through the reticular meshwork, from capillary terminations to nearby venous vessels, as well as by short routes from marginal sinus or marginal zone to venous vessels. In addition, direct connections of arterial capillaries to venous

sinuses were found in contracted spleens of dog. In dilated spleens many more capillary terminations in the reticular meshwork of the red pulp were filled with casting material, whereas direct connections to venous sinuses were not filled. The picture that emerges is that flow through the reticular meshwork of the red pulp is minimized in contracted spleens but predominates in dilated spleens.

What control mechanisms are responsible for this switching of flow pathways? One factor would be contraction of arteriolar smooth muscle, and in spleens injected with norepinephrine abundant evidence of this is present. In the region where an arteriole becomes reduced to an arterial capillary, the contraction of discontinuous bands of vascular smooth muscle produces a series of constrictions, some of which appear as particularly narrow, deep impressions on the cast (Figure 4.37a). An example of extreme arteriolar constriction is seen in Figure

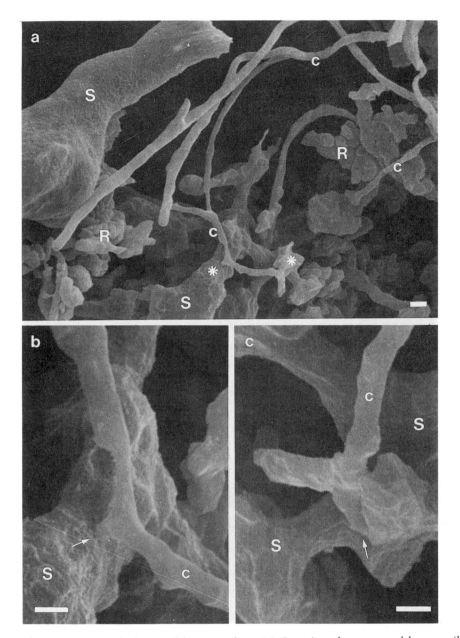

Figure 4.35 Microcorrosion cast of normal human spleen. (a) Overview shows several long capillaries (c), one giving off two short branches that connect directly (*) to adjacent venous sinuses (S). Some filling of reticular meshwork (R) is seen. Bar = 10 μm. (b,c) Magnified views from (a) show continuity between capillary branches (c) and venous sinuses (→). Incomplete filling of capillary resulted from injection of only small amounts of casting material. Bars = 5 μm. (Reproduced with permission from Schmidt, MacDonald and Groom (1988), *American Journal of Anatomy*, **181**, 253–66.)

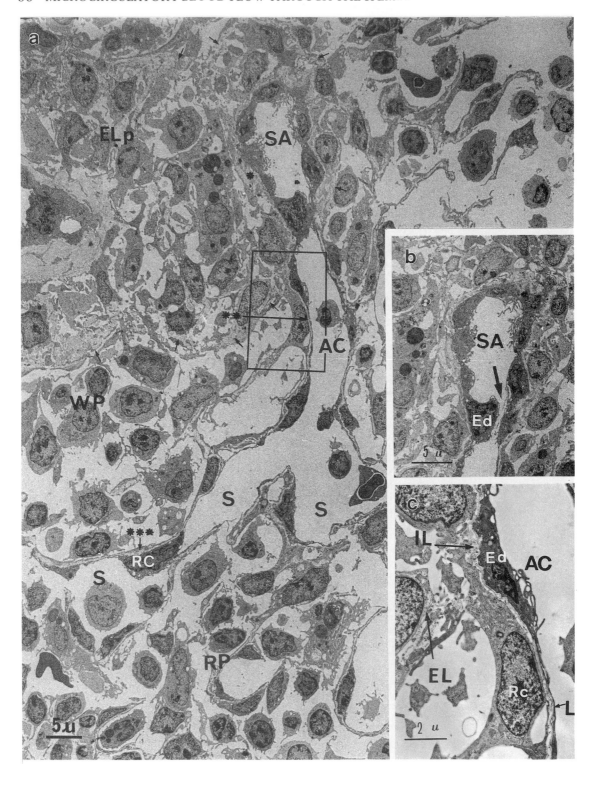

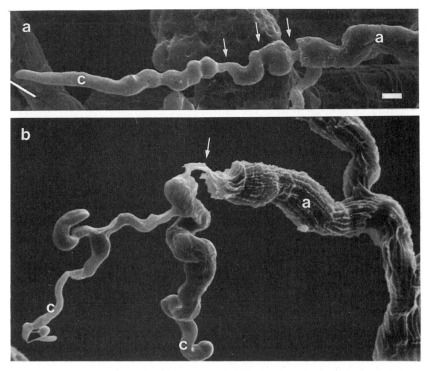

Figure 4.37 (a) Microcorrosion cast of dog spleen contracted by injection of norepinephrine. In the region where an arteriole (a) becomes reduced to an arterial capillary (c), the contraction of discontinuous bands of vascular smooth muscle (corroded away) produces a series of constrictions, some of which appear as particularly narrow, deep impressions on the cast (→). Bar = 15 μm. (b) Microcorrosion cast of cat spleen contracted by norepinephrine, showing extremely constricted region (→) in an arteriole (a) just before it branches into two capillaries (c). Only a fine thread of material supports the cast downstream. Casts of capillaries end blindly because of incomplete filling, due to the increased resistance to flow at the constriction. (Reproduced with permission from Schmidt, MacDonald and Groom (1983c) *Cell Tissue Research*, **228**, 33–41.)

Figure 4.36 Micrographs from chicken spleen demonstrating endothelial continuity from arterial capillary to venous sinuses ('closed' circulation). (a) Sheathed artery (SA) branches into arterial capillary (AC), which connects directly with venous sinuses (S). Internal elastic laminae of sheathed artery (*), arterial capillary (**), and sinuses (***) are continuous. Rod-shaped endothelial cells (RC) line the sinuses. WP, white pulp; RP, red pulp; ELp, ellipsoid. (×1970). (b) Continuity (→) between sheathed artery (SA) and arterial capillary is shown in this section serial to that of (a). Ed, endothelial cell of artery. (×2060). (c) Higher magnification of area in rectangle of (a) showing wall structure of arterial capillary (AC): flattened endothelial cells (Ed) with thin lamina (L), internal lamina (IL), and external lamina (EL) of ellipsoid sheath. (×4300). (Reproduced with permission of the authors and publishers from Miyamoto, Seguchi and Ogawa (1980) *Journal of Electron Microscopy*, **29**, 158–72.)

4.37(b), in which the lumen is almost completely closed and a fine thread of casting material 4–5 μm in diameter precariously supports the weight of the cast downstream. Due to the increased resistance to flow, the capillaries distal to the constrictions (Figure 4.37a,b) are incompletely filled, and therefore appear to end blindly. Taken together with the minimal filling of the reticular meshwork in these casts, the results suggest a shunting of flow to the fast pathway.

Further control of blood flow could be mediated by strategically placed 'sphincters' at the level of the venous sinuses. Knisely's (1936) transillumination studies suggested the presence of such sphincters at both the entrances and exits of venous sinuses, but conclusive morphological evidence of their existence has yet to be obtained. Several observations from microcorrosion casts also suggest that constrictions (perhaps temporary) at the two ends of the venous sinuses may play a part in controlling flow. An extreme narrowing of the 'neck' leading to a venous sinus is sometimes seen (Figure 4.38a), and a ring of impressions, probably made by endothelial cell nuclei, often occurs around the entrance to a sinus (Figure 4.38b). In addition, sphincter-like constrictions of venous sinuses are sometimes observed at points where these sinuses connect with larger sinuses (Figures 4.39a, b and c). The appearance of these constrictions suggests that a ring of vascular smooth muscle may have been their cause, but we know of no histological evidence that would support this conclusion. In contrast, the narrowing at the entrance to venous sinuses

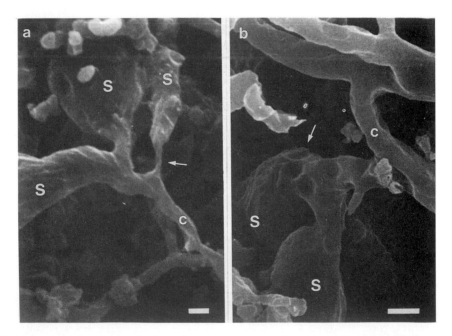

Figure 4.38 Microcorrosion casts of dog spleen showing possible sites for control of flow from arterial capillaries (c) directly into venous sinuses (S). (a) Extreme narrowing of the 'neck' ($\rightarrow$) leading to one venous sinus is seen, whereas the entrances to two adjacent sinuses are more widely open. Bar = 10 μm. (b) A ring of impressions ($\rightarrow$), possibly made by endothelial cell nuclei, is seen around the entrance to a venous sinus (i.e. where the localized constriction was found in (a)). This Figure is a high magnification view of a region in Figure 4.33. Bar = 10 μm. (Reproduced with permission from Schmidt, MacDonald and Groom (1982) *Cell Tissue Research*, **225**, 543–55.)

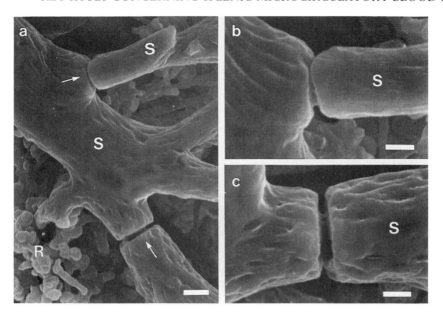

Figure 4.39 Microcorrosion cast of rat spleen. (a) Sphincter-like constrictions (→) of venous sinuses (S) at junctions with larger sinuses. Reticular meshwork (R) has just begun to fill. Bar = 20 μm. (b,c) Higher magnification views of constrictions shown in (a). S, venous sinus. Bars = 10 μm. (Reproduced with permission from Schmidt, MacDonald and Groom (1985a) *Journal of Morphology*, **186**, 1–16).

(Figures 4.38a and b) could conceivably be the result of the contraction of specialized endothelial cells, as seen in other tissues (Lübbers *et al.*, 1979; Weigelt, 1982) as well as in spleen (Drenckhahn and Wagner, 1986). Recent evidence obtained by *in vivo* microscopy suggests that endothelial contractility may also modify red cell flow at the arterial capillary level in the spleen (Ragan *et al.*, 1988). Spontaneous cyclic contractions of the capillary wall were quantitatively analyzed in relaxed spleens (rat, mouse) and it was found that during 50% of the contractions luminal diameter was reduced to less than 1 μm, stopping red cell flow in that capillary. Regression analysis showed that the vessel narrowing was due primarily to bulging of endothelial cells into the lumen, and not to bulging of pericytes or closure caused by changes in transmural pressure. Reduction of flow in such arterial capillaries would decrease red cell supply to the reticular meshwork.

In summary, results from kinetic and morphological studies show that redistribution of intrasplenic blood flow can occur, away from the slow pathways of the reticular meshwork to the fast pathways described earlier (section 4.3.1) and vice versa. The functional significance of this switching of microcirculatory flow paths is not yet clear, but a reduction in flow through the reticular meshwork would presumably reduce the filtration of abnormal red cells by the spleen.

4.3.13 DIFFERENCES BETWEEN MICROCIRCULATORY PATHWAYS IN NORMAL HUMAN SPLEEN AND THOSE IN OTHER SPECIES. CHANGES IN DISEASE

Confusion regarding microcirculatory pathways in normal human spleen has arisen due to extrapolation from other mammalian spleens and from human pathological material. In addition, it has been difficult to trace 3-dimensional routes through the spleen simply from the study of thin sections or cut surfaces of tissue. Microcirculatory pathways have recently been studied from microcorrosion casts (section 4.2.3) of normal human spleens freshly obtained from organ transplant donors (Schmidt, MacDonald and Groom, 1988), as well as casts of surgically removed spleens from patients with various diseases (Schmidt, MacDonald and Groom, unpublished observations). The results have shown several differences between pathways in human spleen and those in other species, as well as changes in disease.

A vascular structure that seems to be unique to the human spleen is the perimarginal cavernous sinus (PMCS), a large blood space bordering the white pulp. The PMCS was unknown until Yamamoto *et al.* (1979), using scanning electron microscopy, presented evidence of its existence in human spleens and named it the 'perimarginal cavernous sinus plexus'. These investigators showed that (1) the PMCS is located between the marginal zone (MZ) and the red pulp, except in areas where the MZ is not well developed and the PMCS borders the white pulp directly; (2) the PMCS is lined by thin endothelial cells with flattened nuclei, in contrast to venous sinuses in which the endothelial nuclei protrude into the lumen; (3) sinuses of the PMCS plexus communicate with each other through narrow channels; (4) many thin endothelial cells and their processes bridge opposite walls of the PMCS; (5) the PMCS communicates with the reticular meshwork of the MZ. They were unable to elucidate the vascular connections between PMCS and other structures. However, the microcorrosion casts obtained in our investigation (Schmidt, MacDonald and Groom, 1988) have now provided 3-dimensional views of the PMCS and its vascular connections.

The PMCS is different in appearance from any other structure in the casts. Large flattened masses of casting material are seen, up to $300 \times 1000~\mu m$ in area and $30-100~\mu m$ in thickness (Figures 4.40a and b). The PMCS may be situated either outside the MZ or directly adjacent to the lymphatic nodule itself, in an area devoid of marginal sinus (Figure 4.40a). The surface of the PMCS cast is smooth and flat, except for small 'pock-marks' and shallow impressions (Figures 4.40a, b and c). A considerable volume of casting material may reach the PMCS even when minimal filling of adjacent vascular spaces is evident, as shown in Figure 4.40(a). Flow of material into the PMCS occurs through direct connections with arterial capillaries (Figure 4.40c), *via* ellipsoid sheaths (Figure 4.41a), and through points of continuity with the MZ (Figure 4.41b). Drainage from the PMCS occurs directly into venous sinuses (Figure 4.41c). Thus, the casts confirm Yamamoto's observations (1), (3) and (5) above, provide evidence consistent with (2) and (4), and furnish new information regarding the flow pathways into and out of the PMCS. The function of the PMCS is not yet known, but clearly it forms part of the fast pathway in human spleen; blood passing through it into the venous sinuses would bypass the reticular meshwork of the red pulp and the interendothelial slits in sinus walls, thus avoiding the sites at which abnormal red cells are filtered from the blood.

We are not aware of any structures other than the PMCS which are unique to the human spleen. In mammals there appears to be a basic common pattern of splenic microvascular structure; however, many species differences are found in terms of the pattern of arterial branching, the configuration of the marginal sinus, the presence or absence of ellipsoid sheaths, the presence of venous sinuses or pulp venules, and the frequency of direct arteriovenous connections. A brief summary of some of the differences between microcirculatory pathways in the human spleen and those in other species is therefore presented next (see also Schmidt, MacDonald and Groom, 1988).

The degree of arterial branching in human spleen is much greater than that found in other species, and the peculiar branching which forms 'arteriolar-capillary bundles' within lymphatic nodules has been reported only for human and monkey spleens. Other characteristics of the

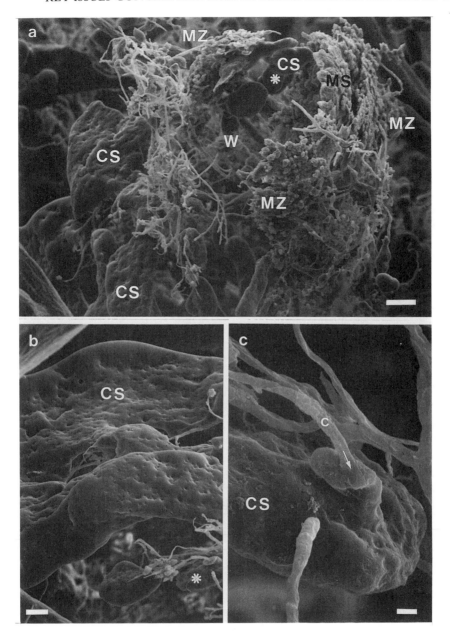

Figure 4.40 Microcorrosion cast of normal human spleen. (a) Perimarginal cavernous sinus plexus (CS) appears as large, flattened masses situated either directly adjacent to white pulp (*, in an area devoid of marginal sinus (MS)), or outside the marginal zone (MZ, at left of figure). W, white pulp corroded away; red pulp is unfilled. Bar = 10 μm. (b) Magnified view of perimarginal cavernous sinus (CS) from (a) (seen at different angle). Surface of CS is smooth and flat, except for small pockmarks and shallow impressions. (*, region shown at higher magnification in (c)). Bar = 50 μm. (c) Magnified view of perimarginal cavernous sinus (CS) from (b). Arterial capillary (c) connects directly to CS (→). (A second capillary, at bottom of figure, is not continuous with CS cast.) Bar = 10 μm. (Reproduced with permission from Schmidt, MacDonald and Groom (1988), *American Journal of Anatomy*, **181**, 253–66.)

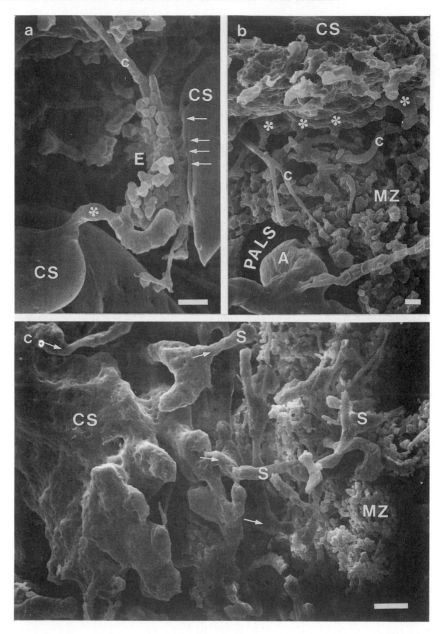

Figure 4.41 Microcorrosion casts of normal human spleen. (a) Two separate areas of perimarginal cavernous sinus (CS) have begun to fill from an ellipsoid sheath (E), either *via* several small lateral channels (→) or *via* a larger channel continuous with one end of the CS (*). c, arterial capillary proximal to ellipsoid sheath. Bar = 20 μm. (b) Perimarginal cavernous sinus (CS) receives flow *via* numerous short, irregular channels (*) from the marginal zone (MZ) surrounding the periarterial lymphatic sheath (PALS). Several arterial capillaries (c) end in MZ. A, central artery. Bar = 20 μm. (c) Perimarginal cavernous sinus (CS) drains directly (→) into the interconnected system of venous sinuses (S) adjacent to marginal zone (MZ). Bar = 50 μm. (Reproduced with permission from Schmidt, MacDonald and Groom (1988) *American Journal of Anatomy*, **181**, 253–66.)

arterial branching in human spleen are the presence of many arterioles curving within the marginal zone around lymphatic nodules, like fingers grasping a ball: this is similar to the arrangement in dog spleen, but differs from that of the rat and mouse. In addition, most follicular capillaries do not originate from branches of the central artery within the nodule, but from arterioles in the marginal zone. Ellipsoid sheaths, which are not present in all species (such as rat and mouse) are present in human spleen. These may be sites where filtration of the blood occurs, but they are certainly not the primary site, although this was implied by Van Krieken *et al.* (1985a).

The existence of the marginal sinus (MS) around lymphatic nodules has been confirmed in normal human spleens (section 4.3.9); however, species differences exist with respect to its 3-dimensional configuration. In human spleen the inner aspect of the MS cast, adjoining the white pulp, appears as a flattened, almost continuous system of anastomosing spaces, similar to those in the dog spleen but different from the small discontinuous spaces found in spleens of rat and mouse. The blood supply to the MS in humans comes primarily from capillaries which end on its outer aspect facing the marginal zone, whereas in many other species the blood supply comes from follicular capillaries terminating on the inner aspect of the MS.

The rarity with which direct connections of arterial capillaries to venous sinuses occur in human spleen (section 4.3.11) is in marked contrast to the abundance of such connections in dog spleen. Direct arteriovenous connections appear to be absent from non-sinusal spleens. Thus, there exists great variability among species with respect to the closed circulation, and extrapolations from animals to man are not

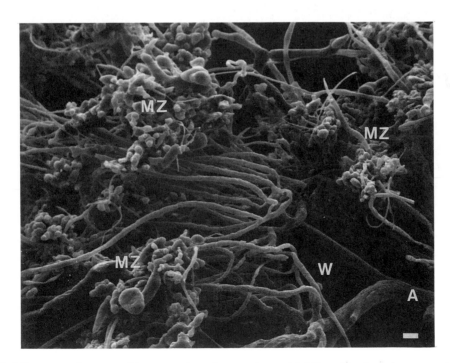

Figure 4.42 Microcorrosion cast of human spleen from patient with idiopathic thrombocytopenia, showing proliferation of arterioles and capillaries within the white pulp (W, corroded away) and marginal zone (MZ). The MZ has just begun to fill (in a few areas only) and the surrounding red pulp is unfilled. A, central artery. Bar = 20 μm.

valid. A major component of the fast pathway for blood flow through sinusal spleens is abundant open-ended venous sinuses beginning in the marginal zone. Such open-ended sinuses are a prominent feature in microcorrosion casts of human spleens as well as those of dog and rat. Flow by this route bypasses the reticular meshwork of the red pulp and interendothelial slits in sinus walls.

When microcorrosion casts of normal human spleens from transplant donors were compared with those of spleens surgically removed from patients with various diseases (idiopathic thrombocytopenia (ITP), carcinoma of the colon, lymphocytic leukemia, hypersplenism, portal hypertension), two consistent differences in the microcirculatory pathways were found in the spleens from diseased subjects (Schmidt, MacDonald and Groom, unpublished observa-

tions). First, a striking proliferation of arterioles and capillaries was found in the white pulp and marginal zone (MZ) and, second, the marginal sinus (MS) was absent. The cast in Figure 4.42, from a patient with ITP, shows a profusion of small vessels branching from the central artery within the white pulp and passing outward through the MZ. In a cast of the region bordering a lymphatic nodule (Figure 4.43) where the MS is found in normal spleens, the knobbly configuration characteristic of MZ filling is seen in the diseased subjects. The appearance of this cast, from a patient with ITP, contrasts markedly with that from the normal spleen (Figure 4.17) where the flattened sheet-like nature of the MS is apparent. The cause of these changes and their functional implications are not yet understood, but it is clear that conclusions regarding microcirculatory pathways in normal

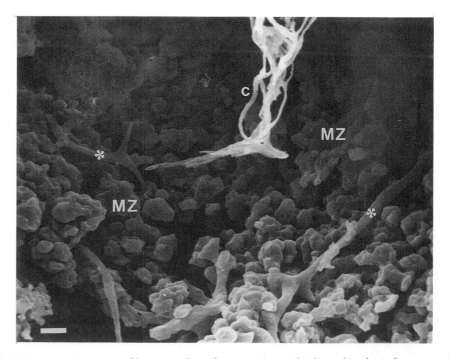

Figure 4.43 Microcorrosion cast of human spleen from patient with idiopathic thrombocytopenia. View of interior of lymphatic nodule (white pulp corroded away) showing region where marginal sinus is found in normal spleen (see Figure 4.17). Note knobbly configuration of the cast characteristic of marginal zone (MZ), which is found bordering the white pulp instead of a marginal sinus. c, follicular capillaries; *, circumferentially oriented capillaries terminate in the MZ. Bar = 20 μm.

human spleen should not be based on material obtained from diseased subjects.

4.4 OVERVIEW OF CURRENT UNDERSTANDING OF MICROCIRCULATORY BLOOD FLOW IN THE HUMAN SPLEEN

Studies of the distribution of intrasplenic blood flow and the morphology of the microcirculatory pathways, using the methods described in section 4.2, have provided much new information which has led to a revision of some commonly accepted concepts of the splenic circulation in man. We have already focused on a number of key issues in detail (section 4.3), and at this point, an overview is presented. The schematic diagram from Bellanti with which we began (Figure 4.1) now needs to be reviewed in the light of the new insights obtained regarding the intermediate circulation between arterial capillaries and the venous channels.

It is now clear that in the normal human spleen a marginal sinus borders the white pulp. This consists of a series of cleft-like, anastomosing, vascular spaces between the white pulp and the surrounding marginal zone. The marginal sinus receives a plentiful blood supply through capillaries terminating on its outer aspect. Microcorrosion casts show that the marginal sinus fills preferentially before filling of the marginal zone and the surrounding red pulp. A uniform distribution of blood from marginal sinus to marginal zone is provided through discontinuities in the outer wall of the marginal sinus; in addition, the marginal zone receives a substantial blood supply from arterial capillaries which terminate directly within its meshwork. From the marginal zone a large proportion of the blood flows into the perimarginal cavernous sinus, or into open-ended venous sinuses originating there, while a small proportion flows radially outward from the marginal zone into the reticular meshwork of the red pulp.

The perimarginal cavernous sinus is a large blood space situated either between the marginal zone and the red pulp or directly adjacent to the white pulp itself. This structure, which appears to be unique to the human spleen, receives blood from direct connections with arterial capillaries, through ellipsoid sheaths, and *via* points of continuity with the marginal zone. Perimarginal cavernous sinus blood drains directly into venous sinuses.

The traditional view has been that venous sinuses begin in the red pulp as blind sacs; blood can enter them, on its way from the reticular meshwork to venous outflow, only by passing through interendothelial slits in sinus walls. However, microcorrosion casts have revealed that many venous sinuses begin as open-ended tubules continuous with the marginal zone (or, in some instances, the marginal sinus), allowing free entry of blood into the venous system and bypassing both the reticular meshwork of the red pulp and the interendothelial slits in venous sinus walls. The extensive filling of venous sinuses seen in microcorrosion casts prepared by injection of very small amounts of material occurs even when the surrounding reticular meshwork is completely unfilled. This indicates that most of the flow enters the interconnected network of venous sinuses through their open ends in the marginal zone. This route forms a major component of the fast pathway for blood flow through the spleen.

Another component of the fast pathway is provided by direct connections of arterial capillaries to venous sinuses ('closed' circulation). Such routes seem to be relatively rare in human spleen, where most of the arterial capillaries in the red pulp terminate in the reticular meshwork ('open' circulation). Ellipsoid sheaths surround many of these capillaries, as well as those ending in the marginal zone, a short distance before the vessel terminations. Flow can occur through fenestrations in the capillary wall radially outward into ellipsoid sheaths and on into the reticular meshwork.

All blood entering the reticular meshwork of the red pulp by the various routes just described, must pass through interendothelial slits in the walls of venous sinuses of sinusal spleens in order to reach the venous outflow. However, the fact that only a small proportion of the total splenic blood flow travels by this particular route has not been recognized until recently. Studies in animal spleens have shown that only 10% of the total flow travels through the slow pathways of the reticular meshwork during a single pass through the organ, whereas 90% reaches the outflow *via* rapid-transit pathways. Furthermore, *in vivo* microscopic studies in rat spleen have shown that red cell velocities in the reticular meshwork are only of the order of 7 μm/s, whereas red cell velocities in venous sinuses may be more than one hundred times greater. Passage of red cells through interendothelial slits was invariably found to be from the reticular meshwork into venous sinuses; red cell flow through individual interendothelial slits occurred in a series of brief, discontinuous bursts separated by periods of zero, or near zero, flow. It was concluded that this behavior was caused primarily by changes in caliber of the interendothelial slits themselves, mediated by contraction of sinus endothelial cells, as has been demonstrated in human spleen. Contrary to the impression gained from scanning electron micrographs showing all interendothelial slits widely open, *in vivo* microscopy showed that only approximately 20% of the total number of slits present anatomically allow passage of red cells during any particular 5-minute period. Because of this, the weighted average flow rate per interendothelial slit is only three red cells per minute. These results from rat spleen provide the only information presently available with respect to the flow rates which might be expected through interendothelial slits in human spleen.

It is in the slow pathways of the spleen through the reticular meshwork of the red pulp, that filtration of abnormal red cells and the concentration of red cells to a hematocrit of approximately 80% take place. Possible mechanisms underlying these functions will be discussed in section 4.5. A salient question remains: 'Since the spleen represents the only lymphatic tissue specialized to filter the blood, why should 90% of the arterial inflow travel through fast pathways which bypass the sites where filtration is carried out?' Either this is an inefficient system, or else the spleen is performing some other function with respect to the blood in the fast pathways. The spleen has important immunological functions, and in this connection it is noteworthy that a large proportion of the blood flowing through the fast pathways passes through the marginal sinus and marginal zone bordering the white pulp, regions which have an important role in the immune response.

4.5 SOME MAJOR UNSOLVED PROBLEMS, AND A HYPOTHESIS

4.5.1 PROBLEM: MECHANISM(S) UNDERLYING SPLENIC FILTRATION OF 'ABNORMAL' RED CELLS FROM THE BLOOD

The traditional view is that filtration of abnormal red cells occurs solely at interendothelial slits in walls of venous sinuses. It is postulated that red cells are unable to traverse the narrow slits when their deformability is reduced; consequently, they are trapped and later phagocytosed. One problem arising from this explanation of the initial trapping event is that venous sinuses are absent from about half of the mammalian species so far examined. In these, the sinuses are replaced by pulp venules, originating as open-ended tubes with walls that show relatively large fenestrations as opposed to narrow interendothelial slits. Nevertheless, filtration of abnormal red cells is carried out effectively in these non-sinusal spleens, in the reticular meshwork itself (see section 4.3.5). It is unlikely that trapping of red cells in the reticular meshwork would be the result of reduced red cell deformability, since the interstices of the reticular meshwork are larger in size than the red cells themselves. Thus, an alternative explanation is needed.

4.5.2 PROBLEM: MECHANISM(S) CAUSING THE DEVELOPMENT OF A HIGH INTRASPLENIC HEMATOCRIT

At present, the mechanism causing the intrasplenic hematocrit to be twice that of arterial blood remains unknown. Various possibilities have been suggested, the most well known being that hemoconcentration is carried out within venous sinuses which are under the control of efferent and afferent sphincters (Knisely, 1936). However, other investigators have not been able to confirm such a mechanism. Furthermore, non-sinusal spleens concentrate red cells to an equally high hematocrit within the reticular meshwork (see section 4.3.2). This argues that the primary mechanism of red cell concentration must be independent of the presence of venous sinuses. The functional significance of the high hematocrit is also not understood: the red cell reservoir function of contractile spleens does not explain the high hematocrit found in species where the spleen is non-contractile. A new hypothesis regarding the mechanism responsible for the high intrasplenic hematocrit is presented below.

4.5.3 HYPOTHESIS: FILTRATION OF 'ABNORMAL' RED CELLS AND DEVELOPMENT OF A HIGH INTRASPLENIC HEMATOCRIT BOTH STEM FROM MICROVASCULAR FLOW CONDITIONS IN THE RED PULP

In the light of our morphological and kinetic studies, including *in vivo* microscopy, we propose a hypothesis for the primary red cell filtration mechanism, based upon adhesion in the reticular meshwork rather than on mechanical filtration at interendothelial slits. Thus, the red cell filtration process would depend primarily on cell membrane surface properties, rather than on deformability. The 'pore size' of the reticular meshwork is several red cell diameters, too large to impede flow on the basis of deformability. However, the meshwork presents an enormous contact surface area for blood cells, and its large cross-sectional area for flow results in very low red-cell velocities (mean: 7 μm/s). As a consequence of the resulting low shear rates abnormal red cells become trapped by adhesion to the meshwork; normal red cells adhere reversibly to each other and to the meshwork, whereas plasma flows on freely. Thus, the mean velocity of red cells is reduced below that of plasma, and intrasplenic hematocrit must rise in consequence. This follows from the law of conservation of mass, and is the inverse of the 'Fåhraeus effect' whereby red cells move towards the axis of flow when blood flows through narrow tubes, and consequently with the velocity of red cells greater than that of plasma, there is a reduction in tube hematocrit below that of the inflowing and outflowing blood.

This hypothesis does not deny that interendothelial slits in venous sinus walls also provide an important mechanism of red cell filtration. However, since such slits are present in spleens of only 50% of mammalian species, the role of interendothelial slits in red cell filtration appears to be secondary to the role of the reticular meshwork. Passage of red cells through interendothelial slits provides a test of red cell deformability; it also provides additional resistance to flow through the reticular meshwork, lowering shear rates yet further and enhancing red cell adhesion within the meshwork. This would appear to give sinusal spleens an advantage over non-sinusal spleens. The presence of ellipsoid sheaths in some species provides yet another site for filtration of the blood. The human spleen possesses both venous sinuses and ellipsoids, in addition to the reticular meshwork giving it every advantage for its task of filtering the cellular elements of the blood.

According to this hypothesis, the high intrasplenic hematocrit is considered to be merely a side effect of the mechanisms for filtration of abnormal red cells. The high hematocrit follows of necessity from the enormous cross-sectional area for flow interposed between the arterial capillaries and the venous channels. This 'intermediate circulation' is necessary in order to provide shear rates low enough for immature or abnormal red cells and possibly senescent red cells to adhere to fine structures of splenic red pulp and be removed from the circulation. At such low shear rates even normal red cells will adhere repeatedly but transiently: this is analogous to the repeated adsorptions of gas molecules which take place when a gas mixture flows through a gas chromatograph column. As a result, the mean red cell velocity through the reticular meshwork falls below that of plasma and, as a biophysical consequence, intrasplenic hematocrit rises above that of the inflowing blood.

Studies with isoproterenol have shown that the process of concentrating red cells in cat spleen is an active one involving smooth muscle endowed with β-adrenergic receptors (Greenway, 1979). Dilatation of splenic arterioles in response to isoproterenol (Reilly and McCuskey, 1977) would increase flow to the reticular meshwork, and thus increase the shear rates to which red cells in the meshwork are subjected. We hypothesize that as a result of these higher shear rates less adhesion of cells to fine structures of the meshwork would occur. This would raise the mean red cell velocity toward that of the plasma and, as Greenway found, reduce the hematocrit of blood in the meshwork toward that of arterial blood.

Blood 'doping' in athletes is a fairly recent innovation, but in some mammalian species the expulsion of high hematocrit intrasplenic blood, in order to raise the O_2 carrying capacity of peripheral blood, is an effective physiological mechanism. Spleens of such species as horse, dog, cat, and diving seal are very contractile and serve as a reservoir of blood at high hematocrit. In times of 'fight or flight', splenic contraction transfers blood from the reservoir into the circulation, and the splenic filtration function is put 'on hold', since all blood flows *via* the fast pathways in contracted spleens, until the organ relaxes again. In the human spleen this reservoir function appears to be lacking and the high intrasplenic hematocrit remains unexploited.

ACKNOWLEDGEMENTS

We thank Mrs Barbara Anderson for typing this manuscript. Our own research reported here was supported by a grant to A.C.G. from the Medical Research Council of Canada.

REFERENCES

Andrew, W. (1946) Age changes in the vascular architecture and cell content in the spleens of 100 Wistar Institute rats, including comparison with human material. *Am. J. Anat.*, **79**, 1–73.

Barcroft, J. and Florey, H. W. (1928) Some factors involved in the concentration of blood by the spleen. *J. Physiol., London*, **60**, 231–4.

Barcroft, J. and Poole, L. T. (1927) The blood in the spleen pulp. *J. Physiol., London*, **64**, 23–9.

Barnhart, M. I., Baechler, C. A. and Lusher, J. M. (1976) Arteriovenous shunts in the human spleen. *Am. J. Hematol.*, **1**, 105–14.

Barnhart, M. I. and Lusher, J. M. (1976) The human spleen as revealed by scanning electron microscopy. *Am. J. Hematol.*, **1**, 234–64.

Barnhart, M. I. and Lusher, J. M. (1979) Structural physiology of the human spleen. *Am. J. Pediatr. Hematol. Oncol.*, **1**, 311–30.

Bellanti, J. A. (1979) *Immunology: Basic Processes.* W. B. Saunders, Philadelphia.

Benbassat, J. (1969) Effect of packing and resuspension on the osmotic fragility and rate of autohaemolysis of incubated red blood cells. *Clin. Sci.*, **37**, 99–107.

Berendes, M. (1959) The proportions of reticulocytes in the erythrocytes of the spleen as compared with those of the circulating blood with special reference to the hemolytic states. *Blood*, **14**, 558–63.

Blue, J. and Weiss, L. (1981a) Periarterial macrophage sheaths (ellipsoids) in cat spleen: an electron microscope study. *Am. J. Anat.*, **161**, 115–34.

Blue, J. and Weiss, L. (1981b) Vascular pathways in nonsinusal red pulp: an electron microscope study of the cat spleen. *Am. J. Anat.*, **161**, 135–68.

Blue, J. and Weiss, L. (1981c) Species variation in the structure and function of the marginal zone: an electron microscope study of cat spleen. *Am. J. Anat.*, **161**, 169–87.

Blue, J. and Weiss, L. (1981d) Electron microscopy of the red pulp of the dog spleen including vascular arrangements, periarterial macrophage sheaths (ellipsoids), and the contractile, innervated reticular meshwork. *Am. J. Anat.*, **161**, 189–218.

Boisfleury, A. De and Mohandas, N. (1977) Antibody-induced spherocytic anemia. II. Splenic passage and sequestration of red cells. *Blood Cells*, **3**, 197–208.

Bowden, T. J. (1978) Storage and transit of red blood cells in skeletal muscle of the cat. PhD thesis. University of Western Ontario, London, Ontario.

Braunbeck, W., Hutten, H. and Vaupel, P. (1973) A contribution concerning the unsettled problem of intrasplenic microcirculation. *Adv. Exp. Med. Biol.*, **37A**, 389–94.

Chen, L. T. (1980) Intrasplenic microcirculation in rats with acute hemolytic anemia. *Blood*, **56**, 737–40.

Chen, L. T. and Weiss, L. (1973) The role of the sinus wall in the passage of erythrocytes through the spleen. *Blood*, **41**, 529–37.

Cho, Y. and DeBruyn, P. P. H. (1975) Passage of red blood cells through the sinusoidal wall of the spleen. *Am. J. Anat.*, **142**, 91–106.

Cilento, E. V. *et al.* (1980) Compartmental analysis of circulation of erythrocytes through the rat spleen. *Am. J. Physiol.*, **239** (*Heart Circ. Physiol.*, **8**), H272–H277.

Crosby, W. H. (1977) Splenic remodeling of red cell surfaces. *Blood*, **50**, 643–5.

Davies, B. N. and Withrington, P. G. (1973) The action of drugs on smooth muscle of the capsule and blood vessels of the spleen. *Pharmacol. Rev.*, **25**, 373–412.

Dintenfass, L. and Burnard, E. (1966) Effect of hydrogen ion concentration on *in vitro* viscosity of packed red cells and blood at high hematocrits. *Med. J. Aust.*, **1**, 1072–4.

Dornfest, B. S., Handler, E. S. and Handler, E. E. (1970) Sequestration of heat-injured erythrocytes in perfused spleens of acute myelogenous leukemic rats as a measure of reticuloendothelial system function. *Cancer Res.*, **30**, 665–73.

Dornfest, B. S., Handler, E. S. and Handler, E. E. (1971) Reticulocyte sequestration in spleens of normal, anaemic and leukaemic rats. *Br. J. Haematol.*, **21**, 83–94.

Drenckhahn, D. and Wagner, J. (1986) Stress fibers in the splenic sinus endothelium *in situ*: Molecular structure, relationship to the extracellular matrix and contractility. *J. Cell Biol.*, **102**, 1738–47.

Emerson, C. P. *et al.* (1956) Studies on the destruction of red blood cells. IX. Quantitative methods for determining the osmotic and mechanical fragility of red cells in the peripheral blood and splenic pulp; the mechanism of increased hemolysis in hereditary spherocytosis (congenital hemolytic jaundice) as related to the function of the spleen. *Arch. Intern. Med.*, **97**, 1–38.

Fujita, T. (1974) A scanning electron microscopy study of the human spleen. *Arch. Histol. Jpn*, **37**, 187–216.

Fujita, T. and Kashimura, M. (1983) Scanning electron microscope studies of human spleen. *Surv. Immunol. Res.*, **2**, 375–84.

Fujita, T., Kashimura, M. and Adachi, K. (1985) Scanning electron microscopy and terminal circulation. *Experientia*, **41**, 167–79.

Ganzoni, A., Hillman, R. S. and Finch, C. A. (1969) Maturation of the macroreticulocyte. *Br. J. Haematol.*, **16**, 119–35.

Goresky, C. A. and Groom, A. C. (1984) Microcirculatory events in the liver and spleen. in *Handbook of Physiology*, Section 2, *The Cardiovascular System*, Vol. IV, *Microcirculation*, Part 2, pp. 689–780. American Physiological Society, Washington, DC.

Greenway, C. V. (1979) Splenic erythrocyte concentration mechanism and its inhibition by isoproterenol. *Am. J. Physiol.*, **236**, (*Heart Circ. Physiol.*, **5**), H238–H243.

Griggs, R. C., Weisman, R., Jr and Harris, J. W. (1960) Alteration in osmotic and mechanical fragility related to *in vivo* erythrocyte aging and splenic sequestration in hereditary spherocytosis. *J. Clin. Invest.*, **39**, 89–101.

Groom, A. C. (1980) Microvascular transit of normal, immature, and altered red blood cells in spleen versus skeletal muscle. in *Erythrocyte Mechanics and Blood Flow* (eds G. R. Cokelet, H. J. Meiselman and D. E. Brooks), Liss, New York, pp. 229–59.

Groom, A. C. (1987) *The Microcirculatory Society Eugene M. Landis Award Lecture*. Microcirculation of the spleen: new concepts, new challenges. *Microvasc. Res.*, **34**, 269–89.

Groom, A. C., Levesque, M. J. and Bruckschweiger, D. (1977) Flow stasis, blood gases and glucose levels in the red pulp of the spleen. *Adv. Exp. Med. Biol.*, **94**, 567–72.

Groom, A. C. and Song, S. H. (1971) Effects of norepinephrine on washout of red cells from the spleen. *Am. J. Physiol.*, **221**, 255–8.

Groom, A. C., Song, S. H. and Campling, B. (1973) Clearance of red blood cells from the vascular bed of skeletal muscle with particular reference to reticulocytes. *Microvasc. Res.*, **6**, 51–62.

Groom, A. C. et al. (1971) Physical characteristics of red cells collected from the spleen. *Can. J. Physiol. Pharmacol.*, **49**, 1092–9.

Groom, A. C. et al. (1985) Does an unfavorable environment for red cells develop within the cat spleen when abnormal cells become trapped? *J. Lab. Clin. Med.*, **105**, 209–13.

Hataba, Y., Kirino Y. and Suzuki, T. (1981) Scanning electron microscopic study of the red pulp of mouse spleen. *J. Electron Microsc.*, **30**, 46–56.

Helly, K. (1902) Zum Nachweise des geschlossenen Gefässsystem der Milz. *Arch. Mikrosk. Anat. Entwicklungsmech.*, **59**, 93–105.

Holzbach, R. T. et al. (1964) Influence of spleen size and portal pressure on erythrocyte sequestration. *J. Clin. Invest.*, **43**, 1125–35.

Irino, S., Murakami, T. and Fujita, T. (1977) Open circulation in the human spleen. Dissection scanning electron microscopy of conductive stained tissue and observation of resin vascular casts. *Arch. Histol. Jpn.*, **40**, 297–304.

Jacob, H. S. and Jandl, J. H. (1962) Effects of sulfhydryl inhibition on red blood cells. II. Studies *in vivo*. *J. Clin. Invest.*, **41**, 1514–23.

Janicik, J. M. et al. (1978) Sequestration of neuraminidase-treated erythrocytes. Studies on its topographic, morphologic and immunologic aspects. *Cell. Tiss. Res.*, **186**, 209–26.

Jandl, J. H. (1960) The agglutination and sequestration of immature red cells. *J. Lab. Clin. Med.*, **55**, 663–81.

Kay, M. M. B. et al. (1982) Antigenicity, storage and aging: physiologic autoantibodies to cell membrane and serum proteins and the senescent cell antigen. *Mol. Cell. Biochem.*, **49**, 65–85.

Kimber, R. J. and Lander, H. (1964) The effect of heat on human red cell morphology, fragility, and subsequent survival *in vivo*. *J. Lab. Clin. Med.*, **64**, 922–33.

Klausner, M. A. et al. (1975) Contrasting splenic mechanisms in the blood clearance of red blood cells and colloidal particles. *Blood*. **46**, 965–76.

Knisely, M. H. (1936) Spleen studies. I. Microscopic observations of the circulatory system of living, unstimulated mammalian spleens. *Anat. Rec.*, **65**, 23–50.

Koyama, S., Aoki, S. and Deguchi, K. (1964) Electron microscopic observations of the splenic red pulp with special reference to the pitting function. *Mie Med. J.*, **14**, 143–88.

Kramer, K. and Luft, U. C. (1951) Mobilization of red cells and oxygen from the spleen in severe hypoxia. *Am. J. Physiol.*, **165**, 215–28.

LaCelle, P. L. (1970) Alteration of membrane deformability in hemolytic anemias. *Semin. Hematol.*, **7**, 355–71.

Leblond, P. F. (1973) Etude, au microscope électronique à balayage, de la migration des cellules sanguines à travers les parois des sinusoides spléniques et médullaires chez le rat. *Nouv. Rev. Fr. Hématol.*, **13**, 771–88.

Levesque, M. J. and Groom, A. C. (1976a) Washout kinetics of red cells and plasma from the spleen. *Am. J. Physiol.*, **231**, 1665–71.

Levesque, M. J. and Groom, A. C. (1976b) pH environment of red cells in the spleen. *Am. J. Physiol.*, **231**, 1672–8.

Levesque, M. J. and Groom, A. C. (1977) Sequestration of heat-treated autologous red cells in the spleen. *J. Lab. Clin. Med.*, **90**, 666–79.

Levesque, M. J. and Groom, A. C. (1980a) A comparative study of the sequestration of 'abnormal' red cells by the spleen. *Can. J. Physiol. Pharmacol.*, **58**, 1317–25.

Levesque, M. J. and Groom, A. C. (1980b) Blood flow distribution within the spleen distended by perfusion at high venous pressure. *J. Lab. Clin. Med.*, **96**, 606-15.

Lewis, O. J. (1957) The blood vessels of the adult mammalian spleen. *J. Anat.*, **91**, 245–50.

Lübbers, D. W. et al. (1979) Contractile properties of frog capillaries tested by electrical stimulation. *Bibl. Anat.*, **17**, 3–l0.

MacDonald, I. C. et al. (1987) Kinetics of red blood cell passage through interendothelial slits into venous sinuses in rat spleen, analyzed by *in vivo* microscopy. *Microvasc. Res.*, **33**, 118–34.

MacKenzie, D. W., Whipple, A. O. and Wintersteiner, M. P. (1941) Studies on the microscopic anatomy and physiology of living transilluminated mammalian spleen. *Am. J. Anat.*, **68**, 397–456.

Matsumoto, N. et al. (1977) An ultrastructural study of the red pulp of the spleen and the liver in unstable hemoglobin hemolytic anemia. *Virchows Arch. Pathol. Anat. Histol.*, **374**, 339–51.

McCuskey, R. S. and McCuskey, P. A. (1977) *In vivo* microscopy of the spleen. *Bibl. Anat.*, **16**, 121–5.

Miescher, P. (1957) The role of the reticuloendothelial system in haematoclasia. in *Physiology of the Reticuloendothelial System*. Blackwell, Oxford, pp. 147–71.

Miyamoto, H., Seguchi, H. and Ogawa, K. (1980) Electron microscope studies of the Schweigger-Seidel sheath in hen spleen with special reference to the existence of a 'closed' microcirculation. *J. Electron Microsc.*, **29**, 158–72.

Mollison, P. L. (1962) The reticulo-endothelial system and red cell destruction. *Proc. Roy. Soc. Med.*, **55**, 915–20.

Motulsky, A. G. *et al.* (1958) Anemia and the spleen. *N. Engl. J. Med.*, **259**, 1164–9.

Murphy, J. R. (1967) The influence of pH and temperature on some physical properties of normal erythrocytes and erythrocytes from patients with hereditary spherocytosis. *J. Lab. Clin. Med.*, **69**, 758–75.

Murphy, J. R. (1969) Erythrocyte osmotic fragility and cell water: influence of pH and temperature. *J. Lab. Clin. Med.*, **74**, 319–24.

Nopanitaya, W., Aghajanian, J. G. and Gray, L. D. (1979) An improved plastic mixture for corrosion casting of the gastrointestinal microvascular system. in *Scanning Electron Microscopy, Part III.* (eds R. P. Becker and O. Johari), SEM, Inc., Illinois. pp. 751–5.

Olah, I. and Glick, B. (1982) Splenic white pulp and associated vascular channels in chicken spleen. *Am. J. Anat.*, **165**, 445–80.

Opdyke, D. F. and Apostolico, R. (1966) Splenic contraction and optical density of blood. *Am. J. Physiol.*, **211**, 329–34.

Pearson, H. A., Spencer, R. P. and Cornelius, E. A. (1969) Functional asplenia in sickle-cell anemia. *N. Engl J. Med.*, **281**, 923–6.

Peters, A. M. (1983) Splenic blood flow and blood cell kinetics. *Clin. Haematol.*, **12**, 421–47.

Pictet, C. L. *et al.* (1969) An electron microscopic study of the perfusion-fixed spleen. II. Nurse cells and erythrophagocytosis. *Z. Zellforsch. Mikrosk. Anat.*, **96**, 400–17.

Piomelli, S., Lurinsky, G. and Wasserman, L. R. (1967) The mechanism of red cell aging. I. Relationship between cell age and specific gravity evaluated by ultracentrifugation in a discontinuous density gradient. *J. Lab. Clin. Med.*, **69**, 659–74.

Prankerd, T. A. J. (1960) Studies on the pathogenesis of haemolysis in hereditary spherocytosis. *Q. J. Med.*, **29**, 199–208.

Prankerd, T. A. J. (1963), The spleen and anaemia. *Br. Med. J.*, **2**, 517–24.

Ragan, D. M. S. *et al.* (1988) Spontaneous cyclic contractions of the capillary wall *in vivo*, impeding red cell flow: a quantitative analysis. Evidence for endothelial contractility. *Microvasc. Res.*, **36**, 13–30.

Reilly, F. D. and McCuskey, R. S. (1977) Studies of the hemopoietic microenvironment. VI. Regulatory mechanisms in the splenic microvascular system of mice. *Microvasc. Res.*, **13**, 79–90.

Rhodin, J. A. G. (1974) Spleen. in *Histology: A Text and Atlas.* Oxford University Press, New York. Chapter 18, pp. 399–415.

Rifkind, R. A. (1966) Destruction of injured red cells *in vivo. Am. J. Med.*, **41**, 711–23.

Sandberg, G. (1972) Splenic blood flow in the guinea pig measured with ^{133}Xe and calculation of the venous output of lymphocytes from the spleen. *Acta Physiol. Scand.*, **84**, 208-16.

Schmidt, E. E., MacDonald, I. C. and Groom, A. C. (1982) Direct arteriovenous connections and the intermediate circulation in dog spleen, studied by scanning electron microscopy of microcorrosion casts. *Cell Tissue Res.*, **225**, 543–55.

Schmidt, E. E., MacDonald, I. C. and Groom, A. C. (1983a) Circulatory pathways in the sinusal spleen of the dog, studied by scanning electron microscopy of microcorrosion casts. *J. Morphol.*, **178**, 111–23.

Schmidt, E. E., MacDonald, I. C. and Groom, A. C. (1983b) The intermediate circulation in the nonsinusal spleen of the cat, studied by scanning electron microscopy of microcorrosion casts. *J. Morphol.*, **178**, 125–38.

Schmidt, E. E., MacDonald, I. C. and Groom, A. C. (1983c) Luminal morphology of small arterial vessels in the contracted spleen, studied by scanning electron microscopy of microcorrosion casts. *Cell Tissue Res.*, **228**, 33–41.

Schmidt, E. E., MacDonald, I. C. and Groom, A. C. (1985a), Microcirculation in rat spleen (sinusal), studied by means of corrosion casts, with particular reference to intermediate pathways. *J. Morphol.*, **186**, 1–16.

Schmidt, E. E., MacDonald, I. C. and Groom, A. C. (1985b) Microcirculation in mouse spleen (nonsinusal) studied by means of corrosion casts. *J. Morphol.*, **186**, 17–29.

Schmidt, E. E., MacDonald, I. C. and Groom, A. C. (1988) Microcirculatory pathways in normal human spleen, demonstrated by scanning electron microscopy of corrosion casts. *Am. J. Anat.*, **181**, 253-66.

Schnitzer, B. *et al.* (1973) An ultrastructural study of the red pulp of the spleen in malaria. *Blood*, **41**, 207–18.

Simon, G. T. and Burke, J. S. (1970) Electron microscopy of the spleen. III. Erythroleukophagocytosis. *Am. J. Pathol.*, **58**, 451–69.

Skutelsky, E. and Danon, D. (1970a) Electron microscopical analysis of surface charge labeled density at various stages of the erythroid line. *J. Membr. Biol.*, **2**, 173–9.

Skutelsky, E. and Danon, D. (1970b) Reduction in surface charge as an explanation of the recognition by macrophages of nuclei expelled from normoblasts. *J. Cell Biol.*, **43**, 8–15.

Snook, T. (1950) A comparative study of the vascular arrangements in mammalian spleens. *Am. J. Anat.*, **87**, 31–61.

Snook, T. (1964) Studies of the perifollicular region of the rat's spleen. *Anat. Rec.*, **148**, 149–59.

Snook, T. (1975) The origin of the follicular capillaries in the human spleen. *Am. J. Anat.*, **144**, 113–17.

Song, S. H. (1972) A study of splenic functions with respect to red blood cells. PhD Thesis, University of Western Ontario, London, Ontario.

Song, S. H. and Groom, A. C. (1971a) Storage of blood cells in spleen of the cat. *Am. J. Physiol.*, **220**, 779–84.

Song, S. H. and Groom, A. C. (1971b) The distribution of red cells in the spleen. *Can. J. Physiol. Pharmacol.*, **49**, 734–43.

Song, S. H. and Groom, A. C. (1971c) Immature and abnormal erythrocytes present in the normal, healthy spleen. *Scand. J. Haematol.*, **8**, 487–93.

Song, S. H. and Groom, A. C. (1972) Sequestration and possible maturation of reticulocytes in the normal spleen. *Can. J. Physiol. Pharmacol.*, **50**, 400–6.

Song, S. H. and Groom, A. C. (1974) Scanning electron microscope study of the splenic red pulp in relation to the sequestration of immature and abnormal red cells. *J. Morphol.*, **144**, 439–452.

Sorbie, J. and Valberg, L. S. (1970) Splenic sequestration of stress erythrocytes in the rabbit. *Am. J. Physiol.*, **218**, 647–53.

Stock, R. J. *et al.* (1983) A compartmental analysis of the splenic circulation in rat. *Am. J. Physiol.*, **245** (*Heart Circ. Physiol.*, **14**), H17–H21.

Suzuki, T. *et al.* (1977) Stereoscopic scanning electron microscopy of the red pulp of dog spleen with special reference to the terminal structure of cordal capillaries. *Cell Tissue Res.*, **182**, 441–53.

Suzuki, T. *et al.* (1978) Three dimensional fine structure of the capillary terminals in the red pulp of the human spleen. in *Electron Microscopy 1978. Ninth International Congress on Electron Microscopy* (Vol. II) (ed. J. M. Sturgess), Toronto: Microscopical Soc. Canada, pp. 468–9.

Tischendorf, F. (1969) Die Milz. in *Handbuch der mikroscopischen Anatomie des Menschen. Band VI, Blutgefäss- und Lymphgefässapparat, innersekretorische Drüsen*, (eds W. Möllendorff and W. Bargmann), Springer Verlag, Berlin, pp. 572–612.

Tischendorf, F. (1985) On the evolution of the spleen. *Experientia*, **41**, 145–52.

Ultmann, J. E. and Gordon, C. S. (1965) The removal of *in vitro* damaged erythrocytes from the circulation of normal and splenectomized rats. *Blood*, **26**, 49–62.

Van Krieken, J. H. J. M. *et al.* (1985a) The splenic red pulp; a histomorphometrical study in splenectomy specimens embedded in methylmethacrylate. *Histopathology*, **9**, 401–16.

Van Krieken, J. H. J. M. *et al.* (1985b) The human spleen; a histological study in splenectomy specimens embedded in methylmethacrylate. *Histopathology*, **9**, 571–85.

Vaupel, P., Ruppert, H. and Hutten, H. (1977) Splenic blood flow and intrasplenic flow distribution in rats. *Pflügers Arch.*, **369**, 193–201.

Wade, L., Jr (1973) Splenic sequestration of young erythrocytes in sheep. *Am. J. Physiol.*, **224**, 265–7.

Wagner, H. N., Jr *et al.* (1962) Removal of erythrocytes from the circulation. *Arch. Intern. Med.*, **110**, 90–7.

Weed, R. I. (1970) The importance of erythrocyte deformability. *Am. J. Med.*, **49**, 147–50.

Weidenreich, F. (1901) Das Gefässystem der menschlichen Milz. *Arch. Mikrosk. Anat. Entwicklungsmech.*, **58**, 247–376.

Weigelt, H. (1982) Die spezialisierte Endothelzelle: erregbare Zelle und mechanischer Effektor der Mikrozirkulation. *Funkt. Biol. Med.*, **1**, 53–60.

Weisman, R. *et al.* (1955) Studies on the role of the spleen in the destruction of erythrocytes. *Trans. Assoc. Am. Physicians*, **68**, 131–40.

Weiss, L. (1962) The structure of fine splenic arterial vessels in relation to hemoconcentration and red cell destruction. *Am. J. Anat.*, **111**, 131–79.

Weiss, L. (1974) A scanning electron microscopic study of the spleen. *Blood*, **43**, 665–91.

Weiss, L., Powell, R. and Schiffman, F. J. (1985) Terminating arterial vessels in red pulp of human spleen: a transmission electron microscopic study. *Experientia*, **41**, 233–42.

Weiss, L. and Tavassoli, M. (1970) Anatomical hazards to the passage of erythrocytes through the spleen. *Semin. Hematol.*, **7**, 372–80.

Wennberg, E. and Weiss, L. (1969) The structure of the spleen and hemolysis. *Ann. Rev. Med.*, **20**, 29–40.

Yamamoto, K. *et al.* (1979) Scanning electron microscopy of the perimarginal cavernous sinus plexus of the human spleen. in *Scanning Electron Microscopy (Part III)*. (eds R. P. Becker and O. Johari), SEM Inc., AMF O'Hare, Illinois, pp. 763–8.

Zetterstrom, B. E. M. (1973) Evaluation of the [133]Xenon clearance method for measurement of blood flow in the dog spleen. *Acta Chir. Scand.*, **139**, 27–33.

THE IMMUNE FUNCTIONS OF THE SPLEEN

William C. Kopp

5.1 INTRODUCTION

The spleen plays a unique role in the clearance of particulate antigens, including pathogenic bacteria, from the peripheral blood. It provides an environment where blood slowly circulates through the cordal channels lined by large numbers of phagocytic cells. Second, the spleen is a true lymphoid organ which contains organized lymphoid compartments. The lymphoid organization of the spleen provides sites for the interaction of immunocompetent cells with antigen, and with each other, to generate effector cells and molecules. Until recently, the importance of the spleen to the integrity of the immune system was underestimated: the anatomical location of the spleen in the circulatory system, and its structural organization, provide a critical opportunity for contact with blood-borne antigens and for participation in the system of circulating lymphocytes. It has been calculated that the traffic of lymphoid cells through the spleen exceeds the combined cell traffic through all the lymph nodes, with a daily exchange rate of about 5×10^{11} lymphocytes (Pabst, 1988).

The predisposition of splenectomized infants to severe and often fatal infections with encapsulated bacteria was first reported by King and Schumaker (1952), and provided the first real evidence that the spleen is important to the maintenance of immunological integrity (see also Chapter 12). Knowledge of the immune functions of the spleen has since expanded greatly: numerous studies, some requiring highly innovative experimental designs, have demonstrated the complexity of the traffic of both lymphoid cells and antigen through the spleen. Furthermore, much has been learnt from immunological studies which utilize the spleen as a convenient source of lymphoid cells for *in vitro* assays of immune cell functions. In some respects, it has proved difficult to relate the results of *in vitro* studies to events which occur within the structurally diverse lymphoid elements of the intact spleen. However, the phenotypic characteristics of subpopulations of cells within the lymphoid compartments of the spleen and other lymphoid organs are now being documented with an expanding array of monoclonal antibodies. These studies have begun to determine anatomically where observed *in vitro* effector functions occur within the intact organ.

It is now clear that the spleen has numerous roles as an immunological organ. The spleen is one of the principal sites of clearance of damaged and effete cells from the blood. It is also involved in the removal of circulating antibody-coated cells generated during autoimmune responses, which may give it a critical role in autoimmune hemolytic disease (Bowdler, 1976). The spleen, together with the liver, is an important site of the fixed macrophages which remove particulate antigens from the blood. The role of the spleen relative to the liver in the clearance of particulates is increased in the absence of opsonins. The spleen appears to have a special role in the elimination of polysaccharide encapsulated bacterial species. It is also an important source of antibody synthesis, particularly of antibody of the IgM class, and in the development of effector T lymphocytes.

The focus of this chapter will be to provide an overview of the spleen as an immunological organ. This will require a discussion of the location of cellular components involved in the generation of immune reactions, how cells travel through the spleen, and where opportunities exist for the cell–antigen and cell–cell contacts essential for development and regulation of immune responses. The discussion will also concern the immunological consequences of splenectomy. Lastly, the role of the spleen in the generation of the immunomodulatory molecule tuftsin will be addressed.

5.2 THE IMMUNOLOGICAL COMPARTMENTS OF THE SPLEEN

5.2.1 OVERVIEW

The spleen can be divided anatomically into three major compartments: the red pulp (RP), the marginal zone (MZ) and the white pulp (WP). These regions are described in greater detail in Chapters 2 and 3. The WP can be further subdivided into the periarteriolar lymphatic sheath (PALS) and the peripheral white pulp which is composed of primary and secondary lymphoid follicles (LF). Each of these anatomically defined regions is involved differently in the immunological functions of the spleen. While the splenic WP shares many characteristics with other lymphoid tissues such as the lymph nodes, structural differences exist which affect the pathways of lymphocyte traffic through the various organs. The spleen lacks the afferent lymphatics which bring both antigen and significant numbers of cells into lymph nodes. In addition, lymph nodes have a specialized high endothelium in the postcapillary venules. These cells possess specific lymphocyte homing receptors to recruit recirculating lym-

phocytes from the peripheral blood (Gowans and Knight, 1964; Woodruff, Clarke and Chin, 1987). High endothelial venules are not present in the spleen, and both cells and antigen enter the parenchyma through interendothelial pores in arterioles and at the arteriolar terminations. Lymphocytes leave lymph nodes through efferent lymphatics: while the spleen also possesses efferent lymphatics, a significant proportion of the lymphoid cells leaving the spleen do so through the venous system.

5.2.2 THE MARGINAL ZONE (MZ)

The MZ marks the anatomical demarcation between WP and RP. Morphometric studies have shown that the MZ compartment of the rat spleen is physically the largest lymphoid zone, and is larger than either the PALS or the LF (Kumararatne, Bazin and MacLennan, 1981). This study showed that although the MZ has a lower cell density than white pulp, the total cellularity of MZ is slightly higher than that of the PALS and is 2.6 times that of the follicles. It is within the MZ that much of the arterial circulation terminates, and this results in a high rate of blood flow into this zone. Studies in experimental animals have shown that the injection of radiolabelled T- and B-cells obtained from thoracic duct lymph leads to initial splenic localization of both cell types in the MZ (Nieuwenhuis and Ford, 1976; Sprent, 1973). This localization is rapid and occurs within 15 minutes of the intravenous injection of labeled cells. Small numbers of typical monocytes and macrophages, presumably derived from peripheral blood, are also found in the MZ (Dijkstra et al., 1985; van Vliet, Melis and van Ewijk, 1985; Hsu, Cossman and Jaffe, 1983). Antigen can be expected to follow this same route to localize in the MZ, and this has been confirmed with both particulate and soluble antigens (Nossal et al., 1966; Mitchell and Abbot, 1971).

The MZ provides an environment with a high potential for promoting the interaction of antigen with cells of the lymphocytic and monocytic lines. In addition, it provides a compartment in which, for periods of at least several hours, the cellular constituents required for the initiation of immune responses are located together. The MZ may serve as a site for the initiation of immune responses where immunomodulatory signals can be generated and transferred between cells of different lineages. Antigen activated B- and T-lymphocytes may then travel to their respective compartments within the white pulp to continue the processes of proliferation and differentiation which lead eventually to the production of effector cell populations.

The influx of circulating cells into the MZ accounts for only part of the lymphoid cells present within this compartment. A population of resident lymphocytes is also found in the MZ. The lymphoid population of the MZ is intact in congenitally athymic nude rodents (Kumararatne, Bazin and MacLennan, 1981; Waksman, Arnason and Jankovic', 1962) and neonatally thymectomized animals (Eikelenboom et al., 1979). The major lymphoid cell population in the MZ has been demonstrated by immunohistochemistry to possess surface immunoglobulin, as well as receptors for both the Fc fragment of immunoglobulin and the C3b (CR1) and C3d (CR2) components of complement (Kumararatne, Bazin and MacLennan, 1981; Gray et al., 1984a). They also express surface Class II MHC proteins and low numbers of receptors for interleukin-2 (IL2 or CD25). Histochemically these lymphocytes have alkaline phosphatase activity (Hsu, 1985). Staining with B lineage-specific monoclonal antibodies such as B1 has established that the resident lymphocyte population in the MZ is composed of B-cells (MacLennan et al., 1982).

Further characterization of the MZ B-cell population has been obtained through studies of mice treated with anti-immunoglobulin antibodies from birth (Kumararatne and MacLennan, 1981; Bazin et al., 1982). The MZ does not become populated with lymphocytes in mice treated from birth with anti-mu, while anti-delta chain specific antibody treatment has no effect on development. This is consistent with the observation that resident MZ B-cells express surface IgM, but are surface IgD negative (MacLennan et al., 1982; Murray, Swerdlow and Habeshaw, 1984; van den Oord et al., 1985). Treatment of rats with 400 mg/m^2 cyclophosphamide results in selective depletion of MZ B-cells (Kumararatne and MacLennan, 1981). B-cell depleted rats have been used to study reconstitution of the MZ. Reconstitution has been obtained with thoracic duct lymphocytes passaged through an irradiated intermediate host. These results suggest that the B-cells which repopulate the MZ are derived from a 'virgin' population of cells which has undergone a considerable period of maturation as recirculating cells before finally localizing in the MZ (Kumararatne and MacLennan, 1981; MacLennan et al., 1982). The MZ does not appear to be a site for B-cell proliferation. The MZ does not label with ^{3}H-thymidine after a five day continuous infusion which would detect proliferating cells (Kumararatne and MacLennan, 1981).

Although resident MZ B-cells are derived from recirculating precursors, evidence indicates that they themselves do not recirculate. Depletion of recirculating lymphocytes by chronic drainage of thoracic duct lymph results in shrinkage of the white pulp while the MZ remains intact. The same result has also been obtained following experimental hemisplenic beta-irradiation (Kumararatne, Bazin and MacLennan, 1981). In this procedure one-half of the spleen of a mouse is exposed to a continuous ^{32}P source of beta-irradiation at short range, while the other half of the organ remains unirradiated. As cells circulate through the ^{32}P-exposed half of the spleen they are lethally irradiated, thereby eliminating any circulating or recirculating lymphocytes. Although the MZ is generally regarded as a region unique to the spleen, van den Oord, de Wolf-Peters and Desmet (1986) reported that immunohistological comparison of spleen and reactive lymph nodes showed the presence of cells within lymph nodes which are phenotypically similar to the cells within the MZ. These cells were found scattered in the lymphocyte corona or forming a peripheral rim around secondary lymphoid follicles.

The marginal zone contains small numbers of phagocytic cells which possess surface markers identifying them as typical peripheral blood monocytes. A second population of non-lymphoid cells has been identified in the MZ of the mouse through reactivity with a monoclonal antibody designated ER-TR9 (Dijkstra *et al.*, 1985; van Vliet, Melis and van Ewijk, 1985). These cells are found in close association with MZ B-cells but, unlike classical antigen-presenting cells, these cells do not express surface Class II MHC proteins (Humphrey and Grennan, 1981; Dijkstra *et al.*, 1985). They constitute a unique population of cells which has been shown to take up neutral polysaccharides selectively (Humphrey and Grennan, 1981). Approximately 80% of these cells have Fc and complement receptors. Isolated neutral polysaccharide-ingesting cells are adherent and phagocytic *in vitro*. During isolation these cells are found associated with adherent B-lymphocytes.

It is not yet clear what role the resident MZ polysaccharide-binding cells and resident B-cells play in the immune response to antigens, especially polysaccharides. The MZ may play a critical role in generating immune responses to polysaccharide encapsulated bacteria. B-cells in the MZ do not appear to be a totally static population. Injection of bacterial endotoxin results in the disappearance of B-cells from the marginal zone, presumably by initiating migration out of the MZ (Gray *et al.*, 1984b). It has been proposed that after activation MZ B-cells may migrate to other regions of the spleen to undergo maturation and differentiation (Mac-Lennan *et al.*, 1982). The polysaccharide-ingesting cells of the MZ may be important to the immune response by providing a splenic reservoir of antigen which is maintained within the spleen in close proximity to B-cells, and which persists long after circulating antigen has been cleared. The immune response to polysaccharide antigens also differs from the response to most other antigens. These antigens comprise a group of antigens known as T-independent antigens, which are capable of generating antibody responses with little or no T-cell help. However, T-cells do regulate the amplitude and immunoglobulin class of the antibodies produced. The antibodies produced in response to T-independent antigens are predominantly of the IgM class.

5.2.3   THE WHITE PULP

(a)   Periarteriolar lymphatic sheath (PALS)

The PALS is the T-lymphocyte compartment of the splenic white pulp. It is deficient in nude mice and in neonatally thymectomized animals, demonstrating that its development is dependent on a functional thymus (Sprent, 1973). The PALS compartment is composed principally of recirculating cells. Elimination of recirculating lymphocytes by cannulation of the thoracic duct for as little as 24 hours results in significant loss of small lymphocytes from the PALS (Sprent, 1973). When normal thoracic duct lymphocytes, which are mainly T-cells, are radiolabeled and injected into syngeneic recipients they localize initially to the MZ, and within several hours can be observed to enter the PALS selectively (Nieuwenhuis and Ford, 1976; Sprent, 1973). Time-course studies show that 24 hours after injection less label is detected in PALS than is detected at an earlier period. This suggests that the cell population which passes through the PALS has a rather brief transit time unless antigen-induced changes in the traffic pattern occur (Sprent, 1973). In the human spleen T-cells predominate in PALS, as shown by the ability of these cells to form E rosettes with sheep red blood cells (Christensen *et al.*, 1978), and by immunohistochemical reactivity with monoclonal antibodies specific for T-cells (Grogan, Jolley and Rangel, 1983; Hsu, Cossman and Jaffe, 1983; Timens and Poppema, 1985). The observation of T-cell mitosis within PALS indicates that this compartment is a site of T-cell clonal expansion (Grogan, Jolley and Rangel, 1983). The distribution of the CD4 and CD8 T-cell subsets in PALS is similar to that in normal peripheral blood with an approximate ratio of 2:1 (Hsu, Cossman and Jaffe, 1983). In the normal spleen only a small percentage of T-cells within the PALS express IL-2 receptors indicative of an activated state (Timens and Poppema, 1985).

The PALS contains a non-lymphoid cell type which is found in close association with T-cells. These cells have been designated interdigitating reticulum cells (IDC) and are mononuclear cells which have numerous branching projections. The IDC are characterized by their intense expression of Class II MHC molecules* (Dijkstra, 1982; Stein *et al.*, 1980). By histological methods Dijkstra (1982) recognized two subsets of rat IDC, based on the presence or absence of acid phosphatase activity. Only those IDC which had acid phosphatase activity were phagocytic as determined by their ability to ingest colloidal carbon. These Class II MHC-positive cells serve as a readily available source of antigen-presenting cells for T-cells during their transit through the PALS.

(b)   Lymphoid follicles (LF)

The LF of the spleen are similar in structure to those in other lymphoid organs and can be differentiated into two distinct types, primary and secondary. The primary follicle consists of an homogeneous aggregate of small B-cells while the structure of the secondary follicle is more complex. Secondary follicles consist of a germinal center of large cells surrounded by a mantle of small B-lymphocytes. The surface phenotype of the small cells in the primary follicle and mantle zone is similar, with these cells expressing surface IgM and IgD, Class II MHC (HLA-DR) and BA-1 (Hsu and Jaffe, 1984a, 1984b; Murray, Swerdlow and Habeshaw, 1984). The majority of these cells are also weakly positive for the B-cell markers B1 and B2 and they also have 5'-nucleotidase

*MHC: Major histocompatibility complex. Each Class II molecule consists of two polymorphic peptides, and these are present on a variety of antigen presenting cells (ed.).

activity (Murray, Swerdlow and Habeshaw, 1984). Cells within the mantle zone are thought to be primarily resting cells which are part of the recirculating lymphocyte population. Depletion of recirculating B-cells by chronic thoracic duct drainage or hemi-splenic beta-irradiation results in depletion of mantle zone cells (Kumararatne, Bazin and MacLennan, 1981). The transit time of B-cells through the normal splenic white pulp appears to be significantly longer than the transit time of T-cells.

The germinal center develops following antigenic stimulation and consists mainly of large, proliferating lymphocytes which are CD20-positive, identifying them as B-cells. They also express surface antigens which identify them as activated B-cells (Hsu, Cossman and Jaffe, 1983; Hsu and Jaffe, 1984b). Cells within the germinal center do express surface immunoglobulin but generally not of the IgD isotype (Timens and Poppema, 1985). Germinal centers undergo discrete stages of maturation and during this process distinguishable light and dark zones of cells appear, which may express different immunoglobulin isotypes (Hsu and Jaffe, 1984b). Germinal center cells in humans bind the lectin peanut agglutinin (PNA) and possess receptors for Fc and C3b. B-cells within germinal centers are not part of the recirculating lymphocyte population. They do not express the surface molecules which allow them to attach to the high endothelium of post-capillary venules. Germinal centers provide a site for rapid proliferation of B-cells where they also undergo isotype switching and affinity maturation. As the germinal center becomes mature cell division stops and the cells differentiate into memory cells or plasma cells, which again acquire the ability to migrate out of the germinal center (Kraal, Weissman and Butcher, 1982; Heinen, Cormann and Kinet-Denoel, 1988).

T-lymphocytes comprise a small minority of the cells found within germinal centers, and are mainly found in the light zone (Stein *et al.*, 1980). They are principally of the CD4 helper/inducer phenotype but differ from typical helper/inducer cells found in PALS. They express the NK cell associated antigen Leu-7 and do not produce IL-2 in response to challenge with anti-CD3 or the lectin phytohemagglutinin (Hsu and Jaffe, 1984b; Velardi *et al.*, 1986). The role of these T-cells in the immune response remains uncertain.

Within lymphoid follicles are found non-lymphoid cell populations which are unique to that splenic compartment. Tingible body macrophages are found in the germinal center. These macrophages do not take up antigen but do actively phagocytose lymphoid cells. Their role may be to eliminate defective lymphoid cells and debris in the germinal center. Small numbers of typical phagocytic macrophages are also present in the germinal center. A third cell population found in the lymphoid follicle is the follicular dendritic cell (FDC). These constitute approximately 2% of germinal center cells and form a network around the lymphocytes. The origin of FDC is not clear but they appear to differentiate from reticular cells. These cells have Fc receptors which allow them to bind immune complexes. They are able to maintain immune complexes on their cell surface for long periods in the absence of phagocytic uptake. They do not bind uncomplexed antigen and are therefore not important in the early stages of a primary B-cell response to antigen. Van Rooijen and Kors (1985) have shown that during a primary response the antibody produced may complex with free antigen in the local environment. The antigen–antibody complexes produced deposit on FDC which are adjacent to secreting B-cells. The FDC appear to play some role in down-regulating the production of plasma cells. It has been proposed that complex deposition in the vicinity of antibody-producing cells may favor differentiation to memory cells of corresponding antigen specificity.

5.2.4   THE RED PULP

Immunohistochemical staining of splenic tissue has shown that the RP is rich in macrophages. Van Furth and Diesselhoff-den Dulk (1984) have shown that murine splenic macrophages are derived both from circulating monocytes and by local production. The relevance of this finding to the human spleen is difficult to assess because local production in the murine system may result from maturation of dividing precursors, since the adult rodent spleen remains a hematopoietic organ. Fc and C3 receptors are found on red pulp macrophages (Christensen *et al.*, 1978). The presence of surface Class II MHC antigens also makes them capable of serving as antigen presenting cells. The red pulp macrophages of the mouse can be differentiated from macrophages in the white pulp by their expression of the F4/80 antigen. A red pulp macrophage isolation procedure has been described by Nusrat *et al.* (1988). Isolated cells were adherent, and shared a characteristic with Kupffer cells of the liver in that they had little if any capacity to synthesize lipoxygenase pathway products and released only low quantities of reactive oxygen intermediates. Isolated splenic macrophages had higher Class II MHC antigen expression than peritoneal macrophages. Unlike peritoneal macrophages, they did not substantially increase Class II expression following culture with recombinant gamma-interferon.

In addition to red pulp macrophages, the sinus endothelial lining cells have significant phagocytic capability (Hirasawa and Tokuhiro, 1970; DeBruyn and Farr, 1980). Phenotypically, these cells have some characteristics of both macrophages and T-lymphocytes (Buckley, Dickson and Walker, 1985). Between one-third and one-half of splenic sinus lining cells express HLA-DR. These cells also react with the monocyte marker OKM5, produce lysozyme and have a non-specific esterase activity which is similar, but not identical, to that produced by monocytes. Other monocyte-associated markers cannot be detected on sinus lining cells. Sinus lining cells are also positive for expression of the T-cell associated antigens CD4 and CD8.

A non-lymphoid cell designated the antigen-laden cell has been described by Bell (1984). This rare cell type was observed at a frequency of approximately 1 in 3000 following incubation of peripheral blood mononuclear cells with soluble antigen. It is also found after *in vivo* antigen challenge and appears to localize to the red pulp of the spleen where it remains detectable for a period of days to weeks. Although these antigen-laden cells ingest large quantities of antigen, their role may be to serve as antigen reservoirs rather than as antigen presenting cells, because they fail to express surface Class II MHC antigens.

Lymphoid cells are found dispersed within the RP. In contrast to observations on T-cell subsets in PALS, a relatively high proportion of $CD8^+$ cells has been observed in RP (Hsu, Cossman and Jaffe, 1983). The percentage of T-cells reactive with antibodies to CD8 ranged from 60 to 80% in the five spleens examined. B-lymphocytes are often found situated about small vessels and are positive in reactions for surface immunoglobulin and for CD19, CD20 and CD21 (Timens and Poppema, 1985).

5.2.5   SPLENIC COLONY FORMING CELLS FOLLOWING BONE MARROW TRANSPLANTATION

Several days after the infusion of histocompatible bone marrow into lethally irradiated mice microscopic colonies of cells can be observed in the spleen (Till and McCulloch, 1961). By 6 to 7 days after infusion these colonies develop into macroscopic nodules on the surface of the spleen. The cells which initiate these colonies have been equated with the hemopoietic stem cell because colonies can be observed to consist of multilineage cells. Only a minority of stem cells appears to localize in the spleen, while the majority go to the bone marrow where similar colonies can be found. Splenic colonies were observed by Antin, Weinberg and Rappeport (1985) in the spleens of 23 of 29 patients who died within 106 days of bone marrow transplantation. They differed from the splenic colonies of mice both in size and location. These colonies were located in PALS and were microscopic. However, as with their mouse counterpart, the human colonies were predominantly multilineage in nature. The ability of the human

spleen to support the development of colonies would suggest that splenic tissues can generate factors which support colony growth. Fabian *et al.* (1985) showed that conditioned media generated by mitogen-stimulated spleen cells contain growth factors for human pluripotent (CFU-GEMM), erythroid (BFU-E) and myeloid (CFU-GM) precursors. Factors responsible for proliferation of the different precursors appeared to be the products of different spleen cell populations.

5.2.6   THE IMPORTANCE OF ANTIGEN PRESENTATION BY B-CELLS IN THE SPLEEN

Ablation of B-cells from lymph nodes results in a marked reduction of lymph node T-cell responses to antigen (Ron *et al.*, 1981). B-cell depletion also reduces lymph node T helper cell responses in primed animals (Malynn and Wortis, 1984). The importance of the B-cell as an antigen presenting cell has been examined in the spleen. Janeway *et al.* (1977) showed that B-cell ablation does not affect the development of splenic T helper cell responses in primed animals. In addition, spleen cells obtained from B-cell depleted animals are able to serve as antigen presenting cells *in vitro* for T-cell clones, while cells from B-depleted lymph nodes cannot (Janeway, Ron and Katz, 1987). These results suggest that the spleen and lymph node rely on different antigen presenting populations for the triggering of antigen-specific T-cell responses.

5.3   ONTOGENY OF SPLENIC LYMPHOID COMPARTMENTS

5.3.1   B-LYMPHOCYTES

Hematopoietic stem cells originate in the fetal yolk sac and from there seed to the fetal liver and bone marrow. These stem cells give rise to precursor cells which may differentiate along distinct and different pathways. The study of B-cell ontogeny has shown that the fetal liver is the most important site of early development of pre-B-cells, which are recognized by the presence of cytoplasmic μ chains in the absence of surface immunoglobulin (Asma, van den Bergh and Vossen, 1984; Gathings, Lawton and Cooper, 1977; Kamps and Cooper, 1982). These cells appear in the liver as early as the eighth week of gestation. As development continues, the relative number of pre-B-cells in the liver decreases. By the fourteenth week pre-B-cells are outnumbered by more mature B-cells. From week 12 to week 20 the bone marrow gradually takes over as the primary site of pre-B-cell development. The main lymphoid cells found in the fetal spleen are of B-cell lineage, but include only a subset of pre-B-cells (Namikawa et al., 1986). In the liver and bone marrow two populations of pre-B-cells can be distinguished by size (Asma, van den Bergh and Vossen, 1984; Gathings, Lawton and Cooper, 1977). Small pre-B-cells are always found in greater numbers than large pre-B-cells and this ratio continues to increase during gestation.

Cells of pre-B-cell phenotype constitute only a small minority of the B lineage cells present in the spleen at all times during gestation (Gathings, Lawton and Cooper, 1977). In the fetal liver and bone marrow there is a progressive increase in the percentage of B-cells, identified by the expression of surface IgM. In addition, the proportion of B-cells expressing a more mature phenotype, represented by co-expression of IgM and IgD, increases with gestational age. In the spleen this mature B-cell phenotype is found in 60–90% of B lineage cells at all times during ontogeny (Gathings, Lawton and Cooper, 1977; Kamps and Cooper, 1982). These observations suggest that large pre-B-cells represent the least mature pre-B-cell phenotype and that these cells are not generated in the fetal spleen. Furthermore, it appears that the spleen is seeded with the more mature small pre-B-cell. The presence of B-cells co-expressing IgM and IgD as the dominant B-cell phenotype provides further evidence that B-cells within the fetal spleen reflect a more mature phenotype than is found in either fetal liver or bone marrow.

The expression of Class II MHC antigens on human B-lymphocytes occurs early in differentiation, with HLA-DR expressed prior to the expression of surface immunoglobulin. B-lymphocytes in the fetal liver have been shown to differentially express the different Class II MHC antigens (Edwards et al., 1985) and this expression has also been studied in the fetal spleen (Edwards et al., 1986). The histological pattern of Class II antigen expression and the number of positive cells in the spleen changes during gestation. Early in development the majority of Class II antigen-positive cells have the morphological appearance of macrophages. Even prior to the development of follicles almost all surface IgM$^+$ B-cells in the spleen express HLA-DR. Smaller percentages of cells express HLA-DP and HLA-DQ respectively. More mature, sIgD-positive, B-cells were shown to express all three types of Class II antigens. The appearance of HLA-DQ expression on B-lymphocytes appeared to be linked to the formation of follicles.

B-lineage cells are found in the fetal spleen prior to week 14 of gestation, distributed throughout the organ; even at this early stage the majority of these cells are of the mature, surface immunoglobulin-positive, phenotype (Kamps and Cooper, 1982). Namikawa et al. (1986) followed the development of the splenic white pulp and observed distinct lymphoid cell accumulations around the arterioles in 14-week fetal tissue. The majority of these cells were positive for B1 (CD20) and expressed surface IgM and IgD. B-cells have been observed to organize into follicles in the absence of detectable FDC. Follicular dendritic cells have been observed as early as week 20 of gestation although other studies have failed to detect FDC prior to week 24 (Bofil et al., 1985).

A subpopulation of B-cells constitutes a high percentage of mouse fetal, but not adult, splenic B-cells. These cells are positive for sIgM and sIgD and also express the Ly-1 (CD5) antigen, a molecule generally recognized as a T-cell antigen. In the mouse these cells have been described as constitutively secreting IgM (Hayakawa et al., 1984) and they can augment suboptimal T cell concentrations in the generation of allotype-restricted antibody production (Okumura, Hayakawa and Tada, 1982). CD5$^+$ B-cells have also been associated with production of IgM autoantibodies in NZB (Hayakawa *et al.*, 1983, 1984) and Mothcatcn (Sidman *et al.*, 1986) mouse strains.

Cells which coexpress B-cell markers and the CD5 antigen were initially observed in cases of centrocytic lymphomas and B-cell-chronic lymphocytic leukemia (B-CLL) in humans. Studies to determine if there was a normal equivalent to these malignant cells which arises during ontogeny determined that CD5$^+$ B-cells are present in the fetal spleen and lymph nodes. The CD5$^+$ B-cell has been the subject of a recent review by Hayakawa and Hardy (1988). These cells are not found in the earliest splenic B-cell accumulations, but they do colonize the spleen by week 22 of gestation. This is four weeks later than their appearance in the lymph nodes. Within the spleen, the CD5$^+$ B-cell is first observed in random distribution, but it later becomes the dominant cell in the primary follicles. Characterization of CD5 expression in spleen cells by flow cytometry shows the presence of both bright and dull populations, with the dull subset representing B-cells (Antin *et al.*, 1986). Both CD5$^+$ and CD5$^-$ B-cell subsets express the surface markers CD19, CD20, HLA-DR, IgM and IgD with equal intensity. Functional studies of splenic CD5$^+$ B-cells isolated by cell sorting have shown that they differ from Ly-1 B-cells of the mouse. They do not constitutively secrete IgM or provide help to antibody-secreting cells in the presence of suboptimal numbers of T-cells (Antin *et al.*, 1986). In the presence of T-cells they are able to secrete suboptimal amounts of IgM, but they are unable to proliferate in the presence of pokeweed mitogen, a lectin which does induce proliferation of other B-cell populations. Antin *et al.* (1986) proposed that the predominance of CD5$^+$ B-cells in primary follicles contributes to the inability of the fetus to mount a mature humoral immune response. Support for this hypothesis includes the observation that even

under optimal conditions these cells respond to stimulation only with production of IgM.

Further characterization of splenic B-cells shows that more than 90% of sIgM-positive B-cells express the CD21 and CD22 antigens. A subpopulation of the B-cells in the fetal spleen expresses an antigen recognized by the monoclonal antibody HB-4 (Tedder, Clement and Cooper, 1985). This antibody appears to recognize an antigen which develops late during B-cell ontogeny, after the expression of IgD; it has been proposed that the cells bearing this antigen represent a subpopulation of mature, resting B-cells. HB-4 identifies between 25 and 48% of B-cells in the fetal spleen. Reactivity with HB-4 declines during maturation of the spleen and other lymphoid organs. In contrast, the HB-4 population becomes the predominant B-cell subset found in peripheral blood.

5.3.2   T-LYMPHOCYTES

The study of T-cell ontogeny in the human spleen has been approached principally by means of immunohistology. T-cell precursors arise in fetal liver and bone marrow and then seed the thymus where maturation occurs. T-cells can be detected in random distribution throughout the spleen at week 14 of gestation, and by 18 weeks there is evidence of organization. Organization of PALS occurs after the appearance of IDC and it has been proposed that these cells may provide a suitable environment for T-cell homing (Namikawa *et al.*, 1986). Immunofluorescence examination of spleen cell suspensions shows that the CD3$^+$ population consists of approximately equal numbers of the CD4$^+$ and CD8$^+$ T-cell subsets (Asma, van den Bergh and Vossen, 1983). A significant number of T-cells in the fetal spleen expresses the OKT-10 (CD38) antigen, which is found on immature and activated T-cells. Evidence that CD38 expression by fetal splenic T-cells represents an immature phenotype is supported by evidence that some CD3-positive lymphocytes in the spleen express the maturation marker OKT6 (CD1a).

5.3.3　MARGINAL ZONE AND SECONDARY FOLLICLES

By week 26 of gestation the basic structure of the mature white pulp is established, and consists of PALS surrounding B-cell areas containing primary follicles (Namikawa *et al.*, 1986). Development of the MZ as a distinct zone demarcating the red pulp from the white pulp appears to occur later in development than the generation of WP. A study of the spleens of three neonates showed that structural demarcation of this region is less evident than in adults (Timens and Poppema, 1985). Germinal centers do not arise during normal fetal development. However, the spleen of a one-year-old infant contains large numbers of germinal centers and primary follicles, and at this time the morphological maturation of lymphoid compartments of the spleen appears complete.

5.4　ANTIGEN CLEARANCE BY THE SPLEEN

The spleen constitutes one of the major sites of fixed phagocytic cells in the body. Although the relative number of phagocytic cells in the spleen is small relative to the liver, the contribution of the spleen to antigen elimination from the blood depends on the nature of the antigen and the presence of opsonizing antibody. There are four major areas of interest relative to antigen clearance by the spleen. The first involves the role of the spleen in the homeostatic process of removal of aged, damaged or chemically modified cells. The second involves elimination of intravenous pathogens, and the relevance of clearance to defense against infection. Clearance of other injected particulates also falls within this category. Third, there is the ability of the spleen to localize and eliminate circulating immune complexes. It is also important to consider the effect of immune complex deposition in the spleen on the ability of phagocytic cells to ingest opsonized particulate antigens. Lastly, there is the ability of the spleen to localize and stimulate immune responses to soluble antigens.

5.4.1　REMOVAL OF AGED, DAMAGED AND MODIFIED CELLS

The spleen is a major site for the removal of damaged and effete cells. The mechanisms whereby these cells are identified for removal are not fully established. The basic abnormality leading to elimination of cells by the spleen may involve their physical structure. Fischer *et al.* (1971) proposed that clearance of heat-damaged red cells is a two-stage event, the first being the rapid removal of sphered cells by the spleen followed by a slow process of removal of the remaining cells by the liver and other sites. Clearance of heat-damaged ^{99m}Technetium-labelled red blood cells by the human spleen is a two-step process (Bowring, Glass and Lewis, 1976). The first step involves rapid clearance by the spleen with a half-time clearance rate of 3 to 7 minutes. This is followed by the slower clearance of the remaining cells, with the spleen accounting for an average total uptake of 75% of labelled cells.

Studies in experimental animals have shown that the spleen is the primary site of clearance of cells modified by treatment with the sulfhydryl-inhibitor N-ethylmaleimide (NEM) (Lawrence, Lockwood and Peters, 1981). Treatment with NEM results in changes in the erythrocyte membrane which in some respects mimic the ageing of red cells. The rate of clearance could be shown to be directly related to the concentration of NEM used and to duration of treatment of target cells.

In addition to the possibility of physical changes inducing splenic uptake of aged cells, a second factor to be considered is the role of autoantibodies. Aged erythrocytes have been shown to expose new antigenic sites which remain cryptic on undamaged cells (Kay and Makinodan, 1981). Exposure of these cryptic antigens could lead to interaction with autoantibodies in serum. Autoantibody-coated, damaged cells would undergo opsonized phagocytic uptake by Fc and C3 receptor-mediated phagocytosis in the spleen and liver.

One factor which may play a significant role in the clearance of antibody-coated erythrocytes is the density of antigenic sites available on the cell surface. A study conducted in rats compared the clearance of antibody-coated erythrocytes obtained from the DA strain and (DA × PVG)F1 progeny (Yousaf, Howard and Williams, 1986c). The (DA × PVG)F1 erythrocytes had only one-half the antigen density of DA cells recognized by the anti-Class I MHC antibody used to coat the cells. The clearance times of antibody-coated erythrocytes from the two sources differed significantly. The half-time of clearance for the DA erythrocytes was 44 minutes whereas the clearance of (DA × PVG)F1 erythrocytes was delayed, with an average half-time of clearance of 82 minutes. (See also Chapter 13.)

5.4.2 CLEARANCE OF PARTICULATES BY THE SPLEEN

Splenic clearance of non-antigenic particulates from the blood stream has been studied using colloidal carbon (Nossal et al., 1966; Mitchell and Abbot, 1971; Burke and Simon, 1970). Phagocytic uptake of colloidal carbon by macrophages within splenic cords has been detected by electron microscopy as early as 20 seconds after intravenous injection. Within one minute of injection there was evidence of platelet aggregation and uptake of carbon. This observation would suggest that platelets may play a role in the sequestration of particulates (Burke and Simon, 1970). Carbon accumulation occurs in both the RP and MZ. Uptake in the RP cords is by macrophages with minimal uptake by endothelial cells. These regions continue to clear and accumulate carbon, maintaining high levels of carbon for extended periods of time. There have been conflicting results with respect to colloidal carbon localization in the white pulp. When it has been seen, white pulp localization has occurred over a period of several days, with diffuse localization within the PALS. In addition, carbon outlined the follicular web of the germinal center 8 hours after

injection and by 5 days this pattern had disappeared; carbon was then found in tingible body macrophages within the germinal center (Nossal et al., 1966; Mitchell and Abbot, 1971).

Detailed studies of particulate protein antigen uptake and the pattern of localization in rat splenic tissue have utilized antigens derived from bacterial flagella (Nossal et al., 1966; Mitchell and Abbot, 1971; Mitchell, 1972). The advantage of this antigen system is that flagellar protein can be prepared in native form, as the soluble protein flagellin and as aggregated flagellin. After intravenous injection there is initially a diffuse distribution of antigen throughout the MZ and RP. Over a period of several hours there is clearing within the RP with increased labelling of the MZ. At this time antigen can also be detected in the white pulp where it localizes as a crescentic cap over the outer aspect of germinal centers. This staining of MZ and germinal center, separated by an antigen-free marginal sinus, produces a localization pattern that Nossal et al. (1966) termed a 'double palisade effect'. The localization of particulate antigen to the germinal center one day after intravenous injection was associated with the dendritic reticular cells (Mitchell and Abbot, 1971). Localization in the primary follicle is detected as a contiguous staining of the entire follicle. The apparent movement of antigen toward germinal centers appears to be a cell-associated event. Transport of antigen to the germinal center is thought to involve antigen-binding lymphocytes which would be expected to be present as a small fraction of the total circulating B-cell population, or as resident B-cells in the MZ. After contacting free antigen, probably in the MZ, these cells would continue their transit through the WP. B-cells normally travel to the germinal center and around the mantle zone, and from there continue their migration out of the spleen. This process involves transit through, but not seeding of, the lymphoid follicles. In contrast, in vitro incubation of lymphocytes with antigen, followed by injection of these antigen-binding cells, results in a progressive increase in the number of antigen-binding cells in the lymphoid follicle. This observation indicates that antigen-binding B-cells both migrate to and seed the follicles.

Polysaccharide antigen localization in the rodent spleen can occur in at least two distinct patterns, depending on the structure of the polysaccharide being tested. Likewise, structure determines the relative proportions of antigen taken up by liver and spleen. Acidic polysaccharides such as pneumococcal polysaccharide type S-III localize predominantly to the RP with relatively less localization to MZ. The greater part of the uptake of this class of polysaccharide antigen is by the liver Kupffer cells. S-III reached the splenic germinal centers 4 to 6 days after injection. In contrast, neutral polysaccharides such as pneumococcal polysaccharide S-XIV, Ficoll and hydroxyethyl starch do not localize to the liver or RP but are confined to the MZ of the spleen (Humphrey, 1981; Humphrey and Grennan, 1981). Within the murine MZ neutral polysaccharides are selectively ingested by the MZ-associated phagocytic cell population identified by the monoclonal antibody ER-TR9 (Dijkstra *et al.*, 1985). It has been proposed that retention of thymus-independent antigens, such as polysaccharides, in the marginal zone favors immunogenicity whereas localization to red pulp macrophages favors tolerance (Humphrey, 1981).

The clearance of viable bacteria has been studied in experimental animal model systems. It has been observed that the liver has a far higher total phagocytic capacity than the spleen due to the relative size of the two organs. The relative contribution of the spleen to phagocytic clearance is, however, greater when the amounts of specific antibody are small. In the absence of antibody the spleen has higher phagocytic activity per unit weight than the liver. In a guinea-pig model of pneumococcal clearance the spleen and liver had different localization patterns depending on the virulence of the organism, with the less-virulent strains localizing to the liver (Brown, Hosea and Frank, 1981).

5.4.3   IMMUNE COMPLEX CLEARANCE

The use of heterologous heat-aggregated immunoglobulin to study splenic clearance of particulate antigens has added another level of complexity to the question of clearance. Aggregated Ig differs from other particulate antigens which had been studied because it is capable of interacting with Fc receptors on cells. In this respect it has similar properties to immune complexes. Liver uptake of aggregated immunoglobulin is greater than uptake by the spleen, although the spleen shows higher specific activity. Clearance of aggregated-Ig by the spleen occurs in two phases: the first appears to involve larger aggregates which are removed by phagocytic uptake by macrophages in the RP and MZ. As the concentration and size of aggregates decreases the uptake is limited to the MZ. Two hours after injection there appeared to be surface staining of cells within the MZ and the mantle layer of the secondary lymphoid follicles. By 24 hours after injection, labeled immunoglobulin is no longer found in the mantle zone, but is isolated to a dendritic staining pattern within the germinal center, which most probably represents Fc receptor-mediated binding to FDC. Germinal center localization is radiosensitive and the transport of aggregated Ig from the MZ to the germinal center has been determined to be the radiosensitive step. Fc receptor-positive noncirculating B-cells in the MZ have been proposed as the cells responsible for transport to the germinal center (Brown *et al.*, 1970, 1973).

The clearance kinetics and tissue distribution of immune complexes prepared at antigen excess have been compared with that of complexes prepared at equivalence which have been complement solubilized (Aguado and Mannik, 1987). Solubilized and antigen-excess complexes were cleared at approximately the same rates after intravenous injection. Molecular-weight fractionation of solubilized complexes showed that larger fractions were cleared more rapidly than unfractionated complexes, whereas lower molecular weight fractions were cleared more slowly. The greater part of the uptake of complexes occurred in the liver. There was evidence that the complement-solubilized complexes were degraded more slowly than antigen-excess complexes in the liver. At nearly all times between 10 minutes and 48 hours after injection there was a relatively higher uptake of complement-solubilized immune complexes by the spleen. The role of Fc-receptor mediated opsonization in immune complexes containing C3 fragments remains unclear, but it appears that opsonizing activity takes place primarily through C3 receptors on phagocytic cells in the spleen.

The ability of phagocytic cells to clear immune complexes has important clinical implications, since complex deposition in other tissues may lead to the generation of immunologically mediated tissue injury. It has been observed that impaired splenic function in patients with nephritis and vasculitis can be improved by plasma exchange. In addition, the finding by Mannik (1980) that the process of removal of immune complexes by mononuclear phagocytic cells could be saturated, led to studies to determine if inhibition of complex clearance altered other splenic phagocytic functions. Studies to examine the effect of immune complexes on the clearance of red blood cells have involved both NEM-modified cells and antibody-coated cells. Lawrence, Lockwood and Peters (1981) observed a decreased rate of clearance of NEM-treated erythrocytes in rabbits after the injection of immune complexes made in 10-fold antigen excess. The degree and duration of the decrease in clearance was related to the dose of complexes injected, but the mechanism was saturable. Studies by Yousaf, Howard and Williams (1986b) were unable to reproduce this observation in rats using 10-fold antigen excess immune complexes, but significant delays in the clearance of NEM-treated erythrocytes were

obtained using complexes prepared at equivalence. This delay could be abolished by treating rats with chlorpheniramine maleate, phentolamine or propranolol which prevented complement-mediated reductions in splenic blood flow. The implication is that, at least in the rat, immune complexes do not have a direct effect on delaying removal of NEM-modified cells. Instead, it appears that delays in clearance are mediated by immune complex-dependent complement activation leading to reduced splenic blood flow.

Immune complexes may have a more direct role in blocking the clearance of cells coated with complement-fixing antibody. Clearance of antibody-coated rat erythrocytes can involve opsonization through either Fc or complement receptors on phagocytic cells. Complement depletion of rats by treatment with cobra venom factor (CVF) increased the clearance time of antibody-coated cells, which suggests that clearance in an intact animal is primarily mediated through receptors for C3 fragments on phagocytes (Yousaf, Howard and Williams, 1986a). Fc receptors do appear to mediate clearance in the absence of complement. The density of antigen sites on target cells is also important in determining rates of clearance of antibody-coated cells (Yousaf, Howard and Williams, 1986c). Infusion of immune complexes into rats delays the clearance of rat erythrocytes coated with complement-fixing antibody (Yousaf, Howard and Williams, 1986b). This delay was observed using complexes prepared at equivalence and at 10-fold antigen excess. The delay was also maintained after treatment with agents which prevented complement-mediated changes in splenic blood flow. CVF-mediated activation of complement during the erythrocyte clearance process produced a significant increase in the clearance time of antibody-coated cells which was not reversed by treatment with chlorpheniramine maleate (Yousaf, Howard and Williams, 1986a). In addition, infusion of rat serum which had been complement activated *in vitro* by zymosan or insolubilized CVF also delayed cell clearance.

5.4.4 CLEARANCE OF SOLUBLE ANTIGENS

Soluble antigens in monomeric form are cleared much less efficiently from peripheral blood than are antigens in aggregated or particulate form. Nossal *et al.* (1966) observed that soluble monomeric bacterial flagellin was minimally retained in the MZ. One hour after injection the heaviest labeling was observed in the red pulp and marginal sinus. Eventually labelling was observed in the marginal zone, and the MZ to germinal center movement of antigen seen with polymerized flagellin occurred. However, labelling of the MZ and germinal center was very light compared to that seen with polymerized antigen. Similar results were obtained in mice given intravenous human gamma globulin (Brown *et al.*, 1970). Measurements indicated that essentially all the antigen which could be detected in the spleen could be accounted for by blood in the organ. Clearance of soluble antigens from blood was much slower than that observed for particulate antigens. These studies show that macrophages are more efficient in the removal of particulate as opposed to soluble antigens.

5.4.5 ANTIGEN-INDUCED CHANGES IN LYMPHOCYTE CIRCULATION

It is well established that lymphocyte recirculation through lymph nodes is altered in the presence of antigen. This is due to the trapping of lymphocytes in the antigen-stimulated lymph node. Similar observations have been made in the spleen following both subcutaneous and intravenous antigenic challenge. Lymphocytes trapped in the antigen-stimulated spleen are not preferentially antigen specific (Black, 1975). Ford (1972) studied splenic trapping of lymphocytes using a complex experimental design involving perfusion of the spleen with antigen and with thoracic duct lymphocytes recovered

from antigen-sensitized donors. The antigens used in this study included tetanus toxoid and the particulate antigen swine influenza virus. An efficient, selective removal of antigen-specific cells by the spleen was observed with tetanus toxoid, but not with swine influenza virus, when perfused in the presence of appropriately sensitized donor cells. A second experiment used cells from two groups of animals sensitized with different antigens, labeled with different radiolabels and injected into an irradiated recipient. The distribution of the two cell populations in the spleen was determined after antigen challenge. The ratio of immune to non-immune cells was 1:1, but there was increased total radioactivity in the spleen 6 hours after challenge. The conclusion was that antigenic stimulation of the spleen results in the transient accumulation of both immune and non-immune lymphocytes in the spleen. This accumulation appears to occur at the expense of brachial and axillary lymph nodes.

5.5 THE IMMUNOLOGICAL CONSEQUENCES OF SPLENECTOMY

A significant body of knowledge about the immunological functions of the spleen has come from the study of the immunological consequences of splenectomy. (See also Chapter 11.) The most severe complication of asplenia is the predisposition to overwhelming infection by encapsulated bacterial species. Susceptibility to infection is not equal for all splenectomized patient populations: the risk of serious infection is significantly higher in infants than in adults, particularly in children splenectomized in the first years of life (King and Schumaker, 1952; Ellis and Smith, 1966; Broberger, Guylai and Hirschfeldt, 1960). In addition, there is an association between the underlying disorder leading to splenectomy and the relative probability of severe infection (Claret, Morales and Montaner, 1975). A review of the incidence of infection in 467 splenectomized children by Eraklis *et al.* (1967) showed an overall mortality from fulminating infection of 5.4%. When mortality was related to the underlying disease it could be shown that children whose primary disorder was not usually associated with severe infection had a mortality rate of only 0.9%. In contrast, the mortality rate of the 124 splenectomized children with primary diseases often associated with severe infection was 18%. The risk of infection in patients splenectomized for trauma, idiopathic thrombocytopenic purpura or localized tumor was not increased. The highest risk of infection was found in patients with histiocytosis, hepatitis, thalassemia major and the Wiscott-Aldrich syndrome.

The risk of post-splenectomy sepsis in children is highest in the first years after splenectomy. However, fulminant pneumococcal sepsis has been reported in adults splenectomized many years earlier during childhood (Hollis *et al.*, 1987). The overall incidence of post-splenectomy sepsis in adults is low. In a retrospective study of 193 residents of Rochester, Minnesota who were splenectomized during the years 1955 to 1979 only two cases of fulminant sepsis were documented during the 1090 person-years of follow up (Schwartz *et al.*, 1982). The incidence of serious infection in these adults was 7.16 per 100 person-years of observation. The lowest incidence was 3.3 cases per 100 person-years, which occurred in patients splenectomized for splenic trauma. The highest rate of infection was in patients who had undergone splenectomy in association with treatment for malignant neoplasm. Many of these patients had received additional therapy which included immunosuppressive therapy or radiation therapy. These treatments may significantly contribute to the increased susceptibility to serious infection seen in this patient population. The greatest risk for infection in this study was during the first year after surgery. (For further discussion, see Chapter 12.)

The risk of sepsis in splenectomized adults who are otherwise normal is generally considered to be very low. However, several cases of fulminant pneumococcal infections have been documented in patients who were splenecto-

mized as adults following traumatic rupture of the spleen (Grinblat and Gilboa, 1975; Gopal and Biano, 1977).

As described above, several factors contribute to the incidence of post-splenectomy infection. Many of these are related to other factors which may have an impact on immune competence. The increased risk associated with infancy is in part due to immaturity of the immune system: not only is the immune system incompletely developed in early childhood, but infants are also more likely than adults to encounter organisms of which they have had no prior immunological experience. In addition, limited exposure to environmental antigens makes infants less likely than adults to have come in contact with antigens which could stimulate a cross-reactive protective response. This lack of immunological experience means that a splenectomized infant is unlikely to have serum opsonins, which are of importance to the clearance of polysaccharide-encapsulated bacteria by the liver. Other risk factors include having primary diseases which are associated with defects in lymphocyte or granulocyte function, and being subjected to other immunosuppressive therapies. The relatively low rate of infection in patients undergoing splenectomy following traumatic rupture of the spleen may, in part, be due to compensatory spleen growth by splenic fragments which remain after surgery (splenosis). A study in rats of compensatory spleen growth showed that the spleen has only a limited capacity for regeneration (van Wyck, Witte and Witte, 1986). Survival after pneumococcal challenge was directly related to the initial size of the remnant, adequacy of vascular flow and age of the subject. Removal of the spleen followed by reimplantation of fragments in an omental pouch provided no increase in protection against bacterial challenge when compared to splenectomized controls.

Studies have been conducted in both experimental animals and humans to determine the effect of splenectomy on the ability to mount primary and secondary immune responses. Claret, Morales and Montaner (1975) performed serial measurements of immunoglobulin levels in 52 children before and after splenectomy. The results obtained were compared to those obtained in a group of normal children, and in 30 children studied before and after appendectomy. Regardless of the primary reason for splenectomy, the splenectomized children had significantly lower levels of IgM and higher levels of IgA than controls. In children with a previous disorder of the reticuloendothelial system, splenectomy led to elevated IgG levels.

A second longitudinal study of 14 splenectomized children was conducted by Andersen, Cohn and Sørensen (1976). Immunological parameters measured included lymphocyte and granulocyte counts, IgM and IgA levels and in vitro lymphocyte transformation responses to antigen and mitogens. Although all of these parameters showed transitory changes during the immediate postoperative period, the only changes observed one year after surgery were a 23% decrease in serum IgM, and increased lymphocyte and eosinophil counts in peripheral blood. Wasi, Wasi and Thongcharoen (1971) measured immunoglobulin levels in 128 patients with thalassemic diseases. The 42 splenectomized patients enrolled in this study had decreased IgM and increased IgA concentrations when compared to non-splenectomized patients. The implication of these studies is that the spleen is particularly important to the generation of IgM responses. Antibodies of the IgM isotype are the first to arise during the initial phase of a humoral immune response. They are also the predominant isotype generated in the immune response to T-independent antigens and this defect may play a role in post-splenectomy sepsis.

The capacity of asplenic patients to respond to intravenous challenge with the particulate antigen bacteriophage ØX174 was studied by Sullivan et al. (1978). This antigen is particularly useful because it represents a particulate antigen of which patients have no prior immunological experience, and which thus permits the study of primary immune responses. In addition, residual bacteriophage in peripheral blood can be directly quantitated: clearance time of the bacteriophage from blood was normal in all patients. Following primary antigenic challenge, the peak antibody response of asplenic patients was significantly lower than the response of normal controls. After secondary challenge the majority of patients had antibody responses within the normal range. Analysis of the isotype of antibody produced after secondary challenge showed that asplenic patients produced significantly lower quantities of anti-ØX174 IgG antibodies than normal controls, with IgM providing the greater part of the antibody produced. Similar results were obtained in a group of severely hyposplenic patients with inflammatory bowel disease (Ryan et al., 1981). In this study both primary and secondary responses were markedly reduced in the hyposplenic population and again the secondary response was principally with IgM.

Because the most demonstrable immunological consequence of splenectomy is increased susceptibility to encapsulated bacteria, a number of studies have directly addressed the question of how splenectomy affects the immune response to deliberate immunization with polysaccharide antigens. In the A/J mouse strain the effect of splenectomy on the response to polysaccharides is dependent on polysaccharide structure. Responses to the acidic pneumococcal polysaccharide type S-III differed significantly from the response to neutral pneumococcal polysaccharide S-XIV in splenectomized animals (Cohn and Schiffman, 1987). The response to S-III is lower in splenectomized than in normal mice, especially at an early period in the response. However, the response to S-XIV is completely lost in splenectomized animals. One factor which may play a role in this differential requirement for the spleen is localization patterns of the respective antigens. As discussed previously, acidic polysaccharides do not localize to the marginal zone whereas neutral polysaccharides do localize to that site. Dependence on MZ localization may mean that there are no equivalent sites which can replace the spleen for stimulating an immune response. In the case of S-III, absence of the spleen may alter the intensity and timing of the response, but extrasplenic sites can substitute to some extent for splenic function in generating an antibody response.

Results of patient studies have been variable in terms of the effect of splenectomy on the ability to generate normal levels of humoral immune responses. Hammarström and Smith (1986) examined the levels of immunoglobulin by class, as well as subclasses of IgG in four children with congenital asplenia or splenectomized prior to bone marrow transplantation, and found normal levels of IgM and the tested IgG subclasses. Antibodies at levels similar to those found in controls were detected against four pneumococcal polysaccharide antigens as well as the protein antigens tetanus toxoid and *Haemophilus influenzae* outer membrane protein. In all but one patient the antibodies measured were thought to have arisen from natural antigenic exposure. The authors concluded that the spleen does not provide a major contribution to the normal background antibody repertoire, and that the main contribution of the spleen to defence against infection is its phagocytic capacity. Sullivan *et al.* (1978) reported that all groups of asplenic patients except those with Hodgkin's disease demonstrated significant seroconversions to pneumococcal capsular antigen given subcutaneously. The patients with Hodgkin's disease had also been treated with combined radiation and chemotherapy, which could have compromised immunity in this patient group. These results lend support to the concept that subcutaneous challenge with antigen circumvents the need for a splenic immune response. Similar results were obtained with meningococcal polysaccharide vaccine (Ruben *et al.*, 1984). Again, patients who underwent splenectomy for trauma or non-lymphoid tumors responded to the vaccine antigens. In contrast, splenectomized patients with lymphoid tumors who had received prior chemotherapy and radiotherapy responded poorly. Other studies have shown defective responses

to direct challenge with polysaccharide antigens. Hosea *et al.* (1981) observed that the IgG and IgM responses of splenectomized patients were markedly impaired to eight of nine pneumococcal polysaccharides found in a commercially available vaccine preparation. This impairment was seen in patients who were not on immunosuppressive therapy. In this patient population the response was less than that of controls in terms of the antibody titre obtained, the kinetics of the rise in titre and in the relative increase in pre- and post-immunization titres. Amlot and Hayes (1985) measured the antibody response of splenectomized patients to the intradermally injected, synthetic, T-independent antigen DNP-Ficoll, to determine the primary and secondary antibody responsiveness to a polysaccharide antigen. The antibody response to DNP-Ficoll in splenectomized patients was approximately 10% of that obtained in controls at 1 to 3 weeks after immunization. In contrast, patients who had received primary immunization prior to splenectomy responded normally to re-immunization 6–28 months after splenectomy. The authors concluded that the spleen is important to the generation of primary antibody responses to certain T-independent antigens, and that failure to detect defective responses to bacterial antigens may result from prior natural exposure and priming, with rechallenge being less dependent on the spleen. They also point out that studies which measure the antibody response several weeks after immunization are relevant to prophylaxis, but not to the pneumococcal infections seen in splenectomized patients. These infections develop rapidly with most deaths occurring in the first 5 days of illness.

The effect of splenectomy on clearance patterns of antibody-coated and NEM-treated cells was studied in the rat by Yousaf, Howard and Williams (1986a). Antibody-coated red blood cells were labelled with ^{99m}Tc or ^{51}Cr to determine tissue localization of injected cells. In normal rats the spleen was principally responsible for the clearance of both antibody-coated and NEM-treated cells. The half-time of clearance of injected NEM-treated cells was increased from 19 minutes to 39 minutes in splenectomized rats. Antibody-sensitized erythrocytes were cleared from the circulation of normal rats more slowly than NEM-treated cells with a half-time of clearance of 38 minutes. Splenectomy had a marked impact on clearance of these cells, increasing the half-time of clearance to more than 180 minutes.

5.6   IMMUNOREGULATION BY THE SPLEEN

The splenic environment plays an important immunoregulatory role for both B- and T-effector cell development. Rapid synthesis of high affinity antibody after re-exposure to antigen is dependent on generation of circulating antigen-specific memory cells during the primary response to antigen. During the immune response antibody produced by maturing B-cells in the germinal center can complex with antigen, and the immune complexes formed bind to follicular dendritic cells. There is evidence that maturation of antigen-specific B-lymphocytes in the presence of FDC-bound immune complexes favours the differentiation of memory B-cells (Klaus et al., 1980).

The B-cell response to T-independent antigens does not require T-lymphocytes to initiate an antibody response. However, the magnitude of the antibody response is influenced by regulatory T-cells with suppressor and amplifying activities. The immune response to pneumococcal polysaccharide S-III has been studied in mice with reference to these T-cell activities (Amsbaugh, Prescott and Baker, 1978; Baker et al., 1981). Suppressor T-cell activity was not impaired by splenectomy, which suggested that suppressor activity in this system is not limited to the spleen. In contrast, amplifier T-cell activity was almost completely lost within 7 days of splenectomy, indicating that the spleen is an important site of amplifier T-cells (Amsbaugh, Prescott and Baker, 1978). Two models of regulation have been proposed to explain the mechanism of T-cell regulation of B-cell responses to T-independent antigens (Baker et al., 1981). Both models involve idiotype–anti-idiotype interactions to induce regulatory T-cell responses. The intact spleen has also been reported to contribute to regulation of autoantibody responses in experimental models (Cox and Finlay-Jones, 1979). Splenectomy results in increased levels of autoantibody production and prolonged persistence of the autoantibody response. Reinfusion of spleen cells alone was not sufficient to restore regulation of the autoantibody response, which suggests that the microenvironment provided by the intact organ plays a significant role in regulation.

The spleen has been shown to be an important source of suppressor cells which can regulate T-dependent antibody production by B-cells (Wu and Lance, 1974; Romball and Weigle, 1977) and T-cell responses to antigens and mitogens (Folch and Waksman, 1974a, 1974b; Gershon, Lance and Kondo, 1974; Sy et al., 1977; Globerson, Abel and Umiel, 1981). Regulation of T-dependent antibody responses appears to involve a T-cell population which requires the splenic microenvironment for development (Wu and Lance, 1974). Following activation and differentiation in the spleen, these suppressor cells migrate out of the spleen to take up residence in other lymphoid organs (Romball and Weigle, 1977).

Suppression of T-cell responses can be mediated by non-T-cells as well as T-cells (Globerson, Abel and Umiel, 1981). T-cell-mediated suppression provides one mechanism for induction of tolerance to antigen. Sy et al., (1977) observed that animals could be induced to tolerate antigen in the absence of the spleen through clonal deletion, but this tolerance could not be transferred to normal recipients. Tolerance mediated by splenic suppressor cells could be transferred. Tolerance could also be transferred if animals were not splenectomized for 3 days after the induction of tolerance, indicating that following induction these suppressor T-cells seed other organs.

5.7 TUFTSIN

The spleen is the normal site of one step in the production of the immunomodulatory molecule tuftsin. Tuftsin was discovered during studies of the kinetics of phagocytic uptake of bacteria in the presence of leukophilic IgG, also known as the leukokinin (Najjar and Nishioka, 1970). A granulocyte surface membrane enzyme, leukokinase, causes the release of a molecular fragment from leukokinin which accounts for the full activity of the leukokinin molecule. Leukokinase was used to isolate the active fragment, which was identified as the tetrapeptide Thr-Lys-Pro-Arg and given the name 'tuftsin'.

Among the numerous immunomodulatory molecules which have been identified, tuftsin is uniquely related to the spleen: tuftsin activity is not found in asplenic individuals. The tetrapeptide which makes up tuftsin is an integral sequence of the IgG molecule. Sequence analysis has determined that tuftsin comprises amino acid residues 289 to 292 in the heavy chain of IgG. This fragment is located in the CH_2 domain of the immunoglobulin Fc fragment, and lies within the segment of the domain which is connected by an intrachain disulfide bond. As the leukokinin IgG passes through the spleen it is acted on by a splenic enzyme, tuftsin-endocarboxypeptidase, which cleaves the immunoglobulin between amino acids 292 and 293 (Najjar, 1974). The nicked IgG molecule, which is now designated leukokinin-S, continues to circulate and enters tissue either free or bound to phagocytic cells through their Fc receptors. Once leukokinin-S is on the phagocytic cell surface leukokinase generates the second nick, which occurs between amino acids 288 and 289 and results in the production of tuftsin (Najjar and Nishioka, 1970).

The tetrapeptide sequence for tuftsin is found in the same location in all four subclasses of IgG, but only IgG1 is susceptible to tuftsin-endocarboxypeptidase and able to generate the active precursor, leukokinin-S. Free tuftsin is the biologically active form of the molecule (Najjar, 1974) and binds to specific receptors found on neutrophil leukocytes, monocytes, macrophages and natural killer cells (Florentin et al., 1983; Bar-Shavit et al., 1979). After tuftsin binds its receptor, it is internalized by the cell where it is susceptible to an aminopeptidase in the cytosol and subsequently degraded. It is for this reason that the phagocytic enhancing potential of leukokinin is rapidly lost.

Among the biological activities attributed to tuftsin, the stimulation of phagocytosis is the best studied (Nishioka et al., 1972; Fridkin et al., 1977; Bar-Shavit et al., 1979). Inactive analogues of tuftsin can inhibit the stimulation of phagocytosis by tuftsin, but have no effect on the basal phagocytic activity of these cells. Other functions which tuftsin has been reported to modulate include: the increased motility of neutrophils (Nishioka et al., 1973), augmentation of antibody formation, the number of antibody forming cells in the spleen (Florentin et al., 1978), and the tumoricidal activity of phagocytic cells (Nishioka, 1979; Bruley-Rosset et al., 1981).

5.8 CONCLUSION

The spleen is a filtration bed which is important in eliminating particulates from the peripheral blood. It is also a lymphoid organ which provides an environment conducive to cellular interactions which lead to the development of antigen-specific immune responses. The spleen has a unique lymphocyte-rich marginal zone which contains a subset of B-lymphocytes with distinctive characteristics, and which is found in association with a non-lymphoid cell population which takes up certain types of polysaccharides. Loss of the spleen results in a decrease in the ability to generate an IgM response and a reduced capacity to respond to polysaccharide antigens. Splenectomy has also been associated with increased risk of severe infection caused by encapsulated bacteria. The spleen may play a critical role in generating a rapid humoral response to the challenge of polysaccharide-encapsulated bacteria which results in efficient opsonin-mediated elimination by the macrophage-lined filtration beds in the liver and spleen. Patients lacking a spleen may retain the capacity to generate an immune response to the bacteria responsible for post-splenectomy sepsis. However, the development of that response in other lymphoid organs, seeded by spleen cells capable of responding to the challenge, may be sufficiently delayed to allow rapidly dividing bacteria an opportunity to overwhelm residual host defences. The marginal zone may prove to be the key region of the spleen which initiates the generation of protective responses against these pyogenic bacterial species.

REFERENCES

Aguado, M. T. and Mannik, M. (1987) Clearance kinetics and organ uptake of complement-solubilized immune complexes in mice. *Immunology*, 60, 255–60.

Amlot, P. L. and Hayes, A. E. (1985) Impaired human antibody response to the thymus-independent antigen, DNP-Ficoll, after splenectomy. Implications for post-splenectomy infections. *Lancet*, i, 1008–11.

Amsbaugh, D. F., Prescott, B. and Baker, P. J. (1978) Effect of splenectomy on the expression of regulatory T cell activity. *J. Immunol.*, 121, 1483–5.

Andersen, V., Cohn, J. and Sørensen, S. F. (1976) Immunological studies in children before and after splenectomy. *Acta Paediatr. Scand.*, 65, 409–15.

Antin, J. H., Weinberg, D. S. and Rappeport, J. M. (1985) Evidence that pluripotential stem cells form splenic colonies in humans after marrow transplantation. *Transplantation*, 39, 102–5.

Antin, J. H. *et al.* (1986) Leu-1+ (CD5+) B cells. A major lymphoid subpopulation in human fetal spleen: Phenotypic and functional studies. *J. Immunol.*, 136, 505–10.

Asma, G. E. M., van den Bergh, R. L. and Vossen, J. M. (1983) Use of monoclonal antibodies in a study of the development of T lymphocytes in the human fetus. *Clin. Exp. Immunol.*, 53, 429–36.

Asma, G. E. M., van den Bergh, R. L. and Vossen, J. M. (1984) Development of pre-B and B lymphocytes in the human fetus. *Clin. Exp. Immunol.*, 56, 407–14.

Baker, P. J. *et al.* (1981) Regulation of the antibody response to pneumococcal polysaccharide by thymus-derived cells. *Rev. Infect. Dis.*, 3, 332–41.

Bar-Shavit, Z. *et al.* (1979) Tuftsin macrophage interaction: Specific binding and augmentation of phagocytosis. *J. Cell. Physiol.*, 100, 55–62.

Bazin, H. *et al.* (1982) Distinct delta+ and delta− B lymphocyte lineages in the rat. *Ann. NY Acad. Sci.*, 399, 157–74.

Bell, E. B. (1984) The migration of antigen-laden cells. *Immunobiology*, 168, 325–37.

Black, S. J. (1975) Antigen-induced changes in lymphocyte circulatory patterns. *Eur. J. Immunol.*, 5, 170–5.

Bofil, M. *et al.* (1985) Human B cell development. II. Subpopulations in the human fetus. *J. Immunol.*, 134, 1531–8.

Bowdler, A. J. (1976) The role of the spleen and splenectomy in autoimmune haemolytic disease. *Sem. Hematol.*, 13, 335–48.

Bowring, C. S., Glass, H. I. and Lewis, S. M. (1976) Rate of clearance by the spleen of heat-damaged erythrocytes. *J. Clin. Pathol.*, 29, 852–4.

Broberger, O., Gyulai, F. and Hirschfeldt, J. (1960) Splenectomy in childhood. A clinical and immunological study of 42 children splenectomized in the years 1951–1958. *Acta Paediatr. (Upps.)* 49, 679–89.

Brown, E. J., Hosea, S. W. and Frank, M. M. (1981) The role of the spleen in experimental pneumococcal bacteremia. *J. Clin. Immunol.*, 67, 975–82.

Brown, J. C. *et al.* (1970) Lymphocyte-mediated transport of aggregated gamma-globulin into germinal centre areas of normal mouse spleen. *Nature*, 228, 367–9.

Brown, J. C. *et al.* (1973) The localization of aggregated human gamma-globulin in the spleens of normal mice. *Immunology*, 24, 955–68.

Bruley-Rosset, M. *et al.* (1981) Prevention of spontaneous tumors of aged mice by immunopharmacologic manipulation: study of immune antitumor mechanisms. *J. Nat. Cancer Inst.*, 66, 1113–19.

Buckley, P. J., Dickson, S. A. and Walker, W. S. (1985) Human splenic sinusoidal lining cells express antigens associated with monocytes, macrophages, endothelial cells and T lymphocytes. *J. Immunol.*, 134, 2310–15.

Burke, J. S. and Simon, G. T. (1970) Electron microscopy of the spleen. II. Phagocytosis of colloidal carbon. *Am. J. Pathol.*, 58, 157–81.

Christensen, B. E. *et al.* (1978) Traffic of T and B lymphocytes in the normal spleen. *Scand. J. Haematol.*, 20, 246–57.

Claret, I., Morales, L. and Montaner, A. (1975)

Immunological studies in the postsplenectomy syndrome. *J. Pediatr. Surg.*, **10**, 59–64.

Cohn, D. A. and Schiffman, G. (1987) Immunoregulatory role of the spleen in antibody responses to pneumococcal polysaccharide antigens. *Infect. Immun.*, **55**, 1375–80.

Cox, K. O. and Finlay-Jones, J. J. (1979) Impaired regulation of erythrocyte autoantibody production after splenectomy. *Br. J. Exp. Pathol.*, **60**, 466–70.

De Bruyn, P. P. H. and Farr, A. G. (1980) Lymphocyte-RES interactions and their fine-structural correlates. in *The Reticuloendothelial System*, Vol. I. (eds I. Carr and W. T. Daems), Plenum Publishing, New York, pp. 499–523.

Dijkstra, C. D. (1982) Characterization of nonlymphoid cells in rat spleen, with special reference to strongly Ia-positive branched cells in T-cell areas. *J. Reticuloendothel. Soc.*, **32**, 167–78.

Dijkstra, C. D. *et al.* (1985) Marginal zone macrophages identified by a monoclonal antibody: characterization of immuno- and enzyme-histochemical properties and functional capacities. *Immunology*, **55**, 23–30.

Edwards, J. A. *et al.* (1985) Differential expression of HLA-class II antigens on human fetal and adult lymphocytes and macrophages. *Immunology*, **55**, 489–500.

Edwards, J. A. *et al.* (1986) Differential expression of HLA class II antigens in fetal human spleen: relationship of HLA-DP, DQ and DR to immunoglobulin expression. *J. Immunol.*, **137**, 490–7.

Eikelenboom, P. *et al.* (1979) Development of T and B cell areas in peripheral lymphoid organs of the rat. *Anat. Rec.*, **194**, 523–38.

Ellis, E. F. and Smith, R. T. (1966) The role of the spleen in immunity. With special reference to the post-splenectomy problem in infants. *Pediatrics*, **37**, 111–19.

Eraklis, A. J. *et al.* (1967) Hazard of overwhelming infection after splenectomy in childhood. *N. Engl. J. Med.*, **276**, 1225–9.

Fabian, I. *et al.* (1985) Human spleen cell generation of factors stimulating human pluripotent stem cell, erythroid, and myeloid progenitor cell growth. *Blood*, **65**, 990–6.

Fischer, J. *et al.* (1971) Clinical value of the functional investigation of the spleen using Cr[51]-labelled heat-damaged erythrocytes. in *Dynamic Studies with Radioisotopes in Medicine*, IAEA, Vienna. pp. 445–62.

Florentin, I. *et al.* (1978) *In vivo* immunostimulation by tuftsin. *Cancer Immunol. Immunother.*, **5**, 211–16.

Florentin, I. *et al.* (1983) Immunopharmacological properties of tuftsin and of some analogs. *Ann. NY Acad. Sci.*, **419**, 177–91.

Folch, H. and Waksman, B. H. (1974a) The splenic suppressor cell. I. Activity of thymus-dependent adherent cells: changes with age and stress. *J. Immunol.*, **113**, 127–39.

Folch, H. and Waksman, B. H. (1974b) The splenic suppressor cell. II. Suppression of the mixed lymphocyte reaction by thymus dependent adherent cells. *J. Immunol.*, **113**, 140–4.

Ford, W. L. (1972) The recruitment of recirculating lymphocytes in the antigenically stimulated spleen. Specific and non-specific consequences of initiating a secondary antibody response. *Clin. Exp. Immunol.*, **12**, 243–54.

Fridkin, M. *et al.* (1977) Tuftsin and some analogs: synthesis and interaction with human polymorphonuclear leukocytes. *Biochim. biophys. Acta*, **496**, 203–211.

Gathings, W. E., Lawton, A. R. and Cooper, M. D. (1977) Immunofluorescent studies of the development of pre-B cells, B lymphocytes and immunoglobulin isotype diversity in humans. *Eur. J. Immunol.*, **7**, 804–10.

Gershon, R. K., Lance, E. M. and Kondo, K. (1974) Immunoregulatory role for spleen localizing thymocytes. *J. Immunol.*, **112**, 546–54.

Globerson, A., Abel, L. and Umiel, T. (1981) Immune reactivity during ageing. III. Removal of peanut-agglutinin binding cells from ageing mouse spleen cells leads to increased reactivity to mitogens. *Mech. Ageing Dev.*, **16**, 275–84.

Gopal, V. and Biano, A. L. (1977) Fulminant pneumococcal infections in 'normal' asplenic hosts. *Arch. Intern. Med.*, **137**, 1526–30.

Gowans, J. L. and Knight, E. J. (1964) The route of recirculation of lymphocytes in the rat. *Proc. Roy. Soc., Lond. (Biol.)*, **159**, 257–81.

Gray, D. *et al.* (1984a) Marginal zone B cells express CR1 and CR2 receptors. *Eur. J. Immunol.*, **14**, 47–52.

Gray, D. *et al.* (1984b) Relation of intra-splenic migration of marginal zone B cells to antigen localization on follicular dendritic cells. *Immunology*, **52**, 659–69.

Grinblat, J. and Gilboa, Y. (1975) Overwhelming pneumococcal sepsis 25 years after splenectomy. *Am. J. Med. Sci.*, **270**, 523–4.

Grogan, T. H. M., Jolley, C. S. and Rangel, C. S. (1983) Immunoarchitecture of the human spleen. *Lymphology*, **16**, 72–82.

Hammarström, L. and Smith, C. I. E. (1986) Development of anti-polysaccharide antibodies in splenic children. *Clin. Exp. Immunol.*, **66**, 457–62.

Hayakawa, K. *et al.* (1983) The 'Ly-1 B' cell subpopulation in normal, immunodefective and autoimmune mice. *J. Exp. Med.*, **157**, 202–18.

Hayakawa, K. *et al.* (1984) Ly-1 B cells: Functionally distinct lymphocytes that secrete IgM autoantibodies. *Proc. Natl. Acad. Sci. USA*, **81**, 2494–8.

Hayakawa, K. and Hardy, R.R. (1988) Normal, autoimmune, and malignant CD5⁺ B cells: the Ly-1 B lineage. *Annu. Rev. Immunol.*, **6**, 197–218.

Heinen, E., Cormann, N. and Kinet-Denoel, C. (1988) The lymph follicle: a hard nut to crack. *Immunology Today*, **9**, 240–3.

Hirasawa, Y. and Tokuhiro, H. (1970) Electron microscopic studies on the normal human spleen: especially on the red pulp and the reticuloendothelial cells. *Blood*, **35**, 201–12.

Hollis, N. *et al.* (1987) Overwhelming pneumococcal sepsis in healthy adults years after splenectomy. *Lancet*, **i**, 110–11.

Hosea, S. W. *et al.* (1981) Impaired immune response of splenectomized patients to polyvalent pneumococcal vaccine. *Lancet*, **i**, 804–7.

Hsu, S. M. (1985) Phenotypic expression of B lymphocytes. III. Marginal zone B cells in the spleen are characterized by the expression of Tac and alkaline phosphatase. *J. Immunol.*, **135**, 123–30.

Hsu, S. M. and Jaffe, E. S. (1984a) Phenotypic expression of B-lymphocytes. 1. Identification with monoclonal antibodies in normal lymphoid tissues. *Am. J. Clin. Pathol.*, **114**, 387–95.

Hsu, S. M. and Jaffe E. S. (1984b) Phenotypic expression of B-lymphocytes. 2. Immunoglobulin expression of germinal center cells. *Am. J. Pathol.*, **114**, 396–402.

Hsu, S. M., Cossman, J. and Jaffe, E. S. (1983) Lymphocyte subsets in normal human lymphoid tissues. *Am. J. Clin. Pathol.*, **80**, 21–30.

Humphrey, J. H. (1981) Tolerogenic or immunogenic activity of hapten-conjugated polysaccharides correlated with cellular localization. *Eur. J. Immunol.*, **11**, 212–20.

Humphrey, J. H. and Grennan, D. (1981) Different macrophage populations distinguished by means of fluorescent polysaccharides. Recognition and properties of marginal-zone macrophages. *Eur. J. Immunol.*, **11**, 221–8.

Janeway, C. A. *et al.* (1977) Evidence for an immunoglobulin-dependent antigen-specific helper T cell. *Proc. Natl. Acad. Sci. USA*, **74**, 4582–6.

Janeway, C. A., Ron, J. and Katz, M. E. (1987) The B cell is the initiating antigen-presenting cell in peripheral lymph nodes. *J. Immunol.*, **138**, 1051–5.

Kamps, W. A. and Cooper, M. D. (1982) Microenvironmental studies of pre-B and B cell development in human and mouse fetuses. *J. Immunol.*, **129**, 526–31.

Kay, M. M. B. and Makinodan, T. (1981) Relationship between ageing and the immune system. *Prog. Allergy*, **29**, 134–81.

King, H. and Schumaker, H. B. (1952) Splenic studies; I. Susceptibility to infection after splenectomy performed in infancy. *Ann. Surg.*, **136**, 239–42.

Klaus, G. G. B. *et al.* (1980) The follicular dendritic cell: its role in antigen presentation in the generation of immunological memory. *Immunol. Rev.*, **53**, 3–28.

Kraal, G., Weissman, I. L. and Butcher, E. C. (1982) Germinal centre B-cells: Antigen specificity and changes in heavy chain expression. *Nature*, **298**, 377–9.

Kumararatne, D. S., Bazin, H. and MacLennan, I. C. M. (1981) Marginal zones: the major B cell compartment of rat spleens. *Eur. J. Immunol.*, **11**, 858–64.

Kumararatne, D. S. and MacLennan, I. C. M. (1981) Cells of the marginal zone of the spleen are lymphocytes derived from recirculating precursors. *Eur. J. Immunol.*, **11**, 865–9.

Lawrence, S., Lockwood, C. M. and Peters, D. K. (1981) Studies on NEM-treated erythrocyte clearance in the rabbit, with special reference to the effects of circulating immune complexes. *Clin. Exp. Immunol.*, **44**, 433–9.

Lockwood, C. M. *et al.* (1979) Reversal of impaired splenic function in patients with nephritis or vasculitis (or both) by plasma exchange. *N. Engl. J. Med.*, **300**, 524–30.

MacLennan, I. C. M. *et al.* (1982) The lymphocytes of splenic marginal zones: A distinct B-cell lineage. *Immunology Today*, **3**, 305–7.

Malynn, B. A. and Wortis, H. H. (1984) Role of antigen-specific B cells in the induction of SRBC-specific T cell proliferation. *J. Immunol.*, **132**, 2253–8.

Mannik, M. (1980) Physicochemical and functional relationships of immune complexes. *J. Invest. Dermatol.*, **74**, 333–8.

Mitchell, J. (1972), Antigens in immunity. XVII. The migration of antigen-binding, bone-marrow-derived and thymus-derived spleen cells in mice. *Immunology*, **22**, 231–245.

Mitchell, J. and Abbot, A. (1971) Antigens in immunity. XVI. A light and electron microscope study of antigen localization in the rat spleen. *Immunology*, **21**, 207–24.

Murray, L. J., Swerdlow, S. H. and Habeshaw, J. A. (1984) Distribution of B lymphocyte subsets in normal lymphoid tissue. *Clin. Exp. Immunol.*, **56**, 399–406.

Najjar, V. A. (1974) The physiological role of γ-globulin. *Adv. Enzymol. D*, **41**, 1229–78.

Najjar V. A. and Nishioka, K. (1970) Tuftsin–a physiological phagocytosis stimulating peptide. *Nature*, **228**, 672–3.

Namikawa, R. *et al.* (1986) Ontogenic development of T and B cells and non-lymphoid cells in the white pulp of human spleen. *Immunology*, **57**, 61–9.

Nieuwenhuis, P. and Ford, W. L. (1976) Comparative migration of B- and T-lymphocytes in the rat spleen and lymph node. *Cell. Immunol.*, **23**, 254–67.

Nishioka, K. (1979) Anti-tumour effect of the physiological tetrapeptide tuftsin. *Br. J. Cancer*, **39**, 342–5.

Nishioka, K. *et al.* (1972) The characteristics, isolation and synthesis of the phagocytosis-stimulating peptide tuftsin. *Biochem. Biophys. Res. Commun.*, **47**, 172–9.

Nishioka, K. *et al.* (1973) Characteristics and isolation of the phagocytosis stimulating peptide-Tuftsin. *Biochim. Biophys. Acta*, **310**, 217–29.

Nossal, G. J. V. *et al.* (1966) Antigens in immunity. XII. Antigen trapping in the spleen. *Int. Arch. Allergy*, **29**, 368–83.

Nusrat, A. R. *et al.* (1988) Properties of isolated red pulp macrophages from mouse spleen. *J. Exp. Med.*, **168**, 1505–10.

Okumura, K., Hayakawa, K. and Tada, T. (1982) Cell-to-cell interaction controlled by immunoglobulin genes. Role of Thy-1⁻, Lyt-1⁺, Ig⁺ (B) cell in allotype-restricted antibody production. *J. Exp. Med.*, **156**, 443–53.

Pabst, R. (1988) The spleen in lymphocyte migration. *Immunology Today*, **9**, 43-5.

Piguet, P-F. *et al.* (1981) Post-thymic T lymphocyte maturation during ontogenesis. *J. Exp. Med.*, **154**, 581–93.

Romball, C. G. and Weigle, W. O. (1977) Splenic role in the regulation of immune responses. *Cell. Immunol.*, **34**, 376–84.

Ron, Y. *et al.* (1981) Defective induction of antigen-reactive proliferating T cells in B cell-deprived mice. *Eur. J. Immunol.*, **11**, 964–8.

Ruben, F. L. *et al.* (1984) Antibody responses to meningococcal polysaccharide vaccine in adults without a spleen. *Am. J. Med.*, **76**, 115–21.

Ryan, F. P. *et al.* (1981) Impaired immunity in patients with inflammatory bowel disease; the response to intravenous ØX174. *Gut*, **22**, 187–9.

Schwartz, P. E. *et al.* (1982) Postsplenectomy sepsis and mortality in adults. *J. Am. Med. Assoc.*, **248**, 2279–83.

Sidman, C. L. *et al.* (1986) Production of immunoglobulin isotypes in Ly-1⁺ B cells in viable Motheaten and normal mice. *Science*, **232**, 1423–5.

Sprent, J. (1973) Circulating T and B lymphocytes of the mouse. I. Migratory properties. *Cell. Immunol.*, **7**, 10–39.

Stein, H. *et al.* (1980) Immunohistologic analysis of the organization of normal lymphoid tissue and non-Hodgkin's lymphomas. *J. Histochem. Cytochem.*, **28**, 746–60.

Sullivan, J. L. *et al.* (1978) Immune response after splenectomy. *Lancet*, **i**, 178–81.

Sy, M-S. *et al.* (1977) A splenic requirement for the generation of suppressor T cells. *J. Immunol.*, **119**, 2095–9.

Tedder, T. F., Clement, L. T. and Cooper, M. D. (1985) Development and distribution of a human B cell subpopulation identified by the HB-4 monoclonal antibody. *J. Immunol.*, **134**, 1539–44.

Till, J. E. and McCulloch, E. A. (1961) A direct measurement of the radiation sensitivity of normal mouse bone marrow cells. *Radiation Res.*, **14**, 213–22.

Timens, W. and Poppema, S. (1985) Lymphocyte compartments in human spleen. An immunohistologic study in normal spleens and noninvolved spleens in Hodgkin's disease. *Am. J. Pathol.*, **120**, 443–54.

van den Oord, K. K. *et al.* (1985) Immature sinus histiocytosis. Light- and electron-microscopic features, immunologic phenotype, and relationship with marginal zone lymphocytes. *Am. J. Pathol.*, **118**, 266–77.

van den Oord, J. J., de Wolf-Peeters, C. and Desmet, V. J. (1986) The marginal zone in the human reactive lymph node. *Am. J. Clin. Pathol.*, **86**, 475–9.

van Furth, R. and Diesselhoff-den Dulk, M. M. C. (1984) Dual origin of mouse spleen macrophages. *J. Exp. Med.*, **160**, 1273–83.

van Rooijen, N. and Kors, N. (1985), Mechanism of follicular trapping: double immunocytochemical evidence for a contribution of locally produced antibodies in follicular trapping of immune complexes. *Immunology*, 55, 31–4.

Van Vliet, E., Melis, M. and van Ewijk, W. (1985) Marginal zone macrophages in the mouse spleen identified by a monoclonal antibody. Anatomical correlation with a B cell subpopulation. *J. Histochem. Cytochem.*, 33, 40–4.

Van Wyck, D. B., Witte, M. H. and Witte, C. L. (1986) Compensatory spleen growth and protective function in rats. *Clin. Sci.*, 71, 573–9.

Velardi, A. *et al.* (1986) Functional analysis of cloned germinal center CD4$^+$ cells with natural killer cell-related features. Divergence from typical helper cells. *J. Immunol.*, 137, 2808–13.

Waksman, B. H., Arnason, B. G. and Jankovic', B. D. (1962) Role of the thymus in immune reactions in rats. III. Changes in the lymphoid organs of thymectomized rats. *J. Exp. Med.*, 116, 187–206.

Wasi, C., Wasi, P. and Thongcharoen, P. (1971) Serum immunoglobulin levels in thalassaemia and the effects of splenectomy. *Lancet*, ii, 237–9.

Woodruff, J. J., Clarke, L. M. and Chin, Y. H. (1987) Specific cell-adhesion mechanisms determining migration pathways of recirculating lymphocytes. *Annu. Rev. Immunol.*, 5, 201–22.

Wu, C-Y. and Lance, E. M. (1974) Immunoregulation by spleen-seeking thymocytes. II. Role in the response to sheep erythrocytes. *Cell. Immunol.*, 13, 1–11.

Yousaf, N., Howard, J. C. and Williams, B. D. (1986a) Studies in the rat of antibody-coated and N-ethylmaleimide-treated erythrocyte clearance by the spleen. I. Effects of *in vivo* complement activation. *Immunology*, 59, 75–9.

Yousaf, N., Howard, J. C. and Williams, B. D. (1986b) Studies in the rat of antibody-coated and N-ethylmaleimide-treated erythrocyte clearance by the spleen. II. Effects of immune complex infusion. *Immunology*, 59, 81–5.

Yousaf, N., Howard, J. C. and Williams, B. D. (1986c) Studies in cobra venom factor treated rats of antibody coated erythrocyte clearance by the spleen: differential influence of red blood cell antigen number on the inhibitory effects of immune complexes on Fc dependent clearance. *Clin. Exp. Immunol.*, 66, 654–60.

THE ROLE OF THE SPLEEN IN HEMOSTASIS AND COAGULATION

W. Jean Dodds

6.1 INTRODUCTION

The reticuloendothelial system, particularly in the liver and spleen, was first implicated in storage, synthesis and regulation of hemostatic components nearly 40 years ago (Penick *et al.*, 1951; Graham *et al.*, 1951; Pool and Spaet, 1954; Webster *et al.*, 1975). An intensive period of research followed and focused on the sites of synthesis of plasma antihemophilic factor (factor VIII) and Christmas factor (factor IX) (Dodds, 1973; Dodds and Hoyer, 1974a; Webster *et al.*, 1975; Bloom, 1979), and the splenic storage of platelets (Penny, Rozenberg and Firkin, 1966). This effort was temporarily abandoned in the late 1970s to await development of the more advanced biotechnology, biochemistry and molecular genetics that have generated definitive answers. Today, the structural genes coding for factors VIII and IX and von Willebrand's factor have been isolated and cloned by recombinant techniques. The respective proteins have been sequenced and cDNA probes have been used to locate and identify the missing or mutant amino acids or sequences in a variety of mutants of hemophilia A and B and von Willebrand's disease (Davie, 1987). The following review summarizes data collected during this four-decade period on the relationship of the spleen to hemostasis and thrombosis.

6.2 COAGULATION FACTORS

6.2.1 FACTOR VIII (ANTIHEMOPHILIC FACTOR)

The search for the site of factor VIII synthesis began in earnest in the early 1950s (Penick *et al.*, 1970; Dodds and Hoyer, 1974a; Bloom, 1979). Investigators at the University of North Carolina utilized normal dogs exposed to total body irradiation, chloroform and carbon tetrachloride (Penick *et al.*, 1951; Graham *et al.*, 1951), and hemophilic dogs (Graham *et al.*, 1951) to show that factor VIII levels were not significantly affected by marrow failure and hepatotoxins. By contrast, platelet counts were severely depressed and prothrombin utilization was impaired. Parallel studies by Pool and Spaet (1954) showed that rats treated with ethionine but not pancreatectomy had decreased factor VIII levels, thereby suggesting the reticuloendothelial system as a possible source of factor VIII. When the chloroform toxicity studies were repeated with an improved method of measuring factor VIII levels, decreased levels were observed. However, blockade of reticuloendothelial phagocytic function with methyl palmitate failed to alter factor VIII levels (Penick *et al.*, 1970).

These conflicting data spawned the hypothesis that the spleen was the organ controlling circulating factor VIII levels (Webster *et al.*, 1975; Bloom, 1979). In the early 1960s, hematologists in Great Britain and France observed elevated factor VIII levels following exercise or adrenaline injection (Goudemand *et al.*, 1964; Libre *et al.*, 1968; Rizza and Eipe, 1971), and these effects appeared to be abolished by splenectomy in some (Goudemand *et al.*, 1964; Libre *et al.*, 1968) but not all (Webster *et al.*, 1975; Rizza and Eipe, 1971) studies. When splenectomized normal dogs were cross-circulated with hemophilic dogs (Weaver, Price and Langdell, 1964), the factor VIII levels of the normal dogs dropped to about 50%. Similarly, factor VIII levels in the counterpart intact hemophilic parabiosis rose to about 60%. Splenectomized hemophilic heterozygotes (carrier female dogs) had a transient change in their factor VIII levels from around 50% prior to surgery to as low as 5% afterwards. The normal control dogs treated in a similar fashion showed essentially no change in activity. Thus the spleen was somehow involved in regulating or maintaining factor VIII levels, although it was not the sole source of factor VIII because splenectomy of normal humans or animals did not produce a hemophilic state (Weaver, Price and Langdell, 1964; Webster *et al.*, 1975).

Pool (1966) provided direct evidence of the prominent role of the spleen in controlling factor VIII levels. In her studies, extracts of splenic (but not other) tissue slices generated factor VIII activity. The following year two other groups independently corroborated her findings using isolated organ perfusion techniques (Norman *et al.*, 1967; Webster *et al.*, 1967b). This technology was adopted by our own laboratory and by others from the late 1960s to the mid-1970s (Dodds, 1969a, b; Kelly, Pechet and Eiseman, 1970; Dodds and Hoyer, 1974a, b; Webster *et al.*, 1975). The studies by Webster and colleagues at the University of North Carolina showed that the amount of factor VIII activity produced by perfusion of normal dog spleens with hemophilic dog blood was about five times greater than that observed for hepatic perfusion (Webster *et al.*, 1967b, 1975). Very

little activity was generated by perfusion of the hind limb and none was obtained from normal perfused lungs or kidneys or hemophilic dog spleens. Norman *et al.* (1967) in Boston perfused normal pig spleens with hemophilic human blood and generated about 18% of normal activity after four hours; activity was also produced from perfused livers. In 1968, the North Carolina group showed that peptidase extracts of dog kidneys contained factor VIII activity, and suggested that a monomeric form of the protein was synthesized by this organ (Webster *et al.*, 1975).

Our laboratory, meanwhile, had developed the isolated perfused rabbit organ model (Dodds, 1969a) and demonstrated production of both factors VIII and IX activity by the liver, spleen and kidney. The appearance of these activities was greatest in the spleen and was prevented by addition of inhibitors of protein synthesis (puromycin, cycloheximide, actinomycin D) to the perfusate. The production of clotting factor activity by the liver and spleen was regulated by negative feedback (Dodds, 1973; Dodds and Hoyer, 1974a, b), and hepatic perfusates contained independent stimulators of the factors VIII and IX produced by perfused spleens (Dodds, 1969b, 1973). These findings indicated that the liver produced specific precursor proteins that enhanced splenic synthesis and/or release of factors VIII and IX. The factor VIII stimulator had a molecular weight between 115 000 and 300 000 daltons, whereas the factor IX stimulator was smaller, around 30 000–100 000 daltons (Dodds *et al.*, 1972). These data are compatible with what is known today about the sizes of the structural subunits of each of these coagulation proteins (Davie, 1987).

Kelly, Pechet and Eiseman (1970) reported that perfused pig spleens generated puromycin-sensitive factor VIII activity with a half-life of about 10 hours. This was followed by the work of Ponn *et al.*, (1971) demonstrating that cultured rabbit splenic macrophages produced factor VIII activity for up to nine days. Similar culture studies with leukocytes and fibroblasts recovered a factor VIII-like activity but it was not decreased by incubation with antifactor VIII antibody (Dodds, 1973). This procoagulant activity was later shown to be tissue factor which shortened the endpoint in clotting assays (Webster *et al.*, 1975).

The discovery that procoagulant activity generated by tissue culture systems or perfused organs could reflect production of non-specific thromboplastic material, or activation in the test system or assay, confirmed long-standing concerns plaguing this area of research. Thus, the question of whether the coagulation activity produced by *in vitro* systems represented *de novo* biosynthesis or storage and release of preformed activity remained unresolved.

More definitive studies of the site(s) of factor VIII (and factor IX) synthesis involved organ transplantation (Webster, Penick and Mandel, 1973; Webster *et al.*, 1975). Orthotopic and heterotopic transplantation of liver, spleen, kidney and bone marrow were performed. These studies showed that the liver was the primary organ site of factors VIII and IX production, and that extrahepatic production of factor VIII but not factor IX also occurred. This conclusion was firmly established when transplantation of livers from dogs with either hemophilia A (factor VIII deficiency) or B (factor IX deficiency) into normal dogs produced a reduction in circulating factor VIII levels to about 20% of normal but not lower, whereas factor IX levels became less than 1% after the counterpart hemophilia B transplant. Furthermore, neither the kidney nor bone marrow transplants were able to correct the defect in hemophilic dogs.

With respect to the spleen, transplants were performed between normal and hemophilic dogs and normal and hemophilic human patients. The first of these landmark experiments was undertaken by Webster *et al.* (1967a), whereby normal dog spleens were transplanted into two hemophilic dogs that survived for only 52 and 72 hours respectively. During this time factor VIII activity increased from <1% prior to transplantation to 5–10% in one animal and 3–7% in the other. Because of the short dura-

tion of these preliminary studies, a distinction between release of stored factor VIII and new biosynthesis could not be made. However, Norman, Covelli and Sise (1968) successfully transplanted normal spleens into three dogs with a more mild form of hemophilia, and one survived for six months. The authors reported sustained factor VIII activity based on assays using human rather than canine plasma controls and concluded that the spleen synthesized factor VIII. This was followed rapidly by seven more studies in dogs (Marchioro *et al.*, 1969; McKee *et al.*, 1970; Penick *et al.*, 1970; Sise *et al.*, 1970; Webster *et al.*, 1971; Hampton *et al.*, 1973; Groth *et al.*, 1974) and one in humans (Hathaway *et al.*, 1969) that failed to demonstrate anything beyond a transient rise in factor VIII activity. Thus, splenic transplants in hemophilic recipients released sufficient stored factor VIII to maintain hemostasis during the postoperative period, but levels never exceeded 20% and were not sustained. It was concluded that the spleen serves as a storage site of factor VIII which is released at times of stress or hemostatic demand (Webster *et al.*, 1975).

Following this work, other lymphatic tissues (vascularized lymph node grafts) have been transplanted into hemophilic dogs with short-term graft viability and transient factor VIII production (Groth *et al.*, 1974). Similarly, human splenic cell suspensions or homogenates failed to sustain factor VIII production when administered to hemophiliacs (Hathaway *et al.*, 1969). The disappointing results overall of these complicated and expensive experiments caused this approach to be abandoned in the mid-1970s.

Interest in identifying the cell site(s) of synthesis of factor VIII has not waned. Since that time Bloom and his colleagues in Wales have localized production of factor VIII to several human tissues by antibody neutralization (Bloom and Giddings, 1972; Bloom, 1979); and recently Kelly, Summerfield and Tuddenham (1984) and Hoyer and Dodds (1985) have detected factor VIII immunologically in tissue extracts and perfused organs from the liver, spleen, lung, and kidney of guinea pigs. Additional evidence that factor VIII is synthesized by several different tissues comes from work of Van der Kwast, Stel and Veerman (1983) and Wion, Kelly and Summerfield (1985) who used specific immunohistochemical staining techniques and mRNA to localize factor VIII in human hepatic sinusoidal endothelial cells, and mononuclear, non-lymphoid cells of the spleen, lung, and lymph nodes.

In conclusion, the cell source of plasma factor VIII is still not established. Several cell types and organs, including the spleen, are still considered to be likely candidates. Interestingly, synthesis of von Willebrand factor, the companion protein of the circulating plasma factor VIII complex, is known to take place in endothelial cells and megakaryocytes (Davie, 1987). It seems highly probable that the 'missing link' with respect to antihemophilic factor synthesis will be supplied in the near future.

6.2.2 FACTOR IX (CHRISTMAS FACTOR)

Interest in the site of factor IX synthesis developed in parallel to that of factor VIII, but was not as actively pursued because the mutation of hemophilia B is much less common than that of hemophilia A in man and other species (Webster *et al.*, 1975). Early observations in the late 1950s from studies of coumarin-induced deficiency states and hepatic disease implicated the liver as the major site of factor IX production. Factor IX was produced by rat liver slices *in vitro*, and by isolated perfused rat and rabbit livers (Dodds, 1969a; Webster *et al.*, 1975) and rabbit kidneys and spleens (Dodds, 1969a). The latter studies performed in our laboratory suggested that organs other than the liver could be involved in synthesis, release, and regulation of factor IX, as was shown to pertain to factor VIII and discussed earlier. A similar negative feedback control of factor IX production in perfused organs was found, and an independent hepatic stimulator of factor IX production from perfused spleens was identified (Dodds, 1969b;

Dodds *et al.*, 1972; Dodds and Hoyer, 1974a, b).

The evidence for extrahepatic production of factor IX has come solely from isolated organ perfusion and tissue extraction studies. Failure to confirm these findings by subsequent organ transplantation studies between normal and hemophilia B dogs (Webster *et al.*, 1975) indicates that the coagulation activity produced in these *in vitro* systems resulted from release of preformed activity in tissue stores.

Webster *et al.* (1975) showed that two normal canine recipients of livers from hemophilia B dogs could not maintain their circulating factor IX levels after transplantation. Levels fell to less than 1% of normal and remained undetectable for the length of the experiment (up to 53 days). Thus the liver is the sole source of factor IX, and the cell site of synthesis is likely to be the hepatocyte.

6.2.3 OTHER COAGULATION FACTORS

Most of the other plasma coagulation factors are synthesized solely in the liver with the exception of factors V and XIII (fibrin stabilizing factor). At one time factor V was believed to be produced by the liver but influenced by the spleen, because the low circulating factor V levels of cirrhotics rebounded if the patients were splenectomized for associated hypersplenism (Vergoz *et al.*, 1967). Current information has identified the sites of factor V production as endothelial cells, megakaryocytes, and hepatocytes (Davie, 1987). Factor XIII is synthesized by hepatocytes, peripheral blood monocytes, and monocytes and macrophages from other tissues (Weisberg *et al.*, 1987).

6.3 PLATELETS

With respect to hemostasis and thrombosis, the spleen has been assigned many roles in the control of platelet kinetics in health and disease (Penny, Rozenberg and Firkin, 1966; Shulman and Jordan, 1987). In hypersplenism, thrombocytopenia has been attributed to excessive platelet sequestration, inhibition of thrombopoiesis, and pooling within the enlarged organ (Aster, 1965; Penny, Rozenberg and Firkin, 1966). In the latter study more than two decades ago, the increase in platelet pool size in splenomegaly was the sole reason for thrombocytopenia in most of their patients. In myeloproliferative disorders, on the other hand, the spleen may be the site of platelet production.

Plateletpheresis in normal and asplenic humans and animals has been performed for therapeutic reasons and to evaluate platelet reserve. The exchangeable platelet pool in the spleen has been calculated to be about one-third of the total number of circulating platelets, by this and other techniques using radiolabelled platelets (Shulman and Jordan, 1987). Platelet production is normal or even slightly enhanced in asplenic subjects after plateletpheresis. However, temporary platelet pooling after platelet depletion may delay entrance of newly formed platelets into the circulation. In rabbits and dogs, the larger younger platelets are preferentially retained by the spleen, whereas after splenectomy the number of large platelets circulating is increased (Shulman and Jordan, 1987).

Platelets leaving the circulation permanently during physiological turnover are taken up equally by the liver and spleen. However, the relative number of platelets sequestered by each organ in pathologic situations varies with the degree of platelet injury (Shulman and Jordan, 1987).

Platelet survival is usually normal or only slightly reduced in the thrombocytopenia of hypersplenism. The nearly normal total platelet mass in the presence of low peripheral platelet counts suggests that total mass rather than concentration is the factor controlling feedback regulation of thrombopoiesis (Shulman and Jordan, 1987).

Recent studies of platelet kinetics suggest that splenic pooling is probably caused by delay during the transit of platelets through the spleen. Splenic transit time of platelets is about 10 minutes and appears to be independent of splenic size or blood flow (Peters et al., 1980).

The thrombocytopenia of hypersplenism may or may not be of sufficient severity to cause spontaneous bruising or bleeding. Conversely, the thrombocytosis of myeloproliferative disorders can produce either bleeding or thrombotic tendencies, the mechanism of which is still poorly understood (Shulman and Jordan, 1987).

6.4 FIBRINOLYTIC COMPONENTS

The major precursor zymogen of the fibrinolytic system is plasminogen. Despite years of intensive studies in animals (Highsmith, 1980), identification of the specific cell sites of plasminogen synthesis in humans was a recent event (Robbins, 1987). Both the liver and kidney are sites of plasminogen synthesis in humans and other species, although considerable species variation exists and multiple sites have been implicated in plasminogen storage and regulation (Highsmith, 1980).

Eosinophils, especially of the bone marrow, and other types of granulocytes have been reported in early studies to produce and release plasma and tissue plasminogen and its activators (Shulman and Jordan, 1987). These findings could not be substantiated, however, by more recent experiments using sophisticated molecular techniques.

Highsmith (1980) reported the kidney to be the primary source of plasminogen following acute depletion studies in cats. As in the earlier work with granulocytes, the spleen was not among other tissues implicated in the metabolic regulation or fate of plasminogen.

6.5 ANTICOAGULANTS (COAGULATION AND FIBRINOLYTIC INHIBITORS)

Of the six major protease inhibitors of blood, four have inhibitory action against one or more clotting factors. These are antithrombin III, CI activator, α_2-macroglobulin, and α_1-antitrypsin; each is synthesized in the liver. The spleen is not known to play a role in the synthesis, regulation or metabolic fate of the inhibitors.

In some patients with systemic lupus erythematosus, the spleen has been implicated in the production of the thromboplastic globulin known as the 'lupus anticoagulant' (Walsh and Schmaier, 1987).

6.6 CLINICAL MANIFESTATIONS

6.6.1 BLEEDING

As the spleen is not a primary organ for production of coagulation proteins, depletion of clotting activity and bleeding are not usually associated with splenic disease or removal. The significant role of the spleen as a source of platelet reserve, however, places patients at risk of bleeding when thrombocytopenia becomes moderate to severe in the absence of a spleen or normal splenic function (Shulman and Jordan, 1987). Similarly the thrombocytopenia associated with hypersplenism may be clinically expressed as a bleeding tendency if some other factor or condition compromising hemostasis is also present (such as von Willebrand's disease, coumadin therapy, hyperfibrinolysis of cryptogenic splenomegaly).

In immune thrombocytopenic states, the spleen is often the focal organ of platelet destruction and splenectomy may be advisable. While this may well induce remission of the immunologic disorder, removal of the spleen has also taken away the splenic platelet pool as a future reserve to protect the patient in the event of recurrence (Penny, Rozenberg and Firkin, 1966).

6.6.2 THROMBOSIS

Thrombosis is a more common manifestation than bleeding during the course of splenic disease. Myeloproliferative disorders, hypersplenism, and other neoplasms, especially of hemato-

logical or vascular origin (lymphoma–leukemia complex, hemangiosarcomas), that involve the spleen are often associated with a thrombotic tendency (Colman *et al.*, 1987).

REFERENCES

Aster, R. H. (1965) Splenic platelet pooling as a cause of 'hypersplenic' thrombocytopenia. *Trans. Assoc. Am. Physicians*, 78, 362–73.

Bloom, A. L. (1979) The biosynthesis of factor VIII. *Clin. Haematol.*, 8, 53–77.

Bloom, A. L. and Giddings, J. C. (1972) Factor VIII (antihaemophilic factor) in tissues detected by antibody neutralization. *Br. J. Haematol.*, 23, 157–65.

Colman, R. W. *et al.* (eds) (1987) Section A. Pathogenesis of thrombosis. in *Hemostasis and Thrombosis*, 2nd edn. Lippincott Company, Philadelphia, pp. 1063–184.

Davie, E. W. (1987) The blood coagulation factors: their cDNA's, genes, and expression. in *Hemostasis and Thrombosis*, 2nd edn (eds R. W. Colman, J. Hirch, V. J. Marder and E. W. Salzman), Lippincott Company, Philadelphia, pp. 242–67.

Dodds, W. J. (1969a) Storage, release and synthesis of coagulation factors in isolated perfused organs. *Am. J. Physiol.*, 217, 879–83.

Dodds, W. J. (1969b) Hepatic influence of splenic synthesis of coagulation factors in isolated perfused organs. *Science*, 166, 882–3.

Dodds, W. J. (1973) Organ perfusion studies in hemophilia. in *Haemophilia* (eds F. Ala and K. W. E. Denson), Excerpta Medica, Amsterdam, pp. 39–49.

Dodds, W. J. and Hoyer, L. W. (1974a) Factors regulating the production of coagulation activities in perfused organs. in *Proceedings, National Conference on Research Animals in Medicine*, National Institutes of Health, Washington, DC, pp. 463–72.

Dodds, W. J. and Hoyer, L. W. (1974b) Coagulation activities in perfused organs: regulation by addition of animal plasmas. *Br. J. Haematol.*, 26, 497–509.

Dodds, W. J. *et al.* (1972) Independent stimulators regulating the production of coagulation factors VIII and IX in perfused spleens. *J. Lab. Clin. Med.*, 79, 770–7.

Goudemand, M. *et al.* (1964) Les variations du taux de factor VIII au cours de l'exercise musculaire. *Nouv. Rev. Fr. Hematol.*, 4, 315–19.

Graham, J. B. *et al.* (1951) Assay of plasma antihemophilic activity in normal and heterozygous (hemophilic) and prothrombinopenic dogs. *Proc. Soc. Exp. Biol. Med.*, **77**, 294–6.

Groth, C. G. *et al.* (1974) Correction of coagulation in the hemophilic dog by transplantation of lymphatic tissue. *Surgery*, **75**, 725–33.

Hampton, J. W. *et al.* (1973) Canine hemophilia in beagles: genetics, site of factor VIII synthesis, and attempts at experimental therapy. in *Haemophilia* (eds F. Ala and K. W. E. Denson), Excerpta Medica, Amsterdam, pp. 26–32.

Hathaway, W. E. *et al.* (1969) Attempted spleen transplants in classical hemophilia. *Transplantation*, **7**, 73–5.

Highsmith, R. F. (1980) Origin of plasminogen and metabolic fate. in *Fibrinolysis* (eds D. L. Kline and K. N. H. Reddy) CRC Press, Boca Raton, FL, pp. 151–64.

Hoyer, L. W. and Dodds, W. J. (1985) Unpublished observations.

Kelly, D. A., Summerfield, J. A. and Tuddenham, E. G. D. (1984) Localization of factor VIIIC:antigen in guinea pig tissues and isolated liver cell fractions. *Br. J. Haematol.*, **56**, 535–43.

Kelly, G., Pechet, L. and Eiseman, B. (1970) Synthesis of antihemophilic globulin by the isolated perfused spleen. *Surg. Gyn. Obst.*, **131**, 473–85.

Libre, E. P. *et al.* (1968) Relationships between spleen, platelets, and factor VIII levels. *Blood*, **31**, 358–68.

Marchioro, T. L. *et al.* (1969) Hemophilia: role of organ homografts. *Science*, **163**, 188–90.

McKee, P. A. *et al.* (1970) Effect of the spleen on canine factor VIII levels. *J. Lab. Clin. Med.*, **75**, 391–402.

Norman, J. C., Covelli, V. H. and Sise, H. S. (1968) Transplantation of the spleen: experimental cure of hemophilia. *Surgery*, **64**, 1–14.

Norman, J. C. *et al.* (1967) Antihemophilic factor release by perfused liver and spleen: relationship to hemophilia. *Science*, **158**, 1060–1.

Penick, G. D. *et al.* (1951) Plasma antihemophilic activity following total body irradiation. *Proc. Soc. Exp. Biol. Med.*, **78**, 732–4.

Penick, G. D. *et al.* (1970) Organ transplantation in animal hemophilia. in *Hemophilia and New Hemorrhagic States* (ed. K. M. Brinkhous), University of North Carolina Press, Chapel Hill, pp. 97–105.

Penny, R., Rozenberg, M. C. and Firkin, B. G. (1966) The splenic platelet pool. *Blood*, **27**, 1–16.

Peters, A. M. *et al.* (1980) Use of [111]indium-labelled platelets to measure spleen function. *Br. J. Haematol.*, **46**, 587–93.

Ponn, R. B. *et al.* (1971) The role of the splenic macrophage in antihemophilic factor (factor VIII) synthesis. *Arch. Surg.*, **103**, 398–401.

Pool, J. G. (1966) Antihemophilic globulin (AHG, factor VIII) activity in spleen. *Fed. Proc.*, **25**, 317.

Pool, J. G. and Spaet, T. H. (1954) Ethionine-induced depression of plasma antihemophilic globulin in the rat. *Proc. Soc. Exp. Biol. Med.*, **87**, 54–7.

Rizza, C. R. and Eipe, J. (1971) Exercise, factor VIII and the spleen. *Br. J. Haematol.*, **20**, 629–35.

Robbins, K. C. (1987) The plasminogen–plasmin enzyme system. in *Hemostasis and Thrombosis*, 2nd edn (eds. R. W. Colman, J. Hirsh, V. J. Marder and E. W. Salzman), Lippincott Company, Philadelphia, pp. 162–81.

Shulman, N. R. and Jordan, J. V., Jr (1987) Platelet kinetics. in *Hemostasis and Thrombosis*, 2nd edn (eds R. W. Colman, J. Hirsch, V. J. Marder and E. W. Salzman), Lippincott Company, Philadelphia, pp. 431–51.

Sise, H. S. *et al.* (1970) Potential of the transplanted spleen in canine hemophilia. in *Hemophilia and New Hemorrhagic States* (ed. K. M. Brinkhous), University of North Carolina Press, Chapel Hill, pp. 106–15.

Van der Kwast, T. H., Stel, H. V. and Veerman, E. C. I. (1983) Localization of VIIIC Ag using different monoclonal antibodies against VIIIC. *Thromb. Haemost.*, **50**, 17.

Vergoz, D. *et al.* (1967) Variations du facteur V au cours des splenectomies dans les cirrhoses. *Rev. Fr. d'Etudes Clin. Biol.*, **12**, 725–31.

Walsh, P. N. and Schmaier, A. H. (1987) Platelet-coagulant protein interactions. in *Hemostasis and Thrombosis*, 2nd edn (eds R. W. Colman, J. Hirsh, V. J. Marder and E. W. Salzman), Lippincott Company, Philadelphia, pp. 689–709.

Webster, W. P., Penick, G. D. and Mandel, S. R. (1973) Orthotopic and heterotopic organ transplantation in hemophilia A. in *Haemophilia* (eds F. Ala and K. W. E. Denson), Excerpta Medica, Amsterdam, pp. 33–8.

Weaver, R. A., Price, R. E. and Langdell, R. D. (1964) Antihemophilic factor in cross-circulated normal and hemophilic dogs. *Am. J. Physiol.*, **206**, 335–7.

Webster, W. P. *et al.* (1967a) Allotransplantation of spleen in hemophilia. *NC. Med. J.*, **28**, 505–7.

Webster, W. P. *et al.* (1967b) Release of factor VIII (antihaemophilic factor) from perfused organs and tissues. *Nature*, **213**, 1146–7.

Webster, W. P. *et al.* (1971) Plasma factor VIII

synthesis and control as revealed by canine organ transplantation. *Am. J. Physiol.*, **220**, 1147–54.

Webster, W. P. *et al.* (1975) Biosynthesis of factors VIII and IX: organ transplantation and perfusion studies. in *Handbook of Hemophilia,* Part I (eds K. M. Brinkhous and H. C. Hemker) Excerpta Medica, Amsterdam, pp. 149–63.

Weisberg, L. J. *et al.* (1987) Identification of normal peripheral blood monocytes and liver as sites of synthesis of coagulation factor XIII a-chain. *Blood,* **70**, 579–82.

Wion, K. L., Kelly, D. and Summerfield, J. A. (1985) Distribution of factor VIII mRNA and antigen in human liver and other tissues. *Nature,* **317**, 725–8.

PART TWO
CHARACTERISTICS OF THE DISORDERED SPLEEN

THE PATHOLOGY OF THE SPLEEN

Stebbins B. Chandor

7.1 INTRODUCTION

The human spleen was long accepted by pathologists as Galen's 'organ of mystery', in that it was rarely examined in life, rarely 'normal' at the time of death, and rarely the primary site of a disease process. Consequently it has received no more than a modicum of attention: as long as two centuries ago, the classic text on morbid anatomy by Mathew Baillie (1793) proved to be the forerunner of most pathology texts in giving the spleen only a few pages of description. Nevertheless, Dr Baillie described alterations in its surface appearance, including hyperemia, adhesions and cartilage formation, together with the more obvious changes in the general texture and size of the organ itself. He provided an accurate description of acute splenitis; conversely, he pointed out that when the spleen was found to be very hard, this was to be considered the result of congestion rather than scarring, since the scirrhous changes characteristic of scarring in other organs were not seen in the spleen. Enlargement was found more commonly than in other viscera, and Baillie pointed out that the large size of the spleen caused more clinical problems than the primary pathological process itself. Among rarer conditions of the spleen he noted cysts and stony concretions, and 'wasting' of the spleen. It is evident that by 1793 many of the abnormalities described in today's texts had already been recognized, and in part their significance realized.

In a recent edition of a classic text on surgical pathology, the chapter on the spleen is still relatively brief, consisting of only 21 pages of a total of more than 1700 (Rosai, 1986). In a major textbook of general pathology, only eight pages are dedicated to the organ, of which two are of references (Robbins, Cotran and Kumar, 1989). In monographs on malignant lymphomas, the organ is frequently omitted from the index, and texts dealing with immunodeficiency diseases may have only 'splenomegaly' as a specific reference to the spleen.

The third edition of one of the more complete manuals of laboratory immunology refers to the spleen only once, and then only to list the types of lymphocytes found in the organ (Rose, Friedman and Fahey, 1986); likewise a text on pathophysiology has eight pages devoted to the spleen (Sodeman and Sodeman, 1979).

The fact that the organ is rarely identified as the primary site of disease has made it necessary to study splenic pathology by referring extensively to other disciplines, and especially by the study of other organs involved primarily with its disease processes. In this context it is of interest that a recent algorithmic approach to the determination of the etiology of splenomegaly makes no mention of the examination of the organ directly, but does recommend the biopsy of several other organs as an integral part of the evaluation (Eichner and Whitfield, 1981). However, in each of the last three decades there has been an attempt to bring together the pathology of the spleen under a single cover (Blaustein, 1963; Macpherson, Richmond and Stuart, 1973; Wolf and Neiman, 1988). These have made it clear that splenic pathology is of considerable breadth and is in some respects unique; consequently this chapter will not attempt a comprehensive coverage, as much of significance is included in later chapters to which reference can be made for additional discussion of individual subjects.

7.2   PATHOLOGIC EXAMINATION OF THE SPLEEN

Pathologic examination of the spleen requires a systematic technique such as that outlined in detail by Schmidt (1983). First, the weight and size need to be measured and compared with normal values, which vary both with age and sex of the subject. Studies through the years have shown considerable variation in the weight of the spleen in a normal adult population, with one recent study showing a range from 35 g in black females to 280 g in white males (Myers and Segal, 1974; see section 7.3). As a consequence, pathological variations in size, suggesting atrophy or splenomegaly, must be assessed with some caution; as in the evaluation of any organ, the normal range needs a clear definition.

The normal configuration and external appearance have already been described (Chapter 1). Accessory spleens and lymph nodes should be sought in the hilar fat, which usually accompanies the spleen in its removal from the abdominal cavity. After weighing, measuring, describing the outer surface and removing the fat, the spleen should be sliced with a sharp knife at about l cm intervals across its long axis. Each slice should be viewed and palpated: the cut surface is generally firm with discernible malpighian corpuscles, and a knife blade drawn across the surface scrapes little tissue from the pulp. Much has been written about the need to view spleen slices carefully when screening for involvement by lymphoma; some authorities advocate the use of a meat slicer on thick slices of fixed splenic tissue. Because of the dense cellularity of the spleen, care must be taken to have adequate fixative for the amount of tissue; perfusion with a fixative via the splenic artery may improve examination of the red pulp. Delayed or inadequate fixation may not only compromise routine histology, but immunohistologic studies may be rendered invalid. To prepare for possible added studies, touch imprints should be made from several areas and tissue put aside for frozen section and electron microscopy. The number of blocks to be taken will vary from about four in a spleen not obviously diseased, to several more when there is splenic enlargement or when lesions are noted.

In many parts of the world, splenic aspiration is part of the customary examination of the organ *in vivo* and as Lampert (1983) points out, it is usually a relatively safe procedure with clinical relevance. The smears obtained from the aspirate should be air-dried and stained with Wright-Giemsa (Romanowsky) stains. It may be that with the current interest in fine-needle aspiration, examination of the spleen by aspiration will again become more commonplace.

7.3   THE WEIGHT OF THE NORMAL SPLEEN

Enlargement of the spleen continues to be the most important single finding indicating the probability of abnormality in the organ. For the clinician this is detected principally by showing that the boundaries of the organ by palpation or percussion extend beyond certain defined anatomical limits (sections 10.1.1 and 10.1.2). More accurate estimates of volume can be made radiographically in the living subject, especially by means of computed tomography, using the sum of the areas of contiguous radiographic sections. Alternatively a relatively accurate radiographic assessment of enlargement can again be made in relation to extension of the organ beyond explicit anatomical boundaries (section 17.5.2).

Because of its significance as a screening test for splenic disease, the size of the spleen is also important to the pathologist: unfortunately there is no simple and highly accurate baseline value which is generally applicable to spleen size, although a mean weight between 120 g and 200 g is often quoted (McCormick and Kashgarian, 1965; Whitley, Maynard and Rhyne, 1966; Blendis, Williams and Kreel, 1969; Miale, 1971). Boyd (1933) studied spleen weight at autopsy in subjects dying within one day of terminal trauma: she showed that (1) spleen weight has a non-Gaussian distribution, with markedly positive skewness to the distribution curve, (2) normal weights are higher in men than in women for a specific age group, and (3) there is a definite secular trend, with spleen weight declining with age (Table 7.1).

Myers and Segal (1974) also studied spleen weight in 366 cases of sudden traumatic death, in which disorders affecting spleen weight were, as far as possible, excluded. They confirmed that spleen weight is higher in the young and in males, and also that white subjects have larger spleens than blacks. Representative values are given in Table 7.1.

7.4 NORMAL ANATOMIC VARIATION

The normal spleen may still show evidence of fetal lobulation, which can produce a surface contour resembling infarction; however, infarction can be distinguished by the associated thickening of the capsule. Accessory spleens are present in approximately 10–15% of the population; they are found more commonly in younger subjects, probably because they become less prominent with the involutional effect of ageing on lymphoid tissue. These spleens (spleniculi; splenculi; see Chapter 1) are functional and have a similar morphology to that of the primary spleen; consequently the outcome of therapeutic splenectomy may be compromised if the accessory splenic tissue is not identified and removed at the same time. Splenculi are single in 90% of cases, but they may also be multiple; their more common locations are at the splenic hilum, in the lienorenal

Table 7.1 The weight of the spleen

The Secular Trend in Spleen Weight (g)*		
Age	Males	Females
3rd decade	96–364	65–300
8th decade	66–234	70–195

	Variables in Spleen Weight (g)†			
	Mean age(yrs)	Median weight(g)	Mean weight(g)	Range weight(g)
Males, white	54	140	145	75–245
Males, black	38	100	105	40–200
Females, white	54	115	115	55–190
Females, black	39	90	95	35–190

*From Boyd (1933). The range of weights is given as the 2.5 to 97.5 percentile range in grams.
†From Myers and Segal (1974). The range of weights is given as the 5 to 95 percentile in grams.

and gastrosplenic ligaments, in the jejunal wall and the tail of the pancreas, and in the mesentery and omentum. The term 'polysplenia complex' is sometimes used for the condition when multiple splenculi are present, and as many as ten have been found in one subject. This is sometimes associated with congenital malformations of the cardiovascular and gastrointestinal systems: Raff and Schwartz (1983) describe a case of the complex with duodenal atresia. Cardiovascular anomalies have included dextrocardia, atrial and ventricular septal defects and anomalous pulmonary venous drainage.

The structure of the accessory spleen is virtually identical to that of the principal spleen, with the exception of size (Figure 7.1). The normal structure of the capsule is an important feature distinguishing an accessory spleen from the splenic remnants of splenosis (section 7.5).

Splenic tissue may also be found in ectopic locations due to a more profound disturbance of embryonic development. One rare form is splenogonadal fusion which usually produces splenic tissue in the scrotum; between weeks 5 and 8 of embryonic life the spleen lies close to the mesonephros, and fusion may lead to splenic tissue being drawn inferiorly during descent of the gonad. The condition occurs predominantly in males. Wick and Rife (1981) describe such a case and discuss the clinical significance of the condition, which has two principal variants. In one form, the discontinuous, there is no evident connection between the spleen and the accessory splenic tissue associated with the gonad. In the second type, the continuous, there is a cord-like structure composed of fibrous connective tissue and spleen-like tissue between the spleen and the gonad. Other congenital defects, including micrognathia, testicular ectopia, peromelia and inguinal hernia may also be found. All cases so far described have been on the left side. Rarer forms of fusion may link the spleen to the liver or kidney.

It is especially important to be able to distinguish an accessory spleen present in the scrotum from other masses found at this site: splenculi are firm, blue–red encapsulated masses, and consequently distinctive.

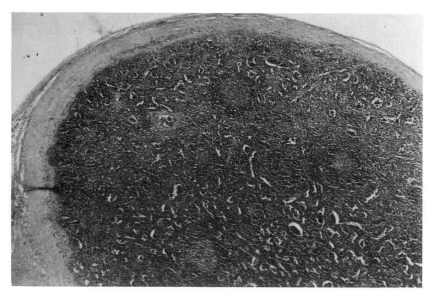

Figure 7.1 Accessory spleen. A well-formed capsule distinguishes this from splenosis. The presence of malpighian corpuscles enables it to be identified, despite similarity to a vascular neoplasm.

7.5 SPLENOSIS

A second form of ectopic splenic tissue results from the regeneration of splenic fragments implanted at suitably supportive sites for growth, usually following traumatic rupture of the organ, but also less commonly following splenic surgery. This appears to be a form of autotransplantation, and its extent is broadly related to the extent of the trauma to the organ (Stovall and Ling, 1988). By far the commonest site of regrowth is the peritoneal cavity, but other cases have involved the pleural and pericardial cavities.

Unlike the accessory spleen, these ectopic nodules are usually multiple, and indeed may be numerous. Generally there is no hilum, and the capsule and fibrous trabecula lack muscle and elastic tissue, so that the individual nodule is less well defined than an accessory spleen. The red pulp is histologically similar to that of the normal spleen, but there is generally a decreased amount of poorly defined white pulp.

There is some residual functional capacity in the nodules of splenosis, and their capacity to take up radionuclide during liver–spleen scanning indicates that they have phagocytic function. However, their capacity to compensate effectively for the loss of the filtration function following splenectomy is in some doubt: their deficiency probably results from abnormality of the vascular structures which evolve during regeneration (see also Chapter 10).

The splenic remnants are rarely symptomatic, but pedunculated forms may undergo torsion with infarction (Fleming, Dickson and Harrison, 1976). Turk, Lipson and Brandt (1988) describe a case of splenosis presenting as a renal mass, and review the further complications of this condition. It is also clear that the nodules of splenosis may be involved in disease processes comparable to those affecting the structurally normal spleen: this is usually seen in relation to the hematological sequelae of hereditary spherocytosis, hypersplenism and immune thrombocytopenia, but it has been observed in other disorders such as malaria.

7.6 PATHOLOGICAL PROCESSES AFFECTING THE SPLEEN

The range of disorders recognized as affecting the spleen is now so wide that it will be necessary to select a relatively short series to illustrate how pathological processes affect the organ. The two principal changes occur (a) in structure, which results usually in enlargement of the organ (splenomegaly), or less commonly in a decrease in size, and (b) in the activity of the organ, which may be expressed either as a decrease ('hyposplenism') or an apparent increase in activity, as in the syndrome of 'hypersplenism' (Chapters 10 and 11). A number of conditions affecting the spleen is shown in Table 7.2, which outlines those which result in enlargement of the organ.

A decrease in spleen size is usually accompanied by a reduction in the expression of splenic function. This may result in diminished efficiency of the filtration of abnormal particles (such as red cells made abnormal by heat treatment, sulfhydryl-blocking agents or warm antibodies), ineffective 'pitting' of intracellular inclusions such as Howell–Jolly bodies, phagocytosis (as shown by the intensity of radionuclide uptake in liver–spleen scanning) and overall by an increased susceptibility to bacterial infection, especially with polysaccharide-encapsulated bacteria.

An increase in spleen size may or may not result in one or more forms of cytopenia in the peripheral blood. If it does, and there is accompanying evidence of adequate production of the relevant blood cells in the bone marrow, then it may be appropriate to presume that 'hypersplenism' is present; this can be confirmed if splenectomy is shown to correct the deficit. It is now clear that 'hypersplenism' is essentially a descriptive term, and does not imply a single specific mechanism: blood cell pooling, increased blood volume and shortened cell lifespans may all contribute in varying degrees to the syndrome. Examples of concurrent changes in the size of the spleen and its functional activity are given in the following sections.

Table 7.2 The causes of splenomegaly*

Infections
1. Acute.
   Infectious mononucleosis; viral hepatitis; septicemia (including tuberculous); salmonelloses; relapsing fever; tularemia; splenic abscess; cytomegalovirus infection; toxoplasmosis.

2. Subacute and chronic.
   Chronic septicemias; tuberculous splenomegaly; leprosy; Yersinia; subacute bacterial endocarditis; brucellosis; syphilis; malaria; leishmaniasis; schistosomiasis; systemic fungal diseases; inflammatory pseudotumor.

Immune proliferations and non-infectious granulomatous disorders
Angioimmunoblastic lymphadenopathy; angiofollicular hyperplasia; systemic lupus erythematosus; rheumatoid arthritis; Still's disease; rheumatic fever; Behçet's syndrome; serum sickness; sarcoidosis; berylliosis; necrotizing splenic granulomas.

Vasculitides
Polyarteritis nodosa; leukocytoclastic angiitis; peliosis.

Congestive splenomegaly
1. Intrahepatic.
   Portal cirrhosis; post-necrotic scarring; biliary cirrhosis; Wilson's disease; hemochromatosis; veno-occlusive disease; congenital fibrosis; bilharziasis.

2. Portal vein obstruction.
   Thrombosis, stenosis, atresia; cavernous malformation; arteriovenous aneurysm; obstructive lesions at porta hepatis.

3. Splenic vein obstruction.
   Thrombosis, stenosis, atresia; angiomatous malformation; obstruction by pancreatic disease, splenic arterial aneurysm and retroperitoneal fibrosis.

4. Hepatic vein occlusion.
   Budd–Chiari syndrome.

5. Cardiac.
   Acute, chronic or recurrent congestive cardiac failure; constrictive pericarditis (Banti's syndrome).

Hematological disorders
1. Hemolytic disorders.
   Hereditary red cell membrane disorders; thalassemia; sickle-thalassemia; sickle cell disease (early stages); hemoglobin-SC disease.

2. Myeloproliferative disorders.
   Primary (agnogenic) myeloid metaplasia; polycythemia vera (variable); essential thrombocythemia (variable).

3. Miscellaneous.
   Primary splenic hyperplasia; megaloblastic anemias; iron deficiency.

Neoplasm
1. Hematological.
   Acute leukemias; chronic leukemias; prolymphocytic leukemia; hairy cell leukemia; malignant lymphomata; malignant histiocytosis; systemic mastocytosis; myelomatosis.

2. Intrinsic.
   Primary lymphosarcoma; plasmacytoma; fibrosarcoma; angiosarcoma; endothelial cell sarcoma; lymphangiosarcoma; malignant fibrous histiocytoma.

3. Metastatic.
   Carcinoma, especially lung and breast; melanoma; neuroblastoma; malignant teratoma; choriocarcinoma.

4. Benign.
   Hamartoma (single, multiple); hemangioma (capillary, cavernous); lymphangioma; lipoma.

Miscellaneous
1. Storage diseases.
   Gaucher's disease; Neimann–Pick disease; Histiocytosis X; ceroid histiocytosis; Tangier disease; Hurler's syndrome; Hunter's syndrome.

2. Cysts.
   Pseudocyst; epidermoid (epithelial) cyst; echinococcal (hydatid) cyst.

3. Others.
   Amyloidosis; Albers–Schönberg disease; hereditary hemorrhagic telangiectasia; hyperthyroidism.

*Adapted from Bowdler (1983).

7.7 DIMINISHED SPLEEN ACTIVITY WITH SMALL TO NORMAL SPLEEN SIZE

Conditions with diminished splenic activity are described further in Chapter 11. They include both congenital and acquired conditions, and also disorders in which the spleen is involved as part of a more generalized immune deficiency.

7.7.1 CONGENITAL DISORDERS WITH HYPOSPLENISM

Congenital absence of the spleen (asplenia) is rare: it may be seen as an isolated defect, but more commonly it is part of a syndrome that may include partial or complete situs-inversus viscerae, severe cardiovascular abnormalities, especially severe conotruncus anomalies, and pulmonary malformations, including accessory lobes. Putschar and Manion (1956) have reviewed the subject and discussed the various combinations reported in the literature and eight cases not previously reported. It is more commonly seen in males and presents clinical problems in and of itself because of increased susceptibility to infection. Hypoplasia is less uncommon and may be associated with other signs of a lack of normal development of mesenchymal organs, and with Fanconi's anemia. Kevy *et al.* (1968) report three such cases, and describe one with a small spleen weighing 1 g, with the white pulp seen only at one pole. Other lymphoid structures were 'normal'.

7.7.2 IMMUNODEFICIENCY DISORDERS

The immunodeficiency disorders are systemic diseases of the immune system, and are principally expressed in the spleen as disorders of the white pulp. The red pulp appears to remain unaffected. Much is now known of the function of the spleen in these disorders, but less has been described of the detailed structural changes. In the severe combined immunodeficiency states the spleen is generally small, and grossly without discernible malpighian corpuscles or white pulp microscopical-

ly. There are scattered mononuclear cells about the central follicular arteries, but these may represent the monocyte–macrophage system simply 'filling a void'. In T-cell disorders the major feature is the lack of lymphocytes in the periarteriolar sheaths; but nodules of small lymphocytes may be seen near the vessels, often along one side of the trabecula and without germinal follicle formation. In B-cell disorders, the periarteriolar sheath may exist and extend out from the trabecula and vessels in a diffuse manner, but there is no evidence of germinal follicle formation.

In several immune-deficiency states, epithelioid cells may be present and these occasionally form distinct granulomata (Neiman, 1977). In some of the less common immunologic deficiencies, a mixed splenic pathology has been described. In the initial case of the syndrome that carries his name, Nezelof (1964, 1968) described the spleen of a 14-month-old male dying with thymic dysplasia. The spleen was slightly reduced in size and grossly consisted of red pulp. The malpighian bodies were visible but consisted essentially of large reticular cells, without germinal follicle formation. Scattered plasma cells were in the red pulp. In the same text, de Vries, Dooren and Cleton (1968) describe splenic histology in two brothers with the Swiss type of agammaglobulinemia and illustrate a spectrum of white pulp changes. In the older sibling there was severe depletion of the white pulp with only a few cells left showing nuclear pyknosis and karyorrhexis, while in the younger boy there was a normal number of follicles, some of which were enlarged, with germinal centers cuffed by lymphocytes. The illustrations show the difference but do not clearly illustrate germinal center formation.

In a review of another uncommon immune deficiency, Snover *et al.* (1981) describe the histologic findings in the Wiskott–Aldrich syndrome. As others have noted in other deficiencies, 'the findings in the spleen tended to parallel those in the lymph nodes'. The only consistent finding was the lymphoid depletion about the arterioles: a reticulum stain demonstrated the collapse of the support structure about the vessels secondary to the cell loss. The next most common finding was extramedullary hematopoiesis, and a few cases showed hemophagocytosis and sequestration of red cells. There was no consistent relationship between these two findings. Eosinophilia was seen in over half the cases and was prominent in most of these. Occasionally plasmacytosis with atypia was seen. As noted in other deficiencies, the germinal follicles revealed a spectrum of changes, ranging from hyperplasia with mitoses and active macrophages, to depletion and predominance of epithelioid cells and PAS-positive extracellular material. The terminal stage of the acquired immune deficiency syndrome shows similar histology and this end stage is illustrated in Figures 7.2 and 7.3. (The spectrum seen in AIDS is discussed more fully below.)

One type of immune deficiency recently described may in fact represent a specific defect in splenic function (Ambrosino *et al.*, 1987). A 30-year-old male showed decreased immune responsiveness to polysaccharides, resulting in repeated infections with *H. influenzae*. Upon challenge with polysaccharide antigens there was essentially no response, yet other immune responses appeared to be intact. Timens and Poppema (1987) have emphasized that the marginal zone of the splenic white pulp may be a unique structure which is important to the host's ability to respond to this type of antigen. This concept is based on their earlier work (Timens and Poppema, 1985) in which normal spleens were examined by immunocytochemistry: splenic lymphoid tissue proved to be similar in lymphocyte phenotyping to other lymphoid organs except for the marginal zone between the white and red pulp. This zone differs in containing circulating and non-circulating B-cells and helper T-cells, and most are medium-sized lymphocytes. It may be that failure to form this zone normally may be responsible for increased susceptibility to certain organisms in neonates, and in congenital immunologic deficiencies.

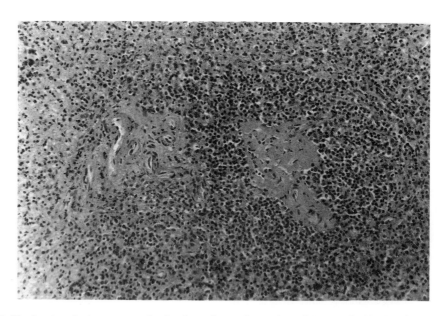

Figure 7.2 Follicular involution – atrophy in the spleen of a patient dying with AIDS. There is loss of the follicular structures except for residual hyalinized material and small numbers of lymphocytes and plasma cells.

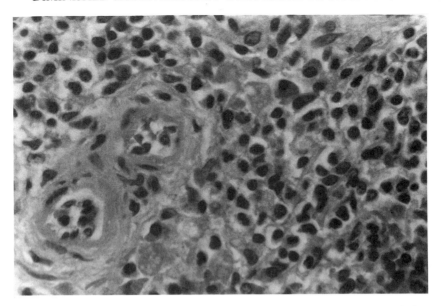

Figure 7.3 Higher power of a field from the case in Figure 7.2. There are lymphocytes and plasma cells but no activated cells.

7.7.3 ACQUIRED SPLENIC ATROPHY AND INFARCTION

Atrophy and infarction are the principal causes of a small spleen. Atrophy occurs in many disorders and is sometimes found in idiopathic form in elderly individuals. The configuration of the spleen is normal, but the capsule is diffusely wrinkled and the tissue 'falls away' from the cut surface. Infarction results in an organ which is irregular in shape and shows focal thickening of the capsule; the loss of tissue can be related in most instances to occlusion of a vessel. In sickle cell disease the end arteries are obstructed by the sickled cells (Chapter 16). In essential thrombocythemia the occluding material is the platelet, while in the rare case of malaria it is the parasite or thrombi. Infarcts may be seen in leukemic and myeloproliferative conditions, but here it is thought that vessels are compressed rather than occluded. In rare instances a localized or systemic arteritis may produce thrombosis and subsequent infarction (Figure 7.4); this generally does not produce a significant loss of spleen size or diminished function. Infarcts vary in number and size but are fairly constant in form, being wedge-shaped with the base at the capsule, and occupying the volume of distribution of the affected vessel. They are well delineated, and in the early stages bulge from the surface and are firm and dark red. The capsule may show loss of its usual glistening character and present a dull shaggy appearance. Later the infarct develops central pallor and softening, with the formation of a distinct red border. Resolution comes in the form of a scar, with white firm retracted tissue being visible on the external and cut surface. Microscopically there is early diffusion of red cells and subsequent necrosis and repair. If an infection supervenes, as may occur with an infected vegetation, the area will be grossly less red and softer from the outset. If small branches of the arterial system are involved, as with *in situ* infectious thrombosis, the areas will appear more like spots, an appearance termed a 'Fleck-milz spleen'.

Atrophy occurs as a complication of several

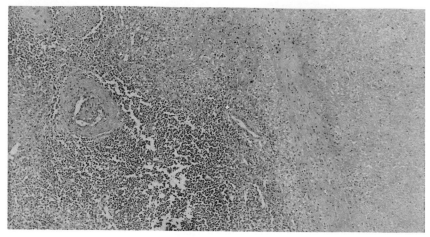

Figure 7.4 Vasculitis with infarction. The vessel on the left is partially occluded by an old thrombus, but occlusion of another vessel has produced the infarct on the right side of the micrograph.

disorders including idiopathic steatorrhea, dermatitis herpetiformis, and autoimmune disorders (see Chapter 11). It may also follow radiation therapy and cytotoxic chemotherapy.

7.7.4 FUNCTIONAL HYPOSPLENISM WITHOUT A DECREASE IN SPLEEN SIZE

This is a commonly found situation, although relatively few disorders contribute to it. The basic pathophysiologic mechanism is the infiltration of the spleen, either by cells or noncellular substances, which can both interfere with its function and cause enlargement (Steinberg, Gatling and Tavassoli, 1983).

(a) Neoplasms

Lymphoid neoplasms have the capacity to diminish the functional activity of the spleen because of their potential for diffuse replacement of the organ. This may occur in leukemias, lymphomata and, less commonly, in myelomatosis. Leukemic spleens have an irregularly thickened capsule and a bulging grey–red cut surface. Microscopically there is a diffuse infiltration by leukemic cells with loss of the definition between red and white pulp. A similar picture may be seen in the aggressive form of multiple myeloma, although splenomegaly occurs in only 5–10% of cases. In malignant lymphoma there may be multiple small tumor masses or a large single lesion (section 7.9.2).

(b) Sarcoidosis

Sarcoidosis may present a similar picture with non-caseating granulomata acting as cell infiltrates; when the process is severe, hypofunction can occur (Guyton and Zumwalt, 1975). The sarcoid spleen weighs up to 800 g and the cut surface is often dark-red with large gray nodules. The nodules of the epithelioid granulomata tend to be localized to the white pulp.

(c) Germinal center hypoplasia

A cellular disorder of genetic origin is the recently described entity showing paucity of splenic germinal centers (Weisdorf and Krivit,

1982). This was present in three generations of a family in which most members had splenomegaly. The spleens were often 'massive', and poorly developed or absent lymphoid follicles and hyperplasia of the red pulp were present on microscopy. Recurrent bacterial sepsis and autoimmune phenomena are also part of the clinical picture. The immunologic findings are similar to those of bursectomized chickens.

McKinley, Kwan and Lam-Po-Tang (1987) describe a similar disorder in a family with splenomegaly and germinal center hypoplasia, apparently inherited as an autosomal dominant trait. In one case the spleen weighed 1750 g, and microscopically there was an expanded white pulp but without germinal centers. Plasma cells were present. Immunoperoxidase stains revealed B- and T-cells in their usual location, as well as dendritic cells. The initial pancytopenia resolved after splenectomy; there appeared to be an overall defect in the helper T-cell population.

(d) Acquired immmunodeficiency syndrome

The acquired counterpart to the inherited hypoplasia of germinal centers is the acquired immunodeficiency syndrome (AIDS). The spleen is often enlarged but the lymphocyte population declines significantly during the course of the disease. In two recent reviews, the mean spleen weight was 315 g (Reichert *et al.*, 1983; Niedt and Schinella, 1985). As in the lymph nodes, initially there is follicular hyperplasia, but later the gross appearance of the cut surface is red and meaty without discernible malpighian corpuscles, reflecting the loss of the lymphoid tissue. Initially the germinal follicles show active centers and there is evidence of active cell turnover with numerous tingible body macrophages. The centers then start to lose cells and gain eosinophilic amorphous materials. There is gradual loss of the cells in the periarteriolar sheaths with replacement by fibrous tissue (Figures 7.2 and 7.3). Erythrophagocytosis and foci of hematopoiesis are seen. In the red pulp there is congestion and an increase in cells,

predominantly plasma cells, immunoblasts, and histiocytes. Hemosiderin may be present, both intra- and extracellularly. The red pulp also shows an increase in vascularity, which is possibly one factor increasing the potential for spontaneous rupture, which is noted later. Lastly, in patients with thrombocytopenia, there are described regressive follicular changes and an increase in CD8 cells, particularly in the germinal centers (Rousselet *et al.*, 1988). Electron microscopic examination shows the retroviral-like particles between dendritic cell extensions. The cells themselves may show edematous vacuolated changes in their processes. Except for a few subtle changes in the CD8 population and the findings of virus particles, some of the changes seen in the spleen in AIDS are not unlike those of idiopathic thrombocytopenic purpura.

(e) Amyloidosis

Amyloidosis occasionally infiltrates the spleen to a degree sufficient to cause hyposplenism; it is probably the commonest substance to produce a large hypofunctioning spleen (Gertz, Kyle and Greipp, 1983). The minimal lesion occurs as a subintimal deposit of the pulp arteries (Figure 7.5). The macroscopic pattern of infiltration ranges from grossly visible small nodular deposits, referred to as a 'sago spleen', to a hard yellow waxy organ produced by diffuse deposits of amyloid throughout the red pulp. It is the extensive involvement of the red pulp which results in hyposplenism. Rarely, amyloid forms a distinct tumor mass, leaving the remaining splenic tissue normal (Chen, Flam and Workman, 1987). The diagnosis is suggested clinically by frequent infections associated with firm splenomegaly. Microscopically the diagnostic feature on light microscopy is the dichroism with polarization on Congo red staining. Electron microscopic examination reveals the distinct beta pleating of the fibrillary pattern. Immunohistochemical analysis can be used to document the presence of light chains or A substance.

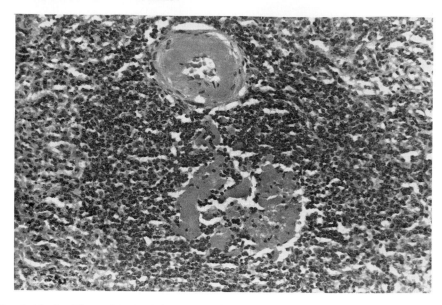

Figure 7.5 Amyloidosis. The subintimal location of the amyloid is demonstrated together with early extension into surrounding white pulp.

7.8 CONDITIONS OF NORMAL SPLENIC FUNCTION WITH DECREASED OR NORMAL SIZE

These conditions of the spleen usually produce little change in the functional activity of the organ, and rarely enlargement, so that they are unlikely to present clinically. Some, however, are accessible to radiological diagnosis and are described further in Chapter 17.

7.8.1 FOLLICULAR LIPIDOSIS

A condition characterized by the presence of clusters of vacuolated cells in or about the white pulp has been known for several decades (Figure 7.6). Both the composition of the substance in the vacuoles and the histologic appearance of the lesions have been subject to much discussion. Cruickshank (1984; Cruickshank and Thomas, 1984) has reviewed the literature and discussed the epidemiologic and histologic aspects: it was concluded that the entity is an acquired condition, which is rare before the age of 20 and unrelated to ethnic factors. At one

time the condition was thought to be principally due to disordered lipid metabolism, but some cases at least appear to be due to ingested mineral oil (Liber and Rose, 1967). There is an increased incidence of lipidosis in patients with peptic ulcer and a decreased incidence in malignant lymphoma.

Histologically the lesions consist of clusters of lipid droplets of varying size within macrophages, lymphocytes, and plasma cells. There is little epithelioid cell or fibroblastic reaction. Wanless and Geddie (1985) drew attention to a wide variability in the incidence of the lesion in autopsy studies, and also to an association between the presence of splenic lesions and similar lesions in the portal areas of the liver. It is more common in males. Some observers have emphasized the occurrence of a sarcoid-like granulomatous lesion, but more recent reports are consistent in finding intracellular lipid droplets only within mononuclear cells.

The lesion is to be distinguished from other lipid lesions such as the reaction to injected radio-opaque substances and Whipple's disease. In rare instances, granulomata related to

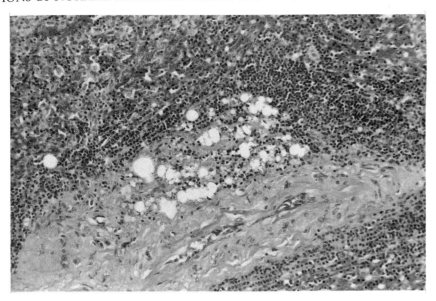

Figure 7.6 Follicular lipogranulomatosis. The variably sized droplets are shown in their periarteriolar location. The usual mononuclear cell population exists in the adjacent tissue.

an infectious agent may contain lipid, but these can be distinguished by the differing pattern of cellular infiltrate.

Haber *et al.* (1988) report the splenic histology of the 'fat overload syndrome'. In this condition intravenous fat emulsion therapy leads to several complications, including splenomegaly. The spleen is a homogeneous salmon pink color with small foci of necrosis noted on the cut surface. Microscopically the red pulp shows distended acellular cords filled with Sudan Black–positive material. Focally fat thrombi occlude small blood vessels, which possibly explains the focal necrosis of the white pulp.

7.8.2 HAMARTOMAS

A hamartoma is defined as a benign tumor composed of the mature tissue normally found in the affected organ. In the spleen the usual mature tissue to become neoplastic is in the red pulp, and the gross and microscopic features are those of a hemangioma or lymphangioma. They are most commonly found in the elderly. The incidence is low: Lee *et al.* (1987) report

about 100 cases in their literature review. On gross examination hamartomas are round and appear well circumscribed, as they compress the surrounding tissue; their size varies from one to several centimeters in diameter and they can weigh more than 1 kg. In most instances the lesion is solitary. Microscopically they consist of vascular spaces with prominent endothelial cells and fibrous stroma, with cells having ovoid nuclei and indistinct cytoplasm. There is no capsule, and trabeculae are not evident. Silverman and LiVolsi (1978) point out that there may be fibrosis, lymphocytes and eosinophils associated with these tumors, potentially causing confusion with Hodgkin's disease. Red cells are usually found in the vascular slits, and hemosiderin is seen in the periphery of some hamartomas. The surrounding parenchyma is normal except for the compression and occasional foci of extramedullary hematopoiesis. As noted earlier, some hematomas become symptomatic and can cause detectable splenomegaly. Splenomegaly may occur because of the relatively uncommon feature of multiple hamartomas as well as growth of one tumor

(Morgenstern *et al.*, 1984). Rarely the spleen may rupture resulting in an acute abdomen. Because most hamartomas consist of red pulp components, an increase in function of the pulp can produce another clinical problem as reported by Iozzo, Haas and Chard (1980). Two children presented with pancytopenia, bone marrow hyperplasia, and enlarged spleens. In these cases the channels in the hamartoma were filled with mononuclear cells, some classified as immunoblasts. Since the hematologic abnormalities resolved following splenectomy, the hamartomas in this case produced the clinical syndrome of 'hypersplenism'.

7.8.3 PELIOSIS

Peliosis is another lesion that is often found incidentally, and like lipidosis may be associated with liver changes, and like the hamartoma is vascular in nature. This condition may cause enlargement of the spleen, but this is generally slight and it does not produce physical signs or symptoms. The lesion is visible on the cut surface of the organ as multiple, small, round to oval, dark-red cystic spaces. The lesion may be localized or spread diffusely throughout the red pulp; conversely it may be so small that it is not seen grossly (Tada, Wakkabayashi and Kishimoto, 1983). Microscopically the cystic spaces are more common in the parafollicular areas, often in the marginal zone, but they can be found throughout the red pulp. The spaces initially are round and lined by distinct splenic cords with intact ring fibers and lining cells. The lumina are filled with erythrocytes and leukocytes at this stage. As the spaces enlarge the lining cells may disappear and some organization of the contents will occur. The cavities may exist either separately or in clusters with no more than a thin reticulum separating them. Occasionally a communication is seen between a space and a venous channel, although this probably has no pathogenetic significance. If the process is extensive, there may be a decrease in the extent of the white pulp. The condition must be distinguished from simple dilatation of

the red pulp sinuses, which is commonly seen in various forms of splenic congestion. However, the parafollicular location of peliosis is distinctive, and congestive dilatation is interfollicular. Usually there are similar lesions in the liver which help to distinguish peliosis from other vascular lesions, but cases confined to the spleen do occur (Warfel and Ellis, 1982). Peliosis, the Greek for 'livid spot, or black and blue', has been associated with several diseases and therapeutic modalities. Naeim, Copper and Semion (1973) proposed anabolic steroids as a possible etiologic agent; it has been found in patients with malignancy, tuberculosis, and cirrhosis (Bleiweiss, Thung and Goodman, 1986). Toxic factors and congenital defects have also been suggested as etiologic factors.

Some reported cases have shown that peliosis can be clinically significant: because of its vascularity, it can lead to splenic rupture with intra-abdominal bleeding, requiring emergency medical attention (Garcia, Khan and Berlin, 1982; Chen and Felix, 1986). Rarely, peliosis can produce hypersplenism, leading to a decrease in blood components including thrombocytopenia (Taxy, 1978; Lacson, Berman and Neiman, 1979).

7.9 CONDITIONS OF NORMAL SPLENIC ACTIVITY, WITH NORMAL OR INCREASED SIZE

7.9.1 CONGESTION

The various causes for splenic enlargement due to congestion are listed in Table 7.2. Regardless of the cause of the congestion, the principal change is the enlargement of the red pulp by red cells without these being significantly abnormal. This may be due to increased pressure in the venous system as a whole, the portal system, or obstruction to venous outflow at the level of the splenic vein. The organ is generally firm, and the capsule thickened. The cut surface is meaty, firm, and dark grey–red, and the white pulp is indistinct. In long-standing congestion, small firm brown-grey nodules, the Gandy-

Gamna bodies, may be noted in the red pulp. Microscopically the venous walls are thickened and cellular with a proliferation of lining cells and fibroblasts. The sinusoids are compressed. The trabeculae are thickened by collagen or fibrous tissue. In areas where congestion has led to hemorrhage, red cells and hemosiderin are present at an early stage; but with the process of organization, there is an increase in fibrous tissue with incrustation with iron and calcium salts on the elastic fibers and connective tissue. In the later stages, hematopoiesis may be seen.

7.9.2 NEOPLASMS

Since the spleen consists principally of vascular channels and lymphoid tissue, the majority of primary neoplasms seen in the organ arise from these two tissues. Benign and malignant vascular tumors make up the majority of splenic neoplasms. There has been debate in the past concerning the existence of a primary lymphoid neoplasm, but there are sufficient cases now to accept this as an entity. Malignant neoplasms may also be primary or secondary.

(a) Benign neoplasms: vascular

The most common benign tumor of the spleen is the hemangioma (Rappaport, 1966). This tumor generally occurs in the younger age group and in males, without racial preference. Like the hamartomas, these tumors do not in most cases produce clinical signs or symptoms, and a high percentage are seen as incidental findings at autopsy (Garvin and King, 1981). They are generally only a few centimeters in diameter and single. They appear red, spongy, and well circumscribed unless infarction, thrombosis, or fibrosis occurs. The microscopic pattern can be either capillary or cavernous, or a combination of both. The vascular spaces are lined by flattened endothelial cells and filled with erythrocytes and proteinaceous material. In some cases hemangiomata are very large or multiple and produce the picture of 'hyper-splenism' with anemia or thrombocytopenia (Harris, 1985). Splenic hemangiomas may be part of a systemic process in which organs such as the liver and skin are also involved (Kagalwala et al., 1987).

A less common vascular tumor is the lymphangioma which produces a 'Swiss cheese' pattern on radiologic examination (Ellison, 1980). Grossly the lesion is spongy, cystic, or occasionally solid, and the spaces are filled with serous fluid. A subcapsular location is more common than with the hemangioma (Hamoudi, Vassay and Morse, 1975). The channels are lined by flattened endothelial cells, and the lumina contain proteinaceous material but very few cells. Like hemangiomata they may be capillary, cavernous or cystic, depending upon the size of the channels. The lymphangioma may be multiple (Pistoia and Markowitz, 1988), and can be present also in other organs (Marymount and Knight, 1987).

(b) Benign neoplasms: cellular

Essentially two types of lesion fall into this category, the one consisting of a lymphoid nodule and the other an inflammatory pseudotumor. Burke and Osborne (1983) describe four cases of localized lymphoid growth in which a single nodule is found in a normal sized spleen. These are up to 1 cm in diameter, and in appearance are fleshy and white to grey–white. Microscopically they are composed of germinal centers or sheets of small and large lymphocytes and plasma cells, forming a round to oval lesion. Away from these distinctive areas, the spleen may show reactive changes or sarcoid-like granulomas.

Inflammatory pseudotumors were first described in other organs such as lung, but recently have been seen in the spleen (Sheahan, Wolf and Neiman, 1988; McMahon, 1988). The process is usually associated with splenomegaly, and on gross examination single or multiple 0.5–1.5 cm nodules are present in or near malpighian corpuscles. The microscopic appearance varies from a very heterogeneous cellular

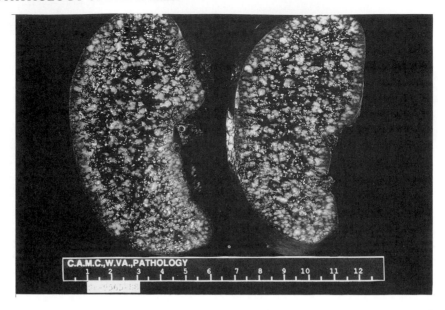

Figure 7.7 Malignant lymphoma. This diffuse small nodular form is one type of presentation of neoplasms in the spleen. (Courtesy of Pathology Department, Charleston Area Medical Center, West Virginia.)

lesion to one showing active fibrosis. Plasma cells are usually prominent, with some atypia. Necrosis and granulomata with giant cells may be present. There is no capsule, but the lesion compresses the surrounding parenchyma. Culture and special stains are negative. The benign nature is substantiated by the polyclonal staining of the B-cell population (McMahon, 1988).

Other elements of the spleen have rarely been the source of a benign tumor. Easler and Dowlin (1969) report such an example of a large yellow lobulated demarcated lipoma found within the splenic capsule.

(c) Malignant neoplasms: lymphomas

Primary lymphomas of the spleen are relatively uncommon and comprise about 1% of all lymphomas (Spier *et al.*, 1985). Various types have been reported but the small lymphocytic lymphoma is the most common. Grossly this presents as multiple small to large firm tan–pink nodules in a spleen weighing from 300 to 4000 g (Figure 7.7). The small cell types tend to have numerous small nodules whereas the large

cell types have fewer and larger tumor masses, which broadly recapitulates the difference in diffuse and localized disease presentation at the two ends of the spectrum of lymphocytic lymphomas. This difference in gross presentation and histologic type was noted by Hara (1985) in a review based on the Japanese experience. Audouin *et al.* (1988) discuss three gross appearances of the primary lymphoma, including the diffuse faintly nodular, the micronodular diffuse, and the micronodular focal. Some cases present as one large tumor mass, more typical of primary Hodgkin's disease of the spleen (Niv, Abu-Avid and Oren, 1986). The surrounding lymph nodes may be involved, and on rare occasions there may be direct extension into adjacent tissues. The principal criterion used to designate a lymphoma as primary to the spleen is one of exclusion, in that there is lack of lymph node or blood involvement; however, some cases can show rather extensive disease.

Microscopically the changes usually show an expansion of the white pulp with malignant cells producing confluent islands and distinct nodules.

(d)   Malignant neoplasms: leukemias

Nearly all leukemias are expressed in the spleen, either structurally or functionally (Chapters 14 and 15). The prominent change pathologically is enlargement which tends to be diffuse, with a cut surface which is homogeneous except for areas of hemorrhage or infarction. The myeloid leukemias in general produce more splenic abnormalities than the lymphoid; however, there are exceptions. In prolymphocytic leukemia the spleen may be very large, and the cut surface is deep red with a diffuse small nodular pattern (Bearman, Pangales and Rappaport, 1978). Microscopically, cells which mark as B-lymphocytes are seen in the grossly defined nodules, in both the white and red pulp. On occasion other leukemias may produce distinct nodules as well as diffuse enlargement (Hogan, Osborne and Butler, 1989). In four cases of myelocytic leukemia small but distinct nodules were noted, varying from dark red, to pink, to brown. The microscopic picture varied from blast transformation to sea-blue histiocytosis.

It has been suggested that hairy cell leukemia (leukemic reticuloendotheliosis) is possibly a primary splenic leukemia. The spleen usually weighs about 2000 g, and the capsule is tense but not thickened. The cut surface is meaty, dark red and without distinct malpighian corpuscles, and may have areas of apparent infarction (Burke, Byrne and Rappaport, 1974). The prominent microscopic feature is a diffuse infiltrate of round to oval cells obscuring the white pulp and filling the red pulp sinusoids and cords (Figure 7.8). The cell population is fairly uniform and without significant mitotic activity. Another diagnostic feature is the presence of ribosomal-lamellar complexes on electron microscopic examination of the spleen (Burke, Byrne and Rappaport, 1974). Additionally, a distinctive feature is the formation of pseudosinuses, which range in size from that of a small dilated sinus to a large sheet of red cells with poorly defined margins, grossly visible on the glass slide. Nanba et al. (1977) demonstrated that these lesions are lined to varying degrees by neoplastic cells, rather than evolved from a defined splenic structure; consequently they are termed pseudosinuses.

Another variant of the leukemic process with

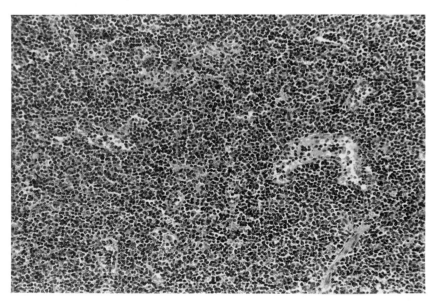

Figure 7.8 Hairy-cell leukemia. The uniform small cell infiltrate blends the white and red pulp into one structure.

prominent involvement of the spleen was described by McKenna *et al.* (1977) as a subtype of chronic lymphocytic leukemia. These cases showed marked neutropenia and splenomegaly in addition to lymphocytosis. This entity has been characterized as a neoplastic proliferation of large granular lymphocytes or 'T8 hyperlymphocytosis', with evidence that the neoplastic cells are probably responsible for the neutropenia (Grillot-Courvalin *et al.*, 1986). The spleen can weigh up to 2000 g and grossly have an intact thinned capsule and a firm smooth red cut surface. Microscopically there is a diffuse infiltration or focal aggregates of the large granular lymphocytes in the red pulp. The lymphoid follicles are present, usually in normal numbers, but they may lack germinal centers. The periarteriolar sheath may show depletion of lymphocytes (Loughran *et al.*, 1985).

Other diseases of cell proliferation also produce splenomegaly. In malignant histiocytosis the spleen may present with tan-colored nodules on the cut surface which consist of histiocytes in the red pulp. In systemic mast cell disease, the spleen is often involved and demonstrates numerous changes, which were reviewed by Travis and Li (1988). The spleen weighs up to 1140 g and capsular thickening is usually seen. The cut surface shows small nodules in a diffuse pattern. Fibrosis involving capsule and parenchyma can be extensive, and calcification may be present. The mast cells are most often seen about the trabecula and follicles, and some degree of fibrosis and eosinophilia is generally present. The authors point out the similarity between this disorder and other hematologic diseases with infiltration.

(e)   Malignant neoplasms: vascular

In contrast to the relative incidence of vascular and cellular benign tumors, malignant primary vascular tumors are less common than malignant tumors originating in the white pulp. Of the mesenchymal tumors, hemangiosarcomas are the least 'rare'; nevertheless they are relatively uncommon as a primary malignancy.

They were first reviewed in 1897, and by 1985 about 56 cases had been reported (Smith, Eisenberg and McDonald, 1985). There is vascular channel formation by sarcomatous tissue. The tumor is either confined to the spleen, or the organ contains the largest tumor mass if multiple organs are involved. Metastatic disease is present in more than three-quarters of cases. Usually the spleen is enlarged, and this may have occurred as a sudden clinical event. These sarcomas appear as a definable red firm nodular mass or as a generalized enlargement of the spleen. Microscopically the appearances are quite variable; vascular spaces may be evident or the stromal sarcomatous element may predominate (Rappaport, 1966). Hemosiderin is generally present, often in significant amounts. Occasionally extramedullary hematopoiesis may be seen in the tumor, and clinically some patients have a microangiopathic hemolytic anemia (Sordillo, Sordillo and Hajdu, 1981). Kaposi's sarcoma may also occur in the spleen, but this is rare even in patients with AIDS (Ziegler and Dorfman, 1988). When present the tumor follows the major blood vessels into the red pulp in a diffuse manner, rather than forming distinct tumor nodules.

(f)   Malignant neoplasms: metastatic

The spleen is a relatively uncommon site for the development of metastatic epithelial tumors; the cause of this resistance is still uncertain. The capsule may be involved in abdominal carcinomatosis, and direct extension can occur from adjacent organs, but a distinct intrasplenic mass is considered rare. In most cases it is an asymptomatic finding and associated with diffuse carcinomatosis, most commonly originating from carcinoma of the breast, bronchus, or ovary. Secondary melanoma also occurs, and rare cases are reported of neuroblastoma and teratoma. It is interesting to note that two cases of metastatic testicular tumors have been reported (Willey, Rodger and Webb, 1982; Carr *et al.*, 1987). The overall autopsy incidence in cases of carcinoma is about 4% but the actual percentage may be higher; its presence in life may become better documented with newer radiologic techniques: up to 50% of melanoma patients have abnormal liver and spleen scans (Klein *et al.*, 1987). Most cases are asymptomatic but painful splenomegaly and cytopenias may occur.

7.9.3 STORAGE DISEASES

Benign infiltrative processes comprise a small portion of cases with splenomegaly but it is an important category as it almost always represents a sign of a systemic disease. The spleen is enlarged because of the accumulation of intra- or extracellular substances. Gaucher's disease (glucosyl ceramide lipidosis) is the commonest, and a classic example of the intracellular type. Like most lipid storage disorders, it is inherited as an autosomal recessive trait. The underlying deficiency is of the enzyme glucocerebrosidase.

In Gaucher's disease the spleen may be large, with a dry, firm and pale grey cut surface, with loss of definition of the pulp compartments. Histiocytes containing glucocerebroside fill the red pulp cords (Lee, Peters and Glew, 1977). The cells have round uniform nuclei, which are occasionally multiple, and abundant cytoplasm which appears vacuolated. In Niemann–Pick disease the same vacuolated appearance is seen, the vacuoles being filled with lipid and sphingomyelin. The sea-blue histiocyte syndrome is due to an accumulation of ceroid in histiocytes which accumulate in liver and spleen (Silverstein, Ellefson and Ahern, 1970). In the spleen, they accumulate in both the splenic cords and sinuses.

7.10 CONDITIONS OF INCREASED SPLENIC ACTIVITY, WITH NORMAL OR DECREASED SIZE

7.10.1 IDIOPATHIC THROMBOCYTOPENIC PURPURA

Idiopathic thrombocytopenic purpura almost invariably presents with a spleen that is not enlarged, but there is increased activity of the spleen in platelet destruction and antibody formation (McMillan *et al.*, 1974). In a review of 12 patients, Tavassoli and McMillan (1975) found that the spleen ranged in weight from 80 to 424 g, but that two weighing over 250 g were enlarged for other reasons. Gross examination is usually unremarkable. Microscopically, the prominent feature is reactive hyperplasia of the white pulp with prominence of the germinal follicles. The 'starry sky' appearance with active histiocytes is seen, and PAS-positive material may be present. If steroid therapy has been given, there may be fewer lymphocytes and more histiocytes than normal. The marginal zone expands into the red pulp, and transformed lymphocytes and plasma cells constitute part of this zone. In the red pulp the phagocytic population is prominent with evidence of phagocytosis of platelet material. The junction of the marginal zone and red pulp is the site of most such activity, as might be expected since this is the first site for antigen and antibody to meet. Periarterial fibrosis is reported to occur in some cases (Berendt, Mant and Jewell, 1986).

7.11 CONDITIONS OF INCREASED SPLENIC ACTIVITY, WITH NORMAL OR INCREASED SIZE

7.11.1 HYPERSPLENISM

The cytopenias of 'hypersplenism' are multifactorial; nevertheless, phagocytic activity often becomes more active in the red pulp in this condition. Of Dameshek's four proposed criteria for the diagnosis of 'hypersplenism', three related to the phagocytic function, and one to size. The increase in size is also evident in circumstances in which the immune function is hyperactive, and sometimes there is evidence of hyperactivity of both functions.

7.11.2 CONGENITAL HEMOLYTIC DISORDERS

In hereditary spherocytosis the spleen is enlarged with a thin tense capsule and few adhesions. The cut surface is red–blue and firm, with little disturbance of the pulp on scraping. The malpighian corpuscles are not prominent, but are still visible as small white specks. Microscopically the white pulp is intact, but dispersed by the widened red pulp. There is marked congestion of Billroth's cords, with an increase in the reticulum fibers. The venous sinuses are patent but empty. Overt phagocytosis of the red cells is usually unimpressive, but hemosiderin is present (Chapter 8). In a related condition, hereditary ovalocytosis, the splenic changes are similar. This pattern also holds true for the hemoglobinopathies, but in thalassemia evidence of perisplenitis may be found. In early sickle cell disease with splenomegaly, the spleen is noted to be more spherical, and the cut section is dark red and dry; the malpighian corpuscles are not prominent. Blaustein (1963) also comments that sickle cell trait spleens from severely hypoxic patients may undergo massive necrosis and hemorrhage so that they come to resemble grossly 'a bag of blood'.

7.11.3 IMMUNE HYPERFUNCTION

In immune hyperfunction, enlargement is generally less, and the prominence of the white pulp is more evident microscopically than grossly. The white pulp tends to go through stages of morphologic change during prolonged stimulation. Unstimulated white pulp is composed of small lymphocytes situated about the arterioles. Early in the course of stimulation the lymphocytes undergo transformation and immunoblasts are seen. In the second stage, germinal centers form with mantle zones, and plasma cells become discernible. These centers gradually enlarge and show the same changes as in lymph nodes, often simulating a 'starry sky' effect because of the histiocytes scattered among the lymphocytes (Figure 7.9). The immune system reaches a height of activity which then starts to decline; at this time there is an influx of epithelioid cells and acellular hyaline material.

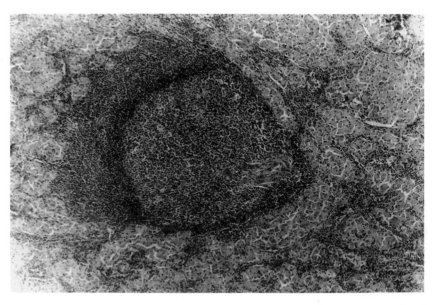

Figure 7.9 Advanced activated immune response. Note the germinal center and mantle zone with polarization which marks it as a reactive process. The spleen is from a patient with Gaucher's disease.

7.11.4 MYELOID METAPLASIA

With the exception of the proliferation of lymphocytes in the stimulated spleen, the adult human spleen does not normally play an active role in blood formation; nevertheless, it is an appropriate environment for the support of hematopoiesis. This is particularly evident in agnogenic (primary) myeloid metaplasia, which is discussed in detail in Chapter 14. In this condition extreme splenomegaly can occur; the surface of the organ is homogeneous except for areas of infarction, and the capsule is smooth and shiny, except for those areas which overlie infarcts. The cut surface is generally dark red–brown and firm, unless the organ is heavily infiltrated with leukocytes, and then it becomes pale red. The malpighian corpuscles are indistinct and dispersed. Microscopically the hematopoietic precursors pervade the tissue, initially predominantly in the sinuses but later in the cords of Billroth. The erythroid precursors are easily detected because of their darkly staining round nuclei, and some authors have proposed that these cells predominate in the sinuses while myeloid precursors locate to the cords. Scattered megakaryocytic precursors are also present, often in prominent numbers. Various splenic cells show reactive changes, and macrophages are usually prominent and contain cells and debris. These cells are particularly prominent with special stains or by electron microscopy (Tavassoli and Weiss, 1973). The reticular structure of the spleen remains intact. Prior therapy may alter the splenic pathology.

7.11.5 INFECTIOUS PROCESSES

The enlarged spleen of acute splenitis has been familiar to physicians for centuries. Acute splenitis presents as a large soft spleen with a thin stretched capsule, and produces the 'acute splenic tumor' (Figure 7.10). The cut surface is grey–pink, and bulges above the capsule; the pulp scrapes away easily, leaving the trabecula easily visible. The white pulp is not discernible grossly, but microscopically it shows varying degrees of hyperplasia, and sometimes germinal centers are clearly formed. The macrophages of the red pulp show active phagocytosis. Neutrophils and eosinophils may be seen in the sinuses; with prolonged infections plasma cells are found.

The spectrum of these non-specific changes in children is described by Gadaleanu (1981) in 221 spleens from children with bronchopulmonary inflammatory diseases. A generalized hyperplasia of follicular and periarteriolar sheath components and plasma cells in the red pulp was noted in about one-third of the cases. The germinal centers were composed either of a mixture of immunoblasts and histiocytes or an immunoblastic core cuffed by smaller lymphocytes. In most cases the hyperplasia was focal and moderate. In about 20% of the cases lymphoid depletion was found to result from a more severe or longer clinical course. A few follicles contained an epithelioid center of histiocytes with abundant eosinophilic cytoplasm.

Some infectious agents produce more distinctive changes, as noted by Blaustein (1963). Streptococcal infections may produce a grey coloration and a very soft spleen. *Clostridium welchii* produces a proliferation of the reticuloendothelial (RE) cells lining the cords so that the sinuses appear empty and the corpuscles spread apart. In brucellosis the RE cells become enlarged and form a pseudosarcoid-like reaction in the red pulp. In spirochetal diseases, there is a spectrum of changes: congenital syphilis produces a large red hyperemic spleen with fibrosis and infiltration of macrophages and plasma cells. Plasma cells are also prominent in secondary syphilis, together with hyperplasia of the white pulp. Gummas can be seen in tertiary syphilis. In louse-borne relapsing fever the large firm spleen shows multiple grey foci on the cut surface which represent microabscesses in the white pulp (Judge *et al.*, 1974). In lyme disease red pulp hyperplasia and spirochetes are seen (Cimmino *et al.*, 1988). Viral diseases such as infectious mononucleosis can also produce areas of necrosis as well as marked reactivity of the white pulp. As in other tissues,

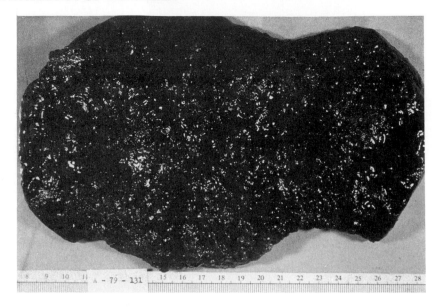

Figure 7.10 Acute splenic tumor. The soft focally pale parenchyma spills over the edge of the capsule.

the immunoblastic reaction can produce cells similar to Reed–Sternberg cells, which can also appear in the spleen in brucellosis.

Tuberculosis is often less active in producing a reaction with enlargement than the diseases already considered, but granulomata are evident as yellow to white irregular nodular areas on the cut surface. Granulomas are found in other infectious diseases, and are also associated with neoplastic conditions like Hodgkin's disease. They may occur non-specifically: Kuo and Rosai (1974) found tuberculosis or a fungal disease in only three of 20 cases with granulomatous inflammation, while others lacking evidence of infectious disease had evidence of hypersplenism.

In drug addicts a variety of splenic changes have been described (Kringsholm and Christoffersen, 1984). Spleen weight increases with the duration of drug addiction: a distinct microscopic feature is the presence of refractile material, the frequency of which increases with the chronicity of drug use, and which is found in the histiocytes near the central arterioles. As in other reactive conditions, germinal centers are prominent.

7.11.6 IDIOPATHIC SPLENOMEGALY, TROPICAL AND NON-TROPICAL

The tropical splenomegaly syndrome (TSS) is characterized by significant splenomegaly, hepatomegaly, elevated ESR, elevation of serum IgM, and often the presence of antibodies to malarial parasites. The patients with TSS are in areas endemic for malaria, but it is clear that there are several etiologies, often dependent on the geographical area, and not all cases of TSS have malaria. The spleen often weighs 4000 g or more, and the capsule is thin and smooth (Geary, Clough and MacIver, 1980). The cut surface is firm and red, although malaria, when present, may produce a dark-brown color in the acute stage due to malarial pigment.

In chronic malaria the spleen has a thick grey–white capsule, and the cut surface is firm and grey–black. Microscopically fibrosis and pigment deposition replaces the reactive lymphoid changes seen in early malaria. Also in early disease the parasites may be visible occluding arterioles.

In TSS the sinuses are dilated and filled with histiocytes which show phagocytic activity. The lymphoid follicles do not show much reaction but in some cases the lymphoid infiltration may be marked. In various endemic forms in different countries the splenomegaly may show different or additional findings. Lowenthal *et al.* (1980) report that TSS spleens in Northern Zambia show marked red cell sequestration, and plasma cells or plasmacytoid lymphocytes are present in the intersinusoidal tissue.

Idiopathic splenomegaly also exists in temperate regions of the world, and the non-tropical variant (Dacie's syndrome)* has been reviewed by Manoharan, Bader and Pitney (1982). In summarizing five cases, they found the spleen to weigh up to 3380 g. The microscopic features are not unlike TSS, except that lymphoid infiltration of the red pulp and erythrophagocytosis are not as prominent. Hemosiderin is more evident. Two of these patients progressed to develop malignant lymphoma. Some patients may have evidence of an antecedent viral infection, but truly idiopathic splenomegaly appears to exist as a distinct entity (Hesdorffer *et al.*, 1986). Some cases have been suggested to have a hereditary basis (Cheng, Williams and Kitahara, 1980).

7.11.7 AUTOIMMUNE DISORDERS

In autoimmune hemolytic anemia of warm-antibody type the spleen is generally enlarged, with a smooth capsule showing focal thickening. The cut surface is smooth and red, and the malpighian corpuscles are dispersed. Microscopically the white pulp shows reactive changes, and the marginal zone is often prominent. The cords of Billroth are congested with red cells; lymphocytes and hemosiderin-laden macrophages are present. Erythrophagocytosis is often present, and occasionally extramedullary hematopoiesis is found.

When Felty's syndrome complicates rheumatoid arthritis (RA), the enlarged hyperactive spleen plays a role in inducing leukopenia. The spleen may be enlarged in uncomplicated RA due to hyperreactive lymphoid tissue with

*Also known to clinicians as 'primary hypersplenism' (ed.).

prominent follicular hyperplasia. The follicular arterioles may show hyaline thickening of their walls with swelling of the endothelial cells. Amyloidosis, particularly of the vessel walls, may occur. In Felty's syndrome, there is expansion of the red pulp as the lining cells proliferate. Furthermore the systemic vasculitis found in severe active rheumatoid disease can involve the spleen.

Vasculitis involving the spleen is found in cases of periarteritis nodosum (PAN) and systemic lupus erythematosus (SLE). In PAN the larger vessels tend to be involved, whereas in SLE it is mainly the arterioles which are affected. The characteristic onion-skin lesion of SLE may be the healed stage of a vasculitis involving the smaller arterial vessels: this change can be very prominent, and lead to obliteration of the follicular structures.

7.11.8 RUPTURE OF THE SPLEEN

This phenomenon can occur regardless of the size or functional status of the spleen, and trauma is the most frequent cause of rupture: it may be the precursor of the development of splenosis (section 7.5). Non-traumatic or spontaneous rupture occurs in many diseases, and Massad *et al.* (1988) have summarized the various causes, which include hematologic disorders, malignant tumors, inflammatory diseases, infections and connective tissue diseases (Table 7.3). Among the more common causes are infectious diseases, and these authors report a case of mumps with splenic rupture. A more commonly predisposing disease is infectious mononucleosis, in which the inflammatory process involves and compromises the integrity of the capsule, making the acutely enlarged spleen prone to rupture. The same process probably underlies the fragility of the spleen in many other disorders, including AIDS (Mirchandani, Mirchandani and Pak, 1985). A recent review reports 10 cases of rupture in splenic amyloidosis (Kozicky *et al.*, 1987). A relatively rare cause of rupture of an unenlarged spleen was described by Wiener and Ong (1989): a spleen of only 76 g ruptured, leading to hemoperitoneum

Table 7.3 Disorders associated with spontaneous rupture of the spleen*

1. Hematological disorders
   Hemoglobin C disease
   Hodgkin's disease
   Polycythemia vera
   Hemolytic anemias
   Hereditary ovalocytosis

2. Malignant tumors
   Leukemias
   Hemangiosarcoma
   Metastatic hepatoma

3. Infections
   Infectious mononucleosis
   Malaria
   Infective endocarditis
   Chickenpox
   Mumps
   Hepatitis A
   Influenza
   Aspergillosis

4. Inflammatory disorders
   Crohn's disease
   Chronic pancreatitis

5. Connective tissue disorders
   Systemic lupus erythematosus
   Rheumatoid disease

6. Miscellaneous
   Sarcoidosis
   Portal hypertension
   Amyloidosis
   Pregnancy
   Acquired immunodeficiency syndrome

*Adapted from Massad *et al.* (1988)

and death, in a patient treated with streptokinase for myocardial infarction. With the increased use of thrombolytic substances, such cases of 'spontaneous' rupture in a normal spleen may be seen more commonly.

Although splenic rupture is usually an acute problem, Prager, Morel and Dex (1971) present cases in which there was significant delay before the subjects presented for medical attention ('chronic' or 'occult' rupture). The abdomen usually shows a palpable mass, but the clinical and pathologic patterns vary. There may be a subcapsular hematoma or free hemorrhage present in the peritoneal cavity, suggesting a delay between rupture and bleeding (Figure 7.11). The hematoma may have developed a capsule, and this is one lesion to be considered in the differential diagnosis of a hemorrhagic mass.

7.11.9 ABSCESS

Like other lymphoid organs, the spleen is not a common site for abscess formation. This may be mimicked by an infected cyst, but Chulay and Lankerani (1976) found only 10 cases in 10 years in a busy hospital. Pain, fever, and left upper quadrant tenderness are part of the symptom complex. Splenomegaly is not always present: but with newer radiologic techniques, the diagnosis may be made antemortem more frequently than a decade ago (Lawhorne and Zuidema, 1976). Johnson and Roff (1984) discuss their experience with fungal splenic abscesses: grossly such an abscess has an apparent capsule and is filled with purulent, foul-smelling material. Microscopically the full range of inflammatory reactions is seen from acute to granulomatous inflammation. With resolution, granulation tissue and fibroblastic proliferation are seen. Three basic pathophysiologic conditions for abscess formation have been proposed: the protective capacity of the spleen may be overwhelmed, internal damage may have occurred, or there may have been extension from adjacent sites of infection. In the first category are cases secondary to infective endocarditis, sepsis, or a depressed immunologic system. Internal damage may be either trauma, hematoma formation or infarction (Epstein and Omar, 1983). Least common is the third, in which external infection penetrates into the spleen. Not all cases are due to infections, as vasculitides and sterile inflammatory reactive conditions can lead to abscess formation. In Weber–Christian disease, Lemley, Chun and Cupps (1987) report sterile abscesses in one patient: grossly the spleen had scattered yellow nodules which consisted of regions of liquefac-

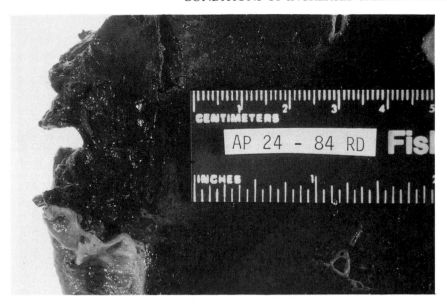

Figure 7.11 Subcapsular hematoma and rupture. There is thickening of the capsule and underlying blood is in various stages of coagulation. (Courtesy of the Pathology Department, Charleston Area Medical Center, West Virginia.)

tion necrosis. The cells in these areas were neutrophils and lipid-laden macrophages, with a peripheral granulomatous reaction. Fibrosis of the capsule and surrounding fat was present.

7.11.10 CYSTS

A variety of cysts is found in the spleen, but basically they are of two types, primary and secondary (Dawes and Malangoni, 1986). The primary form shows two main types, comprising those with an epithelial lining and those due to parasitic infestation. The secondary form of cyst (false cyst, pseudocyst) results from trauma (Chapter 17). In the former there is a definite cyst wall (as in Figure 7.12), or evidence of a parasite such as the *Echinococcus*. The wall of the secondary or false cyst has no distinct lining, grossly or microscopically, and the inner surface is usually shaggy with iron or calcium deposited in the wall. Traumatic cysts tend to occur in younger individuals, due to a congenital defect or trauma leading to the formation of a cyst-like structure. In one large series (Garvin

and King, 1981) trauma generally preceded secondary cyst formation, and this type of cyst made up 80% of the cysts reviewed. There was a male predominance; the mean age at diagnosis was in the range 28–33 years; 75% of patients complained either of an abdominal mass or pain. Cysts may become infected; the contents become purulent and the capsule or surrounding pulp shows an inflammatory response (Didlake and Miller, 1986).

7.11.11 CAPSULAR CHANGES

As shown by Baillie (1793), the splenic capsule occasionally shows fibrosis in the form of a diffuse thickening or plaque formation. Adhesions may be seen if an inflammatory process has been present. Wanless and Bernier (1983) have reviewed the changes in the capsule: normal capsular thickness was found to be about 0.184 mm. Capsules thicker than 0.23 mm, the upper limit of normal variation, were found in 25% of cases. This thickening was more evident with advancing age; other contributory factors

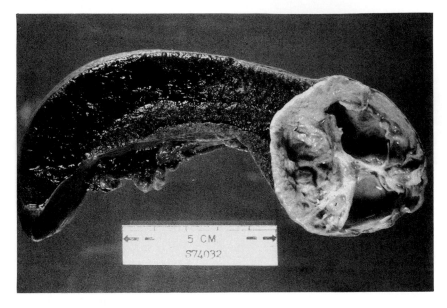

Figure 7.12 Splenic cyst. An epidermoid cyst with a focally thickened but intact capsule. Adjacent spleen shows no significant abnormal characteristics.

were congestive heart failure and intrahepatic sclerosis. Histologically the thickening was usually a dense hyaline band superficial to the elastica of the capsule. In some cases bands of collagen extended internally. Iron was often present, as were small blood vessels, particularly in early lesions.

REFERENCES

Ambrosino, D. M. *et al.* (1987) An immunodeficiency characterized by impaired antibody responses to polysaccharides. *N. Engl. J. Med.*, **316**, 790–3.

Audouin, J. *et al.* (1988) Malignant lymphoplasmacytic lymphoma with prominent splenomegaly (primary lymphoma of the spleen). *J. Pathol.*, **155**, 17–33.

Baillie, M. (1793) *The Morbid Anatomy of Some of the Most Important Parts of the Human Body.* London.

Bearman, R. M., Pangales, G. A. and Rappaport, H. (1978) Prolymphocytic leukemia. Clinical, histopathological, and cytochemical observations. *Cancer*, **42**, 2360–72.

Berendt, H. L., Mant, M. J. and Jewell, L. D. (1986)

Periarterial fibrosis in the spleen in idiopathic thrombocytopenic purpura. *Arch. Pathol. Lab. Med.*, **110**, 1152–4.

Blaustein, A. U. (1963) *The Spleen.* McGraw-Hill, New York.

Bleiweiss, I. J., Thung, S. N. and Goodman, J. D. (1986) Peliosis of the spleen in a patient with cirrhosis of the liver. *Arch. Pathol. Lab. Med.*, **110**, 669–71.

Blendis, L. M., Williams, R. and Kreel, L. (1969) Radiological determination of spleen size. *Gut*, **10**, 433–5.

Bowdler, A. J. (1983) Splenomegaly and hypersplenism. in *The Spleen* (ed. S. M. Lewis), *Clin. Haematol.*, **12**, 467–88.

Boyd, E. (1933) Normal variability in weight of the adult human liver and spleen. *Arch. Pathol.*, **16**, 350–72.

Boyko, W. J., Pratt, R. and Wass, H. (1982) Functional hyposplenism, a diagnostic clue in amyloidosis: Report of six cases. *Am. J. Clin. Pathol.*, **77**, 745–8.

Burke, J. S., Byrne, G. E., Jr and Rappaport, H. (1974) Hairy cell leukemia (leukemic reticuloendotheliosis). I. A clinical pathologic study of 21 patients. *Cancer*, **33**, 1399–410.

Burke, J. S., MacKay, B. and Rappaport, H. (1976)

Hairy cell leukemia (leukemic reticulendotheliosis). II. Ultrastructure of the spleen. *Cancer*, 37, 2267–74.

Burke, J. S. and Osborne, B. M. (1983) Localized reactive lymphoid hyperplasia of the spleen simulating malignant lymphoma. A report of seven cases. *Am. J. Surg. Pathol.*, 4, 373–80.

Carr, A. J., *et al.* (1987) Male choriocarcinoma of the spleen: a case report. *Eur. J. Surg. Oncol.*, 13, 75–6.

Chen, K. T. and Felix, E. L. (1986) Splenic peliosis. *Arch. Pathol. Lab. Med.*, 110, 1122. (Letter)

Chen, K. T., Flam, M. S. and Workman, R. D. (1987) Amyloid tumor of the spleen. *Am. J. Surg. Pathol.*, 11, 723–5.

Cheng, D. S., Williams, H. J. and Kitahara, M. (1980) Hereditary hepatosplenomegaly. *West. J. Med.*, 132, 70–4.

Chulay, J. D. and Lankerani, M. R. (1976) Splenic abscess. Report of 10 cases and review of the literature. *Am. J. Med.*, 61, 513–22.

Cimmino, M. A. *et al.* (1988) Spirochetes in the spleen of a patient with chronic lyme disease. *Am. J. Clin. Pathol.*, 91, 95–7.

Cruickshank, B. (1984) Follicular (mineral oil) lipidosis: I. Epidemiologic studies of involvement of the spleen. *Hum. Pathol.*, 15, 724–30.

Cruickshank, B. and Thomas, M. J. (1984) Mineral oil (follicular) lipidosis: II. Histologic studies of spleen, liver, lymph nodes, and bone marrow. *Hum. Pathol.*, 15, 731–7.

Dawes, L. G. and Malangoni, M. A. (1986) Cystic masses of the spleen. *Am. Surg.*, 52, 333–6.

de Vries, M. J., Dooren, L. J. and Cleton, F. J. (1968) Graft-versus-host or autoimmune lesions in the Swiss type of agammaglobulinemia: their relation to a deficient development of the thymic epithelium. in *Immunologic Deficiency Diseases in Man* (ed. D. Bergsma), The National Foundation, New York, pp. 173–87.

Didlake, R. H. and Miller, R. C. (1986) Epidermoid cyst of the spleen manifested as an abdominal abscess. *South. Med. J.*, 79, 635–7.

Easler, R. E. and Dowlin, W. M. (1969) Primary lipoma of the spleen: A case report. *Arch. Pathol.*, 88, 557–9.

Eichner, E. R. and Whitfield, G. L. (1981) Splenomegaly. An algorithmic approach to diagnosis. *J. Am. Med. Assoc.*, 246, 2858–61.

Ellison, R. B. (1980) Radiologic Seminar CCI: Cystic lymphangioma – a consideration in asymptomatic, massive, cystic splenomegaly. *J. Miss. State Med. Assoc.*, 21, 61–8.

Epstein, B. M. and Omar, G. M. (1983) Infective complications of splenic trauma. *Clin. Radiol.*, 34, 91–4.

Falks, S., Muller, H. and Stutte, H. J. (1988) The spleen in acquired immunodeficiency syndrome. *Pathol. Res. Pract.*, 183, 425–33.

Fleming, C. R., Dickson, E. R. and Harrison, E. G. (1976) Splenosis: autotransplantation of splenic tissue. *Am. J. Med.*, 61, 414–19.

Frank, J. M. and Palomino, N. J. (1987) Primary amyloidosis with diffuse splenic infiltration presenting as fulminant pneumococcal sepsis. *Am. J. Clin. Pathol.*, 87, 405–7.

Gadaleanu, G. (1981) Spleen immunomorphologic behaviour in primary and secondary acute bronchopulmonary inflammations of children. Comparative analysis of the lung and hilar-tracheobronchial lymph node reactions. *Morphol. Embryol.*, 27, 219–25.

Garcia, R. L., Khan, M. K. and Berlin, R. B. (1982) Peliosis of the spleen with rupture. *Hum. Pathol.*, 13, 177–9.

Garvin, D. F. and King, F. M. (1981) Cysts and nonlymphomatous tumors of the spleen. *Pathol. Ann.*, 16, 61–80.

Geary, C. G., Clough, V. and MacIver, J. E. (1980) Tropical splenomegaly. *Br. J. Hosp. Med.*, 24, 419–21.

Gertz, M. A., Kyle, R. A. and Greipp, P. R. (1983) Hyposplenism in primary systemic amyloidosis. *Ann. Intern. Med.*, 98, 475–7.

Grillot-Courvalin, C. *et al.* (1986) The syndrome of T8 hyperlymphocytosis: Variation in phenotype and cytotoxic activities of granular cells and evaluation of their role in associated neutropenia. *Blood*, 69, 1204–10.

Guyton, J. R. and Zumwalt, R. E. (1975) Pneumococcemia with sarcoid-infiltrated spleen. *Ann. Intern. Med.*, 82, 847–8.

Haber, L. M. *et al.* (1988) Fat overload sydrome. An autopsy study with evaluation of the coagulopathy. *Am. J. Clin. Pathol.*, 89, 223–7.

Hamoudi, A. B., Vassay, L. E. and Morse, T. S. (1975) Multiple lymphangioendotheliomata of the spleen in a 13-year-old girl. *Arch. Pathol.*, 99, 605–6.

Hara, K. (1985) Three cases of primary splenic lymphoma: Case report and review of the Japanese experience. *Acta Pathol. Jpn*, 35, 419–35.

Harris, N. (1985) Case Records of the Massachusetts General Hospital. *N. Engl. J. Med.*, 313, 1405–12.

Hesdorffer, C. S. *et al.* (1986) True idiopathic splenomegaly – a distinct entity. *Scand. J. Haematol.*, **37**, 310–15.

Hogan, S. F., Osborne, B. M. and Butler, J. J. (1989) Unexpected splenic nodules in leukemic patients. *Hum. Pathol.*, **20**, 62–8.

Iozzo, R. V., Haas, J. E. and Chard, R. L. (1980) Symptomatic splenic hamartoma: a report of two cases and review of the literature. *Pediatrics*, **66**, 261–5.

Johnson, J. D. and Roff, M. J. (1984) Fungal splenic abscess. *Arch. Intern. Med.*, **144**, 1987–93.

Judge, D. M. *et al.* (1974) Louse-borne relapsing fever in man. *Arch. Pathol.*, **97**, 136–40.

Kagalwala, T. Y. *et al.* (1987) Cavernous hemangiomas of the liver and spleen. *Indian Pediatr.*, **24**, 427–30.

Kevy, S. V. *et al.* (1968) Hereditary splenic hypoplasia. *Pediatrics*, **42**, 752–7.

Klatt, E. C. and Meyer, P. R. (1987) Pathology of the spleen in the acquired immunodeficiency syndrome. *Pathol. Lab. Med.*, **111**, 1050–3.

Klein, B. *et al.* (1987) Splenomegaly and solitary spleen metastasis in solid tumors. *Cancer*, **60**, 100–2.

Kozicky, O. J. *et al.* (1987) Splenic amyloidosis: A case report of spontaneous splenic rupture with a review of the pertinent literature. *Am. J. Gastroenterol.*, **82**, 582–7.

Kringsholm, B. and Christoffersen, P. (1984) Spleen and portal lymph node pathology in fatal drug addiction. *Forensic Sci. Int.*, **25**, 233–44.

Kuo, T. and Rosai, J. (1974) Granulomatous inflammation in splenectomy specimens. *Arch. Pathol.*, **98**, 261–8.

Lacson, A., Berman, L. D. and Neiman, R. S. (1979) Peliosis of the spleen. *Am. J. Clin. Pathol.*, **71**, 586–90.

Lampert, I. A. (1983) Splenectomy as a diagnostic technique. *Clin. Haematol.*, **12**, 535–63.

Lawhorne, T. W., Jr and Zuidema, G. D. (1976) Splenic abscess. *Surgery*, **79**, 686–9.

Lee, J. K. *et al.* (1987) Splenic hamartoma; report of a case and review of the literature. *J. Formosan Med. Assoc.*, **86**, 1125–8.

Lee, R. E., Peters, S. P. and Glew, R. H. (1977) Gaucher's disease: clinical, morphologic and pathogenic considerations. *Pathol. Ann.*, **2**, 309–24.

Lemley, D. E., Chun, B. and Cupps, T. R. (1987) Sterile splenic abscesses in systemic Weber–Christian disease. *Am. J. Med.*, **83**. 567–9.

Liber, A. F. and Rose, H. G. (1967) Saturated hydrocarbons in follicular lipidosis of the spleen. *Arch. Pathol.*, **83**, 116–22.

Loughran, T. P. Jr *et al.* (1985) Leukemia of large granular lymphocytes: association with clonal chromosomal abnormalities and autoimmune neutropenia, thrombocytopenia, and hemolytic anemia. *Ann. Intern. Med.*, **102**, 169–75.

Lowenthal, M. N. *et al.* (1980) Massive splenomegaly in Northern Zambia. I. Analysis of 344 cases. *Trans. Roy. Soc. Trop. Med. Hyg.*, **74**, 91–8.

Macpherson, A. I. S., Richmond, J. and Stuart, A. E. (1973) *The Spleen*. American Lecture Series, No. 893. Charles C. Thomas, Springfield.

Manoharan, A., Bader, L. V. and Pitney, W. R. (1982) Non-tropical idiopathic splenomegaly (Dacie's Syndrome). Report of 5 cases. *Scand. J. Haematol.*, **28**, 175–9.

Marymount, J. V. and Knight, P. J. (1987) Splenic lymphangiomatosis: a rare cause of splenomegaly. *J. Pediatr. Surg.*, **5**, 461–2.

Massad, M. *et al.* (1988) Spontaneous splenic rupture in an adult with mumps: A case report. *Surgery*, **103**, 381–2.

McCormick, W. F. and Kashgarian, M. (1965) The weight of the adult human spleen. *Am. J. Clin. Pathol.*, **43**, 332–3.

McKenna, R. W. *et al.* (1977) Chronic lymphoproliferative disorder with unusual clinical, morphologic, ultrastructural and membrane surface marker characteristics. *Am. J. Med.*, **62**, 588–96.

McKinley, R. A., Kwan, Y. L. and Lam-Po-Tang, P. R. L. (1987) Familial splenomegaly syndrome with reduced circulating T helper cells and splenic germinal center hypoplasia. *Br. J. Haematol.*, **67**, 393–6.

McMahon, R. F. T. (1988) Inflammatory pseudotumor of spleen. *J. Clin. Pathol.*, **41**, 734–6.

McMillan, R. *et al.* (1974) Quantitation of platelet binding IgG produced *in vitro* by spleen from patients with idiopathic thrombocytopenia. *N. Engl. J. Med.*, **291**, 812–7.

Miale, J. B. (1971) Hemopoietic system: reticuloendothelium, spleen, lymph nodes and bone marrow. in *Pathology*, 6th edn (ed. W. A. D. Anderson), C. V. Mosby, St Louis, p. 1302.

Mirchandani, H. G., Mirchandani, I. H. and Pak, M. S. Y. (1985) Spontaneous rupture of the spleen due to acquired immunodeficiency syndrome in an intravenous drug abuser. *Arch. Pathol. Lab. Med.*, **109**, 1114–16.

Morgenstern, L. *et al.* (1984) Hamartomas of the spleen. *Arch. Surg.*, **119**, 1291–3.

Myers, J. and Segal, R. J. (1974) Weight of the spleen. I. Range of normal in a nonhospital population. *Arch. Pathol.*, **98**, 33–5.

Naeim, F., Copper, P. H. and Semion, A. A. (1973)

Peliosis hepatis. Possible etiologic role of anabolic steroids. *Arch. Pathol.*, **95**, 284–5.

Nanba, K. *et al.* (1977) Splenic pseudosinuses and hepatic angiomatous lesions. Distinctive features of hairy cell leukemia. *Am. J. Clin. Pathol.*, **67**, 415–26.

Neiman, R. (1977) Incidence and importance of splenic sarcoid-like granulomas. *Arch. Pathol.*, **100**, 518–21.

Nezelof, C. *et al.* (1964) L'hypoplasie héréditaire du thymus: sa place et sa responsibilité. Une observation d' aplasie lymphocytaire normoplasmocytaire et normoglobulinemique du nourrisson. *Arch. Fr. Pediatr.*, **21**, 897–920.

Nezelof, C. (1968) Thymic dysplasia with normal immunoglobulins and immunologic deficiency: Pure alymphocytosis. in *Immunologic Deficiency Diseases in Man* (ed. D. Bergsma), The National Foundation, New York, pp. 104–5.

Niedt, G. W. and Schinella, R. (1985) Acquired immunodeficiency syndrome. *Arch. Pathol. Lab. Med.*, **109**, 727–34.

Niv, Y., Abu-Avid, S. and Oren, M. (1986) Primary Hodgkin's disease of the spleen. *Am. J. Med.*, **81**, 1120–1.

Pistoia, F. and Markowitz, S. K. (1988) Splenic lymphangiomatosis: CT diagnosis. *Am. J. Radiol.*, **150**, 121–2.

Prager, D., Morel, D. and Dex, W. (1971) The syndrome of chronic occult rupture of the spleen. *J. Am. Med. Assoc.*, **218**, 1824–5.

Putschar, W. G. T. and Manion, W. C. (1956) Congenital absence of the spleen and associated anomalies. *Am. J. Clin. Pathol.*, **26**, 429–70.

Raff, L. J. and Schwartz, S. T. (1983) Polysplenia complex and duodenal atresia. *Arch. Pathol. Lab. Med.*, **107**, 202–3.

Rappaport, H. (1966) Tumors of the hematopoietic system. in *Atlas of Tumor Pathology*, Armed Forces Institute of Pathology, Fascicle 8, Section 3, 357–88.

Reichert, C. M. *et al.* (1983) Autopsy pathology in the acquired immune deficiency syndrome. *Am. J. Pathol.*, **112**, 357–82.

Robbins, S. L., Cotran, R. S. and Kumar, V. (1989) *Pathologic Basis of Disease*. 4th edn. W. B. Saunders, Philadelphia and London.

Rosai, J. (1986) *Ackerman's Surgical Pathology*. 7th edn, C. V. Mosby, St Louis.

Rose, N. R., Friedman, H. and Fahey, J. L. (1986) *Manual of Clinical Laboratory Immunology*, 3rd edn, American Society of Microbiology, Washington, DC.

Rousselet, M-C. *et al.* (1988) Idiopathic thrombocy-topenic purpura in patients at risk for acquired immunodeficiency syndrome. *Arch. Pathol. Lab. Med.*, **112**, 1242–50.

Schmidt, W. A. (1983) *Principles and Techniques of Surgical Pathology.* Maddson-Wesley, Menlo Park, CA, pp. 219–22.

Sheahan, K., Wolf, B. C. and Neiman, R. (1988) Inflammatory pseudotumor of the spleen: a clinicopathologic study of three cases. *Hum. Pathol.*, **19**, 1024–31.

Silverman, M. L. and LiVolsi, V. A. (1978) Splenic hamartoma. *Am. J. Clin. Pathol.*, **70**, 224–9.

Silverstein, M. N., Ellefson, R. D. and Ahern, E. J. (1970) The syndrome of the sea-blue histiocyte. *N. Engl. J. Med.*, **282**, 1–4.

Smith, V. C., Eisenberg, B. L. and McDonald, E. C. (1985) Primary splenic angiosarcoma. Case report and literature review. *Cancer*, **55**, 1625–7.

Snover, D. C. *et al.* (1981) Wiskott–Aldrich syndrome: Histopathologic findings in the lymph nodes and spleens of 15 patients. *Hum. Pathol.*, **12**, 821–31.

Sodeman, W. A. and Sodeman, W. A., Jr (1979) *Pathologic Physiology: Mechanisms of Disease*, 6th edn (eds W. A. Sodeman Jr and T. M. Sodeman), W. B. Saunders, Philadelphia and London.

Sordillo, E. M., Sordillo, P. P. and Hajdu, S. I. (1981) Primary hemangiosarcoma of the spleen: report of four cases. *Med. Pediatr. Oncol.*, **9**, 319–24.

Spier, C. M. *et al.* (1985) Malignant lymphoma with primary presentation in the spleen. *Arch. Pathol. Lab. Med.*, **109**, 1076–80.

Steinberg, M. H., Gatling, R. R. and Tavassoli, M. (1983) Evidence of hyposplenism in the presence of splenomegaly. *Scand. J. Haematol.*, **5**, 437–9.

Stovall, T. G. and Ling, F. W. (1988) Splenosis: report of a case and review of the literature. *Obstet. Gynecol.*, **43**, 69–72.

Tada, T., Wakkabayashi, T. and Kishimoto, H. (1983) Peliosis of the spleen. *Am. J. Clin. Pathol.*, **79**, 708–13.

Tavassoli, M. and McMillan, R. (1975) Structure of the spleen in idiopathic thrombocytopenia purpura. *Am. J. Clin. Pathol.*, **64**, 180–91.

Tavassoli, M. and Weiss, L. (1973) An electron microscopic study of the spleen in myelofibrosis with myeloid metaplasia. *Blood*, **42**, 267–79.

Taxy, J. B. (1978) Peliosis: A morphologic curiosity becomes an iatrogenic problem. *Hum. Pathol.*, **9**, 331–40.

Timens, W. and Poppema, S. (1985) Lymphocyte compartments in the human spleen. An immuno-histologic study in normal spleens and noninvolved spleens in Hodgkin's disease. *Am. J. Pathol.*, **120**, 443–54.

Timens, W. and Poppema, S. (1987) Impaired immune response to polysaccharides. *N. Engl. J. Med.*, **317**, 837–8.

Travis, W. D. and Li, C-Y. (1988) Pathology of the lymph node and spleen in systemic mast cell disease. *Modern Pathol.*, **1**, 4–14.

Turk, C. O., Lipson, S. B. and Brandt, T. D. (1988) Splenosis mimicking a renal mass. *Urology*, **24**, 248–50.

Wanless, I. R. and Bernier, V. (1983) Fibrous thickening of the splenic capsule. *Arch. Pathol. Lab. Med.*, **107**, 595–9.

Wanless, I. R. and Geddie, W. R. (1985) Mineral oil lipogranulomata in liver and spleen. *Arch. Pathol. Lab. Med.*, **109**, 283–6.

Warfel, K. A. and Ellis, G. H. (1982) Peliosis of the spleen. *Arch. Pathol. Lab. Med.*, **106**, 99–100.

Weisdorf, S. A. and Krivit, R. (1982) Paucity of splenic germinal centers: a new and unique splenomegaly syndrome including dysfunctional immune system. *Clin. Immunol. Immunopathol.*, **23**, 492–500.

Whitley, J. E., Maynard, C. D. and Rhyne, A. L. (1966) A computer approach to the prediction of spleen weight from routine films. *Radiology*, **86**, 73–6.

Wick, M. R. and Rife, C. C. (1981) Paratesticular accessory spleen. *Mayo Clin. Proc.*, **56**, 455–6.

Wiener, R. S. and Ong, L. S. (1989) Streptokinase and splenic rupture. *Am. J. Med.*, **86**, 249.

Willey, R. F., Rodger, A. and Webb, J. N. (1982) Seminoma presenting as gross splenomegaly. *Scot. Med. J.*, **27**, 254–5.

Wolf, B. C. and Neiman, R. S. (1988) *Disorders of the Spleen*. W. B. Saunders, Philadelphia and London.

Ziegler, J. L. and Dorfman, R. F. (1988) *Kaposi's Sarcoma: Pathophysiology and Clinical Management*. Marcel Dekker, New York.

SPLENIC POOLING AND THE SURVIVAL OF BLOOD CELLS

8

Anthony J. Bowdler and Aage Videbaek

8.1 INTRODUCTION

The frequency with which deficits in the principal cell lines occur in the blood counts of patients with splenomegaly has indicated a special relationship between the spleen and the composition of the circulating blood. To some investigators this suggested a humoral controlling mechanism whereby the spleen could affect the rates of hemopoietic production and delivery of cells to the circulation (Dameshek and Estren, 1947; Dameshek, 1955): to the present time no convincing evidence has been presented that there is such an effect, at least to the extent that it would be of clinical significance (Bowdler, 1983).

To others the relationship appeared to depend on an increased rate of cell destruction by the spleen (Doan, 1949); this was widely regarded as an exaggeration of the normal splenic function of destroying effete blood cells reaching the end of their normal lifespan. There was an implicit assumption that increased splenic mass would increase the rate of cell destruction, but this left to be explained why hemolysis of detectable degree was so variable among subjects with comparable degrees of splenic enlargement. Furthermore, it did not explain why conditions with active, or even aggressive, hemolysis might be associated with minor degrees of splenomegaly.

A more detailed insight into the relationship between the spleen and circulating blood cells

evolved when effective cell-labeling techniques became available in the decades following 1950. ^{51}Cr-labeling was the most productive (Gray and Sterling, 1950): in the measurement of red cell lifespan it provided only approximate estimates, owing to the elution of radionuclide from cells, for which only approximate corrections could be made. However, the nuclide was detectable at the body surface, and this made it possible to track cells during the various phases of their interaction with the spleen and other organs, and in conjunction with surface counting of ^{131}I-labeled plasma albumin, to determine the relative concentration of red cells and plasma in different regions of the body ('regional hematocrit').

These methods showed that the radionuclide labeling red cells could in various circumstances reflect up to three phases of red cell interaction with the spleen. In normal circumstances the first phase occurs during the first two to three minutes following the injection of labeled cells, during the period in which these are mixing with the cells of the general circulation. There is a rapid rise in the radioactivity detectable over the spleen, with a half-time of one minute or slightly longer, and a simultaneous fall in the radioactivity of venous blood samples (Figure 8.1). These trends terminate in a plateau in both venous and splenic radioactivity when the mixing of injected red cells in the circulation is complete. Following this, on a time-scale of days rather than minutes, there is often a slight but detectable net increase in radioactivity over the spleen, which results from radionuclide adsorbed to the tissues from a fraction of the labeled red cells after their destruction.

In pathological circumstances a further phase in the initial rise in radioactivity over the spleen is often detectable, especially when the spleen is enlarged (Harris, McAlister and Prankerd, 1958; Motulsky *et al.*, 1958; Toghill, 1964; Christensen, 1973). Following the initial rise there is frequently a second and more slowly rising phase with a half-time (T_{50}) of between 5 and 60 minutes or more (Figures 8.1 and 8.2).

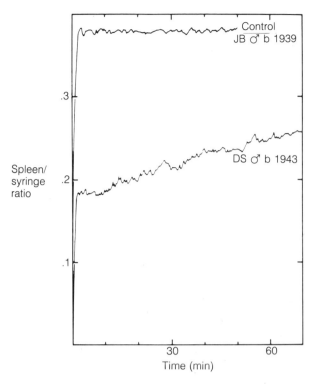

Figure 8.1 Tracings of radioactivity detectable at the body surface over the spleen with a collimated scintillation counter following the intravenous injection of ^{51}Cr-labeled red cells. The control tracing (JB) is from a subject without splenomegaly, and shows a rapid rise to an early plateau. This reflects the mixing of the nuclide-labeled cells with the red cells in the circulation. A single phase tracing of this type is typically found in normal subjects. The lower tracing (DS) is from a subject with warm-antibody autoimmune hemolytic anemia. The surface radioactivity rises in two phases: the first is a rapid rise comparable to that of the normal subject. The slower secondary rise reflects the exchange of red cells with the splenic pool, and is abnormal. *Ordinate*: surface radioactivity in arbitrary units, related to the radioactivity of the syringe containing the labeled red cells, assayed with a standard geometrical relationship to the scintillation counter. *Abscissa*: time in minutes from injection. (Reproduced with permission of the publishers, the American College of Physicians, from Bowdler (1966) *Annals of Internal Medicine*, **65**, Fig. 3, p. 763.)

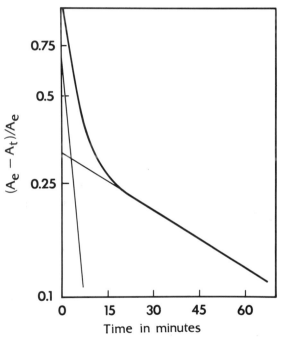

Figure 8.2 The surface radioactivity over the spleen can be separated into two components in cases such as DS in Figure 8.1. Plotting sequentially the radioactivity at time 't' as its difference from the final equilibrial activity, A_e, gives two phases. By semilogarithmic plotting the second phase can be linearized; its regression line can be characterized to give best estimates of the fraction of the radioactivity attributable to the pool and its half-time of development. Subtraction of the slow phase curve from the total curve gives the curve for the initial phase. *Ordinate*: surface radioactivity expressed as ($A_e - A_t$)/A_e. *Abscissa*: time in minutes.

This arises from the mixing of the labeled cells with a splenic pool of red cells which slowly exchanges with the red cells of the general circulation. Comparable pooling has not been described in other organs.

Platelets also show a pooling phenomenon, but in this case the pool is present in the normal spleen and expands as the organ enlarges pathologically. There is also good evidence for the pooling of granulocytes in the normal spleen, the pool being in dynamic equilibruim with circulating granulocytes, and constituting a component of the marginating granulocyte pool (Peters *et al.*, 1985a). The transit times for platelets and granulocytes are similar at approximately 6–12 minutes, which is considerably shorter than is found in most cases of pathologically pooled red cells.

8.2 THE PATHOLOGICAL POOLING OF RED CELLS

8.2.1 THE ANALYSIS OF RADIONUCLIDE UPTAKE BY SURFACE COUNTING

The slowly rising component in surface radioactivity over the spleen after the injection of ^{51}Cr-labeled red cells can be reduced to a simple exponential expression. If A_t is the surface activity at any time t, and A_e is the activity when equilibrium is attained, then $(A_e - A_t)/A_e$ expresses the shortfall in radioactivity from the equilibrium level at any time t, as a fraction of the final level of radioactivity (Figure 8.2). The logarithm of the expression can be plotted graphically against time, most conveniently on semilogarithmic paper, to give a curve which declines in two phases. The second phase reflects the slow secondary rise in splenic radioactivity, and using numerical data from points beyond the primary rise in activity it is possible to define the second phase as the calculated regression line of log $[(A_e - A_t)/A_e]$ against time. This can be extrapolated to the ordinate: the antilog of the point at which it cuts the ordinate gives the fraction of the total radioactivity which can be ascribed to the slow phase. This line can be further characterized by the time taken for its value to fall to half the value at zero time ($T_{1/2}$ or T_{50}). By a conventional 'curve peeling' process, the initial phase of the curve can be corrected by subtracting the values of the extrapolated slow phase regression line from the total curve. The residual values can then be expressed as the 'fast phase' regression line, and characterized as the fraction of total activity and its half-time for disappearance.

8.2.2 PATHOLOGICAL CONDITIONS PRODUCING SPLENIC RED CELL POOLING

Red cell pooling demonstrated by radionuclide studies has been found predominantly in two circumstances: first, it tends to be well marked in conditions characterized by active hemolysis associated with overt abnormalities of the red cells. Second, it occurs in disorders with marked splenic enlargement, but usually with less evidence of accelerated red cell destruction.

In the first group are conditions such as hereditary spherocytosis, hemolytic hereditary elliptocytosis, warm antibody autoimmune hemolytic disease, thalassemia major and pernicious anemia. The properties of the red cell appear to determine the development of pooling, presumably because they impede flow through the pathways of the spleen. With respect to hereditary spherocytosis, and some cases of autoimmune hemolytic anemia, the spherocytic (or more precisely stomatocytic) shape may itself reduce deformability of the cell, and diminish the probability of a normal passage through sites such as the potential interendothelial spaces of the walls of the splenic sinuses. In addition, it is possible that poorly deformable cells are also impeded in passage elsewhere in the splenic circulation, for example in more proximal channels of the red pulp. (See Chapter 4 for a more detailed discussion.) Although red cell shape appears to be the principal characteristic affecting flow through the spleen, other factors may include membrane rigidity (in hereditary spherocytosis), the adherence of cell surface-attached antibody to the F_c-receptors of pulp macrophages (in autoimmune hemolysis), and intraerythrocytic viscosity (in sickle cell syndromes). In these conditions, normal red cells will not pool significantly on infusion into affected subjects, with the exception of a slow splenic uptake in immunohemolytic disorders. Conversely, infusion of the abnormal cells into the circulation of a normal subject produces prompt splenic pooling.

In the second group of conditions, red cell pooling appears to depend on a structural disorder in the affected spleen. Autologous cells have been found to pool in cases of myeloproliferative disorders (especially primary myeloid metaplasia, chronic myeloid leukemia and cases of primary polycythemia with more than slight splenic enlargement), lymphoproliferative disorders (though usually to a lesser degree than in the myeloproliferative disorders), congestive splenomegaly, primary hypersplenism ('nontropical idiopathic splenomegaly') and tropical splenomegaly. Normal red cells infused into subjects with 'structural' splenic pooling will also demonstrate 'slow-phase' accumulation in the spleen, although not necessarily to the same extent as is found with autologous cells.

In both groups of 'pooling' conditions it seems most probable that the principal site of the red cell pool is the red pulp (Stutte, 1970; Pearson, Spencer and Cornelius, 1969) and that the pathological changes in the spleen have interrupted the pathways of flow for blood cells. It is possible that the sinus reticular coat is abnormal and alters the dimensions of the interendothelial slits of the sinuses in conditions such as chronic myelogenous leukemia (Björkman, 1947). In other cases it may be that the arteriolar terminations, which are normally quite close to the external aspects of the sinus walls, have been distracted, so that directed flow towards the sinuses becomes interrupted. Other areas of the pulp flow pathways may be diverted by cellular accumulations, and it is possible to find spleens in which dense pathological cellular infiltrates (as in lymphomata or Gaucher's disease) impair flow to the extent

that no exchangeable pool can be demonstrated.

8.2.3 THE CONCEPT OF THE RED CELL POOL: ITS QUANTITATION

Comparison of the rise in surface radioactivity over the spleen with the corresponding fall in the radioactivity in the blood shows that the loss of red cells to the spleen may greatly exceed the numbers which could be sustainable by red cell production in a steady state. It is clear, therefore, that the secondary rise in splenic radioactivity must reflect an exchange of viable cells rather than a unidirectional loss of cells to the spleen. This suggested the exchange of red cells between two pools, the one present in the general circulation and the other in a splenic pool of viable cells.

The volume of red cells in the exchanging red cell pool in the spleen can be estimated by three principal methods:

1. The volume of distribution of labeled red cells can be measured from blood samples taken by venepuncture at three minutes after injection of the labeled red cells, and again after surface counting over the spleen shows that the pool has equilibrated. The difference in the volumes of distribution approximates to the red cell volume in the pool. The error of the method is increased when the rate of equilibration is high and the $T_{1/2}$ of the slow phase short, as significant pooling may have occurred before the first blood sample is taken.

2. The pool volume may be estimated by measurements of surface radioactivity, calibrated against a phantom (or model) of the spleen with known amounts of activity (Glass *et al.*, 1968; Christensen, 1971). Scanning techniques may be used to provide a more accurate estimate of spleen volume (Rasmussen *et al.*, 1973).

3. A third method of estimating the volume and turnover time is to analyze the fall in circulating red cell activity following the

intravenous injection of labeled red cells. The mathematical model assumes 'first order' exchange kinetics between circulating red cells and the pooled cells, and applies the calculations of two-compartment exchange (Solomon, 1953; Bowdler, 1962).

The structural basis for red cell pooling has been discussed in detail in Chapter 4; radionuclide studies have not provided a unique solution to the question of the required structure, although evidence for a high degree of red cell concentration in the pool suggested a parallel with the storage pool found in many mammals. Harris, McAlister and Prankerd (1958) suggested that the fast-phase of the surface equilibration curve reflected flow through the direct anatomical splenic vascular pathways, whereas the slow-phase was the result of flow through the indirect (pulp) pathways. It has not, however, been possible to define a mechanism whereby cells would be differentially directed into the appropriate pathway when their characteristics were abnormal, and it seems more probable that the spleen functions by passive filtration, rather than by an active

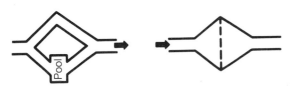

Figure 8.3 Concepts of splenic pooling of red cells. The diagram on the left suggests two routes of blood flow through the spleen, the one providing for unobstructed fast flow, and the second a separate slowly flowing compartment. The diagram on the right suggests a functional barrier to flow, which may permit differential flow, either on the basis of (1) the characteristics of the red cells, or (2) the variable relationships of the afferent arterial capillaries to the efferent vessels (sinuses). (Reproduced with modification by permission of Baillière Tindall Ltd. from *Clinics in Haematology*, 1983, **12**, Figures 1D and 1E, p. 473.)

sorting mechanism (Figure 8.3). This concept holds that the majority of red cells are presented to the same pulp pathway, and that their flow rate is determined either by intrinsic characteristics of the cells, or by the proximity of the arteriolar capillaries to the sinus walls.

The volumes of red cells in the splenic pool are quite variable, and vary from 5% of the total red cell mass to more than 40%, so that in some cases where red cell production is impaired the diversion of cells away from the active circulation may be a supplementary cause of anemia. Taking all causes of splenomegaly together, there is no close correlation between spleen size and the volume of the red cell pool. However, within fairly broad limits there is a tendency for the pool size to increase with spleen weight (Christensen, 1975).

8.2.4   THE CELL ENVIRONMENT IN THE POOLING SPLEEN

Measurements of the 'body hematrocrit', expressed as the percentage of total blood volume which consists of red cells, show that it tends to be lower than the venous hematocrit, which is representative of large vessel blood. The ratio of the body hematocrit to venous hematocrit is normally remarkably constant at about 0.91 ± 0.02 (Mollison, Engelfriet and Contreras, 1987). In the presence of marked splenomegaly the body hematocrit rises in relation to the venous hematocrit, indicating the presence of a region containing blood at a high hematocrit. Surface counting studies with labeled red cells and plasma have shown this to be in the spleen (Bowdler, 1969), where the 'regional hematocrit' is highest. This shows that the splenic red cell environment is one which is plasma poor, and through which the flow is exceptionally slow. It has been suggested that this creates an adverse environment for the red cells, with a tendency to low glucose levels and pH, creating metabolic stress and depletion of intracellular ATP (Jandl and Aster, 1967; Murphy, 1967; Wennberg and Weiss, 1969; see also Chapter 4).

8.2.5 SPLENIC RED CELL POOLING AND HEMOLYSIS

The adverse physical characteristics of the environment of pooled red cells may have a direct influence on the viability of the pooled cells: this has been demonstrated for the red cells in hereditary spherocytosis in which comparable conditions *in vitro* produce accelerated fragmentation of the red cell membrane, and increased sphering of the cells with loss of membrane area in excess of the loss of volume (Weed and Bowdler, 1966.) This appears to be the basis for the conditioning of the red cells to hemolysis in the spleen and elsewhere. However, the red cell membrane is especially vulnerable in this condition, and the extent to which this occurs in other disorders is uncertain.

In immunohemolytic conditions the red cells in the splenic pool remain in close proximity to the macrophages of the spleen, in flow conditions which produce minimal disturbance to the adherence of red cells to the phagocyte surface. This appears to be capable of enhancing partial or complete phagocytosis of sensitized cells. The low volume of plasma in the pool, due to skimming of plasma before blood reaches the cordal environment, may be an additional factor promoting phagocytosis, in that it reduces the inhibitory effect of ambient immunoglobulins.

However, in other conditions, and especially where pooling is due to structural disorders, the degree of red cell concentration is quite variable, and the proportion of the lifespan of the red cell spent in the pool may be quite low. The critical period of retention in the spleen required to produce deleterious changes in the normal red cell remains to be defined. In the majority of cases in which there is significant splenomegaly without a defined red cell defect, the red cell survival tends to be diminished (Ferrant, 1983), often to a lifespan of 20–30 days. However, while this can frequently be corrected by splenectomy, this is not always the case (Bowdler, 1963), and the conditions required to produce the low-grade 'splenopathic'

anemia are clearly not present in all cases of splenic enlargement.

Christensen (1975) has shown that the volume of red cells in the splenic pool tends to correlate positively with the rates of destruction of red cells by the spleen for given disorders. However, the relationship apparently shows marked differences between groups of disorders: for example, the rate of cell destruction is much higher for a given size of red cell pool in myeloproliferative disorders than it is in lymphoproliferative disorders. This indicates that there are properties of the microenvironment of the pool which affect red cell survival which need more detailed definition than is currently available.

8.3 THE POOLING OF PLATELETS IN THE SPLEEN

In 1923 Binet and Kaplan demonstrated that adrenaline (epinephrine) injected intravenously in dogs causes an immediate but transient increase in the platelet count of the peripheral blood; this effect could be repeated 60–90 minutes after the first injection. It was further shown that adrenaline had mobilized platelets from the spleen, since a comparable rise in blood platelet count did not occur in splenectomized dogs. It was, therefore, concluded that there existed a splenic pool of platelets exchangeable with platelets in the bloodstream.

The importance of the spleen to the adrenaline response was confirmed by demonstrating that the increase in platelet count following adrenaline failed to appear in splenectomized human subjects (Wright *et al.*, 1951; Aster, 1966; Kotilainen, 1969; Branehög, Weinfeld and Roos, 1973). Aster (1965) showed that 25–50% of reinjected ^{51}Cr-labeled platelets are pooled in the human spleen, and that entry of platelets into the spleen is delayed by the administration of adrenaline prior to platelet infusion. This finding was confirmed by Freedman and Karpatkin (1975b). Conversely ^{51}Cr-labeled platelets, once pooled in the spleen, can to some extent be mobilized by adrenaline (Figure 8.4):

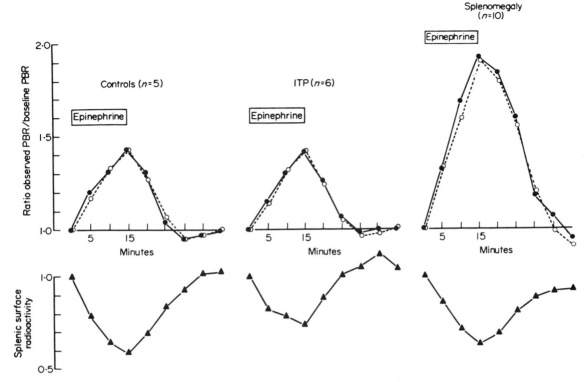

Figure 8.4 The results of epinephrine (adrenaline) tests in five controls, six patients with ITP and ten patients with splenomegaly. Blood samples were drawn for the determination of venous platelet count and platelet bound radioactivity (upper figures), and surface radioactivity over the spleen was recorded during the experiments. Baseline values are given as 1.0, and subsequent values are given in relation to this. Relative platelet counts: ○----○. Relative platelet bound radioactivity: ●——●. Relative splenic surface radioactivity: ▲——▲. (Reproduced by permission of Dr I. Branehög and the publishers of the *British Journal of Haematology* from Branehög, Weinfeld and Roos (1973) *Br. J. Haematol.*, 25, 239–48.)

this was shown by the increase in radioactivity which occurs in the blood following the administration of adrenaline (Aster, 1966; Branehög, Weinfeld and Roos, 1973; Fredén *et al.*, 1978a; Vilén, Fredén and Kutti, 1980) and the concomitant decrease in the platelet radioactivity detectable by surface counting over the spleen (Aster, 1966; Kotilainen, 1969).

When other agents with autonomic effects were investigated, some apparent paradoxes were discovered. The ability of adrenaline to release platelets from the spleen is shared by the beta-1-receptor blocking agent, metoprolol (Kutti *et al.*, 1977), whereas the beta-1-receptor

stimulator, isoprenaline, has the opposite effect and leads to trapping of platelets in the spleen (Olsson *et al.*, 1976; Fredén *et al.*, 1978a, 1978b). Peters and Lavender (1983) suggested that the apparently conflicting results could be explained by the effects of these agents on splenic blood flow, which decreases after adrenaline and increases after isoprenaline. However, adrenaline also diminishes spleen size (Doan and Wright, 1946), and in 13 human subjects Schaffner *et al.* (1985) showed by ultrasound a highly significant correlation between contraction of the spleen and the mobilization of platelets ($r = 0.815$, $P < 0.002$).

Vilén, Fredén and Kutti (1980) observed that a proportion of the platelet pool is located outside the spleen: after having re-infused ^{51}Cr-labeled platelets into three normal and three splenectomized healthy men, adrenaline was given and the blood platelet count and peripheral platelet radioactivity were measured. In the non-splenectomized men, platelet counts increased by 40%; the asplenic men also showed an increase in platelet count and radioactivity, but this was limited to a mean value of only 8%.

Adrenaline and related substances are not the only agents able to mobilize a considerable fraction of the splenic platelet pool. Short-term vigorous physical exercise can induce similar, and sometimes marked, changes which appear immediately after the stress, and disappear after 10–15 minutes rest (Sarajas, Konttinen and Frick, 1961). Dawson and Ogston (1969) investigated 12 intact and 6 splenectomized subjects before and after exercise. Some of the asplenic subjects showed a well-marked transient thrombocytosis, indicating the existence of an extrasplenic exchangeable platelet pool. In humans undertaking physical exercise, Freedman, Altszuler and Karpatkin (1977) noted a transient platelet response. The total mobilizable pool of platelets was calculated to be at least 29% of the total platelet mass. However, splenectomized subjects still show a significant platelet response. On the day following re-injection of ^{111}In-oxine labeled platelets, Schmidt and Rasmussen (1984) investigated 15 healthy subjects who then carried out a defined pattern of vigorous physical work. Platelet radioactivity in the blood increased by about 15% and that measured over the spleen showed an equivalent decrease, which confirmed that the splenic platelet pool was mobilizable by exercise. It is clear, therefore, that there is a substantial fraction of the total platelet population which is held in platelet reservoirs located principally but not exclusively in the spleen, and which can be restored to the general circulation by certain definable and reproducible stimuli.

8.3.1 PLATELET RECOVERY

When radionuclide-labeled platelets tagged with ^{51}Cr or ^{111}In are re-infused, they mix with the platelets present in the circulation. The initial mixing takes place within a matter of minutes (Aster, 1965; Kotilainen, 1969) but this is slower than the equilibration of ^{131}I-labeled albumin with plasma. Because of the delay in complete mixing, the hypothetical 'zero time' activity of labeled platelets must be measured indirectly. The disappearance curve of radioactivity can be extrapolated back to a zero-time value. Alternatively the blood radioactivity due to platelets can be estimated after mixing is complete, and this value taken as '100% of initial activity' (Figure 8.5). Later estimations of platelet activity are then expressed in relation to the initial activity. Plotting the remaining blood radioactivity against time will then demonstrate the platelet disappearance curve. The immediate decrease in radioactivity which occurs in the first 3 minutes reflects initial mixing. Following this the curve slowly reaches a minimum; in normal circumstances this occurs within 10 to 20 minutes of the labeled platelets being infused. Surface radioactivity recorded over the spleen will increase and reach a plateau simultaneously with the blood radioactivity curve reaching its minimum (Figure 8.6). Following this there is an equilibrium phase which tends to be more or less constant for some hours, with the exception of circumstances such as acute idiopathic thrombocytopenia. The spleen and blood curves approach stable values with almost identical monoexponential time courses.

Aster (1966) introduced the term 'platelet recovery': this is the percentage of infused radioactively labeled platelets remaining in the peripheral circulation when equilibrium with the splenic pool is complete. 'Platelet recovery' is calculated from the formula:

$$\text{Platelet recovery (\%)} = \frac{\text{Platelet activity in the total blood volume} \times 100}{\text{Platelet activity infused}}$$

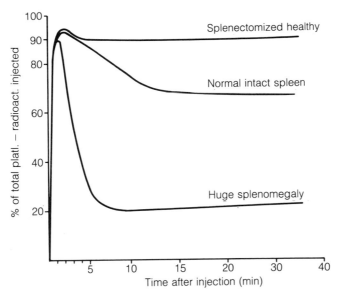

Figure 8.5 ^{51}Cr-platelet radioactivity in the peripheral blood during the first minutes following injection of labeled platelets into normal, splenomegalic and splenectomized human subjects.

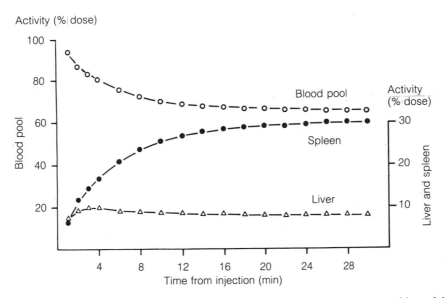

Figure 8.6 Radioactivity curves recorded in relation to the cardiac blood pool, spleen and liver following the injection of autologous ^{111}In-labeled platelets in a normal subject. Ordinate (left): blood pool as percentage of dose. Ordinate (right): liver and spleen activity as percentage of dose. Blood: O——O. Spleen: ●——●. Liver: △——△. (Reproduced by permission of Dr A. M. Peters and the publishers of the *British Journal of Haematology* from Peters, *et al.* (1984) *Br. J. Haematol.*, 57, 637–49.)

In practice this can be calculated as:

$$\frac{\text{Platelet activity/ml blood} \times \text{blood volume (ml)} \times 100}{\text{Infused platelet suspension activity/ml} \times \text{volume infused (ml)}}$$

Platelet recovery has been studied in healthy individuals, splenectomized subjects and patients with splenomegaly from various causes and of differing degrees: an outline of the data is given in Table 8.1. In normal subjects estimates of platelet recovery show a reliable consensus of about 60%, with only slight differences between studies using ^{51}Cr and ^{111}In as the label (*vide infra*). However, individual variation between subjects can be quite considerable. The majority of 'unrecovered' platelets is present in the spleen, with an average calculated value of 27% (Penny, Rozenberg and Firkin, 1966).

^{111}In-oxine, and the later-introduced ^{111}In-tropolonate, offer significant advantages over ^{51}Cr, including higher labeling efficiency, less dependence on available platelet numbers and better external scintigraphic recording (McAfee and Thakur, 1976; Peters and Lavender 1982; Danpure, Osman and Brady, 1982; Kiefel *et al.*, 1985). Since 1979, ^{111}In has largely replaced ^{51}Cr as the platelet label; however, relatively few postsplenectomy platelet recovery studies have been undertaken using this nuclide (Heyns *et al.*, 1980a; Hill-Zobel *et al.*, 1986), and in these recovery values are marginally higher than those obtained by using ^{51}Cr platelets.

In splenectomized subjects (Figure 8.5) the platelet disappearance curve shows no further fall after the initial mixing phase following platelet infusion. This curve lacks the downslope seen when the spleen is present, and platelet recovery is close to 90% in these subjects (Heyns *et al.*, 1980a; Hill-Zobel *et al.*, 1986). These findings indicate that in these circumstances an average of 13% of platelet radioactivity, with a range of 8–20%, is pooled outside the general circulation. Platelet recovery

thus provides an indirect estimate of the splenic platelet pool, since the difference between the total platelet radioactivity infused and platelet recovery represents the sum of the platelet pool in the spleen and the 13% not recovered in asplenic individuals. Since the platelet pools are exchangeable (Aster, 1966; Kotilainen, 1969; Heyns *et al.*, 1980b; Peters *et al.*, 1980) it is apparent that platelets in healthy individuals spend between one-quarter and one-third of their lifespan in the spleen.

The anatomical site of the splenic platelet pool was investigated by scanning electron microscopy (Weiss, 1974): platelets appear to adhere to the surface of the endothelium of the sinuses and reticulum cells of the cords, marginal zone and white pulp.

A special affinity for the spleen is shown by the youngest platelets, which spend the first 1.5 to 2 days after release from the bone marrow in the spleen (Shulman *et al.*, 1965, 1968). This constitutes a platelet pool distinct from the freely exchangeable pool. After splenectomy, no preferential retention of young platelets is found. Adrenaline injection in intact animals mobilizes young platelets (megathrombocytes) from the spleen (Freedman and Karpatkin, 1975b). Likewise, phenylhydrazine-induced hemolysis in the dog and rabbit prevents the retention of megathrombocytes by blockade of the macrophage system (Freedman and Karpatkin, 1975a). This produces a 1.68-fold increase in the total peripheral platelet count, and a 2.08-fold increase in the peripheral megathrombocytes. In splenectomized rabbits macrophage blockade is followed by an equal increase (1.2-fold) in both platelet categories (Karpatkin, 1983). Wichmann and Gerhardts (1981) found that the preferential storage of young platelets fully explains the terminal tail ('sagging') of the physiological platelet survival curve (*cf.* Figure 8.11). Watson and Ludlam (1986) confirmed the heterogeneity of circulating platelets: high density (young) platelets were shown to be preferentially retained in the spleen. It is probable that young platelets in the spleen undergo some late maturation analogous

Table 8.1 Platelet recovery studies at equilibrium in healthy splenomegalic and splenectomized subjects

Author(s)	Normal n mean (%)	Splenomegalic n mean (%)	Splenectomized n mean (%)	Normal pooling	
				Pl. activity not accounted for (% of total)	Splenic platelet pool (% of total)
^{51}Cr-labeling					
Aster (1965)	50 62	14 23	6 92	8	30
Kotilainen (1969)	10 58 (49–76)	16 25	8 85 (51–110)	15	27
Harker and Finch (1969)	15 65	4 12	4 88 (77–99)	12	23
Harker (1970)			10 91 ± 7		
Gehrmann and Elbers (1970)	10 58	8 17	5 83	17	25
Kummer and Bucher (1971)	22 62 ± 61	23 37	4 91	9	29
Kutti and Weinfeld (1971a)	18 52 ± 3		9 80 ± 3	20	28
Abrahamsen (1968b, 1972)	10 58 (45–68)	12 38 (20–63)	12 90	10	32
Gardner (1972)	14 68	8 31	12 88	12	20
Ries and Price (1974)	6 69 (65–74)	8 (8–29)			
Branehög, Weinfeld and Roos (1973)	18 60 ± 2				
Kutti and Safai-Kutti (1975)	10 60		6 90	10	30
Slichter and Harker (1976)	16 59 ± 4				
Heaton et al. (1979)	10 47 ± 7				
Total	209	85	76	66	66
Calculated means	60%	29%	87%	13%	27%
^{111}In-labeling					
Heaton et al. (1979)	10 71 ± 4				
Hawker, Hawker and Wilkinson (1980)	4 69 ± 3				
Heyns et al. (1980a, b)	6 72 ± 16		4 89 ± 13	11	17
Robertson et al. (1981)	5 70 ± 21				
Scheffel et al. (1982)	9 57 ± 11				
Bautista et al. (1984)	12 76				
Schmidt and Rasmussen (1985)	25 56 (42–49)				
Wessels et al. (1985)	28 61 ± 12				
Hill-Zobel et al. (1986)	12 59 ± 9	4 26 ± 6	4 98 ± 9.8	2	39
Total	111	4	8	8	8
Calculated means	63%	26%	94%	7%	28%

to the process of late development of the reticulocyte population in the spleen.

8.3.2   PLATELET RECOVERY IN SPLENOMEGALY

Splenomegaly is accompanied by an increased splenic platelet pool. This is shown by the following

1. The early fall in peripheral ^{51}Cr-labeled platelet radioactivity following infusion is more rapid than in subjects with a spleen of normal size (Aster, 1965; Kotilainen, 1969).
2. In the presence of splenomegaly, the disappearance curve for blood platelet radioactivity finally stabilizes at a lower level than normal (Figure 8.5).
3. With splenomegaly the splenic surface radioactivity following infusion of radioactive platelets reaches equilibrium later, and at a higher level than in normal subjects. The time for equilibrium to occur may be postponed for 1–2 hours following infusion (As-

ter, 1965; Kotilainen, 1969; Abrahamsen, 1972).

4. The mobilization of platelets by adrenaline (Figure 8.4) is greater in subjects with splenomegaly than when the spleen is of normal size (Aster, 1965; Kotilainen, 1969).
5. There is a negative relationship (Figure 8.7) between spleen size and platelet recovery (Penny, Rozenberg and Firkin, 1966; Kutti, Weinfeld and Westin, 1972; Abrahamsen, 1972).
6. Removal of a big spleen results in a greatly increased platelet recovery to the level found in splenectomized but otherwise healthy subjects (Table 8.1).

Calculation of platelet recovery based on the ^{51}Cr method in patients with splenomegaly shows a mean value of 29%, compared to a calculated normal recovery of 60%. It is evident that recovery values of splenomegalic subjects vary principally because of differences in spleen size. In cases of marked splenomegaly, platelet recovery may be as low as 5% (Kotilainen,

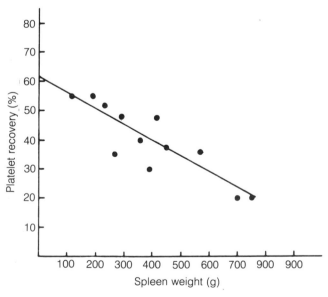

Figure 8.7 ^{51}Cr-platelet recovery in relation to spleen weight in 12 patients with Hodgkin's disease (P < 0.001). (Reproduced by permission of Dr A. Foss Abrahamsen and the publishers of the *Scandinavian Journal of Haematology* from Abrahamsen (1972) *Scand. J. Haematol.*, 9, 153–8.)

Harker and Aster, 1971). In other cases Harker and Finch (1969) reported a platelet recovery of 12% before and 88% after splenectomy, and Abrahamsen (1972) 38% before and 90% after splenectomy (Figure 8.8). A positive relationship between the size of the spleen and that of the platelet pool has also been shown experimentally by investigations of methyl cellulose-induced splenomegaly in rats (Aster, 1967; De Gabriele and Penington, 1967; Harker, 1969; Rolovic and Baldini, 1970).

Even within a fairly narrow range of spleen weights between 110 and 730g (mean 390g; *n*, 12) a highly significant correlation between platelet recovery and spleen weight has been described in patients with Hodgkin's disease (Figure 8.7; Abrahamsen, 1972). Since the mean platelet recovery was as low as 38%, it is possible that in Hodgkin's disease the splenic platelet pool is especially large in proportion to the spleen size. Toghill and Green (1983) investigated 20 biopsy proven cases with ^{111}In-labeled platelets: mean platelet recovery at 1 hour post-infusion was 33%, with a range of 4–90% despite a relatively moderate degree of enlargement (mean 325g, with a range of 118–893g).

In most older patients with sickle cell anemia, the spleen becomes infarcted and atrophic, and therefore loses its pooling effect. Some subjects show a paradoxical situation, with a spleen of normal size which is not able to pool platelets (see also Chapter 16).

In splenomegaly the splenic platelet pool may contain as much as 95% of the total platelet mass (Kotilainen, Harker and Aster, 1971). Consequently a low platelet concentration in the peripheral blood may occur without a decrease in total platelet mass; in such cases the thrombocytopenia is due to maldistribution rather than premature destruction or diminished production. However, in many instances (especially in myeloid metaplasia and the chronic leukemias) reduced platelet production also

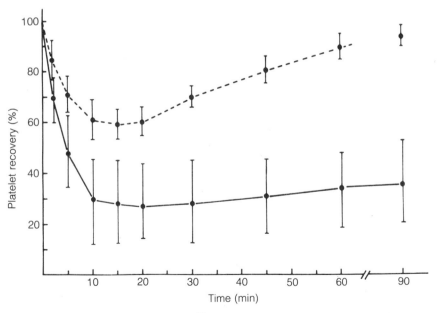

Figure 8.8 Post-infusion clearance of autologous ^{51}Cr-platelets in 12 patients with Hodgkin's disease. Mean and range before splenectomy: solid line. Mean and range after splenectomy: broken line. (Reproduced by permission of Dr A. Foss Abrahamsen and the publishers of the *Scandinavian Journal of Haematology* from Abrahamsen (1972) *Scand. J. Haematol.*, 9, 153–8.)

Table 8.2 Platelet recovery in idiopathic thrombocytopenic purpura*

Authors	Platelet label	Platelet recovery (%)			
		Presplenectomy		Postsplenectomy	
		n	mean	n	mean
Baldini (1966)	^{51}Cr	3	(2–26)		
Solomon and Clatanoff (1967)	^{51}Cr	9	14 (3–54)		
Aster and Keene (1969)	^{51}Cr	15	42	7	93
Harker (1970)	^{51}Cr	14	61 (SD 7)	7	93 (77–98)
Ries and Price (1974)	^{51}Cr	16	49 (1–75)		
Branehög (1975)	^{51}Cr	18	30 (SD3)	18	74 (47–99)
Heyns et al. (1980a)	^{111}In	10	51 (SD 21)		
Gugliotta et al. (1981)	^{51}Cr	197	40 (SD 12)		
Schmidt and Rasmussen (1985)	^{111}In	26	46.5		
Heyns et al. (1986)	^{111}In	10	55 (SD 25)		
Totals: Means		318	41%	32	82%

*Results of platelet recovery are expressed as mean values; in one instance (Baldini, 1966) only a range is given. In four instances, range is available in addition to means. 1 SD values are given in some instances.

contributes to the thrombocytopenia, with an increase in the probability of serious clinical sequelae.

8.3.3   THE SPLENIC PLATELET POOL IN IMMUNE THROMBOCYTOPENIC PURPURA (ITP)

The question of platelet pooling is of special interest in ITP. Table 8.2 presents published results of platelet recovery in ITP; as expected, the majority of cases had spleens of normal size.

In a few instances studies were repeated in the same ITP patients both before and after splenectomy (Branehög, 1975). It is striking that the mean values for platelet recovery vary considerably in the different studies and individual variation is high (Ries and Price, 1974). Platelet recovery, and indirectly the splenic platelet pool, in untreated patients with ITP was considered to be normal by Harker (1970), and Ries and Price (1974) indicated a slightly lower mean value of 49%, but calculated that this was not significantly different from normal. In splenectomized ITP patients the mean recovery values were found to be close to those of the postsplenectomy state in other conditions (Aster and Keene, 1969; Harker, 1970).

The results obtained by Branehög, Weinfeld and Roos (1973) were somewhat different: in six patients with ITP they found a mean ^{51}Cr-platelet recovery of 38% (range 23–49%), which was significantly lower than in five healthy controls (mean 59%, range 58–60%). Likewise, Kutti and Weinfeld (1971a) found a lower platelet recovery in five splenectomized ITP patients (mean 72%, range 46–89%), than in nine splenectomized, otherwise healthy controls (mean 80%, range 65–100%). Branehög, Weinfeld and Roos (1973) had also shown by infusing adrenaline into healthy controls and ITP patients that the mean values of released platelet-bound ^{51}Cr radioactivity for both groups were equal (40%) whereas in non-thrombocytopenic splenomegalic patients there was a two-fold increase in peripheral platelet radioactivity (see Figure 8.4).

It seems most probable that the apparent abnormalities of splenic pooling in ITP are related to the rapid rates of destruction to which the labeled platelets are subjected (Figures 8.9 and 8.10). Branehög (1975) demonstrated a positive relationship between recovery values and the platelet lifespan both before and after splenectomy ($r = +0.80$ and $+0.70$ respectively). Consequently platelet recovery is probably

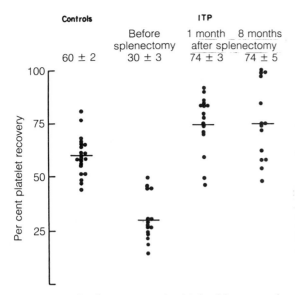

Figure 8.9 Platelet recovery in 21 healthy controls and in ITP patients before splenectomy, 1 month after and 8 months after splenectomy. (Reproduced by permission of Dr I. Branehög and the publishers of the *British Journal of Haematology* from Branehög (1975) *Br. J. Haematol.*, 29, 413–26.)

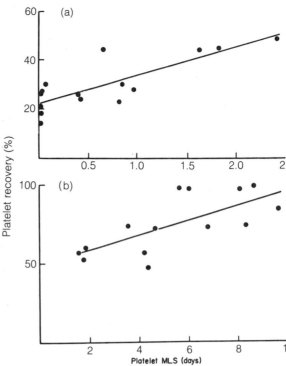

Figure 8.10 (a) The relationship between platelet recovery 15 min after platelet infusion and mean platelet lifespan (MLS) in non-splenectomized patients with ITP. (b) The relationship between platelet recovery 15 min after platelet infusion and platelet MLS in patients with ITP, 8 months after splenectomy. (Reproduced by permission of Dr I. Branehög and the publishers of the *British Journal of Haematology* from Branehög (1975) *Br. J. Haematol.*, 29, 413–26.)

of little value in ITP as an indirect measure of platelet pooling in the spleen, because a steady state may not be achievable. This also vitiates dynamic and recurrent static imaging for the purpose (Peters *et al.*, 1985b).

8.3.4   THE SPLENIC PLATELET POOL IN MYELOPROLIFERATIVE DISORDERS

Kotilainen (1969) investigated seven patients with polycythemia vera, four with and three without a palpable spleen. In both groups, platelet recovery was found to be equal at 58%. Two patients with essential thrombocythemia had a platelet recovery of about 44%, compared to 58% in the controls. Kutti and Weinfeld (1972) investigated 20 patients with polycythemia vera in steady-state conditions. In eight without a palpable spleen, the mean platelet recovery was 39%, in 12 patients with splenomegaly it was 26%, and in 16 controls 53%. As expected, the recoveries were inversely related to the spleen size, but appeared to be independent of the peripheral hematocrit values (Kutti and Weinfeld, 1971b). From these limited studies it appears that platelet recovery is decreased even in the absence of splenomegaly.

8.3.5   THE SURVIVAL OF BLOOD PLATELETS

It is clear, therefore, that the platelet has a special relationship to the spleen even in normal circumstances. The molecular basis for the normal pooling phenomenon is still undefined, but a major factor in pathological platelet pooling appears simply to be the total mass of the spleen, which suggests that there may be an affinity between the platelet and a structural component, probably the reticulum cells and macrophages.

A second factor of possible significance is the effect of pooling on platelet survival. Overtly abnormal platelets, such as those sensitized by autoantibody in ITP, can be shown to be destroyed by macrophages in the spleen and elsewhere. A related question is whether otherwise apparently normal platelets are adversely affected by prolongation of the fraction of their lifespan which is spent in the environment of the enlarged spleen.

(a) Definition and principles

The platelet survival time customarily refers to the total time spent in the blood after the platelet is delivered from the bone marrow or other site of production. The lifespan is longer because it includes the additional time spent by the platelet in the bone marrow before delivery to the peripheral blood.

Platelets obtained from circulating blood, labeled *in vitro* and reinjected are heterogeneous with respect to age and size, and their subsequent disappearance from the blood provides an estimate of the mean survival of platelets in the peripheral circulation. *In vivo* labeling of a cohort of platelets has also been used but the labels available have proved to be expensive or to have unsatisfactory physical properties. Consequently tritiated diisopropyl-fluorophosphate (Adelson et al., 1965), ^{75}Se-labeled methionine (Burger and Schmelczer, 1973) and ^{35}S (Vodopick and Kniseley, 1963) are now seldom used. DF^{32}P was frequently used in the period between 1955 and 1967 (Leeksma and Cohen, 1955; Pollycove, Dal Santo and Lawrence, 1958; Zucker, Ley and Mayer, 1961; Bithell et al., 1967; Cooney and Smith, 1968) but the label is to some extent reutilized. ^{51}Cr was for many years the preferred *in vitro* label. For human studies it was

introduced by Aas and Gardner (1958), since when the method has gradually been improved and applied widely (Aster and Jandl, 1964; Abrahamsen, 1968a, b; Kotilainen, 1969; Aster, 1969; Gardner, 1972; Branehög, Kutti and Weinfeld, 1974; Harker, 1977). Recommendations for standardized ^{51}Cr-platelet survival studies were published by ICSH in 1977, and have recently been further detailed by Snyder et al. (1986).

^{111}In is now considered to be the best available platelet label (Heaton et al., 1979; Hawker, Hawker and Wilkinson, 1980). Subjects investigated by both ^{51}Cr and ^{111}In have shown comparable estimates of platelet survival time (Heaton et al., 1979; Schmidt et al., 1983; Schmidt, Rasmussen and Rasmussen, 1985). However, Joist and Baker (1981) showed that the loss of ^{111}In might be less than that of ^{51}Cr in antibody-induced complement-mediated platelet injury. ^{111}In-platelet survival studies in 91 healthy subjects showed a mean survival of 8.4 days.

A few non-radioisotopic techniques for the estimation of platelet survival have had limited use, in circumstances such as pregnancy (Hirsch and Gardner, 1951; Stouart, Murphy and Oski, 1975; Wallenburg and Van Kessel, 1978; Catalano, Smith and Murphy, 1981).

(b) Survival curves

The rate of platelet clearance from the blood can be calculated in radionuclide studies by plotting the concentration of platelet radioactivity against time (Figure 8.11). After complete early mixing (2–3 min) and equilibrated splenic pooling of the labeled platelets (up to 90 min; phase I), the disappearance curve is mainly rectilinear in arithmetic or semilogarithmic plot (phase II), and ends in a terminal 'tail' of 2 to 3 days duration (phase III). The 'tail' probably represents the small proportion of the youngest and largest of the platelets labeled, and corresponds to about 10% of the total platelet radioactivity injected.

Platelet survival is often expressed as the T_{50}

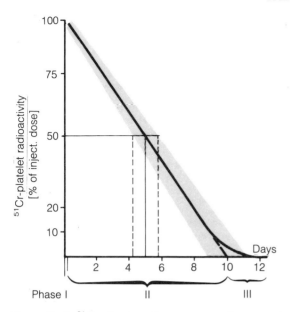

Figure 8.11 ^{51}Cr-platelet disappearance in normal subjects showing the half time of disappearance (T_{50}) and mean lifespan, estimated as the point where the nearly straight extrapolated line of platelet radioactivity crosses the abscissa. The activity of the terminal curve accounts for about 10% of the total platelet radioactivity injected.

(Figure 8.11) which is the time at which platelet radioactivity falls to 50% of the initial (maximum) platelet activity; the mean platelet survival is read as the time at which the extrapolation of the clearance curve crosses the abscissa.

Mean platelet survival shows little variation between subjects; however, Abrahamsen (1968a) demonstrated that platelet survival decreases with age. Kotilainen (1969) has tabulated experimental results obtained up to 1968, which indicate the mean ^{51}Cr-platelet survival time in healthy subjects to be 9.0 ± 0.3 days. His own work showed ^{51}Cr-T_{50} to be 4.01 ± 0.48 days. Mean values of the survival time of ^{111}In-platelets are shown in Table 8.3.

(c) Platelet survival in immune thrombocytopenic purpura (ITP)

In ITP most work has shown platelet survival to be much reduced, often from less than 1 hour to about 1 day (Harker and Finch, 1969; Aster, 1971). However, many studies have not used autologous platelets because of the difficulty of obtaining sufficient numbers from thrombocytopenic subjects, and it remains to be shown conclusively that autologous platelets behave in a manner identical to that of allogenic platelets.

Platelet production is generally increased, sometimes to as much as 8 times normal (Harker, 1970). The platelets are removed and destroyed in the reticuloendothelial system (RES), predominantly in the spleen (Firkin et al., 1969), but also in the liver and bone marrow. Platelet clearance curves are usually linear or exponential, but they may be complex and

Table 8.3 Mean platelet survival time (^{111}In): review of results in normal subjects

Authors	n	Mean (days)
Heaton et al. (1979)	10	8.8 ± 0.2
Hawker, Hawker and Wilkinson (1980)	4	8.4 ± 0.2
Heyns et al. (1980a)	6	9.0 ± 0.7
Robertson et al. (1981)	5	8.3 ± 0.3
Scheffel et al. (1982)	9	8.8 ± 1.1
Bautista et al. (1984)	12	8.1 − 10.4
Schmidt, Rasmussen and Rasmussen (1985)	25	7.7 (5.9–9.4)
Hill-Zobel et al. (1986)	12	8.4 ± 0.8
Vallabhajosula et al. (1986)	8	9.5 ± 0.8
Total	91	8.4

often curvilinear or even biphasic. If linear in an arithmetic or semilogarithmic plot, the mean survival time is read on the abscissa where it is cut by the extrapolated disappearance curve. If the plot is curvilinear, survival is read at the point where the abscissa is cut by the extrapolated tangent to the initial slope.

Baldini (1966) demonstrated a positive correlation between the platelet count and platelet survival. Aster (1969) showed that normally during the 8 days in which ^{51}Cr-labeled platelets are removed from the blood, splenic radioactivity, determined by estimation at the body surface, increased by only 5% whereas hepatic radioactivity increased by 21%. Aster (1971) later demonstrated that in moderately severe ITP, the spleen plays the dominant role in the destruction of platelets, whereas significant hepatic destruction occurs in patients with more severe ITP, in which the platelet T_{50} is very low. This study also emphasized that body surface scanning after the injection of ^{51}Cr-labeled platelets relates closely to the severity of the ITP, but does not precisely predict the benefit of splenectomy. Nevertheless, other investigators have concluded that the surface pattern of the sites of nuclide uptake is a useful predictor: about 90% of 540 ITP patients with a splenic pattern responded well to splenectomy, whereas only a few patients with an hepatic pattern responded (Table 8.4). However, it is also apparent that the hepatic pattern does not preclude improvement by splenectomy; conversely even a pronounced splenic pattern may not be followed by a good response to removal of the spleen. In general, there is a tendency for younger subjects to show a splenic pattern of platelet destruction, and these patients often respond well to corticosteroids or splenectomy.

(d) Sequential quantitation in sites of platelet destruction

When ^{111}In-labeled platelets are combined with computerized dynamic gamma-camera imaging, it is possible to follow the fate of ^{111}In-labeled platelets from the time of equilibrium to the end of their lifespan. Radionuclide accumulation permits platelet destruction to be followed in various organs, while the radioactivity decreases to zero both in the blood and the platelet pool. Klonizakis et al. (1980) showed in normal subjects that at equilibrium the injected ^{111}In-platelet radioactivity was distributed in blood, spleen and liver in the proportion of 58%, 35% and 12% respectively (see Figure 8.6). It was confirmed subsequently that decline of the splenic platelet pool was accompanied by

Table 8.4 Organ localized ^{51}Cr-platelet radioactivity in patients with ITP, who benefited from splenectomy

Author(s)	n	Positive results of splenectomy on thrombocytopenia in relation to site of platelet destruction		
		Spleen	Liver	Liver + Spleen
Gehrmann and Bleifeld (1968)	50	27/31	2/9	4/10
Kotilainen (1969)	11	2/7	0/1	2/2
Seidl and Holtz (1970)	10	5/6		2/4
Najean and Ardaillou (1971)	359	90%		60%
Cooper et al. (1972)	111	78%		20%
Gugliotta et al. (1981)	197	58%	6%	17%
Total	738			

transfer of the splenic platelet ^{111}In to the splenic reticulum cells. By sequential determination of ^{111}In, it was possible to show that at the end of normal platelet survival, the ^{111}In radioactivity in the spleen and liver did not differ appreciably from the values found at equilibrium, and that the bone marrow RES plays a hitherto unsuspected role in platelet destruction (Klonizakis et al., 1980, 1981; Heyns et al., 1982a, 1982b; Scheffel et al., 1982; Hill-Zobel et al., 1983, 1986). In ITP, platelet destruction is accelerated, so that the circulating ^{111}In-labeled platelets have frequently disappeared from the blood within a day. Consequently, splenic ^{111}In radioactivity consists from an early stage of a combination of activity from pooled platelets and ^{111}In-labeled platelets already destroyed (Klonizakis et al., 1981; Peters et al., 1984, 1985b).

(e)   Platelet survival in cases with splenomegaly

Bleifeld (1967) investigated three splenomegalic patients with thrombocytopenia. All had a normal platelet survival. De Gabriele and Penington (1967) found that values of the ^{51}Cr-T_{50} in normal, splenectomized and splenomegalic Wistar rats were almost identical (4.5, 4.5 and 4 days respectively). Cooney and Smith (1968) found in 20 normal, 10 splenomegalic and 9 splenectomized humans that the mean platelet survival time was 11.5, 8.4 and 10.3 days respectively. Aster (1969) demonstrated that the clearance rate of autologous ^{51}Cr-labeled platelets from the blood was the same in 10 healthy and 7 asplenic subjects. Kotilainen (1969) found that the autologous ^{51}Cr-T_{50} values were lower in six patients with congestive splenomegaly (2.8 days) and in eight with proliferative splenomegaly (2.5 days) compared with 4.0 days in ten healthy individuals. Harker (1971, 1977) found the ^{51}Cr-T_{50} to be 4.8 days in normal and asplenic subjects and slightly shorter in splenomegalic patients (4.4 days). Kummer and Bucher (1971) investigated 23 splenomegalic patients and concluded that the size of the splenic platelet pool did not influence the ^{51}Cr-survival time. Abrahamsen (1972) studied the ^{51}Cr-T_{50} before and after splenectomy in 10 patients with Hodgkin's disease. The mean value was 3.2 days in each case but these values were significantly lower than normal. Kutti and Weinfeld (1972) found a slightly reduced ^{51}Cr-platelet survival time in 14 patients with polycythemia vera and splenomegaly (4.6 days). Eight patients without splenomegaly showed a mean platelet survival of 5.3 days, compared to 6.4 days in 16 healthy men matched in age. Toghill and Green (1983) found 12 of 20 patients with chronic liver disease to have a reduced ^{111}In-platelet mean survival. Bautista et al. (1984) demonstrated that 11 patients with primary, and 5 with secondary, thrombocythemia had mean ^{111}In-platelet lifespans which were significantly decreased by comparison with normal values. Schmidt et al. (1985) demonstrated a shortened ^{111}In-platelet mean survival (5.6 days) in 16 patients with various hepatic disorders with splenomegaly and secondary thrombocytopenia, compared to an age-matched normal value of 7.7 days. Hill-Zobel et al. (1986) found a mean ^{111}In-platelet survival of 8.4 days for normals, 9.2 days for asplenic subjects and 6.2 days for splenomegalics.

(f)   Conclusion

Platelet mean survival time has for some years been considered to be nearly equal in normal subjects, splenomegalics and splenectomized individuals. However, the results of studies in recent years have shown convincing evidence that in the presence of splenomegaly, the platelet survival time is significantly reduced. The pathogenesis of the thrombocytopenia which so often accompanies splenomegaly is complex: the distributional effect of the increased splenic platelet pool is usually the major factor, while the reduced platelet survival time plays a lesser role. In some cases reduced platelet production is an additional etiological factor.

8.4 GRANULOCYTE POOLING IN THE SPLEEN

The causes of the granulopenia which accompanies splenomegaly in many cases has been less easily defined than those of anemia and thrombocytopenia. Likewise, the normal relationship of the spleen to the circulating granulocyte has been more obscure. However, Peters *et al.* (1985a) have studied granulocytes labeled with ^{111}In-tropolonate and introduced into the circulation. Hepatic uptake rapidly reaches a plateau, while splenic uptake was in slow monoexponential form, and required 20–40 minutes to reach a plateau. The activity curves were consistent with a dynamically exchanging pool with an intrasplenic transit time of 9.3 ± SE 0.6 minutes. The pool turnover time appears to be accelerated in inflammatory disease.

This granulocyte pool appears to be a major component of the marginating granulocyte pool (Athens *et al.*, 1961; Fieschi and Sacchetti, 1964; Scott *et al.*, 1971).

REFERENCES

Aas, K. and Gardner, F. H. (1958) Survival of blood platelets labeled with chromium[51]. *J. Clin. Invest.*, 37, 1257–68.

Abrahamsen, A. F. (1968a) Survival of Cr[51]-labelled human platelets. Methodological and clinical studies. *Scand. J. Haematol.*, (Suppl. 3), 9–53.

Abrahamsen, A. F. (1968b) A modification of the technique for ^{51}Cr labelling of blood platelets giving increased circulating platelet activity ratio. *Scand. J. Haematol.*, 5, 53–63.

Abrahamsen, A. F. (1970) Platelet survival in Hodgkin's disease. *Scand. J. Haematol.*, 7, 309–313.

Abrahamsen, A. F. (1972) Effects of an enlarged splenic platelet pool in Hodgkin's disease. *Scand. J. Haematol.*, 9, 153–8.

Adelson, E. *et al.* (1965) Platelet tagging with tritium labeled diisopropylfluorophosphate. *Blood*, 26, 744–50.

Aster, R. H. (1965) Splenic platelet pooling as a cause of 'hypersplenic' thrombocytopenia. *Trans. Assoc. Am. Physicians*, 78, 362–73.

Aster, R. H. (1966) Pooling of platelets in the spleen: role in the pathogenesis of 'hypersplenic' thrombocytopenia. *J. Clin. Invest.*, 45, 645–57.

Aster, R. H. (1967) Studies of the mechanism of 'hypersplenic' thrombocytopenia in rats. *J. Lab. Clin. Med.*, 70, 736–51.

Aster, R. H. (1969) Studies of the fate of platelets in rats and man. *Blood*, 34, 117–28.

Aster, R. H. (1971) Sites of platelet destruction in ITP. in *Platelet Kinetics* (ed. J. M. Paulus), North-Holland Publishing Co., Amsterdam and London, pp. 268–73.

Aster, R. H. and Jandl, J. H. (1964) Platelet sequestration in man. I. Methods. *J. Clin. Invest.*, 43, 843–55.

Aster, R. H. and Keene, W. R. (1969) Sites of platelet destruction in idiopathic thrombocytopenic purpura. *Br. J. Haematol.*, 16, 61–73.

Athens, J. W. *et al.* (1961) Leukokinetic studies. IV. The total blood, circulating and marginal granulocyte pools and the granulocyte turnover rate in normal subjects. *J. Clin. Invest.*, 40, 989–95.

Baldini, M. (1966) Idiopathic thrombocytopenic purpura. *N. Engl. J. Med.*, 274, 1245–51.

Bautista, A. P. *et al.* (1984) Measurement of platelet life-span in normal subjects and patients with myeloproliferative disease with indium oxine labelled platelets. *Br. J. Haematol.*, 58, 679–87.

Binet, L. and Kaplan, M. (1923) Mobilisation des plaquettes par l'adrenaline. Plaquettose par spleno-contraction adrenalinique. *C. R. Soc. Biol.*, 97, 1659–60.

Bithell, T. C. *et al.* (1967) Radioactive diisopropyl fluorophosphate as a platelet label: an evaluation of *in vitro* and *in vivo* technics. *Blood*, 29, 354–72.

Björkman, S. E. (1947) The splenic circulation with special reference to the function of the spleen sinus wall. *Acta Med. Scand.*, 128 (Suppl. 191), 7–97.

Bleifeld, W. (1967) Zur Pathogenese der Thrombozytopenie beim Hypersplenismus. *Dtsch. Med. Wochenschr.*, 92, 2149–54.

Bowdler, A. J. (1962) Theoretical considerations concerning measurement of the splenic red cell pool. *Clin. Sci.*, 23, 181–95.

Bowdler, A. J. (1963) Dilution anemia corrected by splenectomy in Gaucher's disease. *Ann. Intern. Med.*, 58, 664–9.

Bowdler, A. J. (1969) Regional variations in the proportion of red cells in the blood in man. *Br. J. Haematol.*, 16, 557–71.

Bowdler, A. J. (1983) Splenomegaly and hypersplenism. *Clin. Haematol.*, 12, 467–88.

Branehög, I. (1975) Platelet kinetics in idiopathic thrombocytopenic purpura (ITP) before and at different times after splenectomy. *Br. J. Haematol.*, 29, 413–26.

Branehög, I., Kutti, J. and Weinfeld, A. (1974) Platelet survival and platelet production in idiopathic thrombocytopenic purpura (ITP). *Br. J. Haematol.*, **27**, 127–43.

Branehög, I., Weinfeld, A. and Roos, B. (1973) The exchangeable splenic platelet pool studied with epinephrine infusion in idiopathic thrombocytopenic purpura and in patients with splenomegaly. *Br. J. Haematol.*, **25**, 239–48.

Burger, T. and Schmelczer, M. (1973) Comparative study of platelet kinetics with ^{75}Se-methionine and ^{51}Cr in ITP and congestive splenomegaly. *Folia Haematol.*, **100**, 278–89.

Catalano, P. M., Smith, J. B. and Murphy S. (1981) Platelet recovery from aspirin inhibition in vivo: differing patterns under various assay conditions. *Blood,* **57**, 99–105.

Christensen, B. E. (1971) A new method for estimating splenic erythrocyte and plasma volumes combined with quantitation of splenic iron incorporation. *Scand. J. Haematol.*, **8**, 245–9.

Christensen, B. E. (1973) Erythrocyte pooling and sequestration in enlarged spleens. Estimations of splenic erythrocyte and plasma volume in splenomegalic patients. *Scand. J. Haematol.*, **10**, 106–19.

Christensen, B. E. (1975) Red cell kinetics. *Clin. Haematol.*, **4**, 393–405.

Cooney, D. P. and Smith, B. A. (1968) The pathophysiology of hypersplenic thrombocytopenia. *Arch. Intern. Med.*, **121**, 332–7.

Cooper, M. R. *et al.* (1972) Platelet survival and sequestration patterns in thrombocytopenic disorders. *Radiology,* **102**, 89–100.

Dameshek, W. (1955) Hypersplenism. *Bull. NY Acad. Med.*, **31**, 113–26.

Dameshek, W. and Estren, I. (1947) *The Spleen and Hypersplenism*. Grune and Stratton, New York and London.

Danpure, H. J., Osman, S. and Brady, F. (1982) The labelling of blood cells in plasma with ^{111}Intropolonate. *Br. J. Radiol.*, **55**, 247–9.

Dawson, A. A. and Ogston, D. (1969) Exercise-induced thrombocytosis. *Acta Haematol.*, *(Basel),* **42**, 241–6.

De Gabriele, G. and Penington, D. G. (1967) Regulation of platelet production: 'hypersplenism' in the experimental animal. *Br. J. Haematol.*, **13**, 384–93.

Doan, C. A. (1949) Hypersplenism. *Bull. NY Acad. Med.*, **25**, 625–50.

Doan, C. A. and Wright, C-T. (1946) Primary congenital and secondary acquired splenic panhematopenia, *Blood,* **1**, 10–26.

Ferrant, A. (1983) The role of the spleen in haemolysis. *Clin. Haematol.*, **12**, 489–504.

Fieschi, A. and Sacchetti, C. (1964) Clinical assessment of granulopoiesis. *Acta Haematol. (Basel),* **31**, 150–62.

Firkin, B. G. *et al.* (1969) Splenic macrophages in thrombocytopenia. *Blood,* **33**, 240–5.

Fredén, K. *et al.* (1978a) The peripheral platelet count in response to adrenergic alpha- and beta-1-receptor stimulation. *Scand. J. Haematol.*, **21**, 427–32.

Fredén, K. *et al.* (1978b) The exchangeable platelet pool in response to intravenous infusion of isoprenaline. *Scand. J. Haematol.*, **20**, 335–40.

Freedman, M., Altszuler, N. and Karpatkin, S. (1977) Presence of a nonsplenic platelet pool. *Blood,* **50**, 419–25.

Freedman, M. L. and Karpatkin, S. (1975a) Heterogeneity of rabbit platelets. IV. Thrombocytosis with absolute megathrombocytosis in phenylhydrazine-induced hemolytic anemia in rabbits. *Thromb. Diath. Haemorrh.*, **33**, 335–40.

Freedman, M. L. and Karpatkin, S. (1975b) Heterogeneity of rabbit platelets. V. Preferential splenic sequestration of megathrombocytes. *Br. J. Haematol.*, **31**, 255–62.

Gardner, F. H. (1972) Platelet kinetics and life span. *Clin. Haematol.*, **1**, 307–24.

Gehrmann, G. and Bleifeld, W. (1968) Lebensdauer und Abbauort menschlicher Thrombozyten bei unterschiedlichen Thrombopenieformen. *Blut,* **17**, 266–75.

Gehrmann, G. and Elbers, C. (1970) Thrombopenischer Hyperspleniesyndrom. *Dtsch. Med. Wochenschr.*, **95**, 1429–32.

Glass, H. T. *et al.* (1968) Measurement of splenic red-blood-cell mass with radioactive carbon monoxide. *Lancet,* **i**, 669–70.

Gray, S. J. and Sterling, K. (1950) The tagging of red cells and plasma proteins with radioactive chromium. *J. Clin. Invest.*, **29**, 1604–13.

Gugliotta, L. *et al.* (1981) Chronic idiopathic thrombocytopenic purpura (ITP): site of platelet sequestration and results of splenectomy. A study of 197 patients. *Scand. J. Haematol.*, **26**, 407–12.

Harker, L. A. (1969) Platelet kinetics in splenomegaly. *Blood,* **34**, 528 (Abstr.).

Harker, L. A. (1970) Thrombokinetics in idiopathic thrombocytopenic purpura. *Br. J. Haematol.*, **19**, 95–104.

Harker, L. A. (1971) The role of the spleen in thrombokinetics. *J. Lab. Clin. Med.*, **77**, 247–53.

Harker, L. A. (1977) The kinetics of platelet production and destruction in man. *Clin. Haematol.*, 6, 671–93.

Harker, L. A. and Finch, C. A. (1969) Thrombokinetics in man. *J. Clin. Invest.*, 48, 963–74.

Harris, I. M., McAlister, J. M. and Prankerd, T. A. J. (1958) Splenomegaly and the circulating red cell. *Br. J. Haematol.*, 4, 97–102.

Hawker, R. J., Hawker, L. M. and Wilkinson, A. R. (1980) Indium (^{111}In)-labelled human platelets: optimal method. *Clin. Sci.*, 58, 243–8.

Heaton, W. A. *et al.* (1979) Indium-111: a new radionuclide label for studying human platelet kinetics. *Br. J. Haematol.*, 42, 613–22.

Heyns, A. du P. *et al.* (1980a) Kinetics, distribution and sites of destruction of [111]Indium-labelled human platelets. *Br. J. Haematol.*, 44, 269–80.

Heyns, A. du P. *et al.* (1980b) Kinetics and fate of [111]Indium-oxine labelled blood platelets in asplenic subjects. *Thromb. Haemost.*, 44, 100–4.

Heyns, A. du P. *et al.* (1982a) Kinetics and sites of destruction of [111]Indium-oxine labeled platelets in idiopathic thrombocytopenic purpura. A quantitative study. *Am. J. Hematol.*, 12, 167–77.

Heyns, A. du P. *et al.* (1982b) Quantification of *in vivo* distribution of platelets labeled with Indium-111-oxine. *J. Nucl. Med.*, 23, 943–4. (Corresp.)

Heyns, A. du P. *et al.* (1986) Platelet turnover and kinetics in immune thrombocytopenic purpura: results with autologous ^{111}In-labeled platelets and homologous ^{51}Cr-labeled platelets differ. *Blood*, 67, 86–92.

Hill-Zobel, R. L. *et al.* (1983) ^{111}In-oxine-labeled rabbit platelets: *in vivo* distribution and sites of destruction. *Blood*, 61, 149–53.

Hill-Zobel, R. L. *et al.* (1986) Organ distribution and fate of human platelets: studies of asplenic and splenomegalic patients. *Am. J. Hematol.*, 23, 231–8.

Hirsch, E. O. and Gardner, F. H. (1951) The life span of transfused human blood platelets. *J. Clin. Invest.*, 30, 649–50.

ICSH (1977) Recommended methods for radioisotope platelet survival studies. *Blood*, 50, 1137–44.

Jandl, J. H. and Aster, R. H. (1967) Increased splenic pooling and the pathogenesis of hypersplenism. *Am. J. Med. Sci.*, 253, 383–97.

Joist, J. H. and Baker, R. H. (1981) Loss of [111]Indium as indicator of platelet injury. *Blood*, 58, 350–3.

Karpatkin, S. (1983) The spleen and thrombocytopenia. *Clin. Haematol.*, 12, 591–604.

Kiefel, V. *et al.* (1985) Platelet survival determined with ^{51}Cr versus [111]In. *Klin. Wochenschr.*, 63, 84–9.

Klonizakis, I. *et al.* (1980) Radionuclide distribution following injection of ^{111}In-labelled platelets. *Br. J. Haematol.*, 46, 595–602.

Klonizakis, I. *et al.* (1981) Spleen function and platelet kinetics. *J. Clin. Pathol.*, 34, 377–80.

Kotilainen, M. (1969) Platelet kinetics in normal subjects and in haematological disorders with special reference to thrombocytopenia and to the role of the spleen. *Scand. J. Haematol.*, (Suppl. 5), 9–97.

Kotilainen, M., Harker, L. A. and Aster, R. H. (1971) Increased platelet pooling. in *Platelet Kinetics* (ed. J. M. Paulus), North-Holland Publishing Co., Amsterdam and London. pp. 300–6.

Kummer, H. and Bucher, U. (1971) Thrombokinetik. Einführing und klinische Anvendung. *Schweiz. Med. Wochenschr.*, 101, 1520–4.

Kutti, J. and Safai-Kutti, S. (1975) *In vitro* labelling of platelets: an experimental study in healthy asplenic subjects using two different incubation media. *Br. J. Haematol.*, 31, 57–64.

Kutti, J. and Weinfeld, A. (1971a) Platelet survival in man. *Scand. J. Haematol.*, 8, 336–46.

Kutti, J. and Weinfeld, A. (1971b) Platelet survival in active polycythaemia vera with reference to the haematocrit level. *Scand. J. Haematol.*, 8, 405–14.

Kutti, J. and Weinfeld, A. (1972) Platelet production and platelet survival in polycythaemia vera with special reference to the spleen size. *Scand. J. Haematol.*, 9, 97–105.

Kutti, J., Weinfeld, A. and Westin, J. (1972) The relationship between splenic platelet pool and spleen size. *Scand, J. Haematol.*, 9, 351–4.

Kutti, J. *et al.* (1977) The exchangeable splenic platelet pool in response to selective adrenergic beta-I-receptor blockade. *Br. J. Haematol.*, 37, 277–82.

Leeksma, C. H. W. and Cohen, J. A. (1955) Determination of the life of human blood platelets using labelled diisopropylfluorophosphate. *Nature*, 175, 552–3.

McAfee, J. G. and Thakur, M. L. (1976) Survey of radioactive agents for in-vitro labelling of phagocytic leukocytes. I. Soluble agents. *J. Nucl. Med.*, 17, 480–7.

Mollison, P. L., Engelfriet, C. P. and Contreras, M. (1987) *Blood Transfusion in Clinical Medicine*, 8th edn. Blackwell Scientific Publications, Oxford and Boston, pp. 80–94.

Motulsky, A. G. *et al.* (1958) Anemia and the spleen. *N. Engl. J. Med.*, 259, 1164–9, 1215–19.

Murphy, J. R. (1967) The influence of pH and temperature on some physical properties of normal erythrocytes and erythrocytes from patients with hereditary spherocytosis. *J. Lab. Clin. Med.*, **69**, 758–75.

Najean, Y. and Ardaillou, N. (1971) The sequestration site of platelets in idiopathic thrombocytopenic purpura: its correlation with the results of splenectomy. *Br. J. Haematol.*, **21**, 153–64.

Olsson, L-B. *et al.* (1976) The peripheral platelet count in response to intravenous infusion of isoprenaline. *Scand. J. Haematol.*, **17**, 213–16.

Pearson, H. A., Spencer, R. P. and Cornelius, E. A. (1969) Functional asplenia in sickle cell anemia. *N. Engl. J. Med.*, **281**, 923–6.

Penny, R., Rozenberg, M. C. and Firkin, B. G. (1966) The splenic platelet pool. *Blood*, **27**, 1–16.

Peters, A. M. and Lavender, J. P. (1982) Factors controlling the intrasplenic transit of platelets. *Eur. J. Clin, Invest.*, **12**, 191–5.

Peters, A. M. and Lavender, J. P. (1983) Platelet kinetics with Indium-111 platelets: comparison with chromium-51 platelets. *Semin. Thromb. Hemost.*, **9**, 100–14.

Peters, A. M. *et al.* (1980) Use of [111]Indium-labelled platelets to measure spleen function. *Br. J. Haematol.*, **46**, 587–93.

Peters, A. M. *et al.* (1984) The interpretation of platelet kinetic studies for the identification of sites of abnormal platelet destruction. *Br. J. Haematol.*, **57**, 637–49.

Peters, A. M. *et al.* (1985a) Splenic pooling of granulocytes. *Clin. Sci.*, **68**, 283–9.

Peters, A. M. *et al.* (1985b) The kinetics of short-lived Indium-111 radiolabelled platelets. *Scand. J. Haematol.*, **34**, 137–45.

Pollycove, M., Dal Santo, G. and Lawrence, J. H. (1958) Simultaneous measurements of erythrocyte, leukocyte, and platelet survival in normal subjects with diisopropylfluorophosphate (DFP[32]). *Clin. Res.*, **6**, 45–6 (Abstr.).

Rasmussen, S. N. *et al.* (1973) Spleen volume determination by ultrasonic scanning. *Scand. J. Haematol.*, **10**, 298–304.

Ries, C. A. and Price, D. C. (1974) [^{51}Cr] platelet kinetics in thrombocytopenia. Correlation between splenic sequestration of platelets and responses to splenectomy. *Ann. Intern. Med.*, **80**, 702–7.

Robertson, J. S. *et al.* (1981) Distribution and dosimetry of ^{111}In-labelled platelets. *Radiology*, **140**, 169–76.

Rolovic, Z. and Baldini, M. (1970) Megakaryocytopoiesis in splenectomized and 'hypersplenic' rats. *Br. J. Haematol.*, **18**, 257–268.

Sarajas, H. S. S., Konttinen, A. and Frick, M. H.

(1961) Thrombocytosis evoked by exercise. *Nature*, **192**, 721–2.

Schaffner, A. *et al.* (1985) The hypersplenic spleen. A contractile reservoir of granulocytes and platelets. *Arch. Intern. Med.*, **145**, 651–4.

Scheffel, U. *et al.* (1982) Human platelets labeled with In-111-8-hydroxyquinoline: kinetics, distribution, and estimate of radiation dose. *J. Nucl. Med.*, **23**, 149–56.

Schmidt, K. G. and Rasmussen, J. W. (1984) Exercise-induced changes in the *in vivo* distribution of ^{111}In-labelled platelets. *Scand. J. Haematol.*, **32**, 159–66.

Schmidt, K. G. and Rasmussen, J. W. (1985) Kinetics and distribution *in vivo* of ^{111}In-labelled autologous platelets in idiopathic thrombocytopenic purpura. *Scand. J. Haematol.*, **34**, 47–56.

Schmidt, K. G., Rasmussen, J. W. and Rasmussen, A. D. (1985) Kinetics of ^{111}In-labelled platelets in healthy subjects. *Scand. J. Haematol.*, **34**, 370–7.

Schmidt, K. G. *et al.* (1983) Comparative studies of *in vivo* kinetics of simultaneously injected [111]In- and ^{51}Cr-labelled human platelets. *Scand. J. Haematol.*, **30**, 465–78.

Schmidt, K. G. *et al.* (1985) Kinetics and *in vivo* distribution of ^{111}In-labelled autologous platelets in chronic hepatic diseases: mechanisms of thrombocytopenia. *Scand. J. Haematol.*, **34**, 39–46.

Schwartz, A. D. (1972) The platelet reservoir in sickle cell anemia. *Blood*, **40**, 678–83.

Scott, J. L. *et al.* (1971) Leukocyte labeling with [51]Chromium. II. Leukocyte kinetics in chronic myelocytic leukemia. *Blood*, **38**, 162–73.

Seidl, S. and Holtz, G. (1970) Die Bestimmung der Thrombozyten-Uberlebenszeit und Oberflächenaktivität bei Patienten mit idiopatisch thrombopenischer Purpura. *Dtsch. Med. Wochenschr.*, **95**, 266–75.

Shulman, N. R. *et al.* (1965) The role of the reticuloendothelial system in the pathogenesis of idiopathic thrombocytopenic purpura. *Trans. Assoc. Am. Physicians*, **78**, 374–90.

Shulman, N. R. *et al.* (1968) Evidence that the spleen retains the youngest and hemostatically most effective platelets. *Trans. Assoc. Am. Physicians*, **81**, 302–13.

Slichter, S. J. and Harker, L. A. (1976) Preparation and storage of platelet concentrates. I. Factors influencing the harvest of viable platelets from whole blood. *Br. J. Haematol.*, **34**, 395–402.

Snyder, E. L. *et al.* (1986) Recommended methods for conducting radiolabeled platelet survival studies. *Transfusion*, **26**, 37–42.

Solomon, A. K. (1953) The kinetics of biological

processes. Special problems connected with the use of tracers. in *Advances in Biological and Medical Physics, III* (eds J. H. Lawrence and C. A. Tobias), Academic Press, New York, p. 65.

Solomon, R. B. and Clatanoff, D. V. (1967) Platelet survival studies and body scanning in idiopathic thrombocytopenic purpura. *Am. J. Med. Sci.*, **254**, 777–84.

Stouart, M. J., Murphy, S. and Oski, F. A. (1975) A simple nonradioisotopic technic for the determination of platelet life-span. *N. Engl. J. Med.*, **292**, 1310–13.

Stutte, H. J. (1970) Die pathologische Anatomie der roten Milzpulpa. Quantitative Analyse mit fermentcytochemischen Methoden. in *Die Milz.* (eds K. Lennart and D. Harms), Springer Verlag, Berlin, pp. 53–6.

Toghill, P. J. (1964) Red cell pooling in enlarged spleens. *Br. J. Haematol.*, **10**, 347–57.

Toghill, P. J. and Green, S. (1973) Factors influencing red cell pooling of erythrocytes in the myelo- and lympho-proliferative syndromes. *Acta Haematol. (Basel)*, **49**, 215–22.

Toghill, P. J. and Green, S. (1983) Platelet dynamics in chronic liver disease using the ^{111}In-oxine label. *Gut*, **24**, 49–52.

Vallabhajosula, S. *et al.* (1986) Indium-111 platelet kinetics in normal human subjects: tropolone versus oxine methods. *J. Nucl. Med.*, **27**, 1669–74.

Vilén, L., Fredén, K. and Kutti, J. (1980) Presence of a non-splenic platelet pool in man. *Scand. J. Haematol.*, **24**, 137–41.

Vodopick, H. A. and Kniseley, R. M. (1963) Sulfur-35 studies in man: platelet survival and urinary radioactivity assayed by beta liquid scintillation spectrometry. *J. Lab. Clin. Med.*, **62**, 109–20.

Wallenburg, H. S. C. and van Kessel, P. H. (1978) Platelet lifespan in normal pregnancy as determined by a nonradioisotopic technique. *Br. J. Obstet. Gynaecol.*, **85**, 33–6.

Watson, H. H. K. and Ludlam, C. A. (1986) Survival of 111-Indium platelet subpopulations of varying density in normal and postsplenectomized subjects. *Br. J. Haematol.*, **62**, 117–24.

Weed, R. I. and Bowdler, A. J. (1966) Metabolic dependence of the critical hemolytic volume of human erythrocytes: relationship to osmotic fragility and autohemolysis in hereditary spherocytosis and normal red cells. *J. Clin. Invest.*, **45**, 1137–49.

Weiss, L. (1974) A scanning electron microscopic study of the spleen. *Blood*, **43**, 665–91.

Wennberg, E. and Weiss, L. (1969) The structure of the spleen and hemolysis. *Ann. Rev. Med.*, **20**, 29–40.

Wessels, P. *et al.* (1985) An improved method for the quantification of the *in vivo* kinetics of a representative population of ^{111}In-labelled human platelets. *Eur. J. Nucl. Med.*, **10**, 522–7.

Wichmann, H. E. and Gerhardts, M. D. (1981) Platelet survival curves in man considering the splenic pool. *J. Theor. Biol.*, **88**, 83–101.

Wright, C. S. *et al.* (1951) Direct splenic arterial and venous blood studies in the hypersplenic syndrome before and after epinephrine. *Blood*, **6**, 195–212.

Zucker, M. B., Ley, A. B. and Mayer, K. (1961) Studies on platelet life span and platelet depots by use of DFP[32]. *J. Lab. Clin. Med.*, **58**, 405–16.

ABNORMALITIES OF BLOOD VOLUME IN DISORDERS OF THE SPLEEN

David Todd and T. K. Chan

9.1 INTRODUCTION

The major components of blood volume are the red cell mass (RCM) and plasma volume (PV). For a normal individual, the former is the more stable and is governed by the need for oxygen transport; plasma volume is more labile and in teleological terms, it changes according to the need 'to fill the vascular space' and to maintain blood pressure. The mechanisms whereby normal control of volume is achieved are therefore different for the two components. Of clinical importance is the fact that anemia, defined as a hemoglobin or hematocrit level less than that normal for the sex and age of the individual, may result either from a decrease in red cell mass or an increase in plasma volume, or from a combination of both effects.

Conditions associated with enlargement of the spleen are frequently accompanied by anemia, contributing to which are several distinct mechanisms which vary in importance depending on the etiology of the splenomegaly.

(a) Spleen-dependent hemolysis

Spleen-dependent hemolysis occurs in which shortened red cell survival is the predominant factor, and which is corrected or improved by splenectomy. The spleen may be the principal site of red cell destruction, or may condition red cells to destruction elsewhere. Hemolysis of this type is frequently associated with overtly abnormal red cells, as in the thalassemias, hereditary and acquired red cell membrane disorders, autoimmune hemolytic anemia and in some anemias associated with inherited red cell enzyme defects (McFadzean, Todd and Tsang, 1958a; Prankerd, 1963; Pryor, 1967a; Richmond *et al.*, 1967; see also Chapter 13). In some cases, red cell pooling adds to the severity of the anemia.

(b) Impaired or ineffective erythropoiesis

This is frequently found in conditions which also show enlargement of the spleen, but without evidence that this is in a strict sense the consequence of the spleen being involved. Consequently there is diminished output of red cells and relative unresponsiveness to red cell loss by hemorrhage and hemolysis. The underlying cause is often obscure, but can sometimes be related to bone marrow infiltration or folate deficiency, and it is unlikely to be affected by splenectomy.

(c) Splenic red cell pooling

Splenic red cell pooling occurs in many conditions with splenomegaly and may result in a significant diversion of red cells from the general circulation (Harris, McAlister and Prankerd, 1958; Motulsky *et al.*, 1958; Bowdler, 1962; Prankerd, 1963; Toghill, 1964; McFadzean and Todd, 1967; Pryor, 1967a). There is a dynamic equilibrium between the pool and the red cells of the extrasplenic circulation which contributes to the disproportion between the total red cell mass and the hematocrit of the peripheral blood (see Chapter 4).

(d)   Expansion of plasma volume

Expansion of plasma volume is overall the most common contributor to anemia in the presence of an enlarged spleen, and results in what is essentially a dilutional anemia: it is not a simple volume expansion compensatory to a reduction in red cell mass, and is usually considerably in excess of the volume required for simple compensation. Excellent reviews of the phenomenon include those of Hess *et al.* (1976), Videbaek, Christensen and Jonsson (1982) and Bowdler (1983). We shall further examine the evidence for this, the mechanisms by which it is produced, and its clinical significance.

9.2   BLOOD VOLUME MEASUREMENT AND THEORETICAL CONSIDERATIONS

The measurement of the components of blood volume has been discussed in detail by Mollison (1983) and will be considered here only in outline.

9.2.1   RED CELL MASS

Red cell mass (RCM) can be accurately measured by the radioactive sodium [^{51}Cr]chromate red cell labeling method (Sterling and Gray, 1950) and detailed recommendations are given in the ICSH report (1973). The principle of isotope dilution is used where:

$$RCM \text{ (ml)} = \frac{\text{Total } ^{51}\text{Cr Radioactivity Injected}}{^{51}\text{Cr Counts per ml RBC}}$$

The accuracy of the estimation depends on the precise measurement of the volume of labeled red cells injected intravenously, and this is obtained by the difference in weight of the syringe before and after the injection of labeled blood. Another important factor is the interval between injection and the time of blood sampling. In normal subjects, mixing *in vivo* is

virtually complete in about 3 minutes, but in patients with abnormal red cells or with massive splenomegaly this may still be incomplete after 30 to 45 minutes or more. Delayed mixing can be demonstrated by continuous monitoring of the radioactivity over the spleen and reflects splenic pooling of red cells (Bowdler, 1962; Prankerd, 1963; Toghill, 1964).

Accuracy of estimation is also improved by correcting the venous hematocrit for plasma trapped in the red cell column: corrections for the hematocrit obtained by the Wintrobe method are given by Chaplin and Mollison (1952), and for the microhematocrit technique by England, Walford and Waters (1972). In samples with morphologically abnormal red cells, the amount of plasma trapped is higher, and with deoxygenated sickle cells this may amount to 20% of the packed cell column; with pathological samples an independent estimate by an alternative method may be necessary.

9.2.2   PLASMA VOLUME

Plasma volume changes more acutely than red cell mass in response to physiological requirements and is subject to variation with posture and physical activity (Besa, 1975). In most studies, plasma volume has been standardized by measurement with the subject recumbent.

A commonly used method employs radioactive ^{131}I- or ^{125}I-labeled human serum albumin (HSA): this is simple and accurate and with ^{131}I has the advantage of permitting surface counting for the determination of regional hematocrit (*vide infra*). However, it is somewhat dependent on the quality of the albumin preparation, since denatured labeled albumin is rapidly lost from the circulation; satisfactory preparations giving consistent results are available commercially (Takeda and Reeve, 1963; Swan and Nelson, 1971). The recommendation for measurement of plasma volume by this method has been published in the ICSH report (1973). When ^{113}In-labeled transferrin (^{113}In-TF) is used, the plasma volume is over-estimated by about 6% when compared with ^{125}I-HSA (Zhang and Lewis, 1987). However, it does provide better quantitative surface scanning of the distribution of radioactivity in the body.

Albumin-binding dyes have also been used for measurement of plasma volume using the dilution principle. The blue azo-dye, Evans Blue or T-1824, has long been known to be satisfactory (Dawson, Evans and Whipple, 1920) and is still used. It binds to plasma albumin promptly and leaves the circulation slowly (Gibson and Evans, 1937; Rawson, 1943) and the zero time value can be easily extrapolated from sequential values or may be calculated from a single 10 minute sample in normal subjects (Mollison, 1983).

9.2.3 BODY HEMATOCRIT/VENOUS HEMATOCRIT RATIO

In normal subjects, the body hematocrit (BH) is lower than the venous hematocrit (VH) so that the ratio BH/VH is less than unity. The difference is due to the flow characteristics of blood: the axial streaming of red cells in small blood vessels produces a shorter transit time than for plasma, and consequently there is a relatively smaller proportion of cells to plasma in small vessels compared to large (Fåhraeus effect). Chaplin, Mollison and Vetter (1953) reported an average BH/VH ratio of 0.910 ± 0.026 and noted its remarkable constancy in subjects with a wide range of VH values produced by anemia and polycythemia. However, in patients with splenomegaly, the ratio differs significantly from normal and approaches or exceeds unity with increasing size of the spleen (Fudenberg et al., 1961). Apart from its theoretical interest, the possibility of a marked deviation of BH/VH ratio from the normal range introduces large errors into the estimation of total blood volume from measurements of RCM or plasma volume alone (Fudenberg et al., 1961; Najean and Deschrymer, 1984).

The increased BH/VH in the presence of splenomegaly is due to a high red cell concentration in the slow-mixing splenic red cell pool. The size of the spleen shows some correlation with the size of this slow-mixing pool and the increase in BH/VH ratio; the degree to which the

cell concentration in the pool is raised is also an important variable. Direct measurement of the hematocrit of splenic blood following splenectomy has unfortunately not contributed greatly to an understanding of this phenomenon as the spleen undergoes contraction upon surgical manipulation (McFadzean and Todd, 1967), and the splenic pool comprises only one component of the total blood content of the organ.

The ratio between red cell mass and plasma volume in situ in the presence of an enlarged spleen has been determined. Using surface counting of ^{51}Cr-labeled autologous red cells and ^{131}I-HSA, Bowdler (1969) measured the regional hematocrit in normal subjects and found this to be highest at the precordium and lowest in the hepatic region. In patients with splenomegaly the ratio of splenic regional hematocrit to venous hematocrit was higher (mean 1.26 ± 0.39) than the normal value for this site (mean 0.86 ± 0.10) and accounted for the raised BH/VH ratio. Christensen (1973), employing similar techniques, reported comparable values with a mean splenic hematocrit/body hematocrit ratio of 1.41 ± 0.25. More recently, Zhang and Lewis (1987), using ^{113}In-TF, which provides better quantitative scanning of plasma within the spleen, and ^{99m}Tc-labeled autologous red cells, reported a mean splenic hematocrit/body hematocrit ratio of 1.30 ± 0.30 in 12 patients with splenomegaly. These studies provide further evidence that enlarged spleens contain plasma-poor (or red cell-rich) blood.

9.3 RED CELL CONTENT OF THE SPLEEN

The normal spleen in humans contains only 20–30 ml of red cells or less than 2% of the red cell mass (Prankerd, 1963). Therefore, it has an insignificant red cell storage function, and in this respect differs from that of mammals such as the horse, dog and sheep. However, in massive splenomegaly, up to 40% of the total RCM may be in the splenic blood volume (Bowdler, 1967). During gastrointestinal bleeding or at splenectomy in cryptogenetic splenomegaly

(Cook, McFadzean and Todd, 1963), or exercise in tropical splenomegaly (Pryor, 1967a), the spleen diminishes in volume and discharges much of its blood to the general circulation. In these disorders, histological examination of the spleen reveals marked hyperplasia and dilatation of the sinuses (Cook, McFadzean and Todd, 1963; Pitney, 1968; Marsden and Crane, 1976); it is likely that most of the red cells are in the red pulp. The remarkable ability of an enlarged spleen to discharge these red cells can be readily demonstrated by infusion of noradrenaline or adrenaline under controlled conditions (Prankerd, 1963; Toghill and Prichard, 1964; Pryor, 1967a).

There is good correlation between the spleen size as measured by its extension below the costal margin or the surface area of an ultrasound scan, with the actual splenic blood volume as measured by quantitative radioisotope scan with [^{11}C]carbon monoxide (Glass et al., 1968). Likewise there is correlation between the size of the spleen and the elevation in BH/VH ratio, as shown by the injection of ^{51}Cr-labeled autologous red cells (Motulsky et al., 1958; Bowdler, 1969). Other studies including those of Blendis, Ramboer and Williams (1970) and Toghill (1964), have shown red cell pooling to be increased in conditions with morphologically abnormal red cells, such as thalassemia and hereditary spherocytosis. In many lymphoproliferative disorders the spleen contains fewer red cells than in myeloproliferative disorders because splenomegaly in the former is the result of proliferation of lymphoid cells with effacement of the structure of the splenic cords and sinuses (Pettit et al., 1971), and pooling is then less prominent.

9.4 SPLENOMEGALY AND PLASMA VOLUME

9.4.1 PLASMA VOLUME IN THE PRESENCE OF AN ENLARGED SPLEEN

It has been known for many years that plasma volume is increased in patients with splenomegaly (Rowntree, Brown and Roth, 1929). Rothschild et al. (1954) found the plasma volume to be expanded in six patients with splenomegaly, while the red cell mass was normal or even increased, despite the venous hematocrit being depressed. Furthermore, there was prolongation of the mixing time of ^{51}Cr-labeled red cells and the BH/VH ratio was above normal, indicating the presence of a volume of red cell-rich blood in the spleen. In a larger series of patients with cryptogenetic splenomegaly, McFadzean, Todd and Tsang (1958b) reported that there was a consistent increase in plasma volume which contributed to the anemia. Following splenectomy in such patients, the VH rose, mainly as a result of the decrease in the plasma volume. Thus the anemia was to a large extent due to hemodilution. Similar observations were reported by Bowdler (1963) in a detailed study of a patient with Gaucher's disease and massive splenomegaly. Many subsequent reports (Table 9.1) have confirmed the presence of increased plasma volume and dilutional anemia in patients with moderate to massive splenomegaly. As anemia is associated with a compensatory increase in the plasma volume (Mollison, 1983), individual patients with a low red cell mass have been excluded from this Table. Also excluded are patients with polycythemia vera and those with red cell defects such as thalassemia major, as (with few exceptions) plasma volume is normal in the former, and there is a large increase in the volume of bone marrow contributing to the higher plasma and blood volumes in the latter (vide infra). It can be seen that the plasma volume is commonly increased in the presence of a normal RCM, and that this is independent of the etiology of the splenomegaly. In the series of patients reported by Bowdler (1970), there was a 12–28% expansion in blood (mainly plasma) volume, but an average of only 2.4% of the total blood volume was present in the splenic pool.

In patients with cirrhosis of the liver, expansion of the plasma volume is common and is not usually closely related to splenic enlargement

(Bateman, Shorr and Elgvin, 1949; Eisenberg, 1956; McFadzean and Todd, 1967; Blendis, Ramboer and Williams, 1970; Donaldson et al., 1970). On the other hand, with moderate to massive splenomegaly the spleen size does play a role as there is a decrease in the plasma volume following splenectomy, although it may remain above normal (McFadzean and Todd, 1967).

9.4.2   POSTSPLENECTOMY STUDIES

Blood volume changes before and after splenectomy have been reported in patients with enlarged spleens associated with cryptogenetic and tropical splenomegaly (McFadzean, Todd and Tsang, 1958b; Hamilton et al, 1967; McFadzean and Todd, 1967; Pryor, 1967b; Crane, Pryor and Wells, 1972), Gaucher's disease (Bowdler, 1963), splenic hyperplasia (Weinstein, 1964), myelo- and lymphoproliferative diseases, other blood dyscrasias and congestive splenomegaly (Bowdler, 1967, 1970; Blendis, Clarke and Williams, 1969; Donaldson et al., 1970; Toghill and Green, 1971; Hess et al., 1971, 1976).

When individual patients in whom the RCM was initially normal are considered, the plasma volume was high in 77 of 83 patients (93%); following splenectomy it decreased to normal levels in 21 (25%), was unchanged or even increased in 9, and decreased but remained higher than normal in the remainder (Table 9.2). In the majority the hemoglobin concentration and/or VH of the peripheral blood rose, and the high BH/VH ratio fell following the disappearance of the splenic pool of red cells. As this red cell pool was not large in many of the patients, the improvement in the anemia after splenectomy was mainly due to the decrease in the plasma volume.

It has been suggested that these changes may be related to a reduction in liver blood flow and portal hypertension following removal of the vascular spleen (Williams et al., 1966; Hess et al., 1971, 1976), with a resulting decrease in efferent renal sympathetic nerve activity and renal sodium retention (vide infra). When postsplenectomy studies were performed serially, the plasma volume tended to decrease further with time but often still remained above normal (McFadzean, Todd and Tsang, 1958b; Crane, Pryor and Wells, 1972). Conversely, when hepatic enlargement increases in the course of time, plasma volume again tends to expand.

On the other hand, in patients with splenomegaly palpable at less than 4 cm below the costal margin, plasma volume often remained unchanged after splenectomy and the VH did not rise. This was also observed in patients with cirrhosis of the liver with relatively minor splenic enlargement (McFadzean and Todd, 1967; Bowdler, 1970) and in several patients in whom the RCM fell after splenectomy as a result of the associated blood dyscrasia (Table 9.2).

From Table 9.1 it can be seen that before splenectomy the RCM was often above normal despite a low hemoglobin or VH value. In many patients the former fell to normal following splenectomy (Table 9.2). This may be attributable to the diminished need for augmented red cell production to maintain a large volume of cells in the expanded vascular bed, notably in the spleen, and the correction of a mild hemolytic state (Prankerd, 1963; Pryor, 1967a, 1967b; Bowdler, 1970).

The low hemoglobin and VH levels in patients with splenomegaly are therefore mainly the result of hemodilution. Further, the plasma volume falls and the peripheral hemoglobin concentration and VH tend to rise after splenectomy (Table 9.2). With the exception of patients with cirrhosis of the liver, there is a positive correlation between the magnitude of splenomegaly and the increase in plasma volume, and an inverse relationship between the peripheral VH level and plasma volume. However, there is no evidence that the excess plasma is contained exclusively in the enlarged spleen (Rothschild et al., 1954; Pryor, 1967a; Blendis, Ramboer and Williams, 1970). Due to variability in plasma volume expansion, the customary correlation between the VH and RCM is lost.

Table 9.1 Plasma volume and splenic red cell pooling in patients with splenomegaly

Authors	No. of patients	Cause of splenomegaly	Spleen size	Low Hb or VH	Increased PV	RCM above normal	Splenic red cell pool (% of RCM)	BH/VH >1.0	Correlation with spleen size	Correlation with VH
Rothschild et al. (1954)	6	Myelo- and lympho-proliferative, cirrhosis of liver	6–25 cm	4/6	6/6	2/6	–	4/6	–	–
McFadzean et al. (1958b)	17	Cryptogenetic	15 ± 3 cm	+*	+	–				
Bowdler (1963, 1967)	14	Various	2–25 cm	+	+	7/14	7%(13) 40%(1)			
Weinstein (1964)	3	Hyperplasia	1.0–2.8 kg	3/3	3/3			0/3		(–) spleen size
McFadzean and Todd (1967)	30	Cryptogenetic with cirrhosis of liver	1–18 cm	+	24/30		59–458 ml	21/30	(+) PV (+) BH/VH (+) Pool	(–) PV (nil) RCM
Pryor (1967a)	62	Tropical	massive	+	62/62	+	3.2–44%	1.23 1.34 (means)	(+) PV	
Richmond et al. (1967)	13	Tropical	15–31 cm	11/13	12/13		6–39% (15–850 ml)	1.07 (mean)	(+) PV (+) Pool (nil) VH	(nil) RCM (nil) Pool
Blendis, Clarke and Williams (1969)	39	Myelo- and lympho-proliferative, Gaucher's, Felty's, Idiopathic	0.12–4.68 kg	31/39	30/39	19/39	9–39%	11/39	(+) PV (+) RCM (–) Pool	(–) PV
Blendis, Ramboer and Williams (1970)	46	Cirrhosis of liver	0.3–1.4 kg	15/46	33/46	23/46		7/46	(nil) PV (nil) RCM	(nil) PV

Reference	N	Disease	Spleen size						Correlation
Bowdler (1970)	13	Myelo- and lymphoproliferative	~15 ± 6 cm	+	+				(+) PV
	3	Hepatic	11 ± 5 cm	+	+				(−) PV
Donaldson et al. (1970)	21	Myelo- and lymphoproliferative, Felty's,	12–34 cm	19/21	19/21	4/21	7.4 ± 5% (includes 7 with hemolytic anemia)	7/21	(+) PV (+) Pool Pool size correlates with PV
	8	Idiopathic Cirrhosis of liver	1–20 cm	5/8	7/8	1/8	10% (0–540 ml)	4/8	(−) PV (with Hb)
Hess et al. (1971, 1976)	11	Myelo and lymphoproliferative	1.5–4.2 kg	11/11	11/11	1/11	6.3% (0–265 ml)	9/11	(+) PV (+) Pool (nil) RCM
Toghill and Green (1971)	8	Myelo- and lymphoproliferative	4–28 cm	4/8	4/8	1/8	13.1%		(+) PV (+) Pool
Crane, Pryor and Wells (1972)	11	Tropical	massive	11/11	11/11	5/11	31.7%		(+) PV
Christensen (1973)	5	Myeloproliferative	960–3273 ml	4/5	4/5	0	21.1%		(+) PV (+) Pool
Pengelly (1977)	18	Myelo- and lymphoproliferative	1–25+ cm	7/18	16/18	7/18		3/18	(+) PV (+) RCM
Lewis et al. (1977)	4	Hairy cell leukemia	7–10 cm	4/14	3/4	0	28.1% (211–726 ml)		(+) RCM
Castro-Malaspina et al. (1979)	29	Hairy cell leukemia	moderate to massive	28/29	25/29				(+) PV (+) Pool
Kesteven, Pullan and Wetherly-Mein (1985)	53	Myelo- and lymphoproliferative	mild to massive	53/53					(+) PV

Hb = hemoglobin gm/dl; VH = venous hematocrit; PV = plasma volume; RCM = red cell mass; BH = body hematocrit; Pool = splenic red cell pool.
*‡: mean value significantly different from controls.
Correlation: (+) positive; (−) inverse; (nil) none.

Table 9.2 Postsplenectomy changes in plasma volume

Authors	Diagnosis	Pre-splenectomy: Increased plasma volume	Postsplenectomy plasma volume			Post-splenectomy VH or hemoglobin	Remarks
			Normal	Decreased but still high	Unchanged		
McFadzean et al. (1958b)	Cryptogenetic splenomegaly	10/10*		10 (at 1 month)		↑	Plasma volume further ↓ at 5 months
Bowdler (1963)	Gaucher's disease	1/1		1 (at 6 months)		↑	RCM ↓ after splenectomy
Weinstein (1964)	Splenic hyperplasia	3/3		3 (at 6–18 wks)		↑	RCM ↓ after splenectomy
Bowdler (1967)	Congestive splenomegaly, myeloproliferative disease	3/3		3 (at 6 wks–17 months)		↑ 2/3†	
Hamilton et al. (1967)	Tropical splenomegaly	5/5	1	4 (at 15 months)		↑	
McFadzean and Todd (1967)	Cryptogenetic splenomegaly with cirrhosis	11/14	5	4 (at 2 years)	5	↑ 10/14	Plasma volume unchanged or ↑ in patients with minor splenomegaly
Pryor (1967b)	Tropical splenomegaly	8/8		8 (at 2–18 months)		↑ 6/7	
Blendis et al. (1969)	Blood dyscrasias	5/5	3	2		↑	RCM ↓ after splenectomy
Donaldson et al. (1970)	Idiopathic splenomegaly, myeloproliferative disease	3/3	2	(at 2–4 months)	1	↑ 2/3†	
Hess et al. (1971)	Myelo- and lympho-proliferative disease	4/4	1	3		↑	
Toghill & Green (1971)	Myelo- and lympho-proliferative disease	5/8	7		1	↑	Chemotherapy or radiotherapy only
Crane et al. (1972)	Tropical splenomegaly	11/11	1	10 (at 9–41 months)		↑	
Hess et al. (1976)	Myelo- and lympho-proliferative disease	8/8	1	5 (at 2–4 months)	2	↑ 6/8†	

*No. of patients; †four patients in total had a marked decrease in red cell mass following splenectomy.

9.4.3 CAUSES OF THE INCREASED PLASMA VOLUME

Garnett et al. (1969) postulated that increased blood flow through an enlarged spleen acts as a functional arterio-venous shunt, the increased venous return to the heart causing a high cardiac output together with an increase in the blood volume. However, Hess et al. (1976) were unable to demonstate major shunting of blood in their patients with splenomegaly.

One suggestion considered in some depth has been that an increase in plasma oncotic pressure may contribute to the hypervolemia in patients with increased levels of serum globulins (Weinstein, 1964; Pryor, 1967a). However, these levels are usually normal in non-tropical splenomegaly, and Blendis, Ramboer and Williams (1970) found no correlation between the plasma volume and the serum albumin, globulin or total protein concentrations in a large series of patients with splenomegaly. A poor correlation between serum globulin concentration and plasma volume has been reported by Kopp, MacKinney and Wasson (1969) in patients with macroglobulinemia and myelomatosis. Hess et al. (1976) reported that the intravascular pool of albumin was increased in their patients with splenomegaly, probably as a result of augmented hepatic albumin synthesis secondary to the expanded plasma volume. The albumin pool fell only gradually after splenectomy, and may have contributed to the slowness of the return of plasma volume to normal (McFadzean and Todd, 1967; Crane, Pryor and Wells, 1972). Increased albumin synthesis is, therefore, to be considered a secondary consequence rather than a primary factor leading to plasma volume expansion.

The increase in plasma volume has also been suggested to be the result of expansion of the intravascular space consequent upon the development of splenomegaly (Bowdler, 1963, 1970). In circumstances in which the capacity for additional erythropoiesis is limited, and when a high proportion of circulating red cells may be pooled in an enlarged spleen, the increase in plasma volume fills that proportion of the increased intravascular space which erythropoiesis is unable to maintain (Bowdler, 1967). In support of this concept is the frequent finding of a greater than normal RCM in these patients, especially when there is marked splenic red cell pooling (Table 9.1). The increase in the RCM may also be related to an increased basal oxygen consumption (basal metabolic rate) which falls after splenectomy (Hess et al., 1976). In keeping with this view is the finding that when the decrease in plasma volume following splenectomy is most pronounced, the red cell mass also commonly falls (Bowdler, 1963, 1970; Weinstein, 1964; Blendis, Clarke and Williams, 1969). However, in many patients with splenomegaly and plasma expansion, the splenic red cell pool is not large and the circulating RCM is normal, so that the stress on erythropoietic reserve does not appear to be excessive (Blendis, Ramboer and Williams, 1970).

In the specific case of patients with cirrhosis of the liver, there is a correlation between the plasma volume and wedged hepatic venous pressure (Lieberman and Reynolds, 1967). There is evidence that intrahepatic hypertension plays an important role in activating hepatic baroreceptors, which increase efferent renal sympathetic nerve activity; this leads in turn to increased renal sodium reabsorption and plasma volume expansion (Di Bona, 1984). Hepatic sinusoidal hypertension also augments hepatic lymph formation, which results in ascites formation and a decrease in the effective vascular volume. Other factors which lead to renal sodium retention include arteriovenous shunting, increased levels of anti-diuretic hormone and aldosterone, and abnormalities in the renal prostaglandin and kinin system (Better and Schrier, 1983; Di Bona, 1984; Rocco and Ware, 1986). In a recent report, patients with cirrhosis of the liver and ascites were found to have increased noradrenaline release from the kidneys, indicating enhanced efferent renal sympathetic nerve activity in this condition (Henriksen et al., 1984).

Increased splenic and portal blood flow with elevation of the portal venous pressure and wedged hepatic vein pressure have been demonstrated in non-cirrhotic patients with splenomegaly (Leather, 1961; Rosenbaum, Murphy and Swisher, 1966; Williams et al., 1966; Blendis et al., 1970; Hess et al., 1971, 1976). Williams et al. (1966) reported that increased blood flow through the enlarged spleen and liver of patients with tropical splenomegaly, together with an unexplained increased presinusoidal resistance, accounted for the portal hypertension. Similar observations have been made in patients with blood dyscrasias and splenomegaly (Blendis et al., 1970; Hess et al., 1971, 1976) in whom the degree of portal hypertension was closely related to the magnitude of splenomegaly and the accompanying increase in splenic blood flow. In general there was significant correlation of both the increased intrasplenic and wedged hepatic venous pressures with the expansion in plasma volume. Thus in patients with enlarged and vascular spleens flow-induced portal and intrahepatic hypertension may play an important role in renal sodium retention and increase in the plasma volume, as in patients with cirrhosis of the liver. The expansion of the anatomical portal vascular bed may also lead to portal venous pooling of blood and activation of the renin–angiotensin–aldosterone system, and the latter may be augmented by the decrease in systemic peripheral resistance which accompanies the hypermetabolic state of massive splenomegaly (Hess et al., 1976).

An analogous phenomenon occurs in normal pregnancy: the average plasma volume increase is 1075 ml, which is equal to a 42% expansion. The RCM increases by an average of 350 ml, which is less than one-third of the increase in plasma volume, and results in dilutional anemia (Chesley, 1972). During pregnancy, metabolic rate and heat production are increased: hemodilution decreases blood viscosity, and increases blood flow, heat dissipation through the skin, and excretion by the kidneys (Hytten, 1985), The increase in plasma volume results from diminished renal sodium excretion mediated by hormone-related elevations of plasma renin activity, angiotensinogen and aldosterone; the effect of arterio-venous shunting in the placenta may also be important (Longo, 1983), but the role of the latter has been questioned (Hytten, 1985). The increase in the red cell mass is probably a response to the increased oxygen demands of pregnancy and is associated with elevated plasma erythropoietin levels (Manasc and Jepsen, 1969; Cotes, Canning and Lind, 1983). The latter was correlated with an increase in human chorionic somatomammotropin, a hormone which may also contribute to the plasma volume expansion by stimulating aldosterone secretion (Jepson and Friesen, 1968).

In summary, it would appear that as the spleen enlarges, there is expansion of the vascular bed, both in the spleen as well as elsewhere in the portal circulation. Plasma volume rises to fill this enlarged intravascular space. However, when splenomegaly further increases, flow-induced portal hypertension with augmented efferent renal sympathetic nerve activity and secondary renal sodium retention becomes an important factor in the expansion of plasma volume.

9.5 PLASMA VOLUME IN SPECIFIC DISORDERS

9.5.1 CRYPTOGENETIC OR TROPICAL SPLENOMEGALY

Splenomegaly of uncertain origin occurs in a variety of different forms, and is frequently designated in relation to the geographical area in which the disorder is found. Associated findings often include chronic infection, such as malaria, excessive immunoglobulin production, macrophage hyperplasia (Fakunle, 1981) and a decrease in suppressor T-lymphocytes (Hoffman et al., 1984). The spleen is often grossly enlarged (Kirk, 1957; Cook, McFadzean and Todd, 1963; Pitney, 1968; Marsden and Crane, 1976; Fakunle, 1981). Relatively homogeneous

Table 9.3 Splenic red cell pooling volumes in cryptogenetic or tropical splenomegaly

Authors	% of RCM	Volume (ml)	Mean BH/VH ratios
Richmond et al. (1967)	6–39 (19.5)	13–850 (367)	–
Pryor (1967a)	3.2–44 (19.4)	–	1.23, 1.34
McFadzean and Todd (1967)	–	108–458 (215)	1.08

( ) = mean value.

groups of patients have been studied, and the effect of splenectomy on the associated anemia and blood volume changes defined.

Anemia is often accompanied by moderate shortening of red cell survival, red cell pooling in the spleen (Table 9.3), increased values of BH/VH, and normal values of red cell mass despite the reduction of hemoglobin and hematocrit levels. Significant improvement in these abnormalities usually follows splenectomy (McFadzean, Todd and Tsang, 1958a; Pryor, 1967a; Richmond et al., 1967; McFadzean and Todd, 1967). In most instances the plasma volume in the unsplenectomized subject is significantly and consistently increased, and falls following splenectomy, although it may not return to normal values (Table 9.4).

In general there is a correlation between the magnitude of splenomegaly and the increase in plasma volume, and an inverse correlation between the VH and the plasma volume. Conversely, there was no correlation between the VH and the volume of the splenic red cell pool.

9.5.2 THALASSEMIA MAJOR

In thalassemia major with splenomegaly, the PV is markedly expanded and this may occur despite a normal RCM (Blendis et al., 1974). Further, these authors found that while the red cell life span and RCM did increase following

splenectomy, the plasma volume remained elevated. The latter was attributed to the gross bone marrow expansion which is present in these patients as a result of normoblastic hyperplasia and ineffective erythropoiesis.

9.5.3 POLYCYTHEMIA VERA

In this disorder, there is an uncontrolled production of red cells and when splenomegaly is slight or moderate, the plasma volume is usually normal in association with a high RCM (Verel, 1961; Donaldson et al., 1970; Bowdler, 1972). This differs from other splenomegalic states in which the expanded intravascular volume is associated with structural or hyperkinetic changes in the portal circulation and the increased volume requirement is met principally by plasma volume expansion. However, when splenomegaly is marked, there may be splenic red cell pooling and a moderate increase in plasma volume.

9.6 CLINICAL CONSIDERATIONS

The clinical importance of the dilutional anemia and splenic pooling of red cells lies in their recognition; otherwise inappropriate therapy for anemia may be instituted. The recognition of dilutional anemia is not difficult when measurement of the RCM and plasma volume

Table 9.4 Blood volumes before and after splenectomy in cryptogenetic or tropical splenomegaly

Authors	No. of patients	Spleen size (cm)	Plasma volume (ml/kg)		Red cell mass (ml/kg)		Remarks
			Before splenectomy	After splenectomy	Before splenectomy	After splenectomy	
McFadzean et al. (1958b)	10	15±2	92.3±11.5	75.5±11.9*			Patients with cirrhosis of liver excluded
Controls		0	45.2± 3.4				
Pryor (1967b)	8	Gross	94.1±13.6	70.3±12.0	35.5± 7.3†		
Controls		0	40–50		25.1±30.3		
Richmond et al. (1967)	13	15–31	68.3±21.2	Decreased when calculated from venous hematocrit	31.2± 5.6		2 patients with low RCM excluded
Controls		0	37.0–45.4		27.4–33.6		

*One month after splenectomy. Further decreased when studied 5 months after splenectomy.
†$n = 12$.

is available. Abnormally high values of the BH/VH ratio suggest splenic red cell pooling, which can also be identified by surface counting for the red cell label over the site of the spleen. When pooling is identified, it becomes important to exclude the presence of primary red cell disorders which can impede flow through the splenic filter.

Since moderate to massive splenomegaly is associated with a wide variety of hematological and non-hematological disorders, in which bone marrow failure or significant red cell destruction occur, treatment should first be directed towards the underlying disorder. It is doubtful whether patients with splenomegaly are symptomatic as a result of the 'hypervolemia' *per se* and splenectomy is not considered for this alone. The indications for splenectomy are beyond the scope of this review. While the increased plasma volume is lowered by splenectomy, and splenic red cell pooling is eliminated, removal of the spleen is usually performed for other indications such as abdominal discomfort, thrombocytopenia, growth retardation, and gastrointestinal bleeding resulting from portal hypertension.

In patients with tropical or cryptogenetic splenomegaly, splenectomy is usually followed by improvement in general health and well being, with better growth and development and a lessened tendency to bleed (Cook, McFadzean and Todd, 1963; Hamilton *et al.*, 1967; Richmond *et al.*, 1967; Crane, Pryor and Wells, 1972). However, there is also a higher risk of severe and even fatal infection following splenectomy (Lowdon, Stewart and Walker, 1966; Cook, McFadzean and Todd, 1963). In malarial areas, attacks can be prevented by appropriate drugs and other measures; however, overwhelming bacterial infections may occur, the majority within 2 years of the operation. Therefore, splenectomy is best considered judiciously for severely incapacitated patients, after other measures have failed to improve nutrition and general health, and attempts to control underlying disorders have failed (Marsden and Crane, 1976).

REFERENCES

Bateman, J. C., Shorr, H. M. and Elgvin, T. (1949) Hypervolemic anemia in cirrhosis. *J. Clin. Invest.,* **28**, 539–47.

Besa, E. C. (1975) Physiological changes in blood volume. *CRC Crit. Rev. Clin. Lab. Sci.,* **6**, 67–79.

Better, O. S. and Schrier, R. W. (1983) Disturbed volume homeostasis in patients with cirrhosis of the liver. *Kidney Int.,* **23**, 303–11.

Blendis, L. M., Clarke, M. B. and Williams, R. (1969) Effect of splenectomy on the haemodilutional anaemia of splenomegaly. *Lancet,* i, 795–8.

Blendis, L. M., Ramboer, C. and Williams, R. (1970) Studies on the haemodilution anaemia of splenomegaly. *Eur. J. Clin. Invest.,* **1**, 54–64.

Blendis, L. M. *et al.* (1970) Spleen blow flow and splanchnic haemodynamics in blood dyscrasia and other splenomegalies. *Clin. Sci.,* **38**, 73–84.

Blendis, L. M. *et al.* (1974) Some effects of splenectomy in thalassaemia major. *Br. J. Haematol.,* **28**, 77–87.

Bowdler, A. J. (1962) Theoretical considerations concerning measurement of the splenic red cell pool. *Clin. Sci.,* **23**, 181–95.

Bowdler, A. J. (1963) Dilution anaemia corrected by splenectomy in Gaucher's disease. *Ann. Intern. Med.,* **58**, 664–9.

Bowdler, A. J. (1967) Dilution anaemia associated with enlargement of the spleen. *Proc. R. Soc. Med.,* **60**, 44–7.

Bowdler, A. J. (1969) Regional variations in the proportion of red cells in the blood in man. *Br. J. Haematol.,* **16**, 557–71.

Bowdler, A. J. (1970) Blood volume changes in patients with splenomegaly. *Transfusion,* **10**, 171–81.

Bowdler, A. J. (1972) Plasma volume and splenomegaly in polycythaemia vera. *Br. J. Haematol.,* **22**, 331–40.

Bowdler, A. J. (1983) Splenomegaly and hypersplenism. *Clin. Haematol.,* **12**, 467–88.

Castro-Malaspina, H. *et al.* (1979) Erythrokinetic studies in hairy-cell leukaemia. *Br. J. Haematol.,* **42**, 189–97.

Chaplin, H. Jr and Mollison, P. L. (1952) Correction for plasma trapped in the red cell volume of the hematocrit. *Blood,* **7**, 1227–38.

Chaplin, H. Jr., Mollison, P. L. and Vetter, H. (1953) The body/venous hematocrit ratio: its constancy over a wide hematocrit range. *J. Clin. Invest.,* **32**, 1309–16.

Chesley, L. C. (1972) Plasma and red cell volumes

during pregnancy. *Am. J. Obstet. Gynecol.*, **112**, 440–50.

Christensen, B. E. (1973) Erythrocyte pooling and sequestration in enlarged spleens. Estimations of splenic erythrocyte and plasma volume in splenomegalic patients. *Scand. J. Haematol.*, **10**, 106–19.

Cook, J., McFadzean, A. J. S. and Todd, D. (1963) Splenectomy in cryptogenetic splenomegaly. *Br. Med. J.*, **2**, 337–44.

Cotes, P. M., Canning, C. E. and Lind, T. (1983) Changes in serum immunoreactive erythropoietin during the menstrual cycle and normal pregnancy. *Br. J. Obstet. Gynaecol.*, **90**, 304–11.

Crane, G. G., Pryor, D. S. and Wells, J. V. (1972) Tropical splenomegaly syndrome in New Guinea. II. Long term results of splenectomy. *Trans. R. Soc. Trop. Med. Hyg.*, **66**, (5), 733–42.

Dawson, A. B., Evans, H. M. and Whipple, G. H. (1920) Blood volume studies. III. Behavior of a large series of dyes introduced into the circulating blood. *Am. J. Physiol.*, **51**, 232–57.

Di Bona, G. F. (1984) Renal neural activity in hepatorenal syndrome. *Kidney Int.*, **25**, 841–53.

Donaldson, G. W. K. *et al.* (1970) Blood volume changes in splenomegaly. *Br. J. Haematol.*, **18**, 45–55.

Eisenberg, S. (1956) Blood volume in patients with Laennec's cirrhosis of liver as determined by radioactive chromium-tagged red cells. *Am. J. Med.*, **17**, 189–95.

England, J. M., Walford, D. M. and Waters, D. A. W. (1972) Re-assessment of the reliability of the haematocrit. *Br. J. Haematol.*, **23**, 247–56.

Fakunle, Y. M. (1981) Tropical splenomegaly. Part I: Tropical Africa. *Clin. Haematol.*, **10**, 963–75.

Fudenberg, H. H. *et al.* (1961) The body hematocrit/venous hematocrit ratio and the 'splenic reservoir'. *Blood*, **17**, 71–82.

Garnett, E. S. *et al.* (1969) The spleen as an arteriovenous shunt. *Lancet*, **i**, 386–8.

Gibson, J. G. and Evans, W. A. Jr (1937) Clinical studies of the blood volume. I. Clinical application of a method employing the azo-dye 'Evans Blue' and the spectrophotometer. *J. Clin. Invest.*, **16**, 301–6.

Glass, H. T. *et al.* (1968) Measurement of splenic red-blood-cell mass with radioactive carbon monoxide. *Lancet*, **i**, 699–70.

Hamilton, P. J. S. *et al.* (1967) Splenectomy in 'Big spleen disease.' *Br. Med. J.*, **3**, 823–5.

Harris, I. M., McAlister, J. M. and Prankerd, T. A. J. (1958) Splenomegaly and the circulating red cell. *Br. J. Haematol.*, **4**, 97–102.

Henriksen, J. H. *et al.* (1984) Splanchnic and renal elimination and release of catecholamines in cirrhosis. Evidence of enhanced sympathetic nervous activity in patients with decompensated cirrhosis. *Gut*, **25**, 1034–43.

Hess, C. E. *et al.* (1971) Dilutional anemia of splenomegaly: an indication for splenectomy. *Ann. Surg.*, **173**, 693–9.

Hess, C. E. *et al.* (1976) Mechanism of dilutional anemia in massive splenomegaly. *Blood*, **47**, 629–44.

Hoffman, S. L. *et al.* (1984) Reduction of suppressor T-lymphocytes in the tropical splenomegaly syndrome. *N. Engl. J. Med.*, **310**, 337–41.

Hytten, F. (1985) Blood volume changes in normal pregnancy. *Clin. Haematol.*, **14**, 601–12.

International Committee for Standardization in Haematology (ICSH) (1973) Standard technique for the measurement of red-cell and plasma volume. *Br. J. Haematol.*, **25**, 801–14.

Jepson, J. H. and Friesen, H. G. (1968) The mechanism of action of human plasma lactogen in erythropoiesis. *Br. J. Haematol.*, **15**, 465–71.

Kesteven, P. J. L., Pullan, J. M. and Wetherly-Mein, G. (1985) Hypersplenism and splenectomy in lymphoproliferative and myeloproliferative disorders. *Clin. Lab. Haematol.*, **7**, 297–306.

Kirk, R. (1957) The pathogenesis of some tropical splenomegalies. *Ann. Trop. Med. Parasitol.*, **51**, 225–34.

Kopp, W. L., MacKinney, A. A. Jr and Wasson, G. (1969) Blood volume and hematocrit value in macroglobulinemia and myeloma. *Arch. Intern. Med.*, **123**, 394–6.

Leather, H. M. (1961) Portal hypertension and gross splenomegaly in Uganda. *Br. Med. J.*, **1**, 15–18.

Lewis, S. M. *et al.* (1977) Splenic red cell pooling in hairy cell leukaemia. *Br. J. Haematol.*, **35**, 351–7.

Lieberman, F. L. and Reynolds, T. B. (1967) Plasma volume in cirrhosis of the liver: its relation to portal hypertension, ascites and renal failure. *J. Clin. Invest.*, **46**, 1297–308.

Longo, L. D. (1983) Maternal blood volume and cardiac output during pregnancy: a hypothesis of endocrinologic control. *Am. J. Physiol.*, **245**, R720–9.

Lowdon, A. G. R., Stewart, R. H. M. and Walker, W. (1966) Risk of serious infection following splenectomy. *Br. Med. J.*, **1**, 446–50.

McFadzean, A. J. S. and Todd, D. (1967) The blood volume in post-necrotic cirrhosis of the liver with splenomegaly. *Clin. Sci.*, **32**, 339–50.

McFadzean, A. J. S., Todd, D. and Tsang, K. C.

(1958a) Observations on the anaemia of cryptogenetic splenomegaly. I. Hemolysis. *Blood*, **13**, 513–23.

McFadzean, A. J. S., Todd, D. and Tsang, K. C. (1958b) Observations on the anemia of cryptogenetic splenomegaly. II. Expansion of the plasma volume. *Blood*, **13**, 524–32.

Manasc, B. and Jepson, J. (1969) Erythropoietin in plasma and urine during human pregnancy. *Can. Med. Assoc. J.*, **100**, 687–91.

Marsden, P. D. and Crane, G. G. (1976) The tropical splenomegaly syndrome. A current appraisal. *Rev. Inst. Med. Trop. Sao Paulo.* **18**, 54–70.

Mollison, P. L. (1983) *Blood Transfusion in Clinical Medicine*, 7th edn, Blackwell, Oxford, Chaper 3.

Motulsky, A. C. *et al.* (1958) Anemia and the spleen. *N. Engl. J. Med.*, **259**, 1164–9.

Najean, Y. and Deschrymer, F. (1984) The body/venous haematocrit ratio and its use for calculating total blood volume from fractional volumes. *Eur. J. Nucl. Med.*, **9**, 558–60.

Pengelly, C. D. R. (1977) The influence of splenomegaly on red cell and plasma volume. *J. R. Coll. Physicians Lond.*, **12**(1), 61–6.

Pettit, J. E. *et al.* (1971) Studies of splenic function in the myeloproliferative disorders and generalized malignant lymphomas. *Br. J. Haematol.*, **20**, 575–86.

Pitney, W. R. (1968) The tropical splenomegaly syndrome. *Trans. R. Soc. Trop. Med. Hyg.*, **62**(5), 717–28.

Prankerd, T. A. J. (1963) The spleen and anaemia. *Br. Med. J.*, **ii**, 517–24.

Pryor, D. S. (1967a) The mechanism of anaemia in tropical splenomegaly. *Q. J. Med.*, **36**, 337–56.

Pryor, D. S. (1967b) Splenectomy in tropical splenomegaly. *Br. Med. J.*, **3**, 825–8.

Rawson, R. A. (1943) The binding of T-1824 and structurally related diazo dyes by plasma proteins. *Am. J. Physiol.*, **138**, 708–17.

Richmond, J. *et al.* (1967) Haematological effects of the idiopathic splenomegaly seen in Uganda. *Br. J. Haematol.*, **13**, 348–63.

Rocco, V. K. and Ware, A. J. (1986) Cirrhotic ascites: pathophysiology, diagnosis and management. *Ann. Intern. Med.*, **105**, 573–85.

Rosenbaum, D. L., Murphy, G. W. and Swisher, S. N. (1966) Hemodynamic studies of the portal circulation in myeloid metaplasia. *Am. J. Med.*, **41**, 360–8.

Rothschild, M. A. *et al.* (1954) Effect of splenomegaly on blood volume. *J. Appl. Physiol.*, **6**, 701–6.

Rowntree, L. G., Brown, G. D. and Roth, G. M. (1929) *The Volume of the Blood and Plasma in Health and Disease*. Saunders, Philadelphia.

Sterling, K. and Gray, S. J. (1950) Determination of the circulating red cell volume in man by radiochromium. *J. Clin. Invest.*, **29**, 1614–19.

Swan, H. and Nelson, A. W. (1971) Blood Volume, I. Critique: spun *vs* isotope hematocrit, ^{125}RIHSA *vs* ^{51}Cr RBC. *Ann. Surg.*, **173**, 481–95.

Takeda, K. and Reeve, E. B. (1963) Clinical and experimental studies of the metabolism and distribution of albumin with autologous ^{131}I albumin in healthy man. *J. Lab. Clin. Med.*, **61**, 183–202.

Toghill, P. J. (1964) Red-cell pooling in enlarged spleens. *Br. J. Haematol.*, **10**, 347–57.

Toghill, P. J. and Green, S. (1971) The influence of spleen size on the distribution of red cells and plasma. *J. Clin. Pathol.*, **25**, 570–3.

Toghill, P. J. and Prichard, B. N. C (1964) A study of the action of noradrenaline on the splenic red cell pool. *Clin. Sci.*, **26**(2), 203–12.

Verel, D. (1961) Blood volume changes in cyanotic congenital heart disease and polycythemia rubra vera. *Circulation*, **23**, 749–53.

Videbaek, A., Christensen, B. E. and Jonsson, V. (1982) *The Spleen in Health and Disease*. Year Book Medical Publishers, Chicago, Chapter 4.

Weinstein, V. F. (1964) Haemodilution anaemia associated with simple splenic hyperplasia. *Lancet*, **ii**, 218–23.

Williams, R. *et al.* (1966) Portal hypertension in idiopathic tropical splenomegaly. *Lancet*, **i**, 329–33.

Zhang, B. and Lewis, S. M. (1987) Splenic haematocrit and the splenic plasma pool. *Br. J. Haematol.*, **66**, 97–102.

PART THREE
CLINICAL ASPECTS OF DISORDERS OF THE SPLEEN

THE SYNDROMES OF SPLENIC DYSFUNCTION: A CLINICAL OVERVIEW

P. J. Toghill

10.1 THE CLINICAL SIGNIFICANCE OF SPLENOMEGALY

10.1.1 THE CLINICAL DETECTION OF SPLENOMEGALY

The principal clinical evidence of abnormality of the spleen is provided by the detection of splenic enlargement, and in adults the most reliable sign of enlargement is that the spleen becomes palpable. In some circumstances, especially in younger subjects and infants, the relationship of palpability to enlargement is sometimes equivocal, but in all cases the palpable spleen directs the clinician towards a series of pathological possibilities, and the need for an explanation. It is, therefore, necessary to know how best to examine the spleen, and to know how confidently splenomegaly can be detected by physical examination alone. The increasing precision of radiological examination of the spleen (Chapter 17) does not diminish the value of accurate bedside evaluation in directing attention towards conditions characterized by splenomegaly.

Clinical examination of the spleen is usually performed from the right side of the supine patient. Palpation is begun in the right iliac fossa, to avoid missing the grossly enlarged spleen, and the right hand is advanced towards the left upper quadrant in order to detect the lower pole or medial border. If the spleen cannot be felt in this way the left hand is placed in the left loin to lift the left lower aspect of the rib cage forwards. This manoeuvre may displace a slightly enlarged spleen forwards sufficiently to make it palpable. A splenic swelling is recognized by its movement downwards and medially on inspiration, its dullness to percussion, and by its characteristic notch in the medial or inferior border. A useful way of recording spleen size is to measure the maximum distance, at right angles from the left costal margin, to the lower pole of the spleen ('splenic axis'). Some clinicians prefer to palpate the spleen with the patient in the right recumbent position facing the examiner. The right hand is placed over the left lower ribs and the thumb used to palpate the lower pole of the spleen as it descends with inspiration: this has the advantage of relaxing the abdominal wall, but in some subjects the spleen may sink away from under the costal margin to a slightly deeper plane.

The detection of minimal degrees of splenic enlargement is a skill learnt by much practice, but percussion over the lower ribs may be a useful adjunct. The long axis of the spleen lies along the length of the 10th rib, and with enlargement it extends medially and downwards along the line of the rib. Splenic dullness to percussion in health rarely extends farther forwards than the mid-axillary line. With the patient supine percussion in the left anterior axillary line over the lower intercostal spaces usually produces a resonant note. Castell (1967) notes that a change to dullness in this

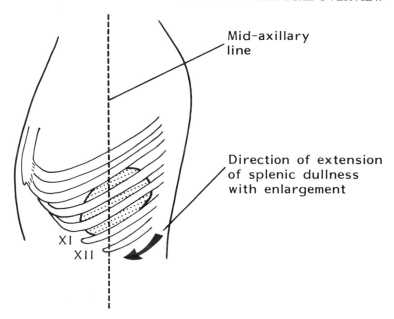

Mid-axillary line

Direction of extension of splenic dullness with enlargement

XI
XII

Figure 10.1 An early physical sign of splenic enlargement; extension of splenic dullness anterior to the mid-axillary line along the line of the 10th rib.

area on inspiration is an early indication that the spleen is enlarged (Figure 10.1). Nixon (1954) examined his patients by placing them in the right recumbent position and percussing over the spleen. He regarded dullness extending to within 8 cm of the costal margin as indicating enlargement.

10.1.2 THE SIGNIFICANCE OF THE PALPABLE SPLEEN

Several authors have challenged the time-honoured concept that the normal spleen is not palpable. McIntyre and Ebaugh (1967) found that 3% of 2000 college freshmen had palpable spleens. Of the 3%, one-third had persistent enlargement after three years, but all students remained well through graduation and on prolonged follow-up. Support for this concept of benign enlargement of the spleen in healthy young adults has recently come from South Africa, where 10 young males were found to have mild splenomegaly for which no significant cause was found, although five had IgG

antibodies specific for cytomegalovirus (Hesdorffer *et al.*, 1986). By correlating ^{99m}Tc sulfur colloid scans with clinical examination, Arkles, Gill and Molan (1986) from Sydney identified 19 patients who had palpable spleens with long axes greater than 13 cm, but who were healthy and remained so on prolonged follow-up.

The age of the patient influences whether or not the normal spleen is palpable. As with lymphoid tissue elsewhere, the spleen tends to atrophy with age. This finding has been corroborated by several autopsy studies (Krumbhaar and Lippincott, 1939; DeLand, 1970; Myers and Segal, 1974). Consequently there is a wide range of normal spleen weight, from 35g in elderly black women to 280g in young white men. It follows that a palpable spleen in an elderly woman is much more likely to be of clinical significance than a marginally palpable spleen in a young man. The oft-quoted comment that the spleen has to be enlarged 2 to 3 times its normal size before it becomes palpable clearly has limitations as a generalization.

Alterations in the position of the spleen may

influence its palpability. A spleen on a long vascular pedicle may vary its position in the upper abdomen, and even descend into the pelvis (Hunter and Haber, 1977; Vermylen *et al.*, 1983). Absence or laxity of the phrenico-colic ligament, poor development of the lieno-renal and lieno-gastric ligaments and loss of tone of the abdominal wall may all contribute to what has been termed the 'wandering spleen' syndrome. Torsion of the long splenic pedicle may lead to ischemia or infarction of the spleen (Simpson and Ashby, 1965). Anomalous orientation of the spleen may also allow the spleen to be palpated more easily, though in reports of the 'upside-down spleen' no abdominal mass was detected (Westcott and Krufky, 1972).

As the spleen enlarges there is less difficulty in estimating spleen size by palpation and observer variation is small (Blendis *et al.*, 1970a). Indeed with gross splenomegaly simple palpation may be more accurate than radiological assessment (Riemenschneider and Whalen, 1965). In their study comparing radionuclide scan size of the spleen with palpation, Arkles, Gill and Molan (1986) regarded a posterior scan length of less than 13 cm as being normal. This figure was derived from examination of 100 patients who subsequently came to autopsy, and whose spleens weighed less than 250g. In other scanning studies 30% of patients had palpable spleens when the posterior spleen length was 14 cm, with 42%, 68%, 80% and 100% having palpable spleens when splenic lengths were 16, 18, 20 and greater than 22 cm respectively. Nevertheless not all clinicians have confirmed such accuracy in palpating large spleens, and in a study of over 4000 patients Fischer (1970) found that 50% of moderately enlarged spleens weighing 600–750g, and 20% of greatly enlarged spleens weighing 900–1600g, could not be palpated.

To summarize, a combination of careful palpation and percussion will identify 90% of enlarged spleens (Sullivan and Williams, 1976), but imaging is necessary to confirm or refute doubtful splenomegaly. In a small proportion of young adults, probably about 3%, the spleen may be palpated without being significant of identifiable disease.

10.2 SYMPTOMS DUE TO SPLENOMEGALY

Symptoms due to the presence of an enlarged spleen are common, but sometimes relatively mild enlargement can cause disproportionate discomfort, and this may be the first symptom to draw attention to a specific disease. Gross enlargement occurs in conditions such as chronic myelogenous leukemia, myelosclerosis and tropical splenomegaly; this may cause dragging pain in the abdomen, gastro-esophageal reflux, discomfort and fullness after meals ('early satiety'), and disturbances of bowel habit. Greater degrees of enlargement of the spleen may cause it to descend into the pelvis, causing vaginal or rectal prolapse.

A common cause of pain in the spleen is infarction. This may be a feature of septicemic illnesses such as bacterial endocarditis in which the spleen is only mildly enlarged. Under these circumstances the infarction becomes clinically important if it causes painful perisplenitis or progresses to splenic abscess. Infarction without embolism occurs frequently in large spleens, and in general the bigger the spleen the greater the risk of infarction. Consequently, patients with primary myeloid metaplasia and chronic myelogenous leukemia are at high risk for ischemic infarction (see Chapter 14). More than one-third of patients dying from chronic myelogenous leukemia show evidence of infarction, and secondary adhesions between the spleen and surrounding structures at autopsy (Krumbhaar and Stengel, 1942). In 'big spleen' syndromes, the symptoms resulting from recurrent infarction may be so severe as to constitute a strong indication for splenectomy.

A high risk of splenic infarction occurs in some patients with hemoglobinopathies. Subjects with sickle-cell hemoglobin C disease may be particularly vulnerable. These patients have hemoglobin levels which are close to normal, so that their blood is of relatively high viscosity. Together with the splenomegaly and large splenic red cell pool of this type of hemoglobinopathy, an ideal setting for anoxic sickling and tissue infarction is produced. Splenic infarction in hemoglobin SC disease has been described during mountain ascents (Diggs, 1965) and on air journeys at low altitude or in unpressurized aircraft (Green, Huntsman and Serjeant, 1971). Even in patients with simple sickle cell trait, episodes of splenic infarction are not uncommon in high altitude flying in unpressurized conditions (Sullivan, 1950; Cooley et al., 1954).

10.3 PORTAL HYPERTENSION IN PATIENTS WITH SPLENOMEGALY

Portal hypertension may result from the complex hemodynamic changes that occur with gross splenomegaly, and may be sufficiently severe to progress to severe gastrointestinal bleeding (Aufses, 1960; Dagradi et al., 1965). It may arise from any form of non-cirrhotic splenomegaly, but is encountered mainly in the myeloproliferative syndromes; in this particular group it may sometimes be due to associated portal or splenic vein thrombosis. Portal hypertension has been reported in other diseases, including chronic lymphatic leukemia (Dal Palu, Ruol and Belloni, 1963), Hodgkin's disease (Lima et al., 1962), Felty's syndrome (Blendis et al., 1970b), Gaucher's disease (Jarett, Kew and Litnaitsky, 1966). Blendis et al. (1970c) measured spleen blood flow and splanchnic hemodynamics in a group of patients with blood dyscrasias; similar changes were described by Williams et al. (1966) in East African patients with idiopathic tropical splenomegaly. The severity of the portal hypertension in both series was closely related to the degree of splenic enlargement, and to the accompanying increase in splenic blood flow. There was an associated increase in liver blood flow. In spite of the high total splenic blood flow, this flow was in fact inversely related to spleen size, when expressed in relation to unit mass of spleen. A proportion of these patients had increased presinusoidal resistance, apparently due to a combination of high liver blood flow and impaired vascular distensibility in the liver because of fibrosis and cellular infiltration.

10.4 THE CONCEPT OF HYPERSPLENISM

The possibility of the spleen being a cause of anemia was first considered by Gretsel (1866), but Osler (1900, 1902) created a more general awareness of it. Guido Banti, the Florentine physician, had described his syndrome earlier, but mistakenly believed the primary pathology to be in the spleen, and regarded the lesions in the liver as purely secondary phenomena (Banti, 1883). The term 'hypersplenism' emerged in 1907 when is was coined by Chauffard, and it has been used extensively since. In a syndromatic sense hypersplenism can be regarded as the association of anemia, leukopenia or thrombocytopenia with active hematopoiesis in the bone marrow, usually in the presence of splenic enlargement. Retrospective confirmation of the syndrome results when splenectomy is followed by remission. It may be noted that many alternative definitions of hypersplenism have been offered: for example, Crosby (1962) simply regarded it as a state in which the patient is improved by losing his spleen!

What is now clear is that in the majority of cases with hypersplenism the anemia, leukopenia and thrombocytopenia are due to a complex of factors, which include cell pooling, destruction of cells within the spleen, and hemodilution due to expansion of plasma volume. Primary functional overactivity of the spleen was once thought to be the dominant factor in hypersplenism, but this in fact proves difficult to define, and less easy to prove, in the sense of a single identifiable pathogenic process. Whatever the nature of the underlying disorder there are three underlying *splenic* mechanisms which contribute to the cytopenias of hypersplenism. These are excessive pooling or sequestration of cells within the spleen, excessive splenic destruction of cells, and intrasplenic production of antibody, aggravating or enhancing splenic or extrasplenic destruction of cells (Corrigan, Van Wyck and Crosby, 1983). These mechanisms may act singly or in combination and in many patients it is difficult to establish their relative significance. A common additional factor is that of plasma expansion. Although of slight importance only in patients with lesser degrees of enlargement of the spleen, it may largely predominate over other mechanisms, particularly when the spleen becomes massively enlarged (Bowdler, 1963, 1967, 1970; McFadzean, Todd and Tsang, 1958).

Studies exploring the role of the hypersplenic spleen in man as a contractile reservoir have emphasized its storage function (Schaffner *et al.*, 1985). Although splenic contraction in man is weak, because of the paucity of trabecular smooth muscle, the spleen may be induced to expel its contents under the influence of epinephrine administered subcutaneously. Reduction in spleen size can be followed sonographically and correlated with changes in leukocyte and platelet levels in the peripheral blood. Mobilization of leukocytes and platelets correlates well with the degree of splenic contraction but not with resting splenic size. Furthermore, hypersplenic patients who mobilize leukocytes and platelets well with adrenaline respond better hematologically after splenectomy than those patients incapable of mobilizing these cells (Schaffner and Fehr, 1981). Similar work has shown that the splenic red cell pool in the 'big spleen' syndromes of myeloid metaplasia and chronic leukemia may be similarly expelled from the spleen by adrenaline (Toghill and Green, 1973). There appear to be functional analogies between the hypersplenic spleen in man and the reservoir spleen found in many mammals.

Earlier hypothetical concepts of the spleen as a source of inhibitors or hormones capable of influencing the release or maturation of precursor cells from the bone marrow has not received experimental support, and such factors have not been shown to be significant in the pathogenesis of the hypersplenic syndrome. While the hematological aspects of hypersplenism have been explored in some detail, the question of such spleens demonstrating excessive immunological activity has not yet been resolved.

At one time, hereditary spherocytosis and immune thrombocytopenias were regarded as forms of hypersplenism, but these have now been excluded, together with diseases associated with immature cells in the circulation. Many of the 'big spleen' syndromes, such as those associated with the chronic leukemias and myeloid metaplasia, fall within the syndromatic definition of hypersplenism, and it would seem both convenient and logical to include appropriate cases of hematological disorders of this type. In practice many patients with hypersplenism have hepatic disease as their primary disorder, and those with portal hypertension (or 'congestive splenomegaly') constitute a significant subset of cases.

Table 10.1 provides a simple schema for hypersplenism with three main groups of cases, namely primary and secondary hypersplenism, and portal hypertension. Primary hypersplenism refers to the small group of diseases in which no recognizable disorder can be detected other than in the spleen. Secondary hypersplenism applies to cases in which the phenomena of hypersplenism are superimposed onto the basic disease. The third group includes those in which the splenic disorder is secondary to liver disease. Some of the more important clinical associations of hypersplenism are described in the following section.

10.5 CONDITIONS ASSOCIATED WITH HYPERSPLENISM

10.5.1 IDIOPATHIC NON-TROPICAL SPLENOMEGALY

Gross enlargement of the spleen with hypersplenism in the absence of systemic disease elsewhere, is uncommon though not exceptionally rare. This condition has been described as nontropical idiopathic splenomegaly (Dacie *et al.*, 1969; Manoharan, Bader and Pitney, 1982),

Table 10.1 Conditions associated with 'hypersplenism'

	Syndrome	*Specific diseases of clinical importance*
Primary	Idiopathic non-tropical splenomegaly	'Dacie's syndrome'
	Cysts and tumours	Hemangioma
		Hemangiosarcoma
Secondary	Acute and chronic infections	Tuberculosis
		Sub-acute bacterial endocarditis
		Kala-azar
	Tropical splenomegaly	Malaria
	Hodgkin's disease	
	Non-Hodgkin's lymphoma	
	Infiltrative disorders	
	(a) Hereditary	Gaucher's disease
	(b) Acquired	Sarcoidosis
		Amyloidosis
	Autoimmune disorders	Felty's syndrome
		Systemic lupus erythematosus
	Hematological 'big spleen' syndromes	Primary myeloid metaplasia
		Chronic leukemia
Portal hypertension	Presinusoidal	Schistosomiasis
	Sinusoidal	Cirrhosis
	Postsinusoidal	Budd–Chiari syndrome
	Portal vein occlusion	
	Splenic vein obstruction	
	('left-sided portal hypertension')	

but it is probable that conditions variously described as primary splenic neutropenia (Wiseman and Doan, 1942), primary hypersplenic pancytopenia (Hayhoe and Whitby, 1955) and simple splenic hyperplasia (Weinstein, 1964) are variants of the same syndrome.

Slight and unremarkable histological changes were found in the excised spleens from Dacie's series. There was variation in the lymphoid follicles with an abnormal configuration of the germinal centers. Some patients had dilatation of the sinuses with an increase in the nucleated cells in the red pulp and erythrophagocytosis was prominent. Four of the patients in the original series died from non-Hodgkin's lymphoma, but the histological findings in the previously removed spleens did not differ from those of other patients who remained well after splenectomy.

The hematological changes in this syndrome have shown variable degrees of anemia, neutropenia and thrombocytopenia with no diagnostic features in blood films. In Dacie's patients four of ten had positive direct antiglobulin (Coombs') tests. Radionuclide studies to define the factors responsible for the anemia have shown variable results, with normal to marked reduction of red cell lifespan, but no excessive splenic uptake of ^{51}Cr-labeled cells by liver or spleen (Dacie *et al.*, 1969; Goonewardene *et al.*, 1979). A major factor contributing to the anemia in many cases was expansion of the plasma volume (Weinstein, 1964; Goonewardene *et al.*, 1979) but the hemoglobin levels in the peripheral blood were further reduced by significant splenic red cell pooling, reaching levels up to 28% of the total red cell mass. Little evidence is available regarding leukocyte and platelet kinetics, but it seems likely that excessive splenic pooling is the major factor responsible for the leukopenia and thrombocytopenia.

This is a syndrome in which the response to splenectomy is likely to be gratifying, and although most authors recommend splenectomy, Coon (1985a) has sounded a note of caution, suggesting that in some younger patients a decision regarding splenectomy could be deferred. Such caution has to be set against the possibility of the spleen being the site of non-Hodgkin's lymphoma, in which case 'diagnostic' splenectomy may be necessary (Long and Aisenberg, 1974). Statistics available for this syndrome suggest that approximately 20% of the patients eventually develop non-Hodgkin's lymphoma (Manoharan, Bader and Pitney, 1982).

The following case history shows the typical hematological changes seen in non-tropical idiopathic splenomegaly.

A 45-year-old farmer presented with a 3-month history of tiredness and night sweats. Examination revealed pallor and gross splenomegaly. A blood count showed hemoglobin 5.3 g/dl, leukocytes $1.9 \times 10^9/l$, and platelets $52 \times 10^9/l$. Bone marrow aspiration and trephine biopsy showed active hematopoiesis. Investigation including lymphangiography yielded no evidence of disease elsewhere. Radionuclide studies using ^{51}Cr-labeled autologous cells revealed a red cell mass of 13.8 ml/kg (normal 25–35 ml/kg), splenic red cell pool 28% of red cell mass, red cell survival (T_{50} ^{51}Cr) 22 days (normal 24–28 days), plasma volume 60 ml/kg (normal 38–42 ml/kg). Surface counting studies showed no excess splenic or hepatic uptake. Histopathology of the excised spleen (1570 g) revealed no specific features. At last review 17 years later the blood count was normal, with hemoglobin 15.7 g/dl, leukocytes $8.3 \times 10^9/l$ and platelets $350 \times 10^9/l$. The patient has remained well apart from the development of insulin-dependent diabetes.

The etiology of the syndrome of non-tropical idiopathic splenomegaly remains unknown. The similarities between the histological features of the spleen and those in tropical splenomegaly and Felty's syndrome led Dacie et al. (1969) to consider the possibility of it being an exaggerated or abnormal reaction to an, as yet, unknown antigenic stimulus. In the 20% of patients who progress to lymphoma no features distinguish the excised spleen from those of

Table 10.2 Reports of patients with idiopathic non-tropical splenomegaly

Author	Title of syndrome	No. of cases	Subsequently developed lymphoma
Hayhoe and Whitby (1955)	Primary hypersplenic pancytopenia	5	No follow-up
Gevirtz et al. (1962)	Primary hypersplenism	1	0 (2 yrs)
Weinstein (1964)	Simple splenic hyperplasia	5 (1 ♂)	No follow-up
Dacie et al. (1969)	Non-tropical idiopathic splenomegaly	10 (2 ♂)	4 (1–7 yrs after Sx)
Goonewardene et al. (1979)	None given (abstracted from a series of 13)	5 (2 ♂)	1 (2 yrs after Sx)
Ellis and Damashek (1975)	Primary hypersplenism	12 (NS)	3 (incomplete follow-up)
Knudson et al. (1982)	None given (abstracted from a series of 28)	2 (2 ♂)	1 (2 yrs)
Manoharan et al. (1982)	Non-tropical idiopathic splenomegaly	5 (3 ♂)	2 (2 and 6 yrs after Sx)

NS, Not stated.
Sx, Splenectomy.

patients who do not progress to malignancy. Table 10.2 summarizes several reports of cases comparable to idiopathic non-tropical splenomegaly.

10.5.2 SPLENIC CYSTS AND TUMORS

Splenic cysts and tumors are extremely rare: they are summarized in Table 10.3 which is modified from Morgenstern, Rosenberg and Geller (1985), and further discussed in Chapters 17 and 18.

In general, benign lesions present with splenomegaly and upper abdominal discomfort, whereas malignant lesions may have in addition fever, cachexia, pleural effusions, and a propensity to rupture either spontaneously or with minimal trauma. Unusual hematological syndromes of hypersplenic type have been described in association with splenic tumors.

One unusual presentation is the hypersplenism associated with splenic cysts. Several such cases have been described with splenic pseudo-

Table 10.3 Splenic cysts and tumors

1. Tumor-like lesions
   A. Non-parasitic cysts
   B. Hamartoma (splenoma)

2. Vascular tumors
   A. Benign
      Hemangioma
      Lymphangioma
      Hemangioendothelioma
   B. Malignant
      Hemangiosarcoma
      Lymphoangiosarcoma
      Hemangioendothelial sarcoma

3. Lymphoid tumors

4. Non-lymphoid tumors
   Lipoma
   Malignant fibrous histiocytoma
   Fibrosarcoma
   Leiomyosarcoma
   Malignant teratoma
   Kaposi's sarcoma

cysts, considered to be secondary to intrasplenic hematomas (Janin *et al.*, 1981; Halvorsen, Semb and Maurseth, 1974; Steidl and Cardy, 1957). The underlying mechanism for the hypersplenism is difficult to discern, unless such patients have an associated and unrecognized splenic vein occlusion. Hypersplenism in patients with true splenic cysts (that is, those with a cellular lining wall) has been described, but this may be no more than coincidental (Qureshi, Hafner and Dorchak, 1964; Marterre and Sugerman, 1986).

Much better recognized has been the relationship between vascular tumors of the spleen and microangiopathic hemolytic anemia, in which erythrocytes are damaged by the irregular vascular endothelium and fibrin strands within the racemose structure of such tumors (Alpert and Benisch, 1970; Toghill, Rigby and Hall, 1972; Smith, 1985). Such lesions may be associated with consumption coagulopathy (Blix and Jacobsen, 1963) in a similar fashion to that seen with giant hemangiomas elsewhere (Zervos, Vlachos and Karpathios, 1967).

Though hamartomas (splenomas) are extremely rare and are mostly found at autopsy, some may be multiple and associated with splenomegaly and hypersplenism (Ross and Schiller, 1971; Videbaek, 1953). These tumors have been shown to cause portal hypertension by creating abnormal anastomotic channels (Bhagwat *et al.*, 1975). The high splenic blood flow with diffuse capillary hemangiomatosis of the spleen may be sufficient to produce portal hypertension (Tada *et al.*, 1972).

10.5.3 ACUTE AND CHRONIC INFECTIONS

In temperate zones infection is rarely responsible for the syndrome of hypersplenism as currently defined. Jandl, Jacob and Daland (1961) described 'hypersplenism' in infective hepatitis, endocarditis, glandular fever, psittacosis and tuberculosis, but their patients had transient splenic hemolysis with the active infective process, and no consistent accompanying leukopenia or thrombocytopenia. True hypersplenism does occur with the occasional case of gross splenomegaly due to tuberculosis (Engelbreth-Holm, 1938) but similar examples are now rare. Kala-azar, which is not necessarily confined to the tropics, is characterized by progressive pancytopenia related to the increasing size of the spleen (Cartwright, Chung and Chang, 1948); the role of the spleen in this disease has been emphasized by the report of near-normal hematology in a previously splenectomized patient infected with leishmaniae (Bada *et al.*, 1979).

10.5.4   TROPICAL SPLENOMEGALY

Splenomegaly is an extremely common finding in tropical regions and there is still truth in the clinical aphorism, 'Most patients in the tropics have enlarged spleens; some are just larger than others' (Geary, Clough and MacIver, 1980). Nevertheless the tropical splenomegaly syndrome (TSS) has emerged as a distinct entity and its close relationship to malaria has been established (Fakunle, 1981; Crane, 1981). Criteria for diagnosis include immunity to malaria, a response to anti-malarial drugs, high serum IgM concentrations and lymphocytic infiltration of the sinusoids on liver biopsy. It must be remembered, however, that not all cases of obscure splenomegaly in the tropics are encompassed by the TSS orbit (de Cock *et al.*, 1983).

Hypersplenism is a common, though not essential, part of the syndrome and is mainly related to the size of the spleen. As with the other 'big spleen' syndromes, red cell pooling and hemolysis, granulocytopenia, thrombocytopenia and plasma expansion have been common features in TSS from East Africa (Richmond *et al.*, 1967), Nigeria (Watson Williams and Allan, 1968), Oceania (Crane, 1981), and Hong Kong (Cook, McFadzean and Todd, 1963). In comparison with other splenomegalic states, the degree of plasma expansion may be gross, amounting to more than 120 ml/kg in some patients and generating a major cause for the anemia (Pryor, 1967). Neutropenia in many other hypersplenic states such as portal cirrhosis may be inconsequential; however, the neutropenia of TSS is often severe and there are often impaired responses to acute bacterial infections (Crane, 1973).

10.5.5   PORTAL HYPERTENSION

It has become conventional to use the somewhat unsatisfactory term 'congestive splenomegaly' to describe a group of diseases in which enlargement of the spleen is associated with portal hypertension. Although most patients with portal hypertension have hepatic cirrhosis, it is essential in diagnosis to consider other causes and to attempt to define the location of the resistance to portal venous flow. This may occur at the following sites:

1. Portal vein obstruction, due to portal vein thrombosis or occlusion at the porta hepatis.
2. Pre-sinusoidal resistance at the level of the portal tracts (e.g. schistosomiasis).
3. Sinusoidal occlusion (as in hepatic cirrhosis).
4. Centrizonal congestion and fibrosis (such as that due to bush-tea drinking).
5. Hepatic vein obstruction (as in the Budd–Chiari syndrome).

Hypersplenism may also complicate splenic vein occlusion, which produces the so-called 'left-sided portal hypertension'. Splenic vein thrombosis may be an isolated phenomenon, or secondary to a local tumor, especially pancreatic carcinoma.

The frequency of hypersplenism in patients with portal hypertension depends on the population studied and the criteria used to define hypersplenism. Taking into account both leukopenia and thrombocytopenia, 24% of a United Kingdom series of 187 patients with various types of cirrhosis had hypersplenism (Toghill and Green, 1979); a comparable incidence was obtained by Soper and Rikkers (1986) in 106 patients from the United States who had bled from varices. Other authors have quoted frequencies between 11 and 55% (Ferrara *et al.*, 1979; Mutchnik, Lerner and Conn, 1975; Fegiz *et al.*, 1983), but comparisons are difficult because of different populations and variable criteria for hypersplenism.

Uncertainty exists with respect to the role of the specific disease causing the hypersplenism. In Australia, Stathers, Ma and Blackburn (1968) studied patients with portal hypertension due to extra-hepatic block, and found 17 of 21 patients to have hypersplenism; this provides a striking contrast with the infrequency of hypersplenism in patients with isolated splenic vein thrombosis (Sutton, Yarborough and Richards, 1970). In presinusoidal portal hypertension due to bilharzia, 66% of patients had leukopenia, though the incidence of thrombocytopenia was not particularly high (Beker and Valencia-Parparcen, 1970). In patients with cirrhosis there seems to be less hypersplenism in the alcoholics than in non-alcoholics (Toghill and Green, 1979; Soper and Rikkers, 1986). This is particularly surprising in view of the depressive effects of alcohol on leukopoiesis and thrombopoiesis. However, non-alcoholic groups may be presumed to contain patients

with cirrhosis secondary to chronic active hepatitis, an autoimmune disorder in which additional reticulo-endothelial activity would be expected. However hypersplenism in chronic active hepatitis itself appears to be relatively infrequent (Gramlich *et al.*, 1970; Toghill and Green, 1975).

Three factors are linked in the pathogenesis of hypersplenism in portal hypertension: spleen size, portal pressure and reticulo-endothelial activity. Of these spleen size seems to be emerging as the dominant factor. Splenomegaly is a well-recognized physical sign in hepatic cirrhosis, so that in the absence of clinical or radiological evidence of enlargement of the spleen, the diagnosis may be questionable. It is often assumed that the splenomegaly is due, at least in part, to the portal hypertension. However, Westaby, Wilkinson and Williams (1978) could find no correlation between spleen size and portal pressure, measured either directly by splenic pulp pressure or indirectly by the radiological assessment of the size of esophageal varices. These results confirm earlier studies which showed that there was no significant difference in hepatic wedge pressure between cirrhotic patients with and without sple-

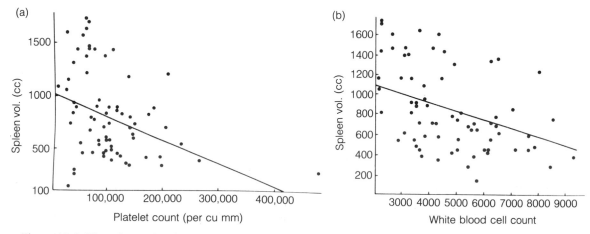

Figure 10.2 The relationship between spleen size and blood counts. (a) Negative correlation between spleen size measured by CT scan and platelet count in 73 patients with portal hypertension and variceal bleeding (*P* < 0.001). (b) Negative correlation between spleen size and white blood count (*P* < 0.001). (Reproduced from el-Khishen *et al.* (1985) *Surg. Gynecol. Obstet.*, **160**, 233–8 by permission of the authors and publisher.)

nomegaly (Krook, 1956). Undoubtedly the splenomegaly in cirrhosis is due mainly to reticulo-endothelial hyperplasia, and hemodynamic studies have shown that the consequent increase in the splenic component of portal blood flow does not contribute to increased portal hypertension (Merkel *et al.*, 1985).

In spite of uncertainty with respect to the cause of splenic enlargement in cirrhosis, it is now apparent that spleen size is of overriding importance in hypersplenism. Both el-Khishen *et al.* (1985) who assessed spleen volume by CT scanning, and Soper and Rikkers (1986) who measured spleen length, found significant negative correlations for both leukocyte and platelet counts (Figure 10.2).

The importance of spleen size in the hypersplenism of chronic liver disease suggests that significant splenic pooling of both granulocytes and platelets occurs. Relatively little work has been performed on granulocyte kinetics in cirrhosis. Although clearance rates are reduced by splenectomy, this does not entirely restore these rates to normal (Uchida and Kariyone, 1973). The large granulocyte pool in the spleen in cirrhosis may be mobilized by epinephrine (Schaffner *et al.*, 1985). More is known about platelet kinetics, although the abnormal platelet count results from the interaction of many factors in alcoholic cirrhotics, including the direct toxic effects of alcohol (Mikhailidis *et al.*, 1986). Platelet kinetic studies using both ^{51}Cr and [111]Indium oxine as labels have confirmed the presence of large platelet pools in cirrhosis (Toghill and Green, 1979) but there was no correlation with spleen size. This contrasts with the well-established positive relationship between spleen size and platelet pool size which exists in the 'hematological' big-spleen syndromes (Branehög, Weinfeld and Roos, 1973). Platelet lifespan is reduced in chronic liver disease, but rarely sufficiently for it to contribute to thrombocytopenia. Platelet-associated immunoglobulins of IgG type are common in both alcoholic and non-alcoholic liver disease, and these may be of importance in the pathogenesis of thrombocytopenia (Barrison *et al.*, 1982).

Among the many causes of anemia associated with liver disease, the spleen plays a relatively minor role. Although measurable splenic red cell pools are present, these are rarely more than 15% of the total red cell mass and have little influence on the hemoglobin level. The mean lifespan of red cells in chronic liver disease is often moderately reduced but surface counting after ^{51}Cr-labeling of autologous cells has not shown grossly increased activity over the spleen (Toghill and Green, 1979). Hypersplenic patients with liver disease do not have unduly large splenic red cell pools or significantly shortened erythrocyte life span. Although in the 'big spleen' syndromes plasma volume expansion is related to spleen size and contributes to anemia by hemodilution, this mechanism does not seem to apply in a wide range of chronic liver diseases (Blendis, Clarke and Williams, 1968). Nevertheless the plasma volume in many cirrhotics may be mildly increased (Lieberman and Reynolds, 1967).

Much has been written about the correction of the pancytopenia of chronic liver disease by splenectomy or procedures to lower portal venous pressure. This stems from earlier concerns related to the hazards of either the leukopenia or the thrombocytopenia, or both factors together. In fact the leukopenia and thrombocytopenia of liver disease are rarely sufficiently severe to be of clinical relevance. Although patients with liver disease unquestionably have an increased susceptibility to infection, this is largely the result of their associated lifestyle, poor nutrition and defective immunological functions (Wyke, 1987). Plasma defects, which differ with the etiology of the cirrhosis, have been shown to lead to impaired neutrophil locomotion or phagocytosis (Campbell *et al.*, 1981) but neutropenia *per se* is rarely the sole factor in infection. Likewise although thrombocytopenia is common, it is an unusual cause of spontaneous bleeding in liver disease. With the stress of major variceal bleeding the contractile splenic reservoir may have a significant role.

It might be expected that surgical operations

Table 10.4 Results of various types of surgery for hypersplenism in chronic liver disease

Author	Material	Criteria for hypersplenism	No. of cases	No. with hypersplenism	Conclusions
Macpherson and Innes (1953)	Patients with portal hypertension	None given	54	N.S.	(a) Hematological improvement in 46 cases treated by Sx, and Sx with LRS (b) No hematological improvement in 3 cases after PCS (c) No hematological improvement in 5 cases after splenic artery ligation
Sullivan and Tumen (1961)	Patients with portal hypertension having PCS	Pl. <150	25	18	PCS may or may not improve thrombocytopenia
Morris et al. (1962)	Patients having PCS	WBC <40 Pl. <150	34	8	Hypersplenism improved in 8 after PCS but relapsed in 2
Rousselot et al. (1963)	Patients with portal hypertension having PCS	Pl. <100	104	15	5 improved. 5 no change. 5 progressive disease
Felix et al. (1974)	Patients with portal hypertension and varices	WBC <5.0 × 3 WBC <4.0 × 1 Pl. <100	277	41	Hypersplenism improved in all patients after PCS. No development of hypersplenism after PCS
Mutchnick et al. (1975)	Patients with portal hypertension	WBC <4.0 Pl. <100	90	N.S.	PCS did not influence pre-existing hypersplenism
Hutson et al. (1977)	Patients having DLRS	WBC <5.0 Pl. <100	66	24	After DLRS average WBC ↑ by 1.0 and platelets ↑ by 40
Soper and Rikkers (1982)	Patients with cirrhosis with bleeding varices Mainly DLRS	WBC <5.0 Pl. <100	76	19	Approximately two-thirds of hypersplenic patients improved
el-Khishen et al. (1985)	Patients having had shunting procedures	WBC <2.5 Pl. <50	563	53	Significant rise in leukocytes + platelets

Sx   = Splenectomy
PCS = Porta-caval shunt
LRS = Lieno-renal shunt
DLRS = Distal lieno-renal shunt
Source: Modified from Toghill and Green (1979).

to reduce portal pressure, or to remove the spleen, might shed some light on the mechanisms of hypersplenism in portal hypertension. A summary of the results of various types of surgery indicates many of the variables in play, and also demonstrates their differing results (Table 10.4). Splenectomy, but not necessarily splenic artery ligation, alone consistently corrects hypersplenism (Macpherson and Innes, 1953); some surgeons recommend that splenectomy should be included as part of the procedure for cirrhotic patients with hypersplenism who require surgical control of variceal hemorrhage (Soper and Rikkers, 1986). The distal lieno-renal shunt popularized by Warren preserves the spleen (Warren, Fomon and Zeppa, 1969); in this operation the splenic vein is divided and its splenic end is anastomosed to the left renal vein. The theoretical advantage is the selective drainage of the esophageal varices *via* the short gastric veins, while preserving blood flow to the liver. Warren's group has suggested that splenectomy is contraindicated for thrombocytopenia secondary to portal hypertension (el-Khishen *et al.*, 1985). In their hands satisfactory improvement in the hematological indices of hypersplenism is achieved by distal lieno-renal shunting alone. However, various groups have produced discrepant results, and porto-caval shunting alone does not invariably improve hypersplenism in patients who suffer variceal bleeding.

The declining popularity of shunting operations for portal hypertension, and the increasing use of sclerotherapy for bleeding varices, has led to a search for more limited and nonsurgical remedies for hypersplenism. Some techniques are discussed further in Chapter 18. Interest in recent years has centered on embolization either by gel foam or steel coils (Alwmark, Bengmark and Gullstrand, 1982; Zannini *et al.*, 1983). Undoubtedly these procedures are effective, although the mortality and risk of complications (including pleural effusion, abdominal pain, splenic abscess, and rupture) are considered by many to be unacceptably high. These risks can be reduced by selec-

tive, repeated embolization, but 75–85% of splenic tissue needs to be infarcted. In view of the small numbers of patients who really have symptomatic hypersplenism the need for embolization in the large number reported seems questionable.

10.5.6 SPLENIC VEIN OCCLUSION

Isolated splenic vein thrombosis causes a rare syndrome characterized by left-sided (sinistral) portal hypertension, upper gastro-intestinal bleeding, splenomegaly and occasionally hypersplenism. The great majority of cases is due to primary pancreatic disease, including acute and chronic pancreatitis and pancreatic tumors (Johnston and Myers, 1973; Salam, Warren and Tyras, 1973; Moossa and Gadd, 1985). If the splenic vein is occluded the preferential path of venous blood is towards the portal vein. This begins with the short gastric veins which cross the fundus of the stomach to enter the right and left gastric veins. This creates a unique form of portal hypertension with gastric varices limited to the fundus of the stomach. Because the portal hypertension is restricted to this area it has been termed left-sided portal hypertension. Upper gastro-intestinal bleeding from these varices is the presenting feature of splenic vein occlusion in 45% of cases and may be notoriously difficult to diagnose endoscopically (Moossa and Gadd, 1985). Splenomegaly is found in approximately one-third of cases, but hypersplenic changes in the blood are relatively unusual and were reported in only four of 53 patients by Sutton, Yarborough and Richards (1970), and in none of the patients reported by Salam, Warren and Tyras (1973).

In this form of portal hypertension more than 90% of patients are relieved of their gastrointestinal bleeding by splenectomy. Nevertheless it must be borne in mind that splenic vein occlusion is usually secondary to primary pancreatic disease for which definitive surgery may also be necessary. Embolization of the splenic artery in attempts to conserve the spleen is a less than satisfactory alternative, since this provides no remedy for the underlying causative disease and may result in splenic abscess (Jones and de Koos, 1984).

10.5.7   FELTY'S SYNDROME

The syndrome described by Felty (1924) is characterized by leukopenia and splenomegaly in patients suffering from rheumatoid arthritis. Between 5 and 10% of patients with rheumatoid arthritis have splenomegaly (Short, Bauer and Reynolds, 1957; Gordon, Stein and Broder, 1973), but Felty's syndrome itself is said to occur in approximately 1% of all patients with rheumatoid arthritis. It may have other features including anemia, thrombocytopenia, pigmentation, leg ulcers, and intercurrent infections. While the syndrome is usually a complication of established rheumatoid disease, the arthropathy may follow the neutropenia, and has even followed splenectomy for previously unexplained hypersplenism (Rodgers and Langley, 1950). In some patients the neutropenia may co-exist with arthritis but with no splenomegaly (Hutchinson and Alexander, 1954).

The principal hematological feature of Felty's syndrome is the leukopenia and the syndrome has been used as a model for studying neutrophil hemodynamics. While pooling of leukocytes has been suggested as the probable cause of the leukopenia (Blendis *et al.*, 1970b) the frequent occurrence of IgG antibodies directed against neutrophils suggests a more complex immunological etiology (Rosenthal *et al.*, 1974; Logue, 1976). After splenectomy the level of IgG antibodies returns to normal. The anemia and thrombocytopenia have received less attention: anemia is common and is probably of multifactorial origin. Occasionally a steroid-responsive hemolytic anemia is seen (Blendis *et al.*, 1970b). Plasma expansion related to the splenomegaly may contribute significantly to the anemia. In one patient shrinkage in spleen size produced by corticosteroid therapy resulted in a 'medical splenectomy', and improved the anemia by reducing the plasma volume (Pengel-

ly, 1966). Platelet counts in Felty's syndrome tend to be between 100×10^9 and $200 \times 10^9/l$ but are rarely reduced as profoundly as the neutrophil counts.

In spite of the severe leukopenia experienced in Felty's syndrome, serious bacterial infection is relatively unusual. Although splenectomy for this condition was performed as long ago as 1932, its place has still to be defined. Earlier reports suggested that the gratifying rise in leukocyte counts after splenectomy led to a reduction in infectious episodes (Riley and Aldrete, 1975; Laszlo *et al.*, 1978). However, in a non-randomized trial, Coon (1985b) found that splenectomized patients fared little better than a similar group not undergoing surgery, the only positive benefit from splenectomy being a greater likelihood of the healing of leg ulcers. It now seems probable that few patients with Felty's syndrome derive appreciable benefit from the operation, and there is no evidence that splenectomy alters the course of the disease.

Some patients with gross splenomegaly may develop portal hypertension, probably in relation to the very high splenic blood flow, which may exceed 1000 ml/minute. Occasionally the portal hypertension is sufficient to cause esophageal varices (Blendis *et al.*, 1970b).

10.5.8   GAUCHER'S DISEASE

Gaucher' disease is the commonest of the non-hematological hereditary diseases in which massive splenomegaly plays a critical role. Three types of disease are described but common to all are deficient β-glucosylceramidase activity, an autosomal recessive inheritance and the presence of Gaucher cells in the bone marrow. The incidence of the disease is particularly high in Ashkenazi Jews. In the common non-neuropathic Type 1 disease progressive accumulation of glucosylceramide causes enlargement of both liver and spleen during late childhood and adolescence. The resulting splenomegaly leads to the development of hypersplenism, abdominal distension and the mechanical difficulties which arise from encroachment of the splenic mass on adjacent organs. In the infantile form of the disease (Type 2) there is rapid neurological deterioration with early death, and in the juvenile form (Type 3) the neurological features again dominate the clinical picture.

The hematological features of adult (Type 1) Gaucher's disease include anemia, leukopenia and thrombocytopenia. The anemia is usually normochromic and normocytic. It is commonly ascribed to marrow infiltration with Gaucher cells; in support of this there are reports of associated extramedullary erythropoiesis and a leukoerythroblastic blood picture. However, this is a disease in which hemodilutional anemia may play an important part. This can be corrected by splenectomy but may relapse years later, relapses appearing to correlate with subsequent enlargement of the liver (Bowdler, 1963). Relatively few studies have been made of the erythrokinetics in Gaucher's disease but the red cell lifespan is reduced (Bowdler, 1963; Lee, Balcerzak and Westerman, 1967) and a hemolytic anemia with spherocytosis and reticulocytosis has been described (Mandelbaum, Berger and Lederer, 1942). It is probable that the leukopenia and thrombocytopenia are principally due to pooling within the spleen but more evidence for this is needed.

Portal hypertension has been documented in several patients with Gaucher's disease (Sales and Hunt, 1970; Kozower, Kaplan and Kanfer, 1974). The most probable cause is the massive portal infiltration of Gaucher cells in the liver; the possibility has been raised (but not proved) that this may be accentuated by increased hepatic deposition after splenectomy. In some patients with portal hypertension the massive splenic blood flow appears to contribute to the development of varices. However, Aderka et al. (1984) have described a 76-year-old patient who succumbed to bleeding esophageal varices, having had a splenectomy 32 years previously.

Many patients with the gross splenomegaly of adult Gaucher's disease are splenectomized because of hypersplenism, or because of the discomfort of the massive splenomegaly. However, the principal single reason for splenectomy is thrombocytopenia; removal of the spleen gives a prompt and lasting increase in the platelet count (Matoth and Fried, 1965). Others have described a complete return to normal of the abnomalities in the blood picture after splenectomy (Salky et al., 1979).

Concern has been expressed that splenectomy may accelerate deposition of glucosylceramide in the liver and bones of Type 1 patients, and even accelerate the central nervous system manifestations of Type 3 patients (Dreborg, Erikson and Hagberg, 1980). There is evidence to suggest that splenectomy worsens the orthopedic complications of Gaucher's disease, including ischemic necrosis, osteolytic areas and coxa vara deformities (Silverstein and Kelly, 1967; Schein and Arkin, 1973; Rose, Graboswki and Desnick, 1982). Certainly young patients who have undergone early splenectomy are more likely to develop orthopedic problems later (Beighton, Goldblatt and Sachs, 1982). Figure 10.3 summarizes the progress of an adolescent boy with Gaucher's disease who was splenectomized for massive splenomegaly and impaired growth. Shortly afterwards he developed bone pains due to ischemic necrosis.

In addition to these reservations, there is a further concern related to postsplenectomy sepsis in children or young adults already affected by a serious disease impairing their immunity. High rates of sepsis have been reported with this disease (Walker, 1976). To offset the potentially serious risk of postplenectomy sepsis, Bar-Maor and Govrin-Yehudain (1985) have performed partial splenectomies in four children with Gaucher's disease and Thanopolous and Frimas (1982) have reported on partial splenic embolization with encouraging initial results. On theoretical grounds, assessing splenic function from the pitting function of splenunculi, 20–30 cm^3 of normal splenic tissue should be adequate to offer some alleviation of risk (Corazza et al., 1984).

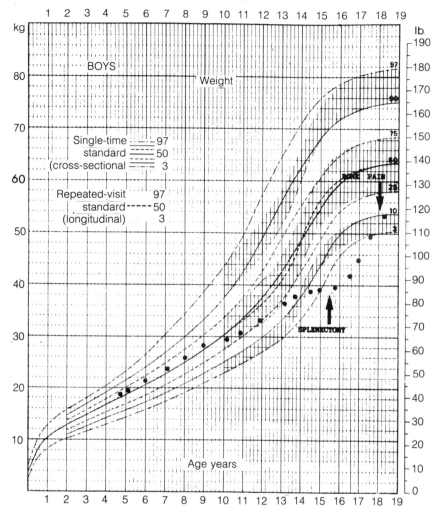

Figure 10.3 The growth chart of a boy with Gaucher's disease. Impaired growth from the age of 13 years onwards was reversed by splenectomy, but bone pain and ischemic necrosis developed 2½ years after splenectomy.

In other storage diseases splenomegaly is only significant in Niemann-Pick disease and in the syndrome of the Sea-Blue histiocyte. In the former, splenectomy has been performed both for diagnosis and for the correction of hematological deficits. In some patients the anemia improved slowly, but the operation did not improve the very limited prognosis of these subjects (Crocker and Farber, 1958). In the latter disease, characterized by aspirates of histiocytes from bone marrow and spleen showing sea-blue staining by the Wright–Giemsa method, splenomegaly is usual and sometimes massive.

10.5.9 THE MALIGNANT LYMPHOMAS

(a) Hodgkin's disease

The adoption of laparotomy and splenectomy for the staging of Hodgkin's disease has expanded knowledge, not only with respect to Hodgkin's disease, but also of the relationship between disease in the spleen and splenomegaly. The recognition of the fact that the spleen may be affected by lymphoma without being enlarged, and that the enlarged spleen may not show disease histologically, has modified the clinician's view of splenomegaly in a significant way. Further consideration of these aspects of Hodgkin's disease and the spleen is given in Chapter 15. The indications for staging splenectomy have become more restricted with time (Table 15.10), and some patients will still experience the syndromes of splenic dysfunction. It may be necessary to consider splenectomy either for splenomegaly of uncertain origin or hypersplenism in diagnosed cases.

Despite the recent developments in radiology including CT and MRI, up to 20% of splenectomies are carried out principally to obtain a tissue diagnosis in patients with unexplained splenomegaly (Goonewardene et al., 1979; Musser et al., 1984; Mitchell and Morris, 1985). Of the diagnostic splenectomies the proportion of spleens containing Hodgkin's tissue has varied from none in 28 in a series from USA (Knudson et al., 1982) to 13 of 34 patients in the United Kingdom (Mitchell and Morris, 1985). In patients splenectomized for the syndrome of idiopathic non-tropical splenomegaly, none has so far developed Hodgkin's disease. By contrast, one-third of such patients eventually develop non-Hodgkin's lymphoma. This suggests that those enlarged spleens removed at staging laparotomy for Hodgkin's disease, which do not show specific diagnostic features of lymphoma, are unrelated (Ell, Britton and Farrer-Brown, 1975).

Hypersplenism remains the commonest reason for therapeutic splenectomy in Hodgkin's disease, although this requirement has declined with the introduction of more effective regimens of chemotherapy and radiotherapy. Correction of hematological deficits may be expected in up to 90% of such cases, despite a proportion who have marrow involvement (Mitchell and Morris, 1985).

(b) The non-Hodgkin's lymphomas (NHL)

Splenomegaly and hypersplenism are common in non-Hodgkin's lymphoma; cell pooling, cell destruction and plasma expansion all play a role in the pathogenesis of cell deficits. Marrow involvement and cytopenias due to radiation and chemotherapy may be additional factors. Each patient with non-Hodgkin's lymphoma and cytopenias requires critical and individual evaluation of their cause. An earlier trend favoring splenectomy in non-Hodgkin's lymphoma has now waned (Meeker et al., 1967; Hyatt et al., 1970; O'Brien et al., 1970) due to improved understanding of the natural history of the disease and its prognosis. There are reports of radiotherapy to the spleen as the sole treatment for hypersplenism in non-Hodgkin's lymphoma: the benefit has tended to be of only a temporary nature (Shukla, Evans and Mittelman, 1976).

Isolated splenomegaly remains a not unusual presentation of non-Hodgkin's lymphoma, for which diagnostic splenectomy may be the only way of achieving a tissue diagnosis. A number of authors have emphasized the value of splenectomy in the initial diagnosis of NHL (Hermann, DeHaven and Hawk, 1968; Hyatt et al., 1970; O'Brien et al., 1970). Undoubtedly NHL presents and is diagnosed much more frequently than Hodgkin's disease with this mode of presentation; in Long and Aisenberg's (1974) series of 15 patients found to have lymphoma none had Hodgkin's disease. Only Mitchell and Morris (1985) have diagnosed significant numbers of patients with Hodgkin's disease at diagnostic splenectomy.

10.5.10 INFILTRATIVE DISEASES WITH HYPERSPLENISM AND HYPOSPLENISM

While there is a general correlation between hypersplenism and enlargement of the spleen and conversely most patients with hyposplenism have small spleens (or no spleen at all), in some disorders there is no clear relationship between spleen size and function. Hematological disorders such as sickle cell disease in crisis, myeloma, and acute leukemia may show evidence of poor splenic function, while the spleen remains either of normal size or enlarged. Some diseases with infiltration of the spleen, such as sarcoidosis and amyloidosis, may manifest either hypersplenic or hyposplenic activity (see also Chapter 7).

Mild splenomegaly is not uncommon in sarcoidosis, and patients with splenomegaly tend to have a higher incidence of constitutional symptoms and more extensive disease (Kataria and Whitcomb, 1980). Occasionally patients present with massive splenomegaly as the first manifestation of the disease (Peter, 1986). Hypersplenism with anemia, leukopenia and thrombocytopenia is not unusual in sarcoidosis and even frank hemolysis may complicate the syndrome (Partenheimer and Meredith, 1950; Maycock et al., 1963; Thadani, Aber and Taylor, 1975). What is of particular interest is that an acquired functional asplenia develops in some patients during the course of the disease (Stone et al., 1986).

Amyloidosis is another disorder in which hyposplenism may co-exist with splenomegaly. Indeed hyposplenic changes in the peripheral blood, with Howell–Jolly bodies, target cells, and Pappenheimer bodies, have provided diagnostic clues to the diagnosis of amyloidosis (Boyko, Pratt and Wass, 1982; Selby, Sprott and Toghill 1987). Presumably the amyloid tissue in the splenic pulp induces sufficient reticuloendothelial blockade to interfere with the 'culling' role of the spleen, and sufficient ridigity of the sinusoidal clefts to interfere with 'pitting'. The extent to which this impairs resistance to infection is uncertain, but 8% of deaths in amyloidosis result from sepsis (Kyle and Bayrd, 1975).

10.6 SPLEEN-PRESERVING ALTERNATIVES TO SPLENECTOMY IN HYPERSPLENIC STATES

Increasing concern about the serious risks of postsplenectomy sepsis in both children and adults (Bohnsack and Brown, 1986) has led to a search for alternative procedures for controlling the deleterious effects of hypersplenism, while preserving some degree of splenic function. Although the risk of postsplenectomy sepsis was originally thought to be restricted to the first 2 to 3 years following splenectomy, it is now clear that the asplenic adult may be vulnerable for many years after the event and perhaps indefinitely (Zarrabi and Rosner, 1986). The critical task is to achieve a balance between ablation and conservation of the spleen (see also Chapter 18).

A possible solution was suggested by Maddison (1973) who first used the technique of embolization of the spleen with autologous blood clots. Unfortunately there was a high risk of complications, and in particular abscess formation, which precluded this from being used as an alternative to surgical splenectomy. Subsequently Witte et al. (1976) showed that hypersplenism could be treated by partial ablation of the splenic mass by segmental embolization of parenchymal arteries with gel foam. Although this method was also associated with complications including pleural effusion, sepsis and splenic abscess, the preservation of a degree of prograde arterial flow does appear to protect against the serious and frequent complication of total splenic infarction. Jonasson, Spigos and Mozes (1985) have used partial splenic embolization in recipients of renal allografts. Earlier work had shown that splenectomy offered early advantages to these grafted patients, presumably because of better tolerance of immunosuppressive drugs producing marrow toxicity (Fryd et al., 1981). This early advantage was offset by late septic complications probably related to the splenectomy. Partial embolization of the spleen was effective in improving the early survival of allograft recipients and also in limiting late sepsis. The ablation of two-thirds of the splenic mass seemed optimal (Mozes et al., 1984).

Partial embolization has also been used successfully to treat myelofibrosis, spherocytosis and thalassemia (Jonasson, Spigos and Mozes, 1985), while others have used it to treat hypersplenism in portal hypertension (Zannini et al., 1983). The latter group utilized Gianturco's coils to occlude the splenic artery and achieved both an improvement in the peripheral cytopenias, and a stable decrease in wedge hepatic vein pressure. Alwmark, Bengmark and Gullstrand (1982) also treated hypersplenism in portal hypertension with partial embolization and achieved hematological improvement. Unfortunately the mortality was high at 12%, but this needs to be evaluated in relation to the poor hepatic function of many of the patients embolized.

A more radical method of addressing the problem of splenic ablation is partial amputation of the spleen; this has now been used in Gaucher's disease (Bar-Maor and Govrin-Yehudain, 1985) and portal hypertension (Witte *et al.*, 1982). Local radiotherapy to the spleen may also prove a temporary alternative to splenectomy and the risk of sepsis in these circumstances.

The problems of limiting the degree of hyposplenism in the treatment of splenic disorders are considered further in Chapter 18.

REFERENCES

Aderka, D. *et al.* (1984) Fatal bleeding from esophageal varices in a patient with Gaucher's disease. *Am. J. Gastroenterol.*, 77, 838–9.

Alpert, L. I. and Benisch, B. (1970) Hemangioendothelioma of the liver associated with microangiopathic hemolytic anemia. *Am. J. Med.*, 48, 624–8.

Alwmark, A., Bengmark, S. and Gullstrand, P. (1982) Evaluation of splenic embolization in patients with portal hypertension and hypersplenism. *Ann. Surg.*, 196, 518–24.

Arkles, L. B., Gill, G. D. and Molan, M. P. (1986) A palpable spleen is not necessarily enlarged or pathological. *Med. J. Aust.*, 145, 15–18.

Aufses, A. H. (1960) Bleeding varices associated with hematologic disorders. *Arch. Surg.*, 80, 655–9.

Bada, J. L. *et al.* (1979) Pancytopenia in kala-azar. *Trans. R. Soc. Trop. Med. Hyg.*, 73, 347–8.

Banti, G. (1883) Dell' anaemia splenica. *Arch. Scul. Anat. Path. Firenze*, 2, 53–122.

Bar-Maor, J. A. and Govrin-Yehudain, J. (1985) Partial splenectomy in children with Gaucher's disease. *Paediatrics*, 76, 398–401.

Barrison, I. G. *et al.* (1982) Is splenomegaly the only cause of thrombocytopenia in chronic liver disease? *Gut*, 23, 447–8.

Beighton, P., Goldblatt, J. and Sachs, S. (1982) Bone involvement in Gaucher's disease. in *Gaucher Disease. A Century of Delineation and Research* (eds R. J. Desnick, S. Gatt and G. A. Grabowski) (Proc. 1st Int. Symposium on Gaucher Disease, New York City, 1981), A. R. Liss, New York, pp. 603–16.

Beker, S. and Valencia-Parparcen, J. (1970) Personal communication quoted by H. J. Tumen. *Ann. NY Acad. Sci.*, 170, 332.

Bhagwat, A. G. *et al.* (1975) Splenoma with portal hypertension. *Br. Med. J.*, 3, 520.

Blendis, L. M., Clarke, M. B. and Williams, R. (1968) Effect of splenectomy on the haemodilutional anaemia of splenomegaly. *Lancet*, i, 795–8.

Blendis, L. M. *et al.* (1970a) Observer variation in the clinical and radiological assessment of hepatosplenomegaly. *Br. Med. J.*, 1, 727–30.

Blendis, L. M. *et al.* (1970b) Liver in Felty's syndrome. *Br. Med. J.*, 1, 131–5.

Blendis, L. M. *et al.* (1970c) Spleen blood flow and splanchnic haemodynamics in blood dyscrasias and other splenomegalies. *Clin. Sci.*, 38, 73–84.

Blix, S. and Jacobsen, C. (1963) The defibrination syndrome in a patient with haemangio-endotheliosarcoma. *Acta Med. Scand.*, 173, 377–83.

Bohnsack, J. F. and Brown, E. J. (1986) The role of the spleen in resistance to infection. *Ann. Rev. Med.*, 38, 48–60.

Bowdler, A. J. (1963) Dilution anaemia corrected by splenectomy in Gaucher's disease. *Ann. Intern. Med.*, 58, 664–9.

Bowdler, A. J. (1967) Dilution anaemia associated with enlargement of the spleen. *Proc. R. Soc. Med.*, 60, 44–7.

Bowdler, A. J. (1970) Blood volume studies in patients with splenomegaly. *Transfusion*, 10, 171–81.

Boyko, W. J., Pratt, R. and Wass, H. (1982) Functional hyposplenism. A diagnostic clue in amyloidosis. *Am. J. Clin. Pathol.*, 77, 745–8.

Branehög, I., Weinfeld, A. and Roos, B. (1973) The exchangeable splenic platelet pool studied with epinephrine infusion in idiopathic thrombocytopenic purpura and in patients with splenomegaly. *Br. J. Haematol.*, 25, 239–48.

Campbell, A. C. *et al.* (1981) Neutrophil function in chronic liver disease. *Clin. Exp. Immunol.*, 45, 81–9.

Cartwright, G. E., Chung, H.-L. and Chang, A. (1948) Studies on kala-azar. *Blood*, 3, 249–75.

Castell, D. O. (1967) The spleen percussion sign. *Ann. Intern. Med.*, **67**, 1265–7.

Chauffard, M. (1907) A propos de la communication de M. Vaqués. *Bulletin de la Societé Hôpitale de Paris*, 1201.

Cock, K. M. de, *et al.* (1983) Obscure splenomegaly in the tropics that is not the tropical splenomegaly syndrome. *Br. Med. J.*, **287**, 1347–8.

Cook, J., McFadzean, A. J. S. and Todd, D. (1963) Splenectomy in cryptogenetic splenomegaly. *Br. Med. J.*, ii, 337–44.

Cooley, J. C. *et al.* (1954) Clinical triad of massive splenic infarction, sicklemia trait and high altitude flying. *J. Am. Med. Assoc.*, **154**, 111–13.

Coon, W. W. (1985a) Splenectomy for splenomegaly and secondary hypersplenism. *World J. Surg.*, **3**, 437–43.

Coon, W. W. (1985b) Felty's syndrome: when is splenectomy indicated? *Am. J. Surg.*, **149**, 272–5.

Corazza, G. R. *et al.* (1984) Return of splenic function after splenectomy. How much tissue is needed? *Br. Med. J.*, **289**, 861–4.

Corrigan, J. J., Van Wyck, D. B. and Crosby, W. H. (1983) Clinical disorders of splenic function: the spectrum from asplenism to hypersplenism. *Lymphology*, **16**, 101–6.

Crane, G. G. (1973) Anaemia in the Upper Watut Valley of New Guinea. *Med. J. Aust.*, **1**, 101–7.

Crane, G. G. (1981) Tropical splenomegaly: Oceania. *Clin. Haematol.*, **10**, 976–82.

Crocker, A. C. and Farber, S. (1958) Niemann-Pick disease: a review of eighteen patients. *Medicine*, **37**, 1–96.

Crosby, W. H. (1962) Hypersplenism. *Ann. Rev. Med.*, **13**, 127–46.

Dacie, J. V. *et al.* (1969) Non-tropical idiopathic splenomegaly (primary hypersplenism). A review of ten cases and their relationship to malignant lymphomas. *Br. J. Haematol.*, **17**, 317–33.

Dagradi, A. E. *et al.* (1965) Bleeding esophageal varices in myelofibrosis. *Am. J. Gastroenterol.*, **44**, 536–44.

Dal Palu, C., Ruol, A. and Belloni, G. (1963) Post-sinusoidal portal hypertension in a patient with chronic lymphatic leukemia. *Am. J. Digest. Dis.*, **8**, 845–51.

DeLand, F. H. (1970) Normal spleen size. *Radiology*, **97**, 589–92.

Diggs, L. W. (1965) Sickle cell crisis. *Am. J. Clin. Pathol.*, **44**, 1–19.

Dreborg, S., Erikson, A. and Hagberg, B. (1980) Gaucher's disease; Norrbottnìan type I. General clinical description. *Eur. J. Pediatr.*, **133**, 107–18.

el-Khishen, M. A. *et al.* (1985) Splenectomy is contraindicated for thrombocytopenia secondary to portal hypertension. *Surg. Gynecol. Obstet.*, **160**, 233–8.

Ell, P. J., Britton, K. E. and Farrer-Brown, G. (1975) An assessment of the value of spleen scanning in the staging of Hodgkin's disease. *Br. J. Radiol.*, **48**, 590–3.

Ellis, L. D. and Damashek, H. L. (1975) The dilemma of hypersplenism. *Surg. Clin. North Am.*, **55**, 277–85.

Engelbreth-Holm, J. (1938) A study of tuberculous splenomegaly and splenogenic controlling of the cell emission from the bone marrow. *Am. J. Med. Sci.*, **195**, 32–40.

Fakunle, Y. M. (1981) Tropical splenomegaly. Part I: Tropical Africa. *Clin. Haematol.*, **10**, 963–75.

Fegiz, G. *et al.* (1983) La valutazione della sopravvivenza piastrinica prima e dopo shunt porto-cavale latero-laterale. *Minerva Medica*, **74**, 205–8.

Felix, W. R. *et al.* (1974) The effect of porta-caval shunt on hypersplenism. *Surg. Gynecol. Obstet.*, **139**, 899–904.

Felty, A. R. (1924) Chronic arthritis in the adult associated with splenomegaly and leucopenia. *Johns Hopkins Hosp. Bull.*, **35**, 16–20.

Ferrara, J. *et al.* (1979) Correction of hypersplenism following D.S.R.S. *Surgery*, **86**, 570–3.

Fischer, J. (1970) Spleen scanning as a method of functional analysis of the spleen. in *The Spleen* (eds K. Lennerts and D. Harms), Springer, Berlin and New York. pp. 11–23.

Fryd, D. S. *et al.* (1981) Results of a prospective randomised study on the effect of splenectomy versus no splenectomy in renal transplant patients. *Transplant. Proc.*, **13**, 48.

Geary, G. C., Clough, V. and MacIver, J. E. (1980) Tropical splenomegaly. *Br. J. Hosp. Med.*, **24**, 417–21.

Gevirtz, N. R., Nathan, D. G. and Berlin, N. I. (1962) Erythrokinetic studies in primary hypersplenism with pancytopenia. *Amer. J. Med.*, **32**, 148–52.

Glatstein, E. *et al.* (1969) The value of laparotomy and splenectomy in the staging of Hodgkin's disease. *Cancer*, **24**, 709–18.

Goonewardene, A. *et al.* (1979) Splenectomy for undiagnosed splenomegaly. *Br. J. Surg.*, **66**, 62–5.

Gordon, D. A., Stein, J. L. and Broder, I. (1973) The extra-articular features of rheumatoid arthritis. *Am. J. Med.*, **54**, 445–52.

Gramlich, F. *et al.* (1970) The spleen in liver disease. in *The Spleen* (eds K. Lennerts and D. Harms), Springer, Berlin and New York. pp. 336–46.

Green, R. L., Huntsman, R. G. and Serjeant, G. R.

(1971) The sickle cell and altitude. *Br. Med. J.*, **4**, 593–5.

Gretsel, G. (1866) Ein Fall von Anaemia splenica bei einem Kind. *Klin. Wochenschr. (Berlin)*, **3**, 212.

Halvorsen, J. F., Semb, B. K. H. and Maurseth, K. (1974) Post-traumatic pseudocyst of the spleen with hypersplenism. *Acta Chir. Scand.*, **140**, 571–5.

Hayhoe, F. G. J. and Whitby, L. (1955) Splenic function. *Q. J. Med.*, NS **XXIV**, 96, 365–91.

Hermann, R. E., DeHaven, K. E. and Hawk, W. A. (1968) Splenectomy for the diagnosis of splenomegaly. *Ann. Surg.*, **168**, 896–900.

Hesdorffer, C. S. *et al.* (1986) True idiopathic splenomegaly is a distinct clinical entity. *Scand. J. Haematol.*, **37**, 310–15.

Hunter, T. B. and Haber, K. (1977) Sonographic diagnosis of wandering spleen. *Am. J. Roentgenol.*, **129**, 925–6.

Hutchinson, H. E. and Alexander, W. D. (1954) Splenic neutropenia in Felty's syndrome. *Blood*, **9**, 986–98.

Hutson, D. G. *et al.* (1977) The effects of the distal splenorenal shunt on hypersplenism. *Ann. Surg.*, **185**, 605–12.

Hyatt, D. F. *et al.* (1970) Splenectomy for lymphosarcoma. *Surg. Gynecol. Obstet.*, **131**, 928–32.

Jandl, J. H., Jacob, H. S. and Daland, G. A. (1961) Hypersplenism due to infection: a study of 5 cases manifesting hemolytic anemia. *N. Engl. J. Med.*, **264**, 1063–71.

Janin, Y. *et al.* (1981) Splenic pseudocyst associated with hypersplenism. *Am. J. Gastroenterol.*, **75**, 289–93.

Jarett, S. N., Kew, M. C. and Litnaitsky, D. (1966) Gaucher's disease with portal hypertension. *J. Pediatr.*, **68**, 810–12.

Johnston, F. R. and Myers, R. T. (1973) Etiologic factors and consequences of splenic vein obstruction. *Ann. Surg.*, **177**, 736–9.

Jonasson, O., Spigos, D. G. and Mozes, M. F. (1985) Partial splenic embolisation: experience in 136 patients. *World J. Surg.*, **9**, 461–7.

Jones, K. B. and de Koos, P. T. (1984) Post-embolization splenic abscess in a patient with pancreatitis and splenic vein thrombosis. *South. Med. J.*, **77**, 390–3.

Kataria, Y. F. and Whitcomb, M. E. (1980) Splenomegaly in sarcoidosis. *Arch. Intern. Med.*, **140**, 35–7.

Knudson, P. *et al.* (1982) Splenomegaly without an apparent cause. *Surg. Gynecol. Obstet.*, **155**, 705–8.

Kozower, M., Kaplan, M. M. and Kanfer, J. N.

(1974) Esophageal varices in a 60 year old man with Gaucher's disease. *Am. J. Dig. Dis.*, **19**, 565–70.

Krook, H. (1956) Circulatory studies in liver cirrhosis. *Acta Med. Scand.*, **156**, Suppl. 318, 6–134.

Krumbhaar, E. B. and Lippincott, S. W. (1939) The post-mortem weight of the 'normal' human spleen at different ages. *Am. J. Med. Sci.*, **197**, 344–58.

Krumbhaar, E. B. and Stengel, A. (1942) The spleen in leukemias. *Arch. Pathol.*, **34**, 117–32.

Kyle, R. A. and Bayrd, E. L. (1975) Amyloidosis. Review of 236 cases. *Medicine*, **54**, 271–99.

Laszlo, J. *et al.* (1978) Splenectomy for Felty's syndrome. *Arch. Intern. Med.*, **138**, 597–602.

Lee, R. E., Balcerzak, S. P. and Westerman, M. P. (1967) Gaucher's disease: a morphologic study and measurements of iron-metabolism. *Am. J. Med.*, **42**, 891–8.

Lieberman, F. L. and Reynolds, T. B. (1967) Plasma volume in cirrhosis of the liver. *J. Clin. Invest.*, **46**, 1297–308.

Lima, J. P. *et al.* (1962) Portal venous pressure in Hodgkin's disease with hepatic involvement and esophageal varices. *Am. J. Med.*, **32**, 618–20.

Logue, G. (1976) Felty's syndrome. Granulocyte-bound immunoglobin G and splenectomy. *Ann. Intern. Med.*, **85**, 437–42.

Long, J. C. and Aisenberg, A. C. (1974) Malignant lymphoma diagnosed at splenectomy and idiopathic splenomegaly: a clinico-pathologic comparison. *Cancer*, **33**, 1054–61.

McFadzean, A. J. S., Todd, D. and Tsang, K. C. (1958) Observations on the anemia of cryptogenetic splenomegaly: II. Expansion of the plasma volume. *Blood*, **13**, 524–32.

McIntyre, O. R. and Ebaugh, F. G. (1967) Palpable spleens in college freshmen. *Arch. Intern. Med.*, **66**, 301–6.

Macpherson, A. I. S. and Innes, J. (1953) Peripheral blood picture after operation for portal hypertension. *Lancet*, **i**, 1120–3.

Maddison, F. E. (1973) Embolic therapy of hypersplenism. *Invest. Radiol.*, **8**, 280–7.

Mandelbaum, H., Berger, L. and Lederer, M. (1942) Gaucher's disease. I. A case with hemolytic anemia and marked thrombocytopenia; improvement after removal of spleen weighing 6822 g. *Ann. Intern. Med.*, **16**, 438–46.

Manoharan, A., Bader, L. V. and Pitney, W. R. (1982) Non-tropical idiopathic splenomegaly (Dacie's syndrome). Report of 5 cases. *Scand. J. Haematol.*, **28**, 175–9.

Marterre, W. F. Jr and Sugerman, H. J. (1986) True

splenic cyst associated with hypersplenism. *Arch. Surg.*, **121**, 859.

Matoth, Y. and Fried, K. (1965) Chronic Gaucher's disease: clinical observations on 34 patients. *Isr. J. Med. Sci.*, **1**, 521–30.

Maycock, R. L. *et al.* (1963) Manifestations of sarcoidosis. Analysis of 145 patients with a review of 9 series selected from the literature. *Am. J. Med.*, **35**, 67–89.

Meeker, W. R. *et al.* (1967) The role of splenectomy in malignant lymphoma and leukemia. *Surg. Clin. North Am.*, **47**, 1163–71.

Merkel, C. *et al.* (1985) Splenic haemodynamics and portal hypertension in patients with liver cirrhosis and spleen enlargement. *Clin. Physiol.*, **5**, 531–9.

Mikhailidis, D. P. *et al.* (1986) Platelet function defects in chronic alcoholism. *Br. Med. J.*, **293**, 715–18.

Mitchell, A. and Morris, P. J. (1985) Splenectomy for malignant lymphomas. *World J. Surg.*, **9**, 444–8.

Moossa, A. R. and Gadd, M. A. (1985) Isolated splenic vein thrombosis. *World J. Surg.*, **9**, 384–90.

Morgenstern, L., Rosenberg, J. and Geller, S. A. (1985) Tumors of the spleen. *World J. Surg.*, **9**, 468–76.

Morris, P. W. *et al.* (1962) Portal hypertension, congestive splenomegaly and porta-caval shunt. *Gastroenterology*, **42**, 555–9.

Mozes, M. F. *et al.* (1984) Partial splenic embolization: an alternative to splenectomy. Results of a prospective randomised study. *Surgery*, **96**, 694–702.

Musser, G. *et al.* (1984) Splenectomy for hematological disease. *Ann. Surg.*, **200**, 40–5.

Mutchnik, M. G., Lerner, E. and Conn, H. O. (1975) Effect of porta-caval anastomosis on hypersplenism in cirrhosis. *Gastroenterology*, **68**, 1070.

Myers, J. and Segal, R. J. (1974) Weight of the spleen. *Arch. Pathol.*, **98**, 33–5.

Nixon, R. K. (1954) The detection of splenomegaly by percussion. *N. Engl. Med. J.*, **250**, 166–7.

O'Brien, P. H. *et al.* (1970) Splenectomy for hypersplenism in malignant lymphoma. *Arch. Surg.*, **101**, 348–52.

Osler, W. (1900) On splenic anemia. *Am. J. Med. Sci.*, **119**, 54.

Osler, W. (1902) Anaemia splenica. *Trans. Assoc. Am. Physicians*, **18**, 429.

Partenheimer, R. C. and Meredith, H. C. (1950) Splenomegaly with hypersplenism due to sarcoidosis. *N. Engl. J. Med.*, **243**, 810–12.

Pengelly, C. D. R. (1966) Felty's syndrome. Good response to adrenocorticosteroids: possible mechanism of the anaemia. *Br. Med. J.*, **2**, 986–8.

Peter, S. A. (1986) Massive splenomegaly as the presenting manifestation of sarcoidosis. *J. Am. Med. Assoc.*, **78**, 243–4.

Peters, A. M. (1981) Measurement of splenic functions in humans using heat-damaged autologous red blood cells. *Scand. J. Haematol.*, **29**, 195–200.

Pryor, D. S. (1967) The mechanism of anaemia in tropical splenomegaly. *Q. J. Med.*, **36**, 337–56.

Qureshi, M. A., Hafner, C. D. and Dorchak, J. R. (1964) Non-parasitic cysts of the spleen. *Arch. Surg.*, **89**, 570–4.

Richmond, J. *et al.* (1967) Haematological effects of idiopathic splenomegaly seen in Uganda. *Br. J. Haematol.*, **13**, 348–63.

Riemenschneider, P. A. and Whalen, J. P. (1965) The relative accuracy of estimation of enlargement of the liver and the spleen by radiologic and clinical methods. *Am. J. Roentgenol. Radiother. Nucl. Med.*, **94**, 462–8.

Riley, S. M. and Aldrete, J. S. (1975) The role of splenectomy in Felty's syndrome. *Am. J. Surg.*, **130**, 51–2.

Rodgers, H. M. and Langley, F. H. (1950) Neutropenia associated with splenomegaly and atrophic arthritis (Felty's syndrome). *Ann. Intern. Med.*, **32**, 745–754.

Rose, J. D., Graboswki, G. A. and Desnick, R. J. (1982) Accelerated skeletal deterioration after splenectomy in Gaucher's Type 1 disease. *Am. J. Roentgenol.*, **139**, 1202–4.

Rosenthal, F. D. *et al.* (1974) White cell antibodies and the aetiology of Felty's syndrome. *Q. J. Med.*, **170**, 187–203.

Ross, C. F. and Schiller, K. F. (1971) Hamartoma of spleen associated with thrombocytopenia. *J. Pathol.*, **105**, 62–4.

Rousselot, L. M. *et al.* (1963) Experiences with porta caval anastomosis: Analysis of 104 elective end to side shunts for the prevention of recurrent hemorrhage from esophageal varices. *Am. J. Med.*, **34**, 297–307.

Salam, A. A., Warren, W. D. and Tyras, D. H. (1973) Splenic vein thrombosis. A diagnostic and curable form of portal hypertension. *Surgery*, **74**, 961–72.

Sales, J. E. L. and Hunt, A. H. (1970) Gaucher's disease and portal hypertension. *Br. J. Surg.*, **57**, 225–8.

Salky, B. *et al.* (1979) Splenectomy for Gaucher's disease. *Ann. Surg.*, **190**, 592–4.

Schaffner, A. and Fehr, J. (1981) Granulocyte demargination by epinephrine in evaluation of hypersplenic states. *Scand. J. Haematol.*, **27**, 225–30.

Schaffner, A. *et al.* (1985) The hypersplenic spleen. A

contractile reservoir of granulocytes and platelets. *Arch. Intern. Med.,* 145, 651–4.

Schein, A. J. and Arkin, A. M. (1973) The classic hip joint involvement in Gaucher's disease. *Clin. Orthopaed.,* 90, 4–10.

Selby, C. *et al.* (1987) Bacteraemia in adults after splenectomy or splenic irradiation. *Q. J. Med.,* 63, 523–30.

Selby, C. D., Sprott, V. M. A. and Toghill, P. J. (1987) Impaired splenic function in systemic amyloidosis. *Postgrad. Med. J.,* 63, 357–60.

Short, G. L., Bauer, W. and Reynolds, W. E. (1957) *Rheumatoid Arthritis.* Harvard University Press, Cambridge, MA.

Shukla, S. S., Evans, J. T. and Mittelman, A. (1976) Splenectomy or radiation and splenectomy for hypersplenism in lymphosarcoma. *J. Surg. Oncol.,* 8, 99–103.

Silverstein, M. N. and Kelly, P. J. (1967) Osteoarticular manifestations of Gaucher's disease. *Am. J. Med. Sci.,* 253, 569–76.

Simpson, A. and Ashby, E. C. (1965) Torsion of wandering spleen. *Br. J. Surg.,* 52, 344–6.

Smith, V. C. (1985) Primary splenic angiosarcoma. *Cancer,* 55, 1625–7.

Soper, N. J. and Rikkers, L. F. (1982) Effect of operations for variceal hemorrhage on hypersplenism. *Am. J. Surg.,* 144, 700–3.

Soper, N. J. and Rikkers, L. F. (1986) Cirrhosis and hypersplenism. Clinical and haemodynamic correlates. *Curr. Surg.,* 43, 21–4.

Stathers, G. M., Ma, M. H. and Blackburn, C. R. B. (1968) Extra-hepatic portal hypertension: the clinical evaluation, investigation and results of treatment of 28 patients. *Aust. Ann. Med.,* 17, 12–19.

Steidl, R. M. and Cardy, J. D. (1957) Solitary cyst of the spleen associated with hypersplenism. *Lancet,* ii, 45.

Stone, R. W. *et al.* (1986) Acquired functional asplenia in sarcoidosis. *J. Natl. Med. Assoc.,* 930, 935–6.

Sullivan, B. H. (1950) Dangers of airplane flight to patients with sicklemia. *Ann. Intern. Med.,* 32, 338–42.

Sullivan, B. H. and Tumen, H. J. (1961) The effect of portacaval shunt on thrombocytopenia associated with portal hypertension. *Ann. Intern. Med.,* 55, 598–603.

Sullivan, S. and Williams, R. (1976) Reliability of clinical techniques for detecting splenic enlargement. *Br. Med. J.,* 2, 1043–4.

Sutton, J. P., Yarborough, D. Y. and Richards, J. T. (1970) Isolated splenic vein occlusion. Review of literature and report of additional case. *Arch. Surg.,* 100, 623–6.

Tada, S. *et al.* (1972) Diffuse capillary hemangiomatosis of the spleen as a cause of portal hypertension. *Radiology,* 104, 63–4.

Thadani, U., Aber, C. P. and Taylor, J. J. (1975) Massive splenomegaly, pancytopenia and haemolytic anaemia in sarcoidosis. *Acta Haematol.,* 53, 230–40.

Thanopolous, B. D. and Frimas, C. A. (1982) Partial splenic embolisation in management of hypersplenism secondary to Gaucher's disease. *J. Pediatr.,* 101, 740–3.

Toghill, P. J. and Green, S. (1973) Factors influencing splenic pooling of erythrocytes in the myelo- and lympho-proliferative syndromes. *Acta Haematol.,* 49, 215–22.

Toghill, P. J. and Green, S. (1975) Haematological changes in active chronic hepatitis with reference to the role of the spleen. *J. Clin. Pathol.,* 28, 8–11.

Toghill, P. J. and Green, S. (1979) Splenic influences on the blood in chronic liver disease. *Q. J. Med.,* 48, 613–25.

Toghill, P. J., Rigby, C. C. and Hall, G. F. M. (1972) Haemangiosarcoma of the spleen. *Br. J. Surg.,* 59, 406–8.

Uchida, T. and Kariyone, S. (1973) Intravascular granulocyte kinetics and spleen size in patients with neutropenia and chronic splenomegaly. *J. Lab. Clin. Med.,* 82, 9–19.

Vermylen, C. *et al.* (1983) The wandering spleen. *Eur. J. Paediatr.,* 140, 112–15.

Videbaek, A. (1953) Hypersplenism associated with hamartomas of spleen. *Acta Med. Scand.,* 146, 276–80.

Walker, W. (1976) Splenectomy in childhood: A review in England and Wales 1960–64. *Br. J. Surg.,* 63, 36–43.

Warren, W. D., Fomon, J. J. and Zeppa, R. (1969) Further evaluation of the selective decompression of varices by distal spleno-renal shunt. *Ann. Surg.,* 169, 652–60.

Watson Williams, E. J. and Allan, N. C. (1968) Idiopathic tropical splenomegaly syndrome in Ibadan. *Br. Med. J.,* iv, 739.

Weinstein, V. F. (1964) Haemodilutional anemia associated with simple splenic hyperplasia. *Lancet,* ii, 218–23.

Westaby, S., Wilkinson, S. P. and Williams, R. (1978) Spleen size and portal hypertension in cirrhosis. *Digestion,* 17, 63–8.

Westcott, J. L. and Krufky, E. L. (1972) The upsidedown spleen. *Radiology,* 105, 517–21.

Williams, R. *et al.* (1966) Portal hypertension in idiopathic tropical splenomegaly. *Lancet,* i, 329–33.

Wiseman, B. K. and Doan, C. A. (1942) Primary splenic neutropenia; a newly recognized syndrome, closely related to congenital hemolytic icterus and essential thrombocytopenic purpura. *Ann. Intern. Med.,* 16, 1097–117.

Witte, C. L. *et al.* (1976) Ischemic therapy in thrombocytopenia from hypersplenism. *Arch. Surg.,* 111, 1115–21.

Witte, C. L. *et al.* (1982) Ischaemia and partial resection for control of splenic hyperfunction. *Br. J. Surg.,* 69, 531–5.

Wyke, R. J. (1987) Problems of bacterial infection in patients with liver disease. *Gut,* 28, 623–41.

Zannini, G. *et al.* (1983) Percutaneous splenic artery occlusion for portal hypertension. *Arch. Surg.,* 118, 897–900.

Zarrabi, M. H. and Rosner, F. (1986) Rarity of failure of penicillin prophylaxis to prevent post-splenectomy sepsis. *Arch. Intern. Med.,* 146, 1207–8.

Zervos, N., Vlachos, J. and Karpathios, T. (1967) Giant hemangioma of the spleen with thrombocytopenia and fibrinogen deficiency. *Acta Pediatr. Scand.,* Suppl. 172, 206.

Peter N. Foster and M. S. Losowsky

11.1 INTRODUCTION

The term 'hyposplenism' was introduced to describe the condition which follows splenectomy (Eppinger, 1913) and its use was extended subsequently to include states of impaired splenic function regardless of etiology (Schilling, 1924; Dameshek, 1955). Although hyposplenism is most commonly due to splenectomy, it may also result from agenesis or atrophy of the spleen, or may be 'functional'. The concept of functional hyposplenism arose from the observation that Howell–Jolly bodies can occur in the peripheral blood of patients with no prior history of splenectomy, and whose spleens are of normal size or even enlarged (Pearson, Spencer and Cornelius, 1969). Furthermore, in some conditions the hematological features are transient, indicating that hyposplenism can be reversible (Lockwood *et al.*, 1979). Customarily hyposplenism has been detected by hematological rather than by immunological methods, the principal hallmark of the hyposplenic state being the presence of Howell–Jolly bodies in the red cells of the peripheral blood (see below).

11.2 THE ASSESSMENT OF SPLENIC FUNCTION

11.2.1 THE PERIPHERAL BLOOD FILM

Evidence for hyposplenism is most easily obtained by light microscopy of a peripheral blood film, the most characteristic feature being the presence of Howell–Jolly bodies, which are small intraerythrocytic inclusions consisting of nuclear remnants, ordinarily removed by the spleen's pitting process; other red cell abnormalities include the presence of acanthocytes and target cells (Figure 11.1). While none of these abnormalities is individually diagnostic, their appearance together is virtually pathognomonic of hyposplenism. When the presence of these features was compared with the clearance of heat-damaged erythrocytes in patients with hyposplenism and celiac disease (Robertson *et al.*, 1983a) it was found that Howell–Jolly bodies occurred only when splenic function was markedly impaired, whereas acanthocytes and target cells were found with milder degrees of hyposplenism. Other abnormalities of red cells which are not diagnostic, but have been observed in association with hyposplenism, include circulating siderocytes and cells containing Heinz bodies (Acevedo and Mauer, 1963).

11.2.2 PITTED ERYTHROCYTES

Differential interference contrast microscopy gives red cells a three-dimensional appearance which allows detailed examination of the cell surface: indentations in the surface membrane, with the appearance of craters or pits, were observed in two thalassemic patients after splenectomy (Nathan and Gunn, 1966) but were not found in unsplenectomized subjects (Figure 11.2). Similar membrane changes had been noted previously, using chromium shadowing techniques (Koyama *et al.*, 1962). Further detailed examination of these pits, using transmission and scanning electron microscopy, has revealed that they are in fact vacuoles

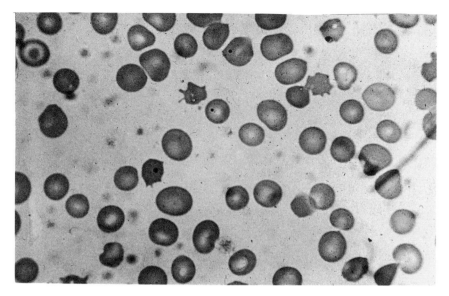

Figure 11.1 Peripheral blood film showing the typical features of hyposplenism: Howell–Jolly bodies, acanthocytes and target cells.

containing the so-called intracellular 'rubbish', including ferritin, hemoglobin and remnants of mitochondria or membranes (Schnitzer *et al.*, 1971; Nathan, 1969). It appears to be a normal function of the spleen to remove these pits: normal erythrocytes acquire pits when transfused into an asplenic subject, whereas pits disappear from erythrocytes of a splenectomized subject when transfused into a normal recipient (Holroyde and Gardner, 1970; Bucha-

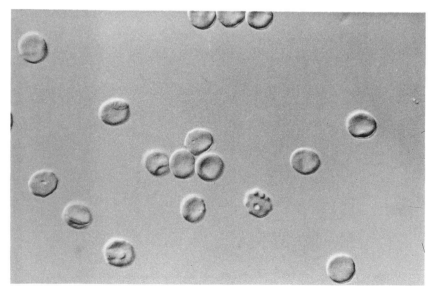

Figure 11.2 Erythrocytes from a splenectomized subject viewed with direct interference contrast microscopy, showing surface craters or pits.

nan, Holtkamp and Horton, 1987). The number of erythrocytes with pits begins to rise a few days after splenectomy, reaching about 50% of their maximum numbers by day 20 post-splenectomy and a constant level after 2–3 months (Zago *et al.*, 1986). Interestingly, the red cells of some families with hereditary spherocytosis exhibit impaired formation of pits after splenectomy, possibly due to a specific membrane defect which limits the cells' ability to form vacuoles; this has also been postulated to explain the reduction in drug-induced vacuole formation in such families (O'Grady *et al.*, 1984a; Kvinesdal and Jensen, 1986; Schrier *et al.*, 1974).

The pitted erythrocyte count is determined on red cells from fresh venous blood fixed with 3% glutaraldehyde buffered to pH 7.4, and examined as a wet preparation using an interference phase microscope fitted with Nomarski optics (Holroyde and Gardner, 1970). The counts are reproducible provided that sufficient cells are examined: 2000 has been recommended (Corazza *et al.*, 1981). In the majority of series, less than 2% of erythrocytes from normal subjects have been found to bear surface pits, which are usually single. The simplicity of the technique has led to the widespread use of counting pitted erythrocytes to study residual function after splenectomy and in the quantitative assessment of the functional hyposplenism associated with a variety of disorders.

11.2.3 CLEARANCE OF RADIOLABELED, DAMAGED ERYTHROCYTES

The ability of the spleen to recognize damaged erythrocytes, and to remove them from the circulation, is utilized to provide a sensitive and quantitative measure of splenic function in which the clearance of radiolabeled, damaged red blood cells is determined (Marsh, Lewis, and Szur, 1966a; Armas, 1985).

Erythrocytes can be damaged chemically, thermally or immunologically but, regardless of the method used, insufficient damage results in little or no splenic uptake whereas excessive damage causes hemolysis or sequestration in the liver. Controlling erythrocyte damage is the most difficult and critical step in the preparation of a spleen-specific probe. All the methods are laborious and require meticulous attention to detail. Heat is probably the most widely used physical agent, whereas mercury-based sulfhydryl-blocking compounds are effective chemical agents. The uptake of chemically damaged cells by the spleen is slower than that of heat-damaged cells. Methods in which cells sensitized with IgG anti-Rh(D) antibody are employed provide a probe for splenic Fc-receptor-specific phagocytic function. In normal volunteers, infusion of IgG-sensitized erythrocytes is followed by progressive clearance of the cells from the circulation. Specific radionuclide counting over the liver and spleen show that these cells are cleared by the spleen and phagocytosed, never reappearing in the circulation. If this experiment is performed with the F(ab)$_2$ antibody fragment, with the Fc portion of the molecule removed, there is no clearance whatsoever; this demonstrates that clearance depends on the interactions of the IgG Fc-fragment with the receptor on phagocytic cells specific for that fragment of the molecule (Frank *et al.*, 1983). ^{51}Chromium and sodium[^{99m}Tc] pertechnetate are the isotopes most commonly used as red cell labels. Technetium is more widely used because the radiation dose to the spleen is less, but some investigators have claimed that the technetium label is unstable and inferior to chromium-51 for quantitative work (Desai and Thakur, 1985).

The method used in our laboratory is as follows: autologous red cells are labeled with 52 MBq (1.4mCi) sodium[^{99m}Tc] pertechnetate (Dacie and Lewis, 1975) then incubated at 50°C for exactly 20 minutes. The cells are reinjected intravenously and samples of blood obtained at intervals. After saponin lysis the radioactivity of the samples is measured in an automatic well scintillation counter. The time to reach 50% remaining radioactivity in normal subjects (the half clearance time) ranges between 10 and 18 minutes which is in accordance with values obtained by others using similar methods (Marsh, Lewis and Szur, 1966a; Ryan *et al.*, 1978).

11.2.4 SCINTISCANS

Radiolabeled colloids are phagocytosed by reticulo-endothelial cells throughout the body, the site of uptake being dependent in part on the size of the particles. [^{99m}Tc] sulfur colloid, with a particle size of approximately 1μm, is the most widely used for scanning the spleen. Following an intravenous dose, about 10% localizes in the spleen and images may be obtained using a gamma camera positioned to view the posterior left upper quadrant of the abdomen (Armas, 1985; Desai and Thakur, 1985). The uptake of radiocolloid provides an index of the spleen's phagocytic activity and the failure of an anatomically present organ to accumulate sulfur colloid indicates functional hyposplenism (Spencer *et al.*, 1978a). Because of the uniform distribution of reticulo-endothelial cells within the spleen, scintiscans provide information about splenic morphology and if appropriate images are obtained estimates of splenic volume may be made (Roberts *et al.*, 1976; Robinson *et al.*, 1980).

11.2.5 THE CORRELATION OF FUNCTIONS

Each of the above methods assesses different aspects of splenic function. The presence of Howell–Jolly bodies and surface pits reflects impaired pitting function, prolongation of the clearance of damaged erythrocytes indicates a reduction in the spleen's ability to cull cells from the circulation, and the uptake of radiolabeled sulfur colloid provides an index of phagocytic activity. Generally there is a good correlation between these various functions; an increased pitted erythrocyte count is associated with prolonged clearance times and reduced splenic volume as determined by scintigraphy (Corazza *et al.*, 1981; Robinson *et al.*, 1980),

and estimates of splenic volume correlate with clearance times (Robinson *et al.*, 1980; Smart *et al.*, 1978). Occasionally dissociation of functions may occur; for example, cases have been described in which Howell–Jolly bodies were observed in the peripheral blood, but the spleen retained the ability to take up sulfur colloid normally (Spencer and Pearson, 1974; Spencer *et al.*, 1984). Some of these patients show a significant reticulocytosis and thus the spleen's pitting function may have been overloaded by the large number of cells presented for the clearance of intracellular inclusions (Spencer and Pearson, 1974). The converse, in which there is failure to accumulate radiocolloid by the spleen and no features of hyposplenism in the peripheral blood, has been described in patients with acute occlusion of the splenic artery (Dhawan, Spencer and Pearson, 1977). Other patients have been reported in whom the spleen was invisible by scintigraphy following injection of [^{99m}Tc] sulfur colloid, but was visualized with [^{99m}Tc]-labeled heat-damaged red cells (Armas, 1985). However, the normal spleen accumulates only about 10% of an injected dose of sulfur colloid but it traps up to 90% of injected damaged erythrocytes. Thus if splenic function is reduced to 10% of normal, the spleen will receive only 1% of an injected sulfur colloid dose, which is insufficient for visualization; however, it will still trap 9% of damaged cells, which may be enough to allow differentiation from the blood-pool background. Nevertheless, studies in animals emphasize that different mechanisms exist for the clearance of colloidal particles and erythrocytes by the spleen and illustrate that these functions are subject to different influences. For example, corticosteroids inhibit the clearance of colloid particles but have no effect on the removal of red cells (Klausner *et al.*, 1975).

11.2.6 ULTRASOUND AND COMPUTERIZED TOMOGRAPHY

These non-invasive imaging techniques will detect the presence or absence of the spleen and estimates of the organ size may be made, but their value in assessing degrees of splenic atrophy has not been studied. (See also Chapter 17.)

11.3 THE CAUSES OF HYPOSPLENISM

11.3.1 SPLENECTOMY

Some 35 000 patients undergo splenectomy each year in the USA (Dickerman, 1979), but surgical removal of the spleen does not invariably result in the complete absence of functioning tissue. Using the non-invasive methods of isotope scanning and counting pitted erythrocytes, residual splenic function has been detected in between a quarter and two-thirds of patients after splenectomy following trauma (Livingston et al., 1983; Kiroff et al., 1983) and in 16% of patients who had undergone splenectomy for hematological disorders (Neilsen et al., 1981; Spencer et al., 1981).

The frequent finding of residual splenic tissue after splenectomy for trauma is due to splenosis, which occurs when fragments of splenic tissue are seeded in the peritoneal cavity. These autotransplanted nodules range in size from a few millimeters to about 3 cm in diameter. The implants do not have a true vascular pedicle of their own with a branching arterial system; rather they depend on new vessels to grow in from the peritoneal surface on which they are implanted. There are usually no associated surrounding reactive tissue changes. Implants have been found most often on the serosal surface of the small bowel, the greater omentum, the parietal peritoneum, the serosal surface of the colon and under the diaphragm. They have also been described in extra-peritoneal locations, such as the pleural cavity, pericardium and in the subcutaneous tissue of old scars; these result from splenic injury, especially gunshot wounds (Widmann and Laubscher, 1971).

Splenosis should be differentiated from the accessory spleens which have been observed in 10% of the population at necropsy (Bowdler, 1982). Accessory splenic tissue is supplied by branches of the splenic artery, there is usually a well-developed hilar region and the capsule has both muscle and elastic fibers. It is rare for more than five accessory spleens to be found in any one subject. The pattern of distribution is determined by embryonic development and includes the splenic hilum and pedicle, the retroperitoneum and the greater omentum. It is probable that splenic tissue persisting after elective splenectomy is, at least in part, due to the presence of accessory spleens which, because of their small size, were missed at laparotomy.

It is well recognized that the presence of an accessory spleen can result in significant splenic function after splenectomy, but the effect of splenosis is less clear. Certainly the pitting function of the spleen can be restored (Corazza et al., 1984) and the ability to accumulate radiocolloid indicates some phagocytic function, but whether the spleen's immune functions are preserved is uncertain. The low incidence of serious infection in patients splenectomized for trauma may be due to a partial return of splenic function consequent on splenosis (Pearson et al., 1978); however, there are reports of fatal infections in patients with significant residual tissue (Rice and James, 1980), and experimentally induced splenosis offers little protection against infection.

11.3.2 'NON-SURGICAL' HYPOSPLENISM

Hyposplenism not due to surgical removal of the spleen occurs in a wide variety of conditions (Table 11.1). In some disorders such as sickle-cell disease and celiac disease, hyposplenism is a frequent association; in others, hyposplenism is observed only in isolated cases.

(a) Splenic function and age

Developmental immaturity is characteristic of the neonate, so that it is to be expected that splenic function is impaired in premature and term infants (Holroyde, Oski and Gardner, 1969; Freedman et al., 1980). In normal individuals the spleen reaches a maximum weight early in adult life, and after the age of 65 there

Table 11.1 Causes of non-surgical hyposplenism*

Congenital
  Asplenia: Ivemark syndrome
              Isolated anomaly
  Cyanotic heart disease

Hematological
  Sickle cell disorders
  Essential thrombocythemia
  Hodgkin's and non-Hodgkin's lymphoma
  Fanconi's syndrome

Autoimmune
  Systemic lupus erythematosus
  Mixed connective tissue disease
  Rheumatoid arthritis
  Sjögren's syndrome
  Thyroid disease
  Chronic active hepatitis

Gastrointestinal
  Celiac disease
  Dermatitis herpetiformis
  Ulcerative colitis
  Crohn's disease
  Idiopathic ulcerative enteritis
  Tropical sprue
  Whipple's disease
  Intestinal lymphangiectasia

Circulatory
  Occlusion of splenic artery or vein
  Thrombosis of celiac artery

Miscellaneous
  Irradiation
  Amyloidosis
  Sarcoidosis
  Graft versus host disease
  Breast cancer
  Hemangiosarcoma
  Methyldopa administration

*For references see text.

is a rapid loss in the weight of the spleen due to the ageing process, to which an increasing atherosclerotic vascular obstruction and fibrosis of the spleen may contribute (Krumbhaar and Lippincot, 1939). In addition, old age is accompanied by splenic hypofunction, as judged by increased numbers of pitted erythrocytes and delayed clearance of heat-damaged red cells (Zago *et al.*, 1985). Of individuals aged over 60 years 50% have pit counts above the upper limit observed in young adults.

(b) Congenital absence or hypoplasia of the spleen

Congenital absence of the spleen is often associated with severe malformations of the heart and great vessels, partial situs inversus and symmetrical three-lobed lungs, a combination of abnormalities which led to the recognition of a syndrome now known as the asplenia or Ivemark syndrome (Polhemus and Schafer, 1952; Ivemark, 1955; Rose, Izukawa and Moes, 1975). In addition to the cardiovascular and pulmonary abnormalities, a variety of other malformations has been reported in the gastrointestinal, respiratory, genitourinary and musculoskeletal systems (Freedom, 1972; Mishalany, Mahnovski and Wooley, 1982). A few patients with congenital cyanotic heart disease and typical features of hyposplenism in the peripheral blood, but anatomically normal spleens, have been observed (Pearson, Schiebler and Spencer, 1971); these patients with functional hyposplenism should be distinguished from those with the asplenia syndrome. Estimates of the incidence of the asplenia syndrome range from 1 in 40 000 to 1 in 1750 (Rose, Izukawa and Moes, 1975; Majeski and Upshur, 1978) and it is generally agreed that the syndrome occurs about twice as often in males; however in one study this incidence was reversed (Majeski and Upshur, 1978). Possible factors in the pathogenesis of the asplenia syndrome include a developmental disturbance, occurring before the fifth week, and affecting the heart, lungs, spleen and other viscera. The syndrome has been observed in a child born to a mother given warfarin during the first six weeks of pregnancy (Cox, Martin and Hall, 1977) and may be the expression of bilateral right-sidedness, leading to absent or abnormal left-sided structures and organs (Van Mierop, Gessner and Schiebler,

1972). In addition, vascular abnormalities may lead to agenesis of the spleen (Monie, 1982). More rarely, congenital asplenia occurs as an isolated anomaly (Waldman *et al.*, 1977) and in some cases there appears to be an hereditary basis (Kevy, Tefft and Vawter, 1968).

(c) Hyposplenism in disorders of the blood and reticulo-endothelial system

(i)   Splenic function in sickle-cell diseases

Splenomegaly is present consistently in the early years of life in sickle-cell anemia, and is followed by atrophy of the spleen which reduces it to a fibrotic nodule as the result of repeated episodes of infarction. (See also Chapter 16.) Functional hyposplenism occurs when the spleen is still clinically enlarged (Pearson, Spencer and Cornelius, 1969). Analysis of pitted erythrocyte data from over 2000 patients has revealed differences between several sickling disorders in the development of splenic hypofunction (Pearson *et al.*, 1985; Figure 11.3). In general, the pattern of dysfunction parallels the expected rates of intravascular sickling and clinical severity, and correlates with the epidemiology of severe bacterial meningitis and sepsis in these diseases. The functional hyposplenism may be reversed transiently by the transfusion of normal red cells. It has been proposed that the high viscosity of sickle-cell blood causes diversion of splenic blood flow through intrasplenic shunts, thus bypassing the phagocytic elements of the organ and producing functional asplenia; when sickle-cells are replaced by normal red cells, splenic circulation and function are temporarily restored (Pearson *et al.*, 1970).

(ii)   Essential thrombocythemia

In a study of eight patients with essential thrombocythemia, three were found to have delayed clearance of damaged red cells, and Howell–Jolly bodies in the peripheral blood (Marsh, Lewis and Szur, 1966b). Splenic atro-

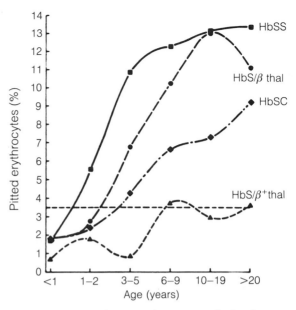

Figure 11.3 Developmental pattern of pitted erythrocytes in several sickle hemoglobinopathies. (Reproduced by permission of *Pediatrics* from Pearson, H.A. *et al.*, *Pediatrics*, 76, 392, 1985.)

phy was noted in three of a series of 23 cases described in the literature (Hardisty and Wolff, 1955). It has been proposed that splenic atrophy results from infarction caused by platelet-initiated vascular occlusion (Crosby, 1963).

(iii)   Malignant lymphoma

Hyposplenism following splenic irradiation in patients with Hodgkin's disease and non-Hodgkin's lymphomas is well recognized (see below). There are also reports of hyposplenism in patients who have not received irradiation, which are presumed to reflect infiltration of the spleen by neoplastic tissue (Pettit *et al.*, 1971; Balchandran, Kumar and Kuo, 1980; Gross *et al.*, 1982).

(iv)   Other disorders

Splenic atrophy has been identified as a feature of the familial form of aplastic anemia, Fanconi's syndrome, and it has been suggested that it results from a generalized dystrophy of mesen-chymal tissue (Garriga and Crosby, 1959). Iso-lated cases of hyposplenism in patients with combined immunodeficiency (Spencer *et al.*, 1978b) and malignant mastocytosis (Roth, Brudler and Henze, 1985) have been reported.

(d) Hyposplenism and autoimmune disorders

Both splenic atrophy and functional hyposplen-ism occur in association with a variety of auto-immune diseases; it is not clear whether the abnormalities of splenic function are a conse-quence of, or contribute to, the development of autoimmunity.

(i) Systemic lupus erythematosus

The reported frequency of hyposplenism in sys-temic lupus erythematosus has varied according to the method used to assess splenic function. Five of 70 (7.1%) patients had Howell–Jolly bodies in the peripheral blood (Dillon, Stein and English, 1982) and a similar proportion (4.6%) was found using counts of pitted erythrocytes in 44 patients (Neilan and Berney, 1983). However, prolongation of the clearance of IgG-sensitized erythrocytes was detected in 13 of 15 (87%) patients (Frank *et al.*, 1979). Impaired splenic Fc-receptor function was observed in most patients with active disease and there was a significant correlation between clinical improvement, improvement of Fc-specific clearance and decreased levels of im-mune complexes (Frank *et al.*, 1979, 1983). Prolonged clearance of heat-damaged red cells, which may be improved by plasmapheresis, was found in patients with active nephritis, but was unusual in patients without renal involvement despite high levels of circulating immune com-plexes (Lockwood *et al.*, 1979; Elkon *et al.*, 1980). These observations suggest that in some patients there is reversible blockade of splenic phagocytic function. Histological examination of atrophic spleens removed at autopsy from two patients revealed marked depletion of lym-phoid tissue but no evidence of involvement by vasculitis (Dillon, Stein and English, 1982; Fos-ter, Hardy and Losowsky, 1984).

(ii) Mixed connective tissue disease

This condition exhibits features of systemic lupus erythematosus, polymyositis and scler-oderma. It is distinguished by the presence of high titers of antibody to extractable nuclear antigen, a ribonucleoprotein moiety. Clinically significant renal disease is uncommon. Defec-tive splenic reticulo-endothelial Fc-specific func-tion, as measured by clearance of IgG-sensitized erythrocytes, was found in four of 18 patients studied, the majority having normal reticulo-endothelial function despite high levels of circu-lating immune complexes (Frank *et al.*, 1983). In addition we have seen a patient with mixed connective tissue disease who developed the typical features of hyposplenism in the peripheral blood and an increased number of pitted erythrocytes, and had a small spleen on computerized tomography (unpublished observations).

(iii) Rheumatoid arthritis

There have been several studies of the clearance of heat-damaged red cells in patients with active rheumatoid arthritis. The number of patients investigated was small in each series and the frequency of prolonged clearance ranged from 21 to 85% (Williams *et al.*, 1979; Gordon *et al.*, 1981; Henderson *et al.*, 1981). In one study there was a significant correlation between the level of circulating immune complexes and the clearance time, but this was not observed in the other series. Fc-receptor specific clearance was measured using IgG-coated erythrocytes in 50 patients with rheumatoid arthritis, and mild or moderate impairment was found in 65% (Frank *et al.*, 1983). There was no correlation with disease activity, titer of rheumatoid factor, immunoglobulin levels or circulating immune complexes. Atrophy of the spleen has been re-ported by Parr, Shipton and Holland (1953) in a patient with juvenile chronic arthritis (Still's disease).

(iv) Sjögren's syndrome

Sjögren's syndrome is characterized by xerophthalmia (with or without lacrimal gland enlargement), xerostomia (with or without salivary gland enlargement) and the presence of various connective tissue disorders. Defective clearance of heat-damaged and IgG-sensitized erythrocytes has been found in patients with this syndrome, but almost invariably in patients with extraglandular disease (Hersey *et al.*, 1983; Hamburger *et al.*, 1979).

(v) Other disorders

Reports of hyposplenism in autoimmune thyroid disease are confined to isolated cases (Wardrop *et al.*, 1975; Brownlie *et al.*, 1975; Jellinek and Ball, 1976). Reversible functional hyposplenism has been described in a patient with autoimmune chronic active hepatitis (Dhawan, Spencer and Sziklas, 1979). There has been no systematic study of splenic function in these disorders.

(e) Hyposplenism in gastrointestinal disorders

(i) Celiac disease

The association of splenic atrophy with intestinal malabsorption was first recognized more than 60 years ago (Blumgart, 1923). Subsequently further cases were reported (Engel, 1939; Martin and Bell, 1965) and for many of these patients it is probable that the malabsorption was due to celiac disease, which more recent studies have shown to be frequently associated with hyposplenism.

There are two components to the impaired splenic function associated with celiac disease: functional hyposplenism and splenic atrophy. The functional hyposplenism fluctuates with disease activity, improves after withdrawal of gluten from the diet (Palmer, Sherriff and Holdsworth, 1979; Corazza *et al.*, 1983; O'Grady *et al.*, 1984b) and appears to be closely related to the morphological state of the jejunal mucosa, whereas splenic atrophy results in irreversible loss of splenic function (Robinson *et al.*, 1980; Trewby *et al.*, 1981). The reported incidence of hyposplenism in celiac disease varies with the diagnostic method used. Splenic atrophy was found in ten of 24 patients at autopsy (Thompson, 1974); evidence of hyposplenism on a peripheral blood film has been found in 16–36% of patients (McCarthy *et al.*, 1966; Marsh and Stewart, 1970; Bullen *et al.*, 1981; Trewby *et al.*, 1981) and elevated pitted erythrocyte counts in 32% and 79% of patients (Corazza *et al.*, 1981; O'Grady *et al.*, 1984b); prolonged clearance of heat damaged red cells occurred in 28–77% of patients studied (Trewby *et al.*, 1981; Robinson *et al.*, 1980; Marsh and Stewart, 1970) and reduction in splenic volume computed from isotope scintigrams was observed in 34–43% (Robinson *et al.*, 1980; Trewby *et al.*, 1981). While differences in the sensitivity of the methods explains some of this variation, another important factor is the effect of gluten withdrawal and the intensity of treatment amongst the patients studied. The frequency and severity of hyposplenism increases with advancing age and duration of exposure to dietary gluten (Corazza *et al.*, 1981; O'Grady *et al.*, 1984b); hyposplenism does not appear to be a feature of the childhood celiac despite autopsy-based case reports of splenic atrophy in two children believed to have celiac disease (Corazza *et al.*, 1982; Macrae and Morris, 1931; Meyer, 1932). It is not clear whether splenic atrophy is a consequence of prolonged functional hyposplenism or is an independent development. There are also reports of hyposplenism progressing despite gluten withdrawal (Szur, Marsh and Pettit, 1972; Trewby *et al.*, 1981).

The mechanism leading to hyposplenism in celiac disease remains obscure. The original reports of splenic atrophy in association with severe malabsorption raised the possibility that hyposplenism might be a consequence of malnutrition, but atrophy of the spleen was not observed amongst severely malnourished inmates of the concentration camps of World War II (de Jongh, 1948) and the presence of hyposplenism in celiac disease does not correlate with the nutritional disturbances (Ferguson, 1976). Rats rendered deficient in folate develop splenic atrophy which can be reversed by administration of the vitamin (Asenjo, 1948). However, the impaired splenic function associated with celiac disease is not correlated with folate deficiency nor does it improve following folic acid administration (Ferguson, 1976; McCarthy et al., 1966). There may be an hereditary component. Marked abnormalities of splenic Fc-receptor function have been found in association with the HLA-B8 antigen (Lawley et al., 1981) which is commonly found in patients with celiac disease, but the results of several studies suggest that splenic hypofunction in celiac disease is independent of the presence of this antigen (Bullen et al., 1981; O'Grady et al., 1984b). However, the observation of increased numbers of pitted erythrocytes in first-degree relatives of patients with celiac disease and with normal small bowel morphology (O'Grady, Stevens and McCarthy, 1985a) is another pointer to a genetic influence on splenic function in celiac disease. Considerable interfamily variation has been found, but the pattern tends to run true within families and is compatible with a recessive mode of inheritance.

In some patients with celiac disease, splenic atrophy occurs in association with atrophy or cavitation of peripheral and mesenteric lymph nodes (McCarthy et al., 1966; Matuchansky et al., 1984), and it has been suggested that hyposplenism is a manifestation of a more widespread atrophy of the lympho-reticulo-endothelial system. However, this concept is not supported by the finding of normal Kupffer cell function in patients with hyposplenism (Palmer et al., 1983).

Increased levels of circulating immune complexes, which could lead to functional blockade of the splenic reticulo-endothelial system, have been detected especially in untreated celiac disease (Doe, Booth and Brown, 1973), but no significant difference in the levels of C1q-binding activity has been found in adult celiac patients with or without hyposplenism (Bullen, Mani and Losowsky, 1980). Furthermore, very high levels of immune complexes are insufficient to induce splenic hypofunction in childhood celiac disease (Corazza, Lazzari and Frisoni, 1983).

Finally, by analogy with animal models, it has been suggested that hyposplenism in celiac disease results from lymphocyte depletion due to chronic loss into the gut (Bullen and Losowsky, 1978). Chronic drainage of the thoracic duct in calves produces lymphoreticular atrophy, and cessation of lymph drainage results in re-population of the spleen with lymphocytes (Fish et al., 1970). The absolute lymphocyte count and T-cell numbers are reduced in untreated celiac disease and tend to return to normal after treatment (Bullen and Losowsky, 1978).

(ii) Dermatitis herpetiformis

Dermatitis herpetiformis is known to be closely related to celiac disease. It is linked to the same histocompatibility antigens, and in most cases gluten-sensitive jejunal lesions are present, similar to those of celiac disease but usually less severe and extensive. Impaired splenic function has been detected by prolonged clearance of heat-damaged erythrocytes in seven out of 24 patients with dermatitis herpetiformis (Pettit et al., 1972) and in three out of seven patients using the pitted cell count (Corazza et al., 1981). Splenic reticulo-endothelial function in dermatitis herpetiformis has also been studied by antibody-coated autologous red cell clearance, which was delayed in half the cases studied, indicating abnormal Fc-receptor function of splenic macrophages (Lawley et al., 1981). The presence of circulating immune complexes may be a significant factor in the development of hyposplenism in this disease (Mowbray et al., 1973).

(iii) Inflammatory bowel disease

Functional hyposplenism is well recognized in association with active ulcerative colitis and tends to improve, or even to return to normal, as the inflammation declines with medical treatment or after colectomy (Ryan *et al.*, 1974, 1978; Palmer *et al.*, 1981; Jewell, Berney and Pettit, 1981); irreversible atrophy also occurs (Ryan *et al.*, 1978; Foster *et al.*, 1982). In a survey of 65 patients with ulcerative colitis, hyposplenism was detected by prolonged clearance of heat-damaged erythrocytes or typical features on a peripheral blood film in 29% of patients (Palmer *et al.*, 1981). In another smaller study, delayed clearance of heat-damaged red cells was observed in 13 of 16 patients with ulcerative colitis (Jewell, Berney and Pettit, 1981). Hyposplenism is detected more frequently in patients with extensive disease. It appears to be less common in patients with Crohn's disease. Delayed clearance of heat-damaged red cells was found in 11 of 42 and 4 of 17 patients in two separate studies (Palmer *et al.*, 1981; Jewell, Berney and Pettit, 1981) and we observed increased pitted erythrocyte counts in only two of 34 patients with Crohn's disease (unpublished observations). It is of interest that impaired splenic function seems to occur only in those patients with colonic involvement, although in a recent study of splenic size in patients who had undergone laparotomy for inflammatory bowel disease, small spleens (<11 cm) were found in seven of 36 patients with Crohn's disease affecting only the small bowel (Pereira, Hughes and Young, 1987). The relationship to disease activity is less clear than with ulcerative colitis, but improvement in splenic function has been reported as the activity of the Crohn's disease abates (Palmer *et al.*, 1981). The mechanisms underlying hyposplenism in inflammatory bowel disease have been less extensively studied than in celiac disease, but as in that condition, raised levels of circulating immune-complexes (Doe, Booth and Brown, 1973) and enteric loss of lymphocytes (Douglas, Weetman and Haggith, 1976; Segal *et al.*, 1981) have been reported which might contribute to the development of splenic hypofunction.

(iv) Chronic idiopathic ulcerative enteritis

This condition is characterized by small intestinal ulceration and malabsorption, but probably represents a spectrum of disorders which bears an inconsistent relationship to gluten sensitivity and small intestinal lymphoma. In two different studies splenic atrophy or Howell–Jolly bodies were observed in 3 of 5 and 3 of 8 patients with small intestinal ulceration (Mills, Brown and Watkinson, 1980; Robertson *et al.*, 1983b). In one of these patients a diagnosis of celiac disease was made, but it is still unclear whether the hyposplenism seen in patients with chronic idiopathic ulcerative enteritis is directly linked to this condition or whether it reflects pre-existing celiac disease.

(v) Tropical sprue

Splenic atrophy proved to be a frequent postmortem finding in a series of 16 patients who died from tropical sprue (Suarez, Spies and Suarez, 1947). Spleen weight varied between 5 and 140 g with an average of 75 g. No *in vivo* measurements of splenic function in tropical sprue have been made, and the relationship between possible reticulo-endothelial dysfunction and other immunological changes in this disease is still unknown.

(vi) Whipple's disease

Splenic atrophy and increased pitted cell counts have been observed in cases of Whipple's disease, which often involves the spleen by infiltration or infarction (Plummer *et al.*, 1950; Haeney and Ross, 1978; Corazza *et al.*, 1982).

(vii) Intestinal lymphangiectasia

The characteristic features of intestinal lymphangiectasia are dilated lymphatics, protein-losing enteropathy and lymphopenia. We have reported a patient with this condition and associated hyposplenism (Foster *et al.*, 1985a). The splenic volume was reduced and there was progressive development of the typical features of hyposplenism in the peripheral blood, and an increase in the number of pitted erythrocytes. The abnormalities of the red cells subsequently returned to normal, suggesting an element of functional hyposplenism in addition to loss of splenic volume. Thrombocytosis was a prominent feature in this case and it is unclear whether the increased platelet count reflected impaired splenic function or contributed to it in a manner analogous to that proposed for essential thrombocythemia (see above). In addition to this case there is a report of splenic atrophy in a patient with lymphangiectasia secondary to lymphoma (Crosby, 1963).

(f) Miscellaneous conditions

(i) Radiation

Splenic atrophy has been reported following external radiation (Dailey, Coleman and Kaplan, 1980; Coleman *et al.*, 1982) or the use of the radiocontrast agent, Thorotrast (Bensinger *et al.*, 1970). The histological changes seen in the irradiated spleens included collapse of the architecture from loss of red pulp, vessel wall thickening and varying degrees of fibrosis with lymphoid depletion. The risk of developing significant splenic atrophy (spleen weight <60 g) has been estimated at 30–40% from the results of a retrospective, necropsy study of patients who had received splenic irradiation for Hodgkin's disease (Dailey, Coleman and Kaplan, 1980), and the majority of patients who have received more than 4000 rads have elevated numbers of pitted erythrocytes (Coleman *et al.*, 1982).

(ii) Amyloidosis

In a retrospective study of 91 patients with systemic amyloidosis, the typical features of hyposplenism were observed in the peripheral blood of 24% (Gertz, Kyle and Griepp, 1983). Palpable splenomegaly was seen in two of the 22 patients with hyposplenism. In a smaller series six of 14 patients had evidence of hyposplenism (Boyko, Pratt and Wass, 1982). Histological examination of spleens removed at autopsy revealed extensive amyloid replacement of splenic cords and Malpighian follicles.

(iii) Sarcoidosis

Although microscopic involvement of the spleen is common in sarcoidosis, reports of hyposplenism are confined to a single case of functional hyposplenism based on the presence of Howell–Jolly bodies and failure to accumulate technetium-labelled sulfur colloid which improved with steroid therapy (Stone *et al.*, 1985). In a case in which the patient died of fulminant pneumococcal sepsis, functional hyposplenism was proposed as a contributory factor, the spleen weighing 300 g and being heavily infiltrated by sarcoid tissue (Guyton and Zumwalt, 1975).

(iv) Other disorders

Impairment of the splenic circulation due to occlusion of the splenic artery or vein, or thrombosis of the celiac artery, has been described as a cause of functional hyposplenism (Spencer, Johnson and Sziklas, 1977; Dhawan, Spencer and Pearson, 1977). Isolated cases of hyposplenism due to direct involvement of the spleen by metastatic breast cancer (Costello, Gramm and Steinberg, 1977) and hemangiosarcoma (Steinberg, Gatling and Tavassoli, 1983) have been reported.

Reversible hyposplenism occurs in patients with graft-versus-host disease following bone marrow transplantation (Demetrakopoulos, Tsokos and Levine, 1982; Al-Eid *et al.*, 1983). It has been suggested that splenic hypofunction results from allogeneic killing of the host lymphoid tissue and that recovery of splenic function is due either to repopulation of the spleen with allogeneic lymphocytes or tolerance of the host's lymphocytes by the engrafted population (Demetrakopoulos, Tsokos and Levine, 1982).

Delayed clearance of IgG-sensitized erythrocytes has been observed in patients taking methyl-dopa for more than one year and it appears that the drug directly depresses the Fc-receptor specific function of splenic reticulo-endothelial cells (Kelton, 1985).

Finally, there has been a preliminary report of abnormal Fc-receptor specific function in patients with the acquired immunodeficiency syndrome (Bender, Quinn and Lawley, 1984), but no evidence of hyposplenism was observed in a series of patients with the syndrome complicated by bacterial pneumonia due to *Streptococcus pneumoniae* and *Haemophilus influenzae* (Polsky *et al.*, 1986).

11.4   THE SEQUELAE OF HYPOSPLENISM

11.4.1   BLOOD

(a) Erythrocytes

Changes in mature erythrocytes after splenectomy have been described above. In addition, there may be a transient normoblastosis and the reticulocyte count is elevated as a consequence of displacement to the peripheral blood of the immature red cells which normally complete maturation within the spleen (Lipson, Bayrd and Watkins, 1959).

(b) Leukocytes

Leukocytosis is a well-recognized sequela of splenectomy. Initially the leukocytosis reflects a neutrophilia which then diminishes and is followed by a more persistent lymphocytosis. A monocytosis and a slight to moderate rise in basophil and eosinophil counts may also occur (Crosby, 1963; Lipson, Bayrd and Watkins, 1959; McBride, Dacie and Shapley, 1968). A marked lymphocytosis is also found in association with hyposplenism not due to splenectomy (Bullen and Losowsky, 1978; Wilkinson, Tang

and Gjedsted, 1983). There is considerable traffic of lymphocytes through the spleen and splenectomy results in loss of this pool, which presumably contributes to the peripheral blood lymphocytosis. In addition animal experiments suggest that the spleen exerts an inhibitory influence on lymphocyte production (Ernstrom and Sandberg, 1970). Lymphocyte populations after splenectomy have been examined in several studies using a variety of marker-techniques and no consistent abnormality in the proportion of B-cells, T-cells and their subsets has been observed, and when the absolute numbers of the different types of cell have been calculated the counts have been normal or increased (Millard and Bannerjee, 1979; Lauria *et al.*, 1981; Grattner, Gullstrand and Hallberg, 1982; Neilsen *et al.*, 1983b; Foster, Heatley and Losowsky, 1985a, b; Durig, Landmann and Harder, 1984).

(c) Platelets

Thrombocytosis is a well-recognized feature of the early post-splenectomy period. The platelet count increases between two- and sixfold during the first two postoperative weeks and tends to return towards normal values after a period of weeks or months; in some patients the thrombocytosis may persist for years (Laufer *et al.*, 1978; Lipson, Bayrd and Watkins, 1959). Chronic elevation of the platelet count was noted particularly in association with continuing anemia and hemolysis (Hirsch and Dacie, 1966), but it is clear that it commonly occurs in splenectomized subjects without anemia (O'Grady *et al.*, 1985; Robertson, Simpson and Losowsky, 1981). Thrombocytosis also occurs in association with splenic atrophy. In some patients with ulcerative colitis or celiac disease both activity of the inflammatory lesion and hyposplenism contribute to the thrombocytosis (Bullen *et al.*, 1977a). Splenic atrophy secondary to thrombocytosis may further increase the platelet count. Platelet volume is increased after splenectomy (Laufer *et al.*, 1978; O'Grady *et al.*, 1985) and the platelets appear hyperactive as judged by their tendency to aggregate (Kenny, George and Stuart, 1980; Zucker and Mielke, 1972). The thrombocytosis is presumably due largely to the loss of the splenic reservoir of platelets, but in addition there is evidence for increased platelet production after splenectomy and it has been postulated that the spleen produces a factor which suppresses platelet formation (Crosby and Ruiz, 1962; Bessler, Mandel and Djaldetti, 1978).

(d) Viscosity

Blood viscosity increases within a few weeks of splenectomy and remains elevated. The hyperviscosity does not appear to be related to thrombocytosis, but rather is consequent on decreased deformability of the red cell (Robertson, Simpson and Losowsky, 1981).

(e) Thrombosis

Venous thrombosis complicating splenectomy was first described by Rosenthal (1925). Subsequently there have been case reports confirming the association and studies of the incidence of postsplenectomy thrombosis; these have, however, been the subject of a critical review (Dawson et al., 1981) in which imperfections in the information have been emphasized. The data have usually been collected without regard for the disorder for which splenectomy was performed and both benign and malignant disorders, in which the incidence of deep vein thrombosis might be expected to differ, have been included. Most studies are retrospective and the methods for detection of venous thrombosis have varied from clinical signs to venography and isotope techniques. Finally, the majority of studies have not included an appropriate or adequately described control group. In the two studies which avoided many of these deficiencies (Butler, Matthews and Irving, 1977; Dawson et al., 1981), no significant increase in deep vein thrombosis was observed after splenectomy. Furthermore, no increase in mortality due to venous thromboembolism was observed in a study of veterans of the Second World War who had undergone splenectomy for trauma (Robinette and Fraumeni, 1977). However, this latter study did reveal an excess mortality from ischemic heart disease, principally myocardial infarction, which raises the possibility that the increase in platelet numbers and activity and hyperviscosity observed after splenectomy, might predispose to coronary artery thrombosis.

11.4.2 IMMUNITY

(a) Immunoglobulins

Immunoglobulin levels after splenectomy have been widely studied with conflicting results, which are probably due to important differences in age, time after splenectomy and the presence of associated disease in the patients investigated. Generally, in older children and adults IgM levels are significantly lower after splenectomy compared with preoperative values or with levels in matched control subjects, IgG levels remain constant or increase, and IgA and IgE levels increase (Schumacher, 1970; Claret, Morales and Montaner, 1975; Andersen, Cohn and Sorensen, 1976; Chaimoff et al., 1978; Constantoulakis et al., 1978; Westerhausen et al., 1981; Chelazzi et al., 1985). Low IgM levels have been found in patients with sickle cell disease and splenic atrophy (Gavrilis, Rothenberg and Roscoe, 1974), but in the few patients with celiac disease and hyposplenism studied immunoglobulin levels were normal (Wardrop et al., 1975).

There is long-standing evidence of an impaired response to intravenously administered antigens (Rowley, 1950). The switch from IgM to IgG production during the secondary response to an intravenous antigen is impaired after splenectomy (Sullivan et al., 1978) and a similar defect has been observed in patients with hyposplenism associated with celiac disease and inflammatory bowel disease (Baker et al., 1975; Bullen et al., 1977b; Ryan et al., 1981). There is increasing evidence that the spleen is necessary for the generation of a normal response to immunization with pneumococcal polysaccharides and that splenectomy results in impaired anti-pneumococcal antibody production (Hosea *et al.*, 1981; Di Padova *et al.*, 1985). It appears that absence of the spleen causes a longlasting B-cell defect characterized by a limited capacity of circulating B-cells to differentiate into antibody secreting cells (Di Padova *et al.*, 1983; Drew *et al.*, 1984; Muller *et al.*, 1984).

(b) Complement

After splenectomy, defective function of the alternative pathway or low levels of particular components of complement have been recorded by some investigators (Carlisle and Saslaw, 1959; Polhill and Johnston, 1975; Corry *et al.*, 1979) but not others (Winkelstein and Lambert, 1975; Ciuttis *et al.*, 1978; Neilsen *et al.*, 1983a). Thus it appears that the spleen makes a contribution to maintaining the integrity of the alternative pathway in man, but the role is not crucial.

(c) Tuftsin

Tuftsin is a naturally occurring tetrapeptide, threonyl-lysil-prolyl-arginine, which stimulates phagocytosis by neutrophils, macrophages and monocytes. It originates from the Fc-fragment of IgG and is released *in vivo* as the free peptide after enzymatic cleavage, one step of which is believed to occur in the spleen, because splenectomy results in low levels of tuftsin (Spirer *et al.*, 1977). Hyposplenism in sickle cell disease is also associated with decreased levels of tuftsin (Spirer *et al.*, 1980b).

(d) Neutrophil function

The function of neutrophils after splenectomy has been studied using various methods and with disparate results (Constantopoulos *et al.*, 1973; Winkelstein and Lambert, 1975; von

Fliedner *et al.*, 1980; Deitch and O'Neal, 1982; Cooper *et al.*, 1982; Falcao, Voltarelli and Bottura, 1982; Hauser, Zakuth and Spirer, 1983; Foster *et al.*, 1985b; Dahl *et al.*, 1986); it appears that there is no intrinsic abnormality of the cells but rather, in some patients, the serum is deficient in opsonic and chemotactic factors which results in impaired neutrophil activity.

(e) Lymphocyte function

No consistent abnormality of the transformation response of lymphocytes to the plant lectins phytohemagglutinin, concanavalin A and pokeweed mitogen, which test T-cell function *in vitro*, has been observed after splenectomy (Andersen, Cohn and Sorensen, 1976; Neilsen *et al.*, 1983b; Cohen and Ferrante, 1982; Ferrante *et al.*, 1985), but in two studies suppressor cell activity was reduced (Melamed *et al.*, 1982; Robertson *et al.*, 1982a). Suppressor cell function is impaired in patients with celiac disease, but it is not related to associated hyposplenism (Robertson *et al.*, 1982a). Natural killer cell activity has been found to be normal or increased after splenectomy (Foster, Heatley and Losowsky, 1985b; Ferrante *et al.*, 1985) and is unaffected by hyposplenism in patients with celiac disease. Antibody-dependent cell-mediated cytotoxicity has been found to be defective in some patients after splenectomy (Kragballe *et al.*, 1981).

(f) Reticulo-endothelial function

The results of studies of reticulo-endothelial function after splenectomy in animals and man suggest that the spleen may have a necessary role in the normal phagocytic activity of other reticulo-endothelial cells throughout the body. In the rat, alveolar macrophage function has been found to be impaired after splenectomy (Chaudry, 1982; Shennib, Chu-Jeng Chiu and Mulder, 1983) and some workers (Chaudry, 1982), but not others (Nashat *et al.*, 1982), have reported reduced Kupffer cell function after splenectomy. Using the clearance of microaggregated albumin from the circulation as a measure of Kupffer cell function, Palmer *et al.* (1983) found significantly reduced rates of clearance in otherwise healthy subjects who had undergone splenectomy, and in patients with hyposplenism associated with celiac disease and ulcerative colitis.

11.4.3 INFECTION

Overwhelming infection is a well-recognized complication of splenectomy, but hyposplenism not due to surgical removal of the spleen may also be complicated by severe infections (Table 11.2). The pneumococcus is the most frequently encountered organism (Selby *et al.*, 1987; Kabins and Lerner, 1970; Torres and Bisno, 1973) but infection with other encapsulated bacteria, in particular *Haemophilus influenzae* and the meningococcus, is well described. The clinical course is usually fulminant and frequently fatal (Balfanz *et al.*, 1976; Gopal and Bisno, 1977). In addition infection with organisms not usually pathogenic in man has been seen in hyposplenic subjects (Archer *et al.*, 1979; Findling, Pohlmann and Rose, 1980; Curti, Lin and Szabo, 1985; Fish, Chia and

Shakir, 1985). The parasitic infection babesiosis is more common in asplenic subjects (Rosner *et al.*, 1984) and there have been reports of fatal malaria developing in patients after splenectomy (Coetzee, 1982; Israeli, Shapiro and Ephros, 1987). Some viral infections may be more frequent and severe after splenectomy (Stone, Stanley and DeJarnette, 1967; Baumgartner *et al.*, 1982; Langenhuijsen and van Toorn, 1982) and there is a recent report suggesting that splenectomy predisposes to the development of clinical acquired immune deficiency syndrome in HIV-positive individuals (Barbui *et al.*, 1987). The relationship of the spleen to infection is further discussed in Chapter 12.

11.4.4 AUTOIMMUNE PHENOMENA

The production of erythrocyte autoantibodies by mice injected with rat red blood cells is enhanced by splenectomy (Cox and Finley-Jones, 1979). Several studies have shown an increased incidence of autoantibodies in splenectomized subjects when compared with normal subjects (Spirer *et al.*, 1980a; Neilsen, Andersen and Ellegaard, 1982; Robertson *et*

Table 11.2 Cases of severe infection complicating non-surgical hyposplenism

Etiology of hyposplenism	References
Congenital	Myerson and Koelle (1956); Kevy, Tefft and Vawter (1968); Waldman *et al.* (1977)
Sickle cell disease	Falter *et al.* (1973)
Celiac disease	O'Donoghue (1986)
Ulcerative colitis	Ryan *et al.* (1978); Foster *et al.* (1982)
Systemic lupus erythematosus	Dillon, Stein and English (1982); Foster, Hardy and Losowsky (1984)
Sarcoidosis	Guyton and Zumwalt (1975)
Amyloidosis	Frank and Palomino (1987)
Irradiation	Bensinger *et al.* (1970); Dailey, Coleman and Kaplan (1980)
Still's disease	Parr, Shipton and Holland (1953)
Ischemia	Whitaker (1969); Grant *et al.* (1970)
Idiopathic	Bisno and Freeman (1970); Hatch, Sibbald and Austin (1983)

al., 1983c) and autoantibodies have been observed to develop within a few months of splenectomy. One study found no increase in the prevalence of autoantibodies in patients splenectomized following trauma (Aaberge and Gaarder, 1986), but no attempt had been made to assess the degree of splenosis which has been shown to be associated with a reduced frequency of autoantibodies (Neilsen, Andersen and Ellegaard, 1982). Whether the development of autoantibodies after splenectomy heralds the onset of clinical autoimmune disease is uncertain. There is a single case report of a patient who underwent splenectomy for idiopathic thrombocytopenic purpura and subsequently developed chronic active hepatitis, antiglobulin-positive hemolytic anemia and pulmonary fibrosis, and in whom it was suggested that splenectomy might have contributed to the development of these autoimmune disorders (Kleiner-Baumgarten, Schlaeffer and Keynan, 1983). An increased prevalence of autoantibodies and autoimmune diseases has been reported among celiac patients with splenic atrophy compared with celiac patients without evidence of hyposplenism (Bullen *et al.*, 1981) and autoimmune thyroid disease occurs more frequently than would otherwise be expected in patients with dermatitis herpetiformis, a condition in which hyposplenism is a frequent association (Cunningham and Zone, 1985; Foster, 1985).

The spleen is a rich source of suppressor cell activity (Sampson *et al.*, 1976) and suppressor cells are believed to play a role in the regulation of immune responses; it is therefore possible that reduced or absent splenic function might lead to impaired suppressor cell activity or an imbalance in immunoregulatory cells, which in turn could explain the increase in autoimmune phenomena associated with hyposplenism. There is some evidence for this hypothesis. Although the numbers of peripheral blood suppressor cells and the ratio of helper-inducer to cytotoxic-suppressor cells appears to be normal in patients with hyposplenism (Foster, Heatley and Losowky, 1985a), decreased suppressor cell function has been reported in two studies of splenectomized patients (Melamed *et al.*, 1982; Robertson *et al.*, 1982a).

Alternatively it may be that defective splenic Fc-receptor specific function, on which the clearance of circulating immune complexes probably depends, contributes to the development of immune complex-mediated autoimmune disease (Frank *et al.*, 1983). The clearance of IgG-sensitized erythrocytes, which is a function of splenic macrophages bearing a receptor specific to the Fc-fragment of IgG, is abnormal in a range of autoimmune disorders. This is also the case in normal subjects with HLAB8-DRw3, which is an HLA type associated with an increased incidence of autoimmune disease.

11.4.5 MALIGNANCY AND HYPOSPLENISM IN CELIAC DISEASE

Splenic atrophy has been observed in patients with celiac disease complicated by lymphoma (Thompson, 1974; O'Grady, Stevens and McCarthy, 1985b) and it has been suggested that it might be a contributory factor to the development of malignancy. However, in a retrospective study of 41 cases of celiac disease complicated by malignancy, the proportion with evidence of hyposplenism in a peripheral blood film was no greater than that of patients without malignancy (Robertson *et al.*, 1982b).

11.5 MANAGEMENT RECOMMENDATIONS

11.5.1 AVOIDING SPLENECTOMY

Given the long-term risk of infection, the need for splenectomy should be considered carefully. The conventional surgical dogma that an injured spleen should be removed has been challenged (Roy, 1984). Alternatives include conservative management, splenorrhaphy, partial splenectomy and splenic autotransplantation (Cooper and Williamson, 1984): some form of splenic salvage was found to be possible in 56%

of 200 patients with splenic injury (Moore *et al.*, 1984). On the basis of animal experiments, it seems that procedures conserving the normal blood supply and more than 25% of normal splenic mass are most likely to preserve normal splenic function (Horton *et al.*, 1982; Van Wyck *et al.*, 1980). The value of autotransplantation is controversial (Oakes, 1981; Kiroff *et al.*, 1985; Rice and James, 1980), and there are reports of fatal overwhelming sepsis occurring in patients with 'functional' autotransplants, as judged by their ability to accumulate radiocolloid (Moore *et al.*, 1983; Tesluk, 1984). Controlled trials with long-term follow-up are needed; surgical aspects of this problem are discussed in Chapter 18.

11.5.2 PENICILLIN PROPHYLAXIS

The rationale for penicillin prophylaxis in hyposplenic subjects is as follows: the pneumococcus is the most frequently encountered bacterium responsible for overwhelming sepsis in these patients, and has been shown usually to be very susceptible to the concentration of penicillin achieved in the blood by twice daily oral administration. The mortality of experimentally induced infection with *Streptococcus pneumoniae* can be reduced by penicillin prophylaxis (Dickerman, 1979; Dickerman, Chalmer and Horner, 1980). The results of a recent controlled trial in children with sickle-cell disease provide strong evidence for the efficacy of penicillin prophylaxis (Gaston *et al.*, 1986). A total of 215 children aged between 3 and 36 months were randomized to receive either oral penicillin twice daily or placebo. The trial was terminated early when it became clear that the frequency of pneumococcal infections in the children taking placebo was high: 13 infections occurred in 110 subjects, and three of these were fatal. Only 2 of 105 subjects on oral penicillin developed infections, and neither was fatal. Uncontrolled studies in splenectomized subjects, and anecdotal reports of overwhelming infection occurring in patients soon after cessation of penicillin prophylaxis, are evidence favor-

ing long-term oral administration of penicillin in this group of patients (Lanzowsky *et al.*, 1976; Lum *et al.*, 1980; Hays *et al.*, 1984). Failure of penicillin prophylaxis to prevent post-splenectomy sepsis appears to be rare. In a recent review of the literature 14 cases of patients who had undergone splenectomy and developed serious infection despite penicillin prophylaxis were identified (Zarrabi and Rosner, 1986). All but one of the patients were under 17 years old and most had their spleens removed during staging laparotomy for Hodgkin's disease. In six patients the sepsis was due to bacteria other than pneumococcus. The risks of penicillin allergy and the emergence of penicillin-resistant strains of pneumococcus appear to be relatively small (Anonymous, 1986), but the problem of poor compliance with long-term oral administration of penicillin is real (Buchanan *et al.*, 1982; Buchanan and Smith, 1986). Unfortunately intra-muscular injections of long-acting penicillin are impractical for prolonged use.

11.5.3 PNEUMOCOCCAL VACCINE

A 23-valent vaccine which contains antigens to the pneumococcal types responsible for approximately 85% of infections with pneumococcus has been developed recently, and replaces the previous octavalent and 14-valent vaccines. There have been no randomized controlled clinical trials of the efficacy of this pneumococcal vaccine in preventing overwhelming infection in hyposplenic subjects, but in a study of the value of octavalent pneumococcal vaccine in 77 patients with sickle cell disease, no infections with *Streptococcus pneumoniae* were observed during a two year follow-up period. This contrasts to the nine infections, two of which were fatal, experienced by a group of 106 non-immunized patients (Ammann *et al.*, 1977). From the results of a study of the distribution of serotypes of pneumococci isolated from patients previously given pneumococcal vaccine, and compared with the distribution of serotypes isolated from unvaccinated persons, the efficacy of vaccination has been calculated to be 85% in adults with hyposplenism due to splenectomy or sickle-cell disease (Bolan *et al.*, 1986). The use of the vaccine is currently recommended in these patients (Ammann, 1982; Health and Public Policy Committee, 1986). However, the antibody response to pneumococcal antigen is blunted in children under the age of two years (Pedersen, Henrickson and Schiffman, 1982; Lawrence *et al.*, 1983), in splenectomized subjects (Hosea *et al.*, 1981; Di Padova *et al.*, 1985) and in patients with concomitant immunodeficiency states (Siber *et al.*, 1978). The majority of reports of true vaccine failures have involved patients who were receiving, or had undergone, immunosuppressive therapy (Ammann, 1982).

In practice we recommend that children under the age of two years should receive oral penicillin prophylaxis, which should be continued at least to the age of five years and perhaps indefinitely. Pneumococcal vaccine should be administered once the child has reached two years. All adults should receive pneumococcal vaccine and penicillin prophylaxis, probably for life. Whenever elective splenectomy or adjuvant immunosuppressive therapy is considered, the vaccine should be administered at least one month beforehand.

11.5.4 GENERAL

Patients should be advised of the risk of serious infection and urged to seek medical assistance immediately in the event of illness or fever. There is a case for issuing patients with a 'splenectomy warning card' to be carried at all times, and a supply of Amoxicillin, or an alternative, for self-administration at the first symptoms of illness or fever. The attending physician should be aware of the dangers of fulminant sepsis in these patients, and be willing to prescribe antibiotics appropriately for any symptoms of infection.

Possibilities for the future include the more widespread use of vaccines against other organisms implicated in overwhelming infection (such as meningococcus) and the administration of tuftsin which can be prepared synthetically; as yet studies of its use in man are still awaited.

REFERENCES

Aaberge, S. I. and Gaarder, P. I. (1986) Autoantibodies in individuals splenectomised because of trauma. *Scand. J. Haematol.*, **37**, 296–300.

Acevedo, G. and Mauer, A. (1963) The capacity for removal of erythrocytes containing Heinz bodies in premature infants and patients following splenectomy. *J. Pediatr.*, **63**, 61–4.

Al-Eid, M. A. *et al.* (1983) Functional asplenia in patients with graft-versus-host disease. *J. Nucl. Med.*, **24**, 1123–6.

Ammann, A. J. (1982) Current status of pneumococcal polysaccharide immunization in patients with sickle cell disease or impaired splenic function. *Am. J. Pediatr. Hemat. Oncol.*, **4**, 301–6.

Ammann, A. J. *et al.* (1977) Polyvalent pneumococcal polysaccharide immunization of patients with sickle cell anemia and patients with splenectomy. *N. Engl. J. Med.*, **297**, 897–900.

Andersen, V., Cohn, J. and Sorensen, S. F. (1976) Immunological studies in children before and after splenectomy. *Acta Paediatr. Scand.*, **65**, 409–15.

Anonymous (1986) Penicillin prophylaxis for babies with sickle cell disease. *Lancet*, **ii**, 1432–3.

Archer, G. L. *et al.* (1979) Human infection from an unidentified erythrocyte-associated bacterium. *N. Engl. J. Med.*, **301**, 897–900.

Armas, R. R. (1985) Clinical studies with spleen-specific radiolabelled agents. *Sem. Nucl. Med.*, **15**, 260–75.

Asenjo, C. F. (1948) Pteroylglutamic acid requirement of the rat and a characteristic lesion observed in the spleen of the deficient animal. *J. Nutr.*, **36**, 601–12.

Baker, P. G. *et al.* (1975) The immune response to ØX174 in man. III. Evidence for an association between hyposplenism and immunodeficiency in patients with coeliac disease. *Gut*, **16**, 538–42.

Balchandran, S., Kumar, R. and Kuo, T. T. (1980) Functional asplenia in the Sézary syndrome. *Clin. Nucl. Med.*, **5**, 149–51.

Balfanz, J. R. *et al.* (1976) Overwhelming sepsis following splenectomy for trauma. *J. Pediatr.*, **88**, 458–60.

Barbui, T. *et al.* (1987) Does splenectomy enhance risk of AIDS in HIV positive patients with chronic thrombocytopenia? *Lancet*, **ii**, 342–3.

Baumgartner, J. D. et al. (1982) Severe cytomegalovirus infection in multiply transfused splenectomised trauma patients. *Lancet*, **ii**, 63–5.

Bender, B. S., Quinn, T. C. and Lawley, T. J. (1984) Acquired immune deficiency syndrome (AIDS): a defect in Fc receptor specific clearance. *Clin. Res.*, **32**, 511A.

Bensinger, T. A. et al. (1970) Thorotrast-induced reticuloendothelial blockade in man. *Am. J. Med.*, **51**, 663–8.

Bessler, H., Mandel, E. M. and Djaldetti, M. (1978) Role of the spleen and lymphocytes in regulation of the circulating platelet numbers in mice. *J. Lab. Clin. Med.*, **91**, 760–8.

Bisno, A. L. and Freeman, J. C. (1970) The syndrome of asplenia, pneumococcal sepsis and disseminated intravascular coagulation. *Ann. Intern. Med.*, **72**, 389–93.

Blumgart, H. L. (1923) Three fatal adult cases of malabsorption of fat with emaciation and anemia, and in two acidosis and tetany. *Arch. Intern. Med.*, **32**, 113–28.

Bolan, G. et al. (1986) Pneumococcal vaccine efficacy in selected populations in the United States. *Ann. Intern. Med.*, **104**, 1–6.

Bowdler, A. J. (1982) The spleen in disorders of the blood. In *Blood and its Disorders* (eds R. M. Hardisty and D. J. Weatherall), Blackwell Scientific Publications, Oxford.

Boyko, W. J., Pratt, R. and Wass, H. (1982) Functional hyposplenism: a diagnostic clue in amyloidosis. *Am. J. Clin. Pathol.*, **77**, 745–8.

Brownlie, B. E. W. et al. (1975) Thyrotoxicosis associated with splenic atrophy. *Lancet*, **ii**, 1046–7.

Buchanan, G. R., Holtkamp, C. A. and Horton, J. A. (1987) Formation and disappearance of pocked erythrocytes; Studies in human subjects and laboratory animals. *Am. J. Hematol.*, **25**, 243–51.

Buchanan, G. R. and Smith, S. J. (1986) Pneumococcal septicemia despite pneumococcal vaccine and prescription of penicillin prophylaxis in children with sickle cell anemia. *Am. J. Dis. Child.*, **140**, 428–32.

Buchanan, G. R. et al. (1982) Oral penicillin prophylaxis in children with impaired splenic function: a study of compliance. *Pediatrics*, **70**, 926–30.

Bullen, A. W. and Losowsky, M. S. (1978) Lymphocyte subpopulations in adult coeliac disease. *Gut*, **19**, 892–7.

Bullen, A. W., Mani, R. W. and Losowsky, M. S. (1980) Circulating immune complexes in coeliac disease. *Gut*, **21**, A915.

Bullen, A. W. et al. (1977a) Mechanisms of thrombocytosis in coeliac disease. *Gut*, **18**, A962.

Bullen, A. W. et al. (1977b) Immunity and the hyposplenism of coeliac disease. *Gut*, **18**, A961–962.

Bullen, A. W. et al. (1981) Hyposplenism, adult coeliac disease and autoimmunity. *Gut*, **22**, 28–33.

Butler, M. J., Matthews, F. and Irving, M. H. (1977) The incidence of post-operative deep vein thrombosis after splenectomy. *Clin. Oncol.*, **3**, 51–6.

Carlisle, H. N. and Saslaw, S. (1959) Properdin levels in splenectomized persons. *Proc. Soc. Exp. Biol. Med.*, **109**, 150–4.

Chaimoff, C. et al. (1978) Serum immunoglobulin changes after accidental splenectomy in adults. *Am. J. Surg.*, **136**, 332–3.

Chaudry, I. H. (1982) Tuftsin restores the depressed reticuloendothelial function after splenectomy and improves survival following splenectomy and sepsis. *J. Reticuloendothel. Soc.*, **32**, 53–4.

Chelazzi, G. et al. (1985) Increased total serum IgE concentration in patients who have undergone splenectomy after trauma. *J. Clin. Pathol.*, **38**, 1309–10.

Ciuttis, A. et al. (1978) Immunologic defect of alternative pathway of complement activation post-splenectomy: a possible relation between splenectomy and infection. *J. Natl. Med. Assoc. NY*, **70**, 667–70.

Claret, I., Morales, L. and Montaner, A. (1975) Immunological studies in the post-splenectomy syndrome. *J. Pediatr. Surg.*, **10**, 59.

Coetzee, T. (1982) Clinical anatomy and physiology of the spleen. *S. Afr. Med. J.*, **61**, 737–46.

Cohen, R. C. and Ferrante, A. (1982) Immune dysfunction in the presence of residual splenic tissue. *Arch. Dis. Child.*, **57**, 523–7.

Coleman, C. N. et al. (1982) Functional hyposplenia after splenic irradiation for Hodgkin's disease. *Ann. Intern. Med.*, **96**, 44–7.

Constantopoulos, A. et al. (1973) Defective phagocytosis due to tuftsin deficiency in splenectomized subjects. *Am. J. Dis. Child.*, **125**, 663–5.

Constantoulakis, M. et al. (1978) Serum immunoglobulin concentrations before and after splenectomy in patients with homozygous beta-thalassaemia. *J. Clin. Pathol.*, **31**, 546–50.

Cooper, M. J. and Williamson, R. C. N. (1984) Splenectomy: indications, hazards and alternatives. *Br. J. Surg.*, **71**, 173–80.

Cooper, M. R. et al. (1982) Does tuftsin alter phagocytosis in human polymorphonuclear neutrophils? *Inflammation*, **6**, 103–12.

Corazza, G. R., Lazzari, R. and Frisoni, M. (1983) C1q binding activity in childhood coeliac disease. *Ital. J. Gastroenterol.*, **15**, 14–16.

Corazza, G. R. et al. (1981) Simple method of assessing splenic function in coeliac disease. *Clin. Sci.*, **60**, 109–13.

Corazza, G. R. *et al.* (1982) Splenic function in childhood coeliac disease. *Gut*, **23**, 415–16.

Corazza, G. R. *et al.* (1983) Effect of gluten-free diet on splenic hypofunction of adult coeliac disease. *Gut*, **24**, 228–30.

Corazza, G. R. *et al.* (1984) Return of splenic function after splenectomy: how much tissue is needed. *Br. Med. J.*, **289**, 861–4.

Corry, J. M. *et al.* (1979) Activity of the alternative pathway of complement after splenectomy: a comparison to activity in sickle cell disease and hypogammaglobulinaemia. *J. Pediatr.*, **95**, 964–9.

Costello, P., Gramm, H. F. and Steinberg, D. (1977) Simultaneous occurrence of functional asplenia and splenic accumulation of diphosphonate in metastatic breast cancer. *J. Nucl. Med.*, **18**, 1237–8.

Cox, D. R., Martin, L. and Hall, B. D. (1977) Asplenia syndrome after fetal exposure to Warfarin. *Lancet*, ii, 1134.

Cox, K. O. and Finlay-Jones, J. J. (1979) Impaired regulation of erythrocyte autoantibody production after splenectomy. *Br. J. Exp. Pathol.*, **60**, 466–70.

Crosby, W. H. (1963) Hyposplenism: an inquiry into normal functions of the spleen. *Annu. Rev. Med.*, **14**, 349–70.

Crosby, W. H. and Ruiz, F. (1962) Evidence of a myeloinhibitory factor in the spleen. *Blood*, **20**, 793.

Cunningham, M. J. and Zone, J. J. (1985) Thyroid abnormalities in dermatitis herpetiformis. *Ann. Intern. Med.*, **102**, 194–6.

Curti, A. J., Lin, J. H. and Szabo, K. (1985) Overwhelming post-splenectomy infection with *Plesimonas shigelloides* in a patient cured of Hodgkin's disease. *Am. J. Clin. Pathol.*, **83**, 522–3.

Dacie, J. V. and Lewis, J. M. (1975) *Practical Haematology*, 5th edn, Churchill Livingstone, London, pp. 438–51.

Dahl, M. *et al.* (1986) Polymorphonuclear neutrophil function and infections following splenectomy in childhood. *Scand. J. Haematol.*, **37**, 137–43.

Dailey, M. O., Coleman, C. N. and Kaplan, H. S. (1980) Radiation-induced splenic atrophy in patients with Hodgkin's disease and non-Hodgkin's lymphoma. *N. Engl. J. Med.*, **302**, 215–17.

Dameshek, W. (1955) Hyposplenism. *J. Am. Med. Assoc.*, **157**, 613.

Dawson, A. A. *et al.* (1981) Thrombotic risks of staging laparotomy with splenectomy in Hodgkin's disease. *Br. J. Surg.*, **68**, 842–5.

Deitch, E. A. and O'Neal, B. (1982) Neutrophil function in adults after traumatic splenectomy. *J. Surg. Res.*, **33**, 98–102.

De Jongh, C. L. (1948) *Malnutrition and Starvation in the Western Netherlands*, 90. General State Printing Office, The Hague.

Demetrakopoulos, G. E., Tsokos, G. C. and Levine, A. S. (1982) Recovery of splenic function after GVHD-associated functional asplenia. *Am. J. Haematol.*, **12**, 77–80.

Desai, A. G. and Thakur, M. L. (1985) Radiopharmaceuticals for spleen and marrow studies. *Sem. Nucl. Med.*, **15**, 229–37.

Dhawan, V., Spencer, R. P. and Pearson, H. A. (1977) Functional asplenia in the absence of circulating Howell–Jolly bodies. *Clin. Nucl. Med.*, **2**, 395–6.

Dhawan, V. M., Spencer, R. P. and Sziklas, J. J. (1979) Reversible functional asplenia in chronic aggressive hepatitis. *J. Nucl. Med.*, **20**, 34–6.

Dickerman, J. D. (1979) Splenectomy and sepsis: a warning. *Pediatrics*, **63**, 938–9.

Dickerman, J. D., Chalmer, B. and Horner, S. R. (1980) The effect of penicillin on the mortality of splenectomised mice exposed to an aerosol of *Streptococcus pneumoniae* type 3. *Pediatr. Res.*, **14**, 1139–41.

Dillon, A. M., Stein, H. B. and English, R. A. (1982) Splenic atrophy in systemic lupus erythematosus. *Ann. Intern. Med.*, **96**, 40–3.

Di Padova, F. *et al.* (1983) Role of the spleen in immune response to polyvalent pneumococcal vaccine. *Br. Med. J.*, **287**, 1829–31.

Di Padova, F. *et al.* (1985) Impaired antipneumococcal antibody production in patients without spleens. *Br. Med. J.*, **290**, 14–16.

Doe, W. F., Booth, C. C. and Brown, D. L. (1973) Evidence for complement-binding immune complexes in adult coeliac disease, Crohn's disease and ulcerative colitis. *Lancet*, i, 402–3.

Douglas, A. P., Weetman, A. P. and Haggith, J. W. (1976) The distribution and enteric loss of ^{51}Cr-labelled lymphocytes in normal subjects and in patients with coeliac disease and other disorders of the small intestine. *Digestion*, **14**, 29–43.

Drew, P. A. *et al.* (1984) Alterations in immunoglobulin synthesis by peripheral blood mononuclear cells from splenectomised patients with and without splenic regrowth. *J. Immunol.*, **132**, 191–6.

Durig, M., Landmann, R. M. and Harder, F. (1984) Lymphocyte subsets in human peripheral blood after splenectomy and auto-transplantation of splenic tissue. *J. Lab. Clin. Med.*, **104**, 110–15.

Elkon, K. B. *et al.* (1980) Splenic function in nonrenal systemic lupus erythematosus. *Am. J. Med.*, 69, 80–2.

Engel, A. (1939) Om sprue och mjaltatrofi. *Nordisk Medicin*, 1, 388–92.

Eppinger, H. (1913) Zur pathologie Milzfunktion. *Klin. Wochenschr.*, 50, 1509–12.

Ernstrom, U. and Sandberg, G. (1970) Influence of splenectomy on thymic release of lymphocytes into the blood. *Scand. J. Haematol.*, 7, 342–8.

Falcao, R. P., Voltarelli, J. L. and Bottura, C. (1982) The possible role of the spleen in the reduction of nitro-blue tetrazolium by neutrophils. *Acta Haematol.*, 68, 89–95.

Falter, M. L. *et al.* (1973) Splenic function and infection in sickle-cell anaemia. *Acta Haematol.*, 50, 154–61.

Ferguson, A. (1976) Coeliac disease and gastrointestinal food allergy. In *Immunological Aspects of the Liver and Gastrointestinal Tract* (eds A. Ferguson and R. N. M. MacSween), MTP Press, Lancaster, pp. 153–202.

Ferguson, A. *et al.* (1970) Adult coeliac disease in hyposplenic patients. *Lancet*, i, 163–4.

Ferrante, A. *et al.* (1985) Elevated natural killer (NK) cell activity: a possible role in resistance to infection and malignancy in immunodeficient splenectomised patients. *Med. Hypoth.*, 16, 133–46.

Findling, J. W., Pohlmann, G. P. and Rose, H. D. (1980) Fulminant gram-negative bacillemia (DF-2) following a dog-bite in an asplenic woman. *Am. J. Med.*, 68, 154–9.

Fish, H. R., Chia, J. K. and Shakir, K. M. (1985) Post-splenectomy sepsis caused by Group B streptococcus (*S. agalactiae*) in an adult patient with diabetes mellitus. *Diabetes Care*, 8, 608–9.

Fish, J. C. *et al.* (1970) Circulating lymphocyte depletion: effect on lymphoid tissue. *Surgery*, 67, 658–66.

von Fliedner, V. *et al.* (1980) Polymorphonuclear neutrophil function in malignant lymphomas and the effects of splenectomy. *Cancer*, 45, 469–75.

Foster, K. J. *et al.* (1982) Overwhelming pneumococcal septicaemia in a patient with ulcerative colitis and splenic atrophy. *Gut*, 23, 630–2.

Foster, P. N. (1985) Thyroid disease, dermatitis herpetiformis and splenic atrophy. *Ann. Intern. Med.*, 130, 157.

Foster, P. N., Hardy, G. J. and Losowsky, M. S. (1984) Fatal salmonella septicaemia in a patient with systemic lupus erythematosus and splenic atrophy. *Br. J. Clin. Pract.*, 38, 434–5.

Foster, P. N., Heatley, R. V. and Losowsky, M. S. (1985a) Hyposplenism and T-lymphocyte sub-populations in coeliac disease and after splenectomy. *J. Clin. Lab. Immunol.*, 17, 75–7.

Foster, P. N., Heatley, R. V. and Losowsky, M. S. (1985b) Natural killer cells in coeliac disease. *J. Clin. Lab. Immunol.*, 17, 173–6.

Foster, P. N. *et al.* (1985a) Development of impaired splenic function in intestinal lymphangiectasia. *Gut*, 26, 861–4.

Foster, P. N. *et al.* (1985b) Defective neutrophil activation after splenectomy. *J. Clin. Pathol.*, 38, 1175–8.

Frank, J. M. and Palomino, N. J. (1987) Primary amyloidosis with diffuse splenic infiltration presenting as fulminant pneumococcal sepsis. *Am. J. Clin. Pathol.*, 87, 405–7.

Frank, M. M. *et al.* (1979) Defective reticuloendothelial system Fc-receptor function in systemic lupus erythematosus. *N. Engl. J. Med.*, 300, 518–23.

Frank, M. M. *et al.* (1983) Immunoglobulin G Fc-receptor mediated clearance in autoimmune diseases. *Ann. Intern. Med.*, 98, 206–18.

Freedman, R. M. *et al.* (1980) Development of splenic reticuloendothelial function in neonates. *J. Pediatr.*, 96, 466–8.

Freedom, R. M. (1972) The asplenia syndrome: a review of significant extracardiac structural abnormalities in twenty-nine necropsied patients. *J. Pediatr.*, 81, 1130–3.

Garriga, S. and Crosby, W. H. (1959) The incidence of leukemia in families with hypoplasia of the marrow. *Blood*, 14, 1008–14.

Gaston, M. H. *et al.* (1986) Prophylaxis with oral penicillin in children with sickle cell anemia. *N. Engl. J. Med.*, 314, 1593–9.

Gavrilis, P., Rothenberg, S. P. and Roscoe, G. (1974) Correlation of low serum IgM levels with absence of functional splenic tissue in sickle-cell disease syndromes. *Am. J. Med.*, 57, 542–5.

Gertz, M. A., Kyle, R. A. and Griepp, P. R. (1983) Hyposplenism in primary systemic amyloidosis. *Ann. Intern. Med.*, 98, 475–7.

Gopal, V. and Bisno, A. L. (1977) Fulminant pneumococcal infections in 'normal' asplenic hosts. *Arch. Intern. Med.*, 137, 1526–30.

Gordon, P. A. *et al.* (1981) Splenic reticuloendothelial function in patients with active rheumatoid arthritis. *J. Rheumatol.*, 8, 491–3.

Grant, M. D. *et al.* (1970) Waterhouse–Friderichsen syndrome induced by pneumococcemic shock. *J. Am. Med. Assoc.*, 212, 1373–4.

Grattner, H., Gullstrand, P. and Hallberg, T. (1982) Immunocompetence after incidental splenectomy. *Scand. J. Haematol.*, 28, 369–75.

Gross, D. J. *et al.* (1982) Functional asplenia in immunoblastic lymphoma. *Arch. Intern. Med.*, **142**, 2213–15.

Guyton, J. R. and Zumwalt, R. E. (1975) Pneumococcemia with sarcoid infiltrated spleen. *Ann. Intern. Med.*, **82**, 847.

Haeney, M. R. and Ross, I. N. (1978) Whipple's disease in a female with impaired cell mediated immunity unresponsive to cotrimoxazole and levamisol therapy. *Postgrad. Med. J.*, **54**, 45–50.

Hamburger, M. I. *et al.* (1979) Sjögren's syndrome: a defect in Fc-receptor specific clearance. *Ann. Intern. Med.*, **91**, 534–8.

Hardisty, R. M. and Wolff, H. H. (1955) Haemorrhagic thrombocythaemia: a clinical and laboratory study. *Br. J. Haematol.*, **1**, 390–405.

Hatch, J. P., Sibbald, W. J. and Austin, T. W. (1983) Overwhelming pneumococcal infection in a hyposplenic adult. *Can. Med. Assoc. J.*, **129**, 851–4.

Hauser, G. J., Zakuth, V. and Spirer, Z. (1983) Normal reduction of nitroblue tetrazolium by neutrophils. *Acta Haematol.*, **70**, 142–3.

Hays, D. M. *et al.* (1984) Complications related to 234 staging laparotomies performed in the Intergroup Hodgkin's Disease in Childhood Study. *Surgery*, **96**, 471–8.

Health and Public Policy Committee, American College of Physicians (1986) Pneumococcal vaccine. *Ann. Intern. Med.*, **104**, 118–20.

Henderson, J. M. *et al.* (1981) Reticuloendothelial function in rheumatoid arthritis: correlation with disease activity and circulating immune complexes. *J. Rheumatol.*, **8**, 486–9.

Hersey, P. *et al.* (1983) Association of Sjögren's syndrome with C4 deficiency, defective reticuloendothelial function and circulating immune complexes. *Clin. Exp. Immunol.*, **52**, 551–60.

Hirsh, J. and Dacie, J. V. (1966) Persistent postsplenectomy thrombocytosis and thromboembolism: a consequence of continuing anaemia. *Br. J. Haematol.*, **12**, 44–53.

Holroyde, C. P. and Gardner, F. H. (1970) Acquisition of autophagic vacuoles by human erythrocytes. Physiological role of the spleen. *Blood*, **36**, 566–75.

Holroyde, C. P., Oski, F. A. and Gardner, F. H. (1969) The 'pocked' erythrocyte: red cell surface alterations in reticuloendothelial immaturity in the neonate. *N. Engl. J. Med.*, **281**, 516–20.

Horton, J. *et al.* (1982) The importance of splenic blood flow in clearing pneumococcal organisms. *Ann. Surg.*, **195**, 172–6.

Hosea, S. W. *et al.* (1981) Impaired immune response of splenectomised patients to polyvalent pneumococcal vaccine. *Lancet*, **i**, 804–7.

Israeli, A., Shapiro, M. and Ephros, M. A. (1987) *Plasmodium falciparum* malaria in an asplenic man. *Trans. R. Soc. Trop. Med. Hyg.*, **81**, 233–4.

Ivemark, B. I. (1955) Implications of agenesis of the spleen on the pathogenesis of cono-truncus anomalies in childhood. An analysis of the heart malformations in the splenic agenesis syndrome with fourteen new cases. *Acta Paediatr.*, **44**, Suppl. 104, 1–110.

Jellinek, E. H. and Ball, K. (1976) Hashimoto's disease, encephalopathy and splenic atrophy. *Lancet*, **i**, 1248.

Jewell, D. P., Berney, J. J. and Pettit, J. E. (1981) Splenic phagocytic function in patients with inflammatory bowel disease. *Pathology*, **13**, 717–23.

Kabins, S. A. and Lerner, C. (1970) Fulminant pneumococcemia and sickle cell anemia. *J. Am. Med. Assoc.*, **211**, 467–71.

Kelton, J. G. (1985) Impaired reticuloendothelial function in patients treated with methyldopa. *N. Engl. J. Med.*, **313**, 596–600.

Kenny, M. W., George, A. J. and Stuart, J. (1980) Platelet hyperactivity in sickle cell disease: a consequence of hyposplenism. *J. Clin. Pathol.*, **33**, 622–5.

Kevy, S. F., Tefft, M. and Vawter, G. F. (1968) Hereditary splenic hypoplasia. *Pediatrics*, **42**, 752–7.

Kiroff, G. K. *et al.* (1983) Splenic regeneration following splenectomy for traumatic rupture. *Aust. NZ. J. Surg.*, **53**, 431–4.

Kiroff, G. K. *et al.* (1985) Lack of effect of splenic regrowth on the reduced antibody responses to pneumococcal polysaccharides in splenectomised subjects. *Clin. Exp. Immunol.*, **62**, 48–56.

Klausner, M. A. *et al.* (1975) Contrasting splenic mechanisms in the blood clearance of red blood cells. *Blood*, **46**, 965–76.

Kleiner-Baumgarten, A., Schlaeffer, F. and Keynan, A. (1983) Multiple autoimmune manifestations in a splenectomized subject with HLA-B8. *Arch. Intern. Med.*, **143**, 1987–9.

Koyama, S. *et al.* (1962) Post-splenectomy vacuole: new erythrocyte inclusion body. *Mie. Med. J.* (Jap.), **11**, 425–43.

Kragballe, K. *et al.* (1981) Monocyte cytotoxicity after splenectomy. *Scand. J. Haematol.*, **27**, 271–8.

Krumbhaar, E. B. and Lippincot, S. W. (1939) The post-mortem weight of the 'normal' human spleen at different ages. *Am. J. Med. Sci.*, **197**, 344–58.

Kvinesdal, B. B. and Jensen, M. K. (1986) Pitted erythrocytes in splenectomised subjects with congenital spherocytosis and in subjects splenectomised for other reasons. *Scand. J. Haematol.*, 37, 41–3.

Langenhuijsen, M. M. and van Toorn, T. W. (1982) Splenectomy and the severity of cytomegalovirus infection. *Lancet*, ii, 820.

Lanzowsky, P. *et al.* (1976) Staging laparotomy and splenectomy: treatment and complications of Hodgkin's disease in children. *Am. J. Hematol.*, 1, 393–404.

Laufer, N. *et al.* (1978) The influence of traumatic splenectomy on the volume of human platelets. *Surg. Gynecol. Obstet.*, 146, 889–91.

Lauria, F. *et al.* (1981) T-lymphocyte subsets in healthy splenectomised patients. *Boll. Ist. Sieroter. Milan*, 60, 417–20.

Lawley, T. J. *et al.* (1981) Defective Fc-receptor functions associated with HLA-B8/DRw3 haplotype: studies in patients with dermatitis herpetiformis and normal subjects. *N. Engl. J. Med.*, 300, 524–30.

Lawrence, E. M. *et al.* (1983) Pneumococcal vaccine in normal children. *Am. J. Dis. Child.*, 137, 846–50.

Lipson, R. L., Bayrd, E. D. and Watkins, C. H. (1959) The post-splenectomy blood picture. *Am. J. Clin. Pathol.*, 32, 526–32.

Livingston, C. D. *et al.* (1983) Incidence and function of residual splenic tissue following splenectomy for trauma in adults. *Arch. Surg.*, 118, 617.

Lockwood, C. M. *et al.* (1979) Reversal of impaired splenic function in patients with nephritis or vasculitis (or both) by plasma exchange. *N. Engl. J. Med.*, 300, 524–30.

Lum, L. G. *et al.* (1980) Splenectomy in the management of the thrombocytopenia of the Wiskott–Aldrich syndrome. *N. Engl. J. Med.*, 302, 892–6.

Macrae, O. and Morris, N. (1931) Metabolism studies in coeliac disease. *Arch. Dis. Child.*, 6, 75–96.

Majeski, J. A. and Upshur, J. K. (1978) Asplenia syndrome: a study of congenital abnormalities in sixteen cases. *J. Am. Med. Assoc.*, 240, 1508–10.

Marsh, G. W. and Stewart, J. S. (1970) Splenic function in adult coeliac disease. *Br. J. Haematol.*, 19, 445–57.

Marsh, G. W., Lewis, S. M. and Szur, L. (1966a) The use of ^{51}Cr-labelled heat-damaged red cells to study splenic function. I. Evaluation of the method. *Br. J. Haematol.*, 12, 161–6.

Marsh, G. W., Lewis, S. M. and Szur, L. (1966b) The use of ^{51}Cr-labelled heat-damaged red cells to study splenic function. II. Splenic atrophy in thrombocythaemia. *Br. J. Haematol.*, 12, 167–71.

Martin, J. B. and Bell, H. E. (1965) The association of splenic atrophy and intestinal malabsorption: report of a case and review of the literature. *Can. Med. Assoc. J.*, 92, 875–8.

Matuchansky, R. *et al.* (1984) Cavitation of mesenteric lymph nodes, splenic atrophy and a flat intestinal mucosa. Report of six cases. *Gastroenterology*, 87, 606–14.

McBride, J. A., Dacie, J. V. and Shapley, R. (1968) The effect of splenectomy on the leucocyte count. *Br. J. Haematol.*, 14, 225–31.

McCarthy, C. F. *et al.* (1966) Lymphoreticular dysfunction in idiopathic steatorrhoea. *Gut*, 7, 140–8.

Melamed, I. *et al.* (1982) Suppressor T-cell activity in splenectomized subjects. *J. Clin. Lab. Immunol.*, 7, 173–7.

Meyer, A. (1932) Uber coeliakie. *Zeit. Klin. Med.*, 1198, 667–86.

Millard, R. E. and Bannerjee, S. K. (1979) Changes in T and B blood lymphocytes after splenectomy. *J. Clin. Pathol.*, 32, 1045–9.

Mills, P. R., Brown, I. L. and Watkinson, G. (1980) Idiopathic chronic ulcerative enteritis. Report of five cases and review of the literature. *Q. J. Med.*, 194, 137–49.

Mishalany, H., Mahnovski, V. and Wooley, M. (1982) Congenital asplenia and anomalies of the gastrointestinal tract. *Surgery*, 91, 38–41.

Monie, I. W. (1982) The asplenia syndrome: an explanation for absence of the spleen. *Teratology*, 25, 215–19.

Moore, F. A. *et al.* (1984) Risk of splenic salvage after trauma. *Am. J. Surg.*, 148, 800–3.

Moore, G. E. *et al.* (1983) Failure of splenic implants to protect against fatal post-splenectomy infection. *Am. J. Surg.*, 146, 413–14.

Mowbray, J. F. *et al.* (1973) Circulating immune complexes in dermatitis herpetiformis. *Lancet*, i, 400–1.

Muller, C. H. *et al.* (1984) Peripheral blood mononuclear cells of splenectomised patients are unable to differentiate into immunoglobulin-secreting cells after pokeweed mitogen stimulation. *Clin. Immunol. Immunopathol.*, 31, 118–23.

Myerson, R. M. and Koelle, W. A. (1956) Congenital absence of the spleen in an adult. Report of a case with recurrent Waterhouse–Friderichsen syndrome. *N. Engl. J. Med.*, 254, 1131–2.

Nashat, K. *et al.* (1982) A method for the study of Kupffer cell function. *Clin. Sci.*, 63, 59P.

Nathan, D. G. (1969) Rubbish in the red cell. *N. Engl. J. Med.*, **281**, 558–9.

Nathan, D. G. and Gunn, R. B. (1966) Thalassemia: the consequence of unbalanced hemoglobin synthesis. *Am. J. Med.*, **41**, 815–30.

Neilan, B. A. and Berney, S. N. (1983) Hyposplenism in systemic lupus erythematosus. *J. Rheumatol.*, **22**, 176–8.

Neilsen, J. L., Andersen, P. and Ellegaard, J. (1982) Influence of residual splenic tissue on autoantibodies in splenectomised patients. *Scand. J. Haematol.*, **28**, 273–7.

Neilsen, J. L. *et al.* (1981) Detection of splenosis and ectopic spleens with ^{99m}Tc-labelled heat damaged autologous erythrocytes in 90 splenectomised patients. *Scand. J. Haematol.*, **27**, 51–6.

Neilsen, J. L. *et al.* (1983a) Complement studies in splenectomised patients. *Scand. J. Haematol.*, **30**, 194–200.

Neilsen, J. L. *et al.* (1983b) The cellular immune response after splenectomy in humans. *Scand. J. Haematol.*, **31**, 85–95.

O'Donoghue, D. J. (1986) Fatal pneumococcal septicaemia in coeliac disease. *Postgrad. Med. J.*, **62**, 229–30.

O'Grady, J. G., Stevens, F. M. and McCarthy, C. F. (1985a) Genetic influences on splenic function in coeliac disease. *Gut*, **26**, 1004–7.

O'Grady, J. G., Stevens, F. M. and McCarthy, C. F. (1985b) Celiac disease; does hyposplenism predispose to the development of malignant disease? *Am. J. Gastroenterol.*, **80**, 27–9.

O'Grady, J. G. *et al.* (1984a) 'Pitted' erythrocytes: impaired formation in splenectomised subjects with congenital spherocytosis. *Br. J. Haematol.*, **57**, 441–6.

O'Grady, J. G. *et al.* (1984b) Hyposplenism and gluten sensitive enteropathy: natural history, incidence and relationship to diet and small bowel morphology. *Gastroenterology*, **87**, 1326–31.

O'Grady, J. G. *et al.* (1985) Influence of splenectomy and the functional hyposplenism of coeliac disease on platelet count and volume. *Scand. J. Haematol.*, **34**, 425–8.

Oakes, D. D. (1981) Splenic trauma. *Curr. Prob. Surg.*, **18**, 346–401.

Orda, R. *et al.* (1981) Post-splenectomy splenic activity. *Ann. Surg.*, **194**, 771–4.

Palmer, K. R., Sherriff, S. B. and Holdsworth, C. D. (1979) Changing pattern of splenic function in coeliac disease. *Gut*, **20**, A920.

Palmer, K. R. *et al.* (1981) Further experience of hyposplenism in inflammatory bowel disease. *Q. J. Med.*, **200**, 463–71.

Palmer, K. R. *et al.* (1983) Reticuloendothelial function in coeliac disease and ulcerative colitis. *Gut*, **24**, 384–8.

Parr, L. J. A., Shipton, E. A. and Holland, E. H. (1953) A fatal case of Still's disease associated with Waterhouse–Friderichsen syndrome due to pneumococcal septicaemia. *Med. J. Aust.*, **1**, 300–4.

Pearson, H. A., Schiebler, G. L. and Spencer, R. P. (1971) Functional hyposplenia in cyanotic congenital heart disease. *Pediatrics*, **48**, 277–80.

Pearson, H. A., Spencer, R. P. and Cornelius, E. A. (1969) Functional asplenia in sickle cell anemia. *N. Engl. J. Med.*, **281**, 923–6.

Pearson, H. A. *et al.* (1970) Transfusion-reversible functional asplenia in young children with sickle cell anemia. *N. Engl. J. Med.*, **283**, 334–7.

Pearson, H. A. *et al.* (1978) The born-again spleen. Return of splenic function after splenectomy for trauma. *N. Engl. J. Med.*, **298**, 1389–92.

Pearson, H. A. *et al.* (1985) Developmental pattern of splenic dysfunction in sickle cell disorders. *Pediatrics*, **76**, 392–7.

Pedersen, F. K., Henrickson, J. and Schiffman, G. (1982) Antibody response to vaccination with pneumococcal capsular polysaccharides in splenectomised children. *Acta Paediatr. Scand.*, **71**, 451–5.

Pereira, J. L. R., Hughes, L. E. and Young, H. L. (1987) Spleen size in patients with inflammatory bowel disease. Does it have any clinical significance? *Dis. Colon Rectum*, **30**, 403–9.

Pettit, J. E. *et al.* (1971) Studies of splenic function in the myeloproliferative disorders and generalised malignant lymphomas. *Br. J. Haematol.*, **20**, 575–86.

Pettit, J. E. *et al.* (1972) Splenic atrophy in dermatitis herpetiformis. *Br. Med. J.*, **2**, 438–40.

Pines, A. *et al.* (1983) Hyposplenism in systemic lupus erythematosus. *Br. J. Rheumatol.*, **22**, 176–8.

Plummer, K. *et al.* (1950) Lipophagic intestinal granulomatosis (Whipple's disease). *Arch. Intern. Med.*, **86**, 280–310.

Polhemus, D. W. and Schafer, W. B. (1952) Congenital absence of the spleen. Syndrome with atrioventricularis and situs inversus. *Pediatrics*, **9**, 696–708.

Polhill, R. B. and Johnston, R. B. (1975) Diminished alternative complement pathway activity after splenectomy. *Pediatr. Res.*, **9**, 333.

Polsky, B. *et al.* (1986) Bacterial pneumonia in patients with the Acquired Immunodeficiency Syndrome. *Ann. Intern. Med.*, **104**, 38–41.

Rice, H. M. and James, P. D. (1980) Ectopic splenic tissue failed to prevent fatal pneumococcal septicaemia after splenectomy for trauma. *Lancet*, i, 565–6.

Roberts, J. G. *et al.* (1976) Prediction of human spleen size by computer analysis of splenic scintigrams. *Br. J. Radiol.*, 49, 151–5.

Robertson, D. A. F., Simpson, F. G. and Losowsky, M. S. (1981) Blood viscosity after splenectomy. *Br. Med. J.*, 283, 573–5.

Robertson, D. A. F. *et al.* (1982a) Suppressor cell activity, splenic function, and HLA-B8 status in man. *J. Clin. Lab. Immunol.*, 9, 133–8.

Robertson, D. A. F. *et al.* (1982b) Coeliac disease, splenic function and malignancy. *Gut*, 23, 666–9.

Robertson, D. A. F. *et al.* (1983a) Blood film appearances in the hyposplenism of coeliac disease. *Br. J. Clin. Pract.*, 37, 19–22.

Robertson, D. A. F. *et al.* (1983b) Small intestinal ulceration: diagnostic difficulties in relation to coeliac disease. *Gut*, 24, 565–74.

Robertson, D. A. F. *et al.* (1983c) Splenectomy causes autoantibody formation. *J. Clin. Lab. Immunol.*, 11, 63–5.

Robinette, C. D. and Fraumeni, J. F. (1977) Splenectomy and subsequent mortality in veterans of the 1939–45 war. *Lancet*, ii, 127–9.

Robinson, P. J. *et al.* (1980) Splenic size and function in adult coeliac disease. *Br. J. Radiol.*, 53, 532–7.

Rose, V., Izukawa, T. and Moes, C. A. F. (1975) Syndrome of asplenia and polysplenia: a review of cardiac and non-cardiac malformations in 60 cases with special reference to diagnosis and prognosis. *Br. Heart J.*, 37, 840–52.

Rosenthal, N. (1925) Clinical and hematological studies on Banti's disease: the platelet factor with reference to splenectomy. *J. Am. Med. Assoc.*, 84, 1887–91.

Rosner, F. *et al.* (1984) Babesiosis in splenectomized adults: review of 22 reported cases. *Am. J. Med.*, 76, 696–701.

Roth, J., Brudler, O. and Henze, E. (1985) Functional asplenia in malignant mastocytosis. *J. Nucl. Med.*, 26, 1149–52.

Rowley, D. A. (1950) The formation of circulating antibody in the splenectomised human being following intravenous injection of heterologous erythrocytes. *J. Immunol.*, 65, 515–21.

Roy, D. (1984) The spleen preserved. *Br. Med. J.*, 289, 70–1.

Ryan, F. P. *et al.* (1974) Hyposplenism in ulcerative colitis. *Lancet*, ii, 318–20.

Ryan, F. P. *et al.* (1978) Hyposplenism in inflammatory bowel disease. *Gut*, 19, 50–5.

Ryan, F. P. *et al.* (1981) Impaired immunity in patients with inflammatory bowel disease and hyposplenism: the response to intravenous ØX174. *Gut*, 22, 187–9.

Sampson, D. *et al.* (1976) Suppressor activity of the human spleen and thymus. *Surgery*, 79, 393–7.

Schilling, V. (1924) Uber die Diagnose einer Milzatrophie durch den Befund von Kernkugeln als Teilerscheinung pluriglandular Insuffizienz. *Klin. Wochenschr.*, 43, 1960–2.

Schnitzer, B. *et al.* (1971) Erythrocytes: pits and vacuoles as seen with transmission and scanning electron microscopy. *Science*, 173, 251–2.

Schrier, S. L. *et al.* (1974) Erythrocyte membrane vacuole formation in hereditary spherocytosis. *Br. J. Haematol.*, 26, 59–69.

Schumacher, M. J. (1970) Serum immunoglobulin and transferrin levels after childhood splenectomy. *Arch. Dis. Child.*, 45, 114–17.

Scully, R. E., Galdabini, J. J. and McNeely, B. U. (1975) Case records of the Massachusetts General Hospital. *N. Engl. J. Med.*, 293, 547–53.

Segal, A. W. *et al.* (1981) Indium-111 tagged leucocytes in the diagnosis of inflammatory bowel disease. *Lancet*, ii, 230–2.

Selby, C. *et al.* (1987) Bacteraemia in adults after splenectomy or splenic irradiation. *Q. J. Med.*, 63, 523–30.

Shennib, H., Chu-Jeng Chiu, R. and Mulder, D. S. (1983) The effects of splenectomy and splenic implantation on alveolar macrophage function. *J. Trauma*, 23, 7–12.

Siber, G. R. *et al.* (1978) Impaired antibody response to pneumococcal vaccine after treatment for Hodgkin's disease. *N. Engl. J. Med.*, 299, 442–8.

Smart, R. C. *et al.* (1978) Relationship between splenic size and splenic function. *Gut*, 19, 56–9.

Spencer, G. R. *et al.* (1981) Spleen scanning with ^{99m}Tc-labelled red blood cells after splenectomy. *Br. J. Surg.*, 68, 412–14.

Spencer, R. P., Johnson, P. M. and Sziklas, J. J. (1977) Unusual scan presentation of splenic vasculature occlusion by tumour. *Clin. Nucl. Med.*, 2, 197–9.

Spencer, R. P. and Pearson, H. A. (1974) Splenic radiocolloid uptake in the presence of circulating Howell–Jolly bodies. *J. Nucl. Med.*, 15, 294–5.

Spencer, R. P. *et al.* (1978a) Causes and temporal sequence of onset of functional asplenia in adults. *Clin. Nucl. Med.*, 3, 17–18.

Spencer, R. P. *et al.* (1978b) 'Reversible' functional asplenia in combined immunodeficiency. *Int. J. Nucl. Med. Biol.*, 5, 125.

Spencer, R. P. *et al.* (1984) Splenic overload syndrome: possible relationship to a small spleen. *J. Nucl. Med. Biol.*, **11**, 291–4.

Spirer, Z. *et al.* (1977) Decreased tuftsin concentrations in patients who have undergone splenectomy. *Br. Med. J.*, **2**, 1574–6.

Spirer, Z. *et al.* (1980a) Autoimmune antibodies after splenectomy. *Acta Haematol.*, **63**, 230–3.

Spirer, Z. *et al.* (1980b) Decreased serum tuftsin concentration in sickle-cell disease. *Arch. Dis. Child.*, **55**, 566–7.

Steinberg, M. H., Gatling, R. R. and Tavassoli, M. (1983) Evidence of hyposplenism in the presence of splenomegaly. *Scand. J. Haematol.*, **31**, 437–9.

Stone, H. H., Stanley, D. G. and DeJarnette, R. H. (1967) Post-splenectomy viral hepatitis. *J. Am. Med. Assoc.*, **199**, 851–3.

Stone, R. W. *et al.* (1985) Acquired functional asplenia in sarcoidosis. *J. Natl Med. Assoc. NY*, **77**, 930–6.

Suarez, R. M., Spies, T. D. and Suarez, R. M. Jr (1947) The use of folic acid in sprue. *Ann. Intern. Med.*, **26**, 643–77.

Sullivan, J. C. *et al.* (1978) Immune response after splenectomy. *Lancet*, **i**, 178–81.

Szur, L., Marsh, G. W. and Pettit, J. E. (1972) Studies of splenic function by means of radioisotope-labelled red cells. *Br. J. Haematol.*, **23**, Suppl., 183–199.

Tesluk, G. C. (1984) Fatal overwhelming post-splenectomy sepsis following autologous splenic transplantation in severe congenital osteopetrosis. *J. Pediatr. Surg.*, **19**, 269–72.

Thompson, H. (1974) Necropsy studies in adult coeliac disease. *J. Clin. Pathol.*, **27**, 710–21.

Torres, J. and Bisno, A. L. (1973) Hyposplenism and pneumococcemia. *Am. J. Med.*, **55**, 851–5.

Trewby, P. N. *et al.* (1981) Splenic atrophy in adult coeliac disease: is it reversible? *Gut*, **22**, 628–32.

Van Mierop, L. H. S., Gessner, I. H. S. and Schiebler, G. L. (1972) Asplenia and polysplenia syndromes. *Birth Defects: Original Article Series*, **8**, 36–44.

Van Wyck, D. B. *et al.* (1980) Critical splenic mass for survival from experimental pneumococcemia. *J. Surg. Res.*, **78**, 14–17.

Waldman, J. D. *et al.* (1977) Sepsis and congenital asplenia. *J. Pediatr.*, **90**, 555–9.

Wardrop, C. A. J. *et al.* (1975) Immunological abnormalities in splenic atrophy. *Lancet*, **ii**, 4–7.

Westerhausen, M. *et al.* (1981) Immunological changes following post-traumatic splenectomy. *Blut*, **43**, 345–53.

Whitaker, A. N. (1969) Infection and the spleen: association between hyposplenism, pneumococcal sepsis and disseminated intravascular coagulation. *Med. J. Aust.*, **1**, 1213–19.

Widmann, W. D. and Laubscher, F. A. (1971) Splenosis: a disease or a beneficial condition? *Arch. Surg.*, **102**, 152–8.

Wilkinson, L. S., Tang, A. and Gjedsted, A. (1983) Marked lymphocytosis suggesting lymphocytic leukemia in three patients with hyposplenism. *Am. J. Med.*, **75**, 1053–6.

Williams, B. D. *et al.* (1979) Defective reticuloendothelial system function in rheumatoid arthritis. *Lancet*, **i**, 1311–14.

Winkelstein, J. A. and Lambert, G. H. (1975) Pneumococcal serum opsonizing activity in splenectomized children. *J. Pediatr.*, **87**, 430–3.

Zago, M. A. *et al.* (1985) Aspects of splenic hypofunction in old age. *Klin. Wochenschr.*, **63**, 590–2.

Zago, M. A. *et al.* (1986) Red cell pits appear preferentially in old cells after splenectomy. *Acta Haematol.*, **76**, 54–6.

Zarrabi, M. H. and Rosner, F. (1986) Rarity of failure of penicillin prophylaxis to prevent post-splenectomy sepsis. *Arch. Intern. Med.*, **146**, 1207–8.

Zucker, S. and Mielke, C. H. (1972) Classification of thrombocytosis based on platelet function tests: correlation with hemorrhagic and thrombotic complications. *J. Lab. Clin. Med.*, **80**, 385–94.

THE RELATIONSHIP OF THE SPLEEN TO INFECTION

12

Geoffrey J. Gorse

12.1 INTRODUCTION

The predisposition to infection experienced by patients with diminished or absent splenic function is now well documented. Currently the commonest cause of hyposplenism is surgical splenectomy, but an increasingly broad range of diseases and disorders is now known to be associated with hyposplenism (Eichner, 1979; Foster, Hardy and Losowsky, 1984): these have been reviewed in Chapter 11.

In addition to the now classical association of infection with splenectomy in infancy, bacteremia has been documented to occur during periods of hyposplenism in ulcerative colitis, in which splenic function waxes and wanes in proportion to the activity of the colitis (Foster *et al.*, 1982). Systemic lupus erythematosus (SLE) shows impaired splenic function, in part due to reticuloendothelial blockade produced by circulating immune complexes and reversed by plasmapheresis. In addition, splenic atrophy in patients with SLE results from lymphocyte depletion, and overwhelming septicemia has been reported in association with splenic atrophy in this disorder (Foster, Hardy and Losowsky, 1984).

Sickle cell anemia is also associated with severe bacterial infections: the child with sickle cell disease is at greatest risk for pneumococcal sepsis when the spleen is enlarged early in life. At a later stage, when the spleen is atrophic, there has been the opportunity for an immuno-logical response to various pneumococcal serotypes, and the resulting production of type-specific antibody enhances the clearance of pneumococci by the reticuloendothelial cells of the liver. (See also section 11.3.2. and Chapter 16.)

In this chapter the pathophysiological mechanisms for the increased risk of infection in the patient with impaired splenic function, and the types of organisms which cause these infections, will be reviewed. The prevention of infectious complications in patients at risk will also be discussed.

12.2 MEASUREMENT OF THE DEGREE OF HYPOSPLENISM

Methods for demonstrating impaired splenic function have been described elsewhere (Chapter 11, section 11.2). They have contributed in large measure to the recognition of hyposplenism and have provided insight into its various degrees of expression. For example, Coleman *et al.* (1982) showed that patients newly diagnosed with lymphoma had a mean pitted red cell count of 0.6%, which rose to 13% after radiation to the spleen of at least 4000 rads, and 33.7% after surgical splenectomy. This indicates that splenic radiation diminishes splenic function, and practically, such patients should be regarded as having a significantly increased risk of infection.

Dailey, Coleman and Kaplan (1980) also

documented splenic atrophy induced by radiation in patients with lymphoma: the mean postmortem weight of the spleen in radiated subjects was 75 g and in subjects not radiated it was 200 g. During life there was demonstrably decreased uptake of ^{99m}Tc in sulfur-colloid spleen scans after radiation; however, chemotherapy differed in not being accompanied by a reduction in spleen size.

The degree to which splenic function is reduced is variable even after splenectomy for trauma to the spleen. Pearson *et al.* (1978) reported a study in which the peripheral blood of normal children showed fewer than 1% of red cells to have pits microscopically. Subjects splenectomized for trauma could be divided into two somewhat disparate groups, based on the proportion of pitted cells. Of 22 children 13 showed 6% or less; the remainder had much higher levels of pitted cells, with a mean of 21%. These were comparable to patients who underwent splenectomy for hematological disorders, and who showed a mean of 20%. Subjects with 6% or less of cells with pits showed

multiple nodules of regenerate splenic tissue in ^{99m}Tc sulfur-colloid spleen scans. These authors attributed the difference to the function of the regenerated tissue ('splenosis'), and ascribed lower rates of infection to these patients.

12.3 CLINICAL MANIFESTATIONS OF OVERWHELMING POSTSPLENECTOMY INFECTION

The syndrome of overwhelming postsplenectomy infection (OPSI) usually begins with a prodrome of influenza-like symptoms followed by an abrupt onset of septicemia with massive bacteremia from an unknown source. Bacteria may be identified using Gram's stain on a buffy coat smear of the peripheral blood. The first report of this syndrome was by King and Shumacker (1952) in five infants splenectomized for congenital hemolytic anemia, four of whom developed meningitis or overwhelming meningococcemia six weeks to three years later. The syndrome commonly comprises fever, chills, abdominal pain, nausea, vomiting, multi-

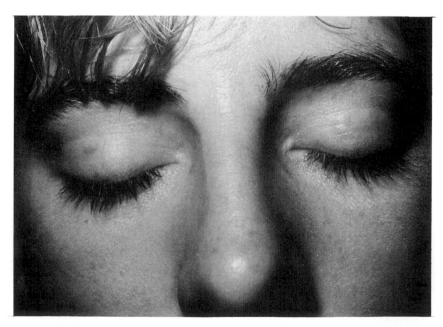

Figure 12.1 Purpura on the face of a patient with fulminant meningococcemia. These lesions are typical of those found in patients with fulminant septicemia and disseminated intravascular coagulation.

ple organ failure, disseminated intravascular coagulation (DIC), adrenal hemorrhage (Waterhouse–Friderichsen syndrome), seizures, and death within 36 hours of onset (Bisno and Freeman, 1970; Kingston and MacKenzie, 1979; Singer, 1973).

Purpuric skin lesions are commonly distributed on the face and extremities in patients with DIC and overwhelming septicemia (Figures 12.1 and 12.2; Kingston and MacKenzie, 1979). The causative organism can be cultured from aspirates of the purpuric skin lesions. Severe hypoglycemia, electrolyte imbalance and shock are frequently noted. Waterhouse–Friderichsen syndrome is usually associated with a fatal outcome, but the incidence of other symptoms and signs in OPSI and their predictive value of outcome are as yet poorly documented.

12.4   MICROORGANISMS ASSOCIATED WITH POSTSPLENECTOMY INFECTIONS

Postsplenectomy infections are known to be caused principally by encapsulated bacteria (*Streptococcus pneumoniae, Haemophilus influenzae* type b, and *Neisseria meningitidis*) and also by non-encapsulated and non-bacterial pathogens such as viruses and protozoa (Table 12.1). The most fulminant infections which occur in the postsplenectomy state are usually due to encapsulated bacteria.

12.4.1   BACTERIAL INFECTIONS

Of the bacterial causes of postsplenectomy infection, the most common organism is *S. pneumoniae*, particularly in patients with OPSI (Table 12.2; Askergren and Björkholm, 1980; Barrett-Connor, 1971; Buchanan *et al.*, 1983; Green *et al.*, 1979; Hitzig, 1985; Rosner and Zarrabi, 1983; Singer, 1973; Wåhlby and Domellöf, 1981). For instance, Askergren and Björkholm (1980) reported that pneumococcal septicemia accounted for 71% of septic episodes among their splenectomized patients, but for only 4.7% of all septic episodes at their institutions. Other bacterial pathogens each account individually for less than 15% of infections reported in splenectomized patients.

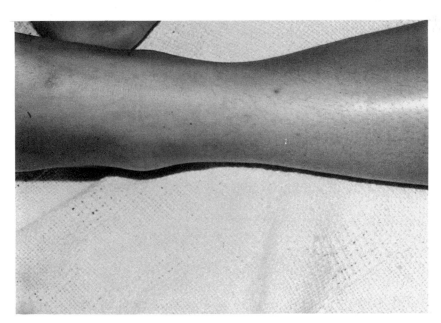

Figure 12.2 Purpura on the anterior aspect of the leg in meningococcemia. (Same patient as in Figure 12.1.)

Table 12.1 Organisms causing severe infections in splenectomized patients

Bacteria
  Streptococcus pneumoniae
  Haemophilus influenzae
  Neisseria meningitidis
  Pseudomonas aeruginosa
  Escherichia coli
  Dysgonic fermenter 2 (DF-2)
  Other bacteria:
    Neisseria gonorrhoea
    Plesiomonas shigelloides
    Other Streptococcal spp.

Viruses
  Cytomegalovirus
  Herpes zoster virus
  Epstein–Barr virus
  Rubeola virus
  Human immunodeficiency virus

Protozoa
  Babesia spp.
  Plasmodium spp.

These include other encapsulated organisms (*H. influenzae* and *N. meningitidis*), other streptococcal species, *Pseudomonas aeruginosa*, *Escherichia coli*, and more unusual bacterial pathogens.

N. meningitidis is a cause of serious post-splenectomy infection, although the incidence is less than that of *S. pneumoniae* (Holmes *et al.*, 1981; Loggie and Hinchey, 1986). Serious meningococcal infection has been reported in patients who required splenectomy for underlying disease (King and Shumacker, 1952), as well as abdominal trauma (Holmes *et al.*, 1981). Loggie and Hinchey (1986) reported that intraperitoneal and intravenous challenge with *N. meningitidis* group B in a murine model did not result in greater mortality among splenectomized mice when compared with normal mice. This supports literature review findings that meningococcal infection is less frequent than pneumococcal in patients who have undergone splenectomy.

One case of fulminant septicemia, shock and adrenal hemorrhage due to *Neisseria gonorrhoeae* was reported by Austin, Sargeant and Warwick (1980). The patient had been splenectomized during a staging laparotomy for Hodgkin's disease and later received radiation therapy. As with the pneumococcus, blood isolates of *N. gonorrhoeae* from persons with disseminated gonococcal infections are resistant to killing by serum alone (Schoolnik, Buchanan and Holmes, 1976). This may contribute to the mechanism for the development of overwhelming infection with this organism in the splenectomized patient. A similar patient with Hodgkin's disease, who underwent splenectomy and radiotherapy, died of fulminant septicemia due to *Plesiomonas shigelloides* and developed DIC and adrenal hemorrhage (Curti, Lin and Szabo, 1985). *P. shigelloides* is an unusual cause of septicemia in the general population and is most commonly associated with a mild diarrheal illness.

Another unusual pathogen first described in 1977 and reported to be the causative agent of severe infections in splenectomized patients is a slow-growing Gram-negative bacillus assigned the name of dysgonic fermenter 2 (DF-2) by the Centers for Disease Control, Atlanta, GA. It is sensitive to penicillin and chloramphenicol, as well as to several other antibiotics. The organism can be confused with other fastidious Gram-negative bacilli, but is distinguishable by routine biochemical laboratory testing. Infections caused by DF-2 have, in general, been characterized by septicemia and a history of a dog bite (Hicklin, Verghese and Alvarez, 1987; Kalb *et al.*, 1985; Martone *et al.*, 1980). The DF-2 organism is most frequently isolated from blood and CSF. DIC has been reported in association with septicemia: fulminant infections and DIC have occurred in 50% of splenectomized patients reported to be septicemic with this organism. Eschariform skin lesions develop at the site of the dog bite. Peripheral blood smears from these patients may show Gram-negative rods. Splenectomized patients should be aware of the association of fulminant infec-

Table 12.2 Etiologic agents which cause sepsis in patients with hyposplenia and asplenia and their relative frequencies of isolation

Ref no.	Reason for hyposplenism or splenectomy	Total no. of patients in study	No. of episodes of postsplenectomy sepsis due to the indicated organism (% of episodes)						
			Total	S. pneumoniae	H. influenzae	N. meningitidis	Salmonella spp	E. coli	Unknown and other
1	Hodgkin's disease	52	8	6 (75)	1 (12.5)	—	—	—	1 (12.5)
2	Hodgkin's disease	115	13*	7 (54)	4 (31)	2 (15)	—	—	—
3	Hodgkin's disease	76	5	5 (100)	—	—	—	—	—
	All others	1072	9	4 (44)	—	—	—	—	5 (56)
4	Trauma	413	10	4 (40)	3 (30)	1 (10)	—	—	2 (20)
5	Sickle cell anemia	166	9	4 (44)	1 (12)	—	2 (22)	2 (22)	—
6	Mainly hematological+ (see text)	2795	72	36 (50)	6 (8)	9 (13)	—	8 (11)	13 (18)
7	Hemoglobin SC disease	51	6	5 (83)	1 (17)	—	—	—	—
	Totals:	4740	132	71 (54)	16 (12)	12 (9)	2 (1)	10 (8)	21 (16)

*Fatal episodes only.
+None with sickle cell anemia.
References: 1, Green *et al.* (1979); 2, Rosner and Zarrabi (1983); 3, Askergren and Björkholm (1980); 4, Wåhlby and Domellöf (1981); 5, Barrett-Connor (1971); 6, Singer (1973); 7, Buchanan *et al.* (1983).

tion and dog bites. The organism appears to be serum-sensitive and it has been postulated that the susceptible host may have a defect in the lytic activity of serum due to a quantitative or qualitative complement abnormality or possibly due to the presence of non-bactericidal blocking antibodies (Hicklin, Verghese and Alvarez, 1987).

In addition to *H. influenzae* type b as a cause of serious postsplenectomy infection, type f was reported to cause meningitis in an asplenic patient with biliary cirrhosis (Meier, Waldvogel and Zwahlen, 1985). The strain isolated from the patient's blood cultures was not cleared as rapidly from the bloodstream of splenectomized rats challenged with the organism, when compared to clearance from normal rats. These findings indicate that *H. influenzae* strains other than type b can cause serious infection in splenectomized patients.

12.4.2   VIRAL INFECTIONS

Viruses which may be associated with increased severity or rates of infection in splenectomized hosts include varicella-zoster virus and cytomegalovirus. Although reported rates vary, varicella-zoster virus infection occurs in approximately 20% of splenectomized patients with Hodgkin's disease, but less frequently in patients splenectomized for non-neoplastic diseases (Green *et al.*, 1979; Green *et al.*, 1986; Monfardini *et al.*, 1975). Other investigators have denied that a higher rate of varicella-zoster occurs after splenectomy (Guinee *et al.*, 1985; Naraqi *et al.*, 1977; Reboul, Donaldson and Kaplan, 1978; Schimpff *et al.*, 1972).

The contributions of radiation treatment and chemotherapy to the increased incidence of viral infections are additional factors which are difficult to separate out from the effect of splenectomy. Splenectomy appeared to be a risk factor for varicella-zoster virus infection independent of Hodgkin's disease in a series of 1130 patients with lymphoma reported by Goffinet, Glatstein and Merigan (1972). Monfardini *et al.* (1975) reported a higher incidence of varicella-zoster in 232 splenectomized patients with Hodgkin's (26 (19%) of 139 patients) and non-Hodgkin's (11 (12%) of 93 patients) lymphomas (16% overall) than in 175 non-splenectomized patients with Hodgkin's (5 (11%) of 45 patients) and non-Hodgkin's (10 (8%) of 130 patients) lymphomas (9% overall). The incidence of varicella-zoster was significantly higher in splenectomized patients who received cyclic chemotherapy with Hodgkin's (27%) and non-Hodgkin's (15%) lymphomas (22% for all chemotherapy recipients) compared to the group which was splenectomized but not treated with chemotherapy with Hodgkin's (8%) and non-Hodgkin's (6%) lymphomas (7% for all who did not receive chemotherapy). Overall, the rate of varicella-zoster in children and adolescents with Hodgkin's disease is reported to be from 12% to 38%; Green *et al.* (1979) reported a trend toward a higher rate of varicella-zoster among splenectomized patients with Hodgkin's disease. The cumulative percentage of patients who had undergone splenectomy and experienced zoster was 42.8%, as opposed to 18.3% of Hodgkin's disease patients who had not undergone splenectomy. Guinee *et al.* (1985) reported attack rates of zoster in patients with Hodgkin's disease using univariate and multiple regression analyses to be the same whether laparotomy (and presumably splenectomy) had been performed or not.

An association between the postsplenectomy state and clinical cytomegalovirus infection has not been firmly established. Severe cytomegalovirus infection characterized by interstitial pneumonia, high fever, and lymphocytosis with atypical forms, has been reported in patients who underwent splenectomy for trauma and received multiple blood transfusions (Baumgartner *et al.*, 1982). Anti-cytomegalovirus IgM antibodies were detected in only one of the three patients in whom tests for these antibodies were done. The authors postulated that the lack of anti-CMV IgM antibody may have been due to the postsplenectomy state. Okun and Tanaka (1978) reported a case of CMV mononucleosis with an associated lymphocyte count greater than 100 000/mm^3 and other authors have reported severe symptomatic post-transfusion CMV infection in splenectomized patients (Adler, 1983). However, Langenhuijsen and van Toorn (1982) reported that four of 26 consecutive patients with cytomegalovirus infection had undergone splenectomy and none of these patients was seriously ill from the cytomegalovirus infection. Peterson *et al.* (1980) reported that the incidence of CMV disease was identical in renal allograft recipients with and without a history of splenecomy. An experimental murine model for cytomegalovirus infection has demonstrated a different effect of splenectomy; Katzenstein, Yu and Jordan (1983) showed that splenectomized mice had lower mortality rates than mice with intact spleens when infected with murine cytomegalovirus. These authors concluded that early replication of murine cytomegalovirus in splenic macrophages augmented virus-induced hepatic injury, and thus contributed to the pathogenesis of lethal murine cytomegalovirus infection. The relevance of these findings to human infection remains to be clarified.

Epstein–Barr and rubeola virus infections have been reported to show unusual manifestations in splenectomized patients (Baumgartner *et al.*, 1982). Jones *et al.* (1975) reported a prolonged course of fever and lymphocytosis in a patient with rubeola infection recently splenectomized for trauma. Purtilo *et al.* (1980) reported severe Epstein–Barr virus infection characterized by profound lymphocytosis, acquired hypogammaglobulinemia and severe hepatitis in a patient who acquired the infection from blood transfusions following splenectomy for trauma. Modification of the immune response to Epstein–Barr virus by splenectomy due to trauma may have led to a Kawasaki disease syndrome in a young adult (Barbour *et al.*, 1979).

Thrombocytopenia in patients with human immunodeficiency virus (HIV) infection is clinically indistinguishable from autoimmune thrombocytopenic purpura (Abrams *et al.*,

1986; Barbui *et al.*, 1987). Patients with HIV-related ITP treated with steroids have a lower rate of progression to acquired immunodeficiency syndrome than do patients with HIV infection and ITP treated with splenectomy (Barbui *et al.*, 1987).

12.4.3 PROTOZOAL INFECTIONS

Plasmodium species and *Babesia* species are associated with more severe and frequent infections in patients who have impaired or absent splenic function. (See also Chapter 3.)

Human babesiosis is a febrile illness characterized by myalgias, fatigue, hemolytic anemia, and hemoglobinuria caused by tick-borne protozoan agents of the genus *Babesia* (Rosner *et al.*, 1984). Frequently it will mimic malaria but is generally milder in severity. In addition to tick-borne spread, it can be acquired by the transfusion of infected blood. The spleen plays an important role in resistance to *Babesia* infections in animals. Mild infections with low levels of parasitemia in animals can be exacerbated by splenectomy. Rosner *et al.* (1984) summarized 22 previously reported cases of human babesiosis among splenectomized patients, ranging in age from 23 to 70 years. Splenectomy had been performed for various indications one month to 36 years prior to the babesia infection; most had moderate to severe clinical disease and 16 (73%) survived. Dammin *et al.* (1981) reported 57 clinical cases of *Babesia microti* infection of which 10 (17%) occurred in splenectomized patients; these were acquired on offshore islands of the northeastern United States (Nantucket Island, Martha's Vineyard, and the eastern tip of Long Island) and Cape Cod. None of these infections was fatal. Other *Babesia* species have caused infection in splenectomized patients and the resultant disease is often more severe in splenectomized patients (Dammin *et al.*, 1981; Rosner *et al.*, 1984; Shute, 1975).

Splenectomy is known to predispose to unusually severe clinical malaria, and to reactivation of latent and subclinical malarial infections in both humans and animals. It has been observed that certain experimental animals not normally susceptible to certain species of *Plasmodium* can be rendered susceptible by splenectomy (Wyler, Oster and Quinn, 1978). However, the effects of splenectomy are not uniform since the species of experimental animal, species of *Plasmodium*, and timing of splenectomy may affect susceptibility to and severity of infection (Nooruddin and Ahmed, 1967). Monkeys splenectomized two to three months after infection with *Plasmodium inui* tolerated their infection without effect on mortality, although these animals rapidly developed the same levels of parasitemia which killed monkeys splenectomized prior to infection (Wyler, Miller and Schmidt, 1977). The spleen limits the magnitude of parasitemia in acute infections and restricts the level of parasitemia in chronic infections (Littman, 1974; Llende, Santiago-Delpiń and Lavergne, 1986; Looareesuwan *et al.*, 1987; Rosner *et al.*, 1984; Shute, 1975; Tapper and Armstrong, 1976; Walzer, Gibson and Schultz, 1974). The spleen exerts other influences on host defense against the intraerythrocytic, asexual stage of plasmodia: it may be important for clinical tolerance early in infection, and it is required as an effector organ in mediating protection induced by vaccines but not for sustaining antibody production in response to these vaccines (Wyler, Oster and Quinn, 1978).

The spleen is important in the reduction of parasitemia, probably because erythrocytes infected with *Plasmodia* spp. are more susceptible to splenic filtration, due to their reduced deformability (Miller, Usami and Chien, 1971). However, the pitting process lacks a recognition system which would provide for the species-specificity of malaria immunity (Wyler, Oster and Quinn, 1978). Sequestration of erythrocytes parasitized with *Plasmodium falciparum* usually limits the observable parasitemia to ring forms and gametocytes. Splenectomy results in the presence of all stages of the intraerythrocytic parasite in the peripheral blood smears (Israeli, Shapiro and Ephros, 1987). Splenectomy appears to have no effect on susceptibility to sporozoite-induced infection or on the development of exoerythrocytic stages (Wyler, Oster and Quinn, 1978). During active experimental infection of rats with *Plasmodium berghei*, the efficiency of the splenic removal of parasitized cells and of heat-treated red cells is much diminished, whereas spontaneous resolution of the parasitemia is associated with a marked increase in the rates of clearance (Wyler, Quinn and Chen, 1981). Splenectomy may result in overwhelming infection and the recurrence of acute symptomatic malaria in patients with chronic asymptomatic *Plasmodium malariae* infection due to a rapid rise in parasitemia after splenectomy (Wyler, Oster and Quinn, 1978). The mechanism for the role of the spleen in the induction of immunity to malaria other than by its non-immunological parasiticidal effects is yet to be determined. One possibility is a cytotoxic effect of a spleen cell population on parasitized erythrocytes (Coleman *et al.*, 1975).

Patients with splenic hypofunction should be cautioned about their susceptibility to more severe illness due to *Plasmodium* spp. and advised to avoid endemic regions. If travel plans cannot be altered, then the standard antimalarial prophylaxis regimens and protective measures against mosquito vectors should be recommended.

A study of the splenic clearance of autologous heat-treated red cells in patients with acute malaria due to *P. falciparum* has been published by Looareesuwan *et al.* (1987). Clearance was enhanced in patients with splenomegaly, but not in those with normal spleen size, suggesting that enlargement of the spleen may itself be an effective means of increasing particle filtration rates. However, within a few days of starting antimalarial therapy, the clearance rates were found to be increased above normal in the patients without splenomegaly as well; in both groups normal clearance rates resumed within six weeks of treatment. (See also Chapter 3.)

12.5 THE RELATIONSHIP OF MICROORGANISMS, CLINICAL OUTCOME AND SITE OF INFECTION TO THE UNDERLYING DISEASE

Rosner and Zarrabi (1983) reported on 115 patients with Hodgkin's disease who experienced 145 episodes of postsplenectomy infection. These infections included pneumonia in 37.2% of 145 episodes, septicemia in 28.3% of episodes, meningitis in 13.8%, urinary tract infection in 2.7%, skin infection in 4.7%, and infection at other sites in 13.2%. Of the 41 (28.3%) patients with an episode of septicemia, 20 had a fulminant course with DIC and adrenal hemorrhage; twelve of these 20 patients with a fulminant course were under 10 years of age. At least 50 of the 115 patients (43%) died as a result of their infections. Among those patients who developed DIC, only two survived, giving an overall mortality in this group of 90%. For those without clinical DIC, the mortality rate was 35%.

The bacteria associated with postsplenectomy infection included S. pneumoniae in 31.7% of episodes, H. influenzae in 7.6%, streptococcal species in 7.6%, and P. aeruginosa in 6.2%; smaller percentages were due to other organisms. The pneumococcus was the most common organism associated with fatal infection in these patients. Barrett-Connor (1971) reviewed retrospectively the infections in sickle cell anemia patients occurring during a period of one year at two hospitals in Dade County, Florida; these were compared with the infections experienced by blacks in the general population living in the same county. The attack rate in patients with sickle cell anemia was higher than in the controls with respect to bacterial meningitis (18.5 versus 0.06 per 1000 patient years), for pneumococcal meningitis (11.6 versus 0.02 per 1000 patient years), and for H. influenzae meningitis (3.5 versus 0.03 per 1000 patient years). Thus, the relative risk for bacterial, pneumococcal and H. influenzae-caused meningitis in patients with sickle cell

anemia ranged from 116 to 570 times higher than in the controls. Other infections such as salmonellosis, shigellosis and tuberculosis were increased in patients with sickle cell anemia when compared to the control group; however, the relative risk was between 7 and 25. The author was uncertain whether this was an artifactual increase or due to better case documentation in the sickle cell anemia patients who were subject to closer medical follow-up.

Splenectomy and chemotherapy in patients who are renal transplant recipients may create a risk for infection which is no greater than that of splenectomy for trauma alone. Bourgault et al. (1979) reported five severe pneumococcal infections in 236 patients (2.1%) who were splenectomized in conjunction with renal transplantation. None of the 57 renal transplant patients with an intact spleen developed severe pneumococcal infection during the same follow-up period, which ranged from one month to 150 months, with a mean of 34.1 months. Despite administration of immunosuppressive drugs such as azathioprine and prednisone to these patients, the rate of pneumococcal infection in the splenectomized renal transplant patients was similar to that reported in patients splenectomized because of trauma.

Other authors have reported the rates of postsplenectomy septicemia in various patient groups who underwent splenectomy for hematological and oncological disorders and trauma. The largest series was a literature review by Singer (1973) of 2795 splenectomized patients, the majority of whom were splenectomized for underlying hematological diseases such as idiopathic thrombocytopenic purpura, hereditary spherocytosis, hemolytic anemia, and thalassemia. Combining these patients with those in reports of sickle cell disease (Overturf, Powars and Baroff, 1977), splenectomized patients with Hodgkin's disease (Chilcote et al., 1976), and patients splenectomized for trauma and in association with miscellaneous abdominal surgery (Wara, 1981), the percentage of patients with postsplenectomy septicemia ranged from 1.5% in those who had suffered trauma, to 25% in patients who had undergone splenectomy for thalassemia. Ten per cent of patients with Hodgkin's disease, 15% of patients with sickle cell disease, 3.5% of patients with the miscellaneous hematological diseases, and 8.2% of those with portal hypertension were reported to have had episodes of septicemia. Mufson (1981) reported an incidence of pneumococcal infection of five to ten per 1000 patients per year in patients splenectomized for trauma. The number of fatalities due to septicemia ranged from 33 to 71% of those patients who developed septicemia. Among the 2795 patients reported by Singer (1973), 119 cases of fulminant sepsis occurred (4.3%). A total of 71 patients (representing 60% of these 119 cases and 2.5% of the total patients reported) died of fulminant septicemia. In comparison, estimated rates of culture-confirmed invasive pneumococcal disease in the general US population range from eight to 16 cases per 100 000 population (Istre et al., 1987). A normal non-splenectomized population would be expected to have an overall mortality of approximately 0.01% due to septicemia (Wara, 1981).

Rates of septicemia and mortality derived from pooled retrospective clinical series must, of course, be interpreted with caution. These figures may not reflect the true incidence rates of fulminant sepsis following splenectomy, because (1) many of the series deal primarily with infants and children who have undergone splenectomy for hematological disease, (2) data were assimilated from a variety of sources, with differing definitions of sepsis and effectiveness of follow-up, (3) the populations studied were mostly at referral hospitals, and (4) the duration of the follow-up was not taken into account in calculating the true incidence of postsplenectomy sepsis.

Schwartz et al. (1982) attempted to document accurate incidence rates of fulminant sepsis in the splenectomized population through a retrospective report of 193 persons who had undergone splenectomy between 1955 and 1979 in Rochester, Minnesota. The mean duration of follow-up was 5.6 years. Two cases of fulminant septicemia occurred during this period and only one patient died as a result of fulminant infection. Fifty-two patients had at least once serious infection in the postsplenectomy period: abscess, bacteremia and pneumonia accounted for 62 of the 78 infections. Gram-negative enteric bacilli outnumbered Gram-positive cocci as causative agents of infection in a ratio of 2.3:1. There was only one pneumococcal infection. Risk factors associated with serious infections in these splenectomized patients included irradiation, immunosuppression, and chemotherapy. These authors felt that their study reflected more accurately the prognosis of patients with a history of splenectomy in a primary care practice. The total of 78 infections resulted in an overall incidence of one infection per 14 patient-years. The infection rate, expressed as the incidence of serious infections per 100 person-years, in patients with hematological disorders was 6.5, in patients splenectomized for trauma 3.3, in patients with incidental splenectomy due to other surgery 9.6, and in patients with incidental splenectomy in association with malignant neoplasm 16.6. The highest relative risk of serious infection after splenectomy was therefore in the group with an underlying malignant neoplasm, who had undergone an incidental splenectomy. The relative distribution of microorganisms, sites of infection and mortality are radically different in this series when compared to the others. Further investigations, including a carefully followed prospective series, will be needed to resolve these differences.

12.6   SUBJECT AGE AND RISK OF INFECTION

Among patients with sickle cell anemia, the risk of infection with encapsulated bacteria appears to be highest in early life. Pearson (1977) reported that 10% of 422 patients with sickle cell anemia experienced one or more severe episodes of infection during the first five years of life. The highest number of episodes of meningitis and septicemia occurred before the age of 5 years. However, cases of osteomyelitis appeared to be equally frequent in age groups from birth to age 25 years. These authors suggested that susceptibility to encapsulated bacteria was greatest during early childhood because of a relative lack of circulating antibodies to specific serotypes of encapsulated bacteria. The development of humoral immunity to these organisms allows these patients to overcome at least partially their functional hyposplenia and opsonophagocytic defects, resulting in a lower rate of infectious episodes.

Heier (1980) summarized the findings of three series of splenectomized patients in the literature and related the age of the patients to the risk of bacterial infection. Children and infants appeared more susceptible to postsplenectomy septicemia than adults. Splenectomy between the ages of one and 16 years was associated with a frequency of serious infections of between 9 and 20%. In one series, 50% of patients splenectomized before the age of 12 months acquired serious bacterial infection, compared with 2.8% of those splenectomized after the age of 12 months (Horan and Colebatch, 1962). In another series, 8.1% of patients splenectomized before the age of 5 years developed fatal septicemia or meningitis compared with 3.3% of those splenectomized after the age of 5 years (Eraklis et al., 1967). Singer (1973) found that 21% of patients splenectomized for hereditary spherocytosis before the age of 12 months acquired serious bacterial infection, compared with 3.5% of those who were splenectomized later in life. Deaths due to infection also appear to be significantly higher in children after splenectomy. Chaikof and McCabe (1985) reported a retrospective study of patients who had undergone splenectomy between 1962 and 1972. Follow-up was available in 1982 on 637 patients: for adults, 10% of deaths overall were due to infection and two cases of fatal overwhelming postsplenectomy infection occurred (0.34%). This was significantly lower than the incidence of fatal OPSI among 53 patients who were under the age of 16 years at the time of splenectomy (3.77%).

12.7 THE RISK OF POSTSPLENECTOMY INFECTION AS A FUNCTION OF INTERVAL AFTER SPLENECTOMY

The risk of fatal overwhelming postsplenectomy infection appears to be greatest in the first two years following splenectomy (Hitzig, 1985). However, sepsis can occur more than 2 years after splenectomy. Wåhlby and Domellöf (1981) reported 10 cases of postsplenectomy sepsis occurring in 413 patients (2.4%), with a mean follow-up period of 5.9 years after splenectomy for blunt abdominal trauma. Three patients developed pneumococcal septicemia more than five years after the splenectomy, and two of these three cases had a fatal outcome. One fatal case of meningococcal septicemia occurred four years after splenectomy, and two non-fatal cases of septicemia due to H. influenzae occurred at three and four years after splenectomy.

Zarrabi and Rosner (1984) reviewed 47 published adult cases of serious bacterial infection following splenectomy for splenic trauma. The mean interval between splenectomy and serious infection was 7.2 years, with a range of six months to 31 years. Eleven patients developed serious infection within two years of the splenectomy. Four patients died of septicemia despite the presence of ectopic splenic tissue, suggesting that splenosis did not fully protect against subsequent infection. In a review of 145 episodes of postsplenectomy infection in 115 patients (53.1% between age 10 and 60 years) with Hodgkin's disease, Rosner and Zarrabi (1983) showed that 35.2% had occurred within two years of the splenectomy and 16.6% developed later; the interval following splenectomy was unknown in 48.2%. The median age at the time of occurrence of the postsplenectomy infection was 19.8 years. The median interval between splenectomy and the infectious episode was 21.9 months. It is clear, therefore, that the splenectomized patient may develop overwhelming infection long after loss of the spleen and continues to require vigilant observation.

12.8 REASONS FOR INCREASED RATES OF INFECTION IN SPLENECTOMIZED PATIENTS

Opsonization, at least in the absence of serotype specific antibody, and clearance of encapsulated bacteria are abnormal in splenectomized patients, and the underlying reasons have been investigated in both human and animal models.

An initial question is, 'What effect does splenectomy have on serum opsonizing activity?'. Winkelstein, Lambert and Swift (1975) investigated phagocytosis of *S. pneumoniae* type 25 by normal polymorphonuclear leukocytes *in vitro* in the presence of serum obtained from 24 splenectomized children, none of whom had sickle cell anemia, and from 23 age-matched controls. Pneumococcal opsonizing activity in the two groups of children was not significantly different. Nevertheless, three of the subjects who had undergone splenectomy developed pneumococcal septicemia despite having normal serum opsonizing activity for pneumococci. The two groups did not have statistically different serum titers of complement factor 3, complement factor 5, and factor B. The authors concluded that fulminant bacterial sepsis observed in children after surgical splenectomy cannot be attributed to deficient pneumococcal serum opsonizing activity. The authors do not report whether or not their subjects were seropositive for the type 25 pneumococcus used in their study. Presumably they had serum antibody to this pneumococcal serotype which resulted in the finding of normal opsonization. An interesting corollary to their findings is that the autosplenectomy which occurs in children with sickle cell anemia probably does not account completely for the decreased pneumococcal serum opsonizing activity seen in sickle cell anemia patients. This decreased activity is due in part to defective

alternative pathway function (Johnston, Newman and Struth, 1973).

Clearance of bacteremia appears in part to be dependent upon an intact alternative complement pathway. In a guinea-pig model, Brown, Hosea and Frank (1983) compared the clearance of an intravenous bolus of *S. pneumoniae* type 7 in normal animals which were non-immune, animals which were complement factor 4 deficient, and animals which had been treated with cobra venom factor, which causes a consumption of the alternative complement pathway and complement factors 3 through 9. They found that in non-immune animals with an intact spleen, alternative pathway activation played a critical role in host defense and clearance of pneumococcal bacteremia. Of the three groups, only the animals which had deficient alternative pathway activity were unable to clear the intravenous pneumococcal challenge. Intravascular clearance of *S. pneumoniae* was then investigated in normal non-immune guinea pigs and those which had been splenectomized. Clearance was significantly impaired in those animals which were splenectomized; however, the clearance deficit was more severe in those animals challenged with a more virulent strain of pneumococcus (serotype 12) than with a less virulent strain (serotype 7). A rough strain of *S. pneumoniae* (unencapsulated) was cleared equally well in those animals which were splenectomized and the normal non-immune guinea pigs. The better clearance of the less virulent strains in splenectomized guinea pigs appears to be related to better hepatic sequestration of the organisms. The more virulent the pneumococcal strain, the more likely the host was to sequester the pneumococcus preferentially in the spleen. Thus, splenectomized animals were less able to clear the most virulent pneumococcal serotype, because the normal host response is to direct the organism to the spleen for removal from the blood stream by filtration and phagocytosis.

Type-specific humoral immunity affects intravascular clearance patterns. Brown, Hosea and Frank (1983) further compared sequestration patterns in non-immune guinea pigs and immune guinea pigs which were intravenously challenged with radiolabeled *S. pneumoniae*. Immunization against the challenge pneumococcal strain resulted in increased hepatic sequestration of the radiolabeled pneumococci in both normal guinea pigs and those deficient in complement factor 4. The change in sequestration patterns, with preferential sequestration in the liver induced by immunization, was blocked by administration of cobra venom factor which consumed the alternative pathway and C3 through C9 complement factors. Other studies by Hosea *et al*.. (1981a) have investigated the differential clearance of particles from the blood by liver and spleen, by measuring the half-life of IgG-sensitized erythrocyte clearance in normal human volunteers, splenectomized patients, and splenectomized patients who received highly sensitized erythrocytes. There was a significant delay in the rate of clearance in splenectomized patients when compared with normal subjects with an intact spleen; however, the use of highly sensitized erythrocytes resulted in a marked improvement in the rate of clearance in the splenectomized patients. Erythrocytes sensitized with IgG antibody are cleared by the reticuloendothelial system rather than by intravascular hemolysis; hepatic clearance must occur with a shorter contact time between the particle and the macrophage than is the case in the spleen, and appears to require a higher concentration of surface antibody on the red cell to be effective. Consequently higher levels of antibody binding are necessary for the hepatic sequestration of blood-borne particles. Splenectomized patients lack the splenic macrophages, which are able to clear bacteria coated with only small amounts of IgG from the blood stream, and they are unable to mount a sufficient antibody response for liver macrophages to overcome the defect (Hosea, 1983).

Pneumococcal polysaccharide encapsulation is anti-phagocytic: the bacterium must be phagocytosed to be killed, but the capsule must be neutralized first. Pneumococcal polysaccharide activates the alternate complement pathway, resulting in C3b binding to the bacterial cell surface and clearance of organisms. Coating of the organisms with C3b, however, does not by itself lead to ingestion of the organisms by phagocytes. Consequently the clearance of these C3b-coated particles is only transient and the organisms are released back into the blood stream in splenectomized, non-immune patients (Hosea, 1983). In patients with pre-existing antibody to specific pneumococcal serotype, antibodies attached to the capsular wall of the pneumococci cause activation of the classical complement pathway and attachment of C3b molecules to the surface of the bacteria. The presence of antibody on the surface of the bacteria improves Fc-mediated hepatic macrophage clearance of the opsonized pneumococci. Thus, the complement system in splenectomized patients and in those patients with splenic hypofunction in the absence of sickle cell anemia, seems to be intact, and in the presence of serotype specific opsonizing antibody, these patients are better able to defend against challenge with encapsulated organisms.

Other encapsulated organisms have been studied in animal models of hyposplenism. Chen and Moxon (1983) investigated the susceptibility of rats to *H. influenzae* type b challenge in the presence of phenylhydrazine-induced hemolytic anemia. This experimental model of hemolytic anemia results in splenic congestion and a decreased filtering capacity of the spleen, probably due to a decrease in both the open pulp circulation and total splenic blood flow. The phenylhydrazine-treated rats developed levels of bacteremia which were ten times greater than those of control rats, after intranasal inoculation of *H. influenzae* type b; the anemic rats also had a higher mortality after intravenous bacterial challenge than controls. Moxon, Goldthorn and Schwartz (1980) challenged surgically splenectomized rats with *H. influenzae* type b and found the LD_{50} after intravenous administration to be $10^{4.6}$ bacteria, and after intranasal inoculation to be $10^{4.7}$ bacteria. Both doses were significantly lower than in sham-operated rats, which were $10^{8.6}$ and $10^{9.0}$ bacteria respectively. The phenylhydrazine-treated rats of Chen and Moxon (1983) all died after intravenous injection of 5×10^7 bacteria at the nadir of their anemia, but an LD_{50} was not determined. As a result, it is difficult to assess the degree of splenic hypofunction induced by splenic congestion during hemolytic anemia as compared to surgical asplenia. These studies support the concept that the spleen is important in the host immune response to *H. influenzae* infection. The phenylhydrazine-induced hemolytic anemia model shows that splenic congestion, such as that seen during sickle cell crisis, is a contributing factor to reduced host resistance to encapsulated bacteria. However, when anemia is not associated with splenic congestion, it does not result in similar degrees of splenic hypofunction.

The effect of splenectomy on the host response to challenge with unencapsulated bacteria, such as *E. coli*, is less well studied in animal models. Almdahl *et al.* (1987) found that bacteremia following intraperitoneal and intravenous injection of *E. coli* was significantly prolonged in splenectomized rats, when compared to the effect in sham-operated control animals.

Another important immunological defect noted in patients splenectomized for various underlying diseases is consistently low serum IgM antibody levels. This has been present in many studies reporting mean serum IgM antibody levels, when compared to the values in normal subjects and in those with the same underlying disease, but with an intact spleen (Krivit, 1977). However, the clinical significance of reduced levels of serum IgM is uncertain at this time, since the efficiency of IgM antibody in opsonizing pneumococci is significantly less than that of IgG.

12.9 THE PROTECTION OF THE SPLENECTOMIZED PATIENT FROM ENCAPSULATED BACTERIAL INFECTIONS

Strategies for protection from, and early treatment of, severe bacterial infection in splenectomized patients have been suggested in the literature (Table 12.3). Vaccination against encapsulated organisms such as *H. influenzae* type b (at least in children, with *Haemophilus* type b polysaccharide-diphtheria toxoid conjugate vaccine), *N. meningitidis* (meningococcal polysaccharide vaccine, Groups A, C, Y, and W-135 combined) and *S. pneumoniae* (23-valent capsular polysaccharide vaccine) is indicated prior to elective splenectomy, and should also be given to those patients who have already undergone splenectomy, if not already administered. The clearest indication for *Haemophilus* type b conjugate vaccine is in children between the ages of 18 months and 5 years (Centers for Disease Control, 1988). However, the conjugate vaccine (20 µg of polyribosephosphate per 0.5 ml IM dose) has been found to be safe and immunogenic in normal healthy adults (Granoff, Boies, and Munson, 1984; Lepow, Samuelson and Gordon, 1984). Administration of conjugate vaccine to hyposplenic adults should be strongly considered.

If chemotherapy is in prospect, vaccination should be given beforehand. Since splenic irradiation with more than 3000 rads results in hyposplenia, vaccination should be accomplished prior to the start of treatment. Chronic oral antibiotic prophylaxis with agents such as penicillin, amoxicillin, or trimethoprim-sulfamethoxazole has been advocated during the

Table 12.3 Measures which may protect the splenectomized patient from overwhelming sepsis

1. Vaccination against:
   Streptococcus pneumoniae
   Haemophilus influenzae type b
   Neisseria meningitidis
2. Oral antibiotic prophylaxis
3. Preservation of splenic tissue
4. Provision of medical identification bracelet
5. Early institution of therapeutic parenteral antibiotics during infection

first two to three years after splenectomy because of the higher number of infections which occur during the early years following splenectomy. However, patients with Hodgkin's disease have developed postsplenectomy sepsis with pneumococcal serotypes contained in the pneumococcal vaccine while receiving penicillin prophylaxis. Poor compliance with the antibiotic regimen, pneumococcal resistance, and failure to cover other causes of overwhelming infection reduce the effectiveness of chronic antibiotic prophylaxis. Surgical preservation of splenic tissue, whenever possible, would be a desirable goal. An identification bracelet alerting health care professionals to the presence of the postsplenectomy state is advisable, as this may help in the institution of appropriately early empirical antibiotic treatment.

Given the high fatality rate of bacterial septicemia in splenectomized patients, it is prudent to institute therapeutic empirical antibiotic treatment early in the course of nondescript febrile illness in the hope that mortality can be reduced. Whether this goal is actually achieved by this form of therapy is unclear. Therapeutic regimens chosen empirically at the time of presentation might include a third generation cephalosporin such as parenterally administered cefotaxime or ceftriaxone. These agents are effective in the treatment of both bacteremia and meningitis, and use of these two antibiotics assures activity against the encapsulated organisms most likely to cause infection in splenectomized patients, including penicillin-resistant pneumococci (with minimum inhibitory concentration >1.0 μg/ml) and moderately susceptible S. pneumoniae (with minimum inhibitory concentration between 0.1 μg/ml to 1.0 μg/ml) as well as β-lactamase producing, ampicillin-resistant H. influenzae (Istre et al., 1987). Once the causative organism is isolated and characterized, a narrower spectrum antimicrobial agent such as penicillin or ampicillin can be substituted, when appropriate. In the patient with significant penicillin allergy, chloramphenicol is empirically the drug of choice.

In subsequent sections, evidence supporting these strategies for protection against overwhelming bacterial sepsis in the splenectomized patient will be described.

12.9.1 IMMUNIZATION AGAINST ENCAPSULATED ORGANISMS

The serological response to pneumococcal polysaccharide vaccine has been studied in both animals and humans. In rabbits and mice, the spleen is the primary site of early antibody formation after immunization with pneumococcal polysaccharide antigen. Splenectomy removes most of the lymphocytes that initially respond to antigenic stimulation by polysaccharide antigens. The magnitude of the response to the polysaccharide antigen is possibly affected in these circumstances by normal T-cell suppressor activity, but abnormally low T-cell helper activity (Hosea et al., 1981b; Jones, Amsbaugh and Prescott, 1976). Hosea et al. (1981b) investigated serum IgM and IgG antibody responses measured by ELISA to pneumococcal vaccine in nine normal and nine splenectomized human volunteers: of the latter, four had no disease, three had idiopathic thrombocytopenic purpura, and there were two with idiopathic hemolytic anemia requiring cytotoxic treatment. It was found that significantly higher post-vaccination serum IgM antibody titers developed to all nine pneumococcal serotypes tested in the normal volunteers, when compared to the splenectomized patients. There were also higher serum IgG antibody titers to seven of the nine tested pneumococcal serotypes, in the normal subjects when compared to splenectomized patients.

Ammann et al. (1977) compared the responses to pneumococcal polysaccharide immunization in young subjects aged 2 to 25 years. Nineteen patients with congenital or surgical asplenia developed serum antibody responses measured by indirect hemagglutination which were not statistically different from those of 38 normal children. A group of 68 patients with homozygous sickle cell disease, seven with sickle cell thalassemia and two with hemoglobin SD disease developed serum antibody responses to the pneumococcal polysaccharide vaccine which were likewise not statistically different from those of 44 healthy African children. In this study, therefore, a humoral response developed to the pneumococcal polysaccharide vaccine antigens in patients with sickle cell disease and in asplenic patients.

The response to pneumococcal polysaccharide vaccine in patients with Hodgkin's disease has also been studied. Siber *et al.* (1978) evaluated the antibody response of patients with Hodgkin's disease to polysaccharide vaccine after splenectomy and completion of radiation therapy and chemotherapy. The antibody response was impaired, but was relatively normal in those given the polysaccharide vaccine three and four years after cessation of chemotherapy. Addiego *et al.* (1980) evaluated the serum antibody response to pneumococcal polysaccharide vaccine in 16 normal controls and 27 patients with Hodgkin's disease prior to radiation and/ or chemotherapy, and either before or after splenectomy. The pneumococcal vaccine was administered 48–72 hours before splenectomy or after staging laparotomy and splenectomy. Serum antibody levels to pneumococcal serotypes were measured using indirect hemagglutination and radioimmunoassay methods. The proportion of fourfold serum antibody responders was not significantly different between the two patient groups. In fact, the mean post-immunization antibody levels to pneumococcal polysaccharide antigen were all greater than 300 ng of antibody nitrogen per ml of serum, which are levels thought to be protective. No significant difference in serum antibody response was noted when stage I and II Hodgkin's disease patients were compared to stage III and IV Hodgkin's disease patients. Also, there was no significant difference in response when the vaccine was administered 48–72 hours prior to splenectomy compared to administration during the three to five day period post-splenectomy.

Sullivan *et al.* (1978) investigated the route of immunization in patients who had been splenectomized in comparison to normal controls and patients with Hodgkin's disease. Intravenously administered bacteriophage ØX174 produced a good primary and secondary serum antibody response in normal controls; however, the primary response was not adequate in the five asplenic patients with Hodgkin's disease. The secondary response was better in these patients, but still abnormal when compared to the normal controls, except in the one Hodgkin's disease patient who had stage IA disease and had not received chemotherapy. Among patients who were asplenic but did not have Hodgkin's disease, there was significantly decreased serum IgG antibody formation after secondary immunization with bacteriophage compared to the normal controls. This suggested to the authors that switching of the antibody class from IgM to IgG production was not normal in their asplenic patients. These results confirmed previous studies showing deficient antibody response to intravenously administered heterologous red blood cells in anatomically and functionally asplenic individuals (Rowley, 1950; Schwartz and Pearson, 1972).

The geometric mean antibody response (by radioimmunoassay) to subcutaneously injected capsular polysaccharide antigens in 26 asplenic individuals without Hodgkin's disease was not significantly different from the response of 27 normal control patients with intact spleens. The geometric mean antibody titer in the four patients with Hodgkin's disease who had received chemotherapy and radiotherapy did not rise significantly compared to preimmunization levels; however, the antibody response in the one Hodgkin's disease patient who had not received chemotherapy was comparable to normal controls and significantly higher than preimmunization antibody level (Sullivan *et al.*, 1978).

These studies support the concept that the spleen is necessary for normal immune response to blood-borne antigens, but that other parenteral routes of immunization, such as the subcutaneous, circumvent the need for the splenic immune response. They also support the concept that chemotherapy significantly reduces the response to subsequent immunization with parenteral polysaccharide antigen vaccines.

Siber *et al.* (1986) investigated the serum antibody response to immunization with various capsular polysaccharide antigens in patients with Hodgkin's disease who received chemotherapy and between 3500 and 4000 rads to the spleen, as well as mantle and para-aortic node distributions. The serum antibody response in these patients was compared to that of asplenic controls who did not receive chemotherapy and did not have Hodgkin's disease, and also to healthy controls. All patients received 14-valent pneumococcal polysaccharide vaccine, *H. influenzae* type b capsular polysaccharide vaccine, and meningococcal group C vaccine. Three to four weeks after vaccination, serum antibody levels to meningococcal group C polysaccharide antigen were significantly lower in patients with Hodgkin's disease whether they had received radiation, chemotherapy or both, when compared to the asplenic controls and healthy normal controls. The serum antibody response to capsular polysaccharides of *H. influenzae* type b and *S. pneumoniae* were not significantly different in patients with Hodgkin's disease compared to asplenic controls and healthy controls. These authors found that only the interval between immunization and the start of chemotherapy correlated with the antibody response. Those patients who began bimodal therapy or chemotherapy alone less than 10 to 14 days after immunization had a lower mean serum antibody response to pneumococcal antigen.

Timing of immunization relative to splenectomy had no apparent effect on serum antibody levels (Siber *et al.*, 1986). In patients with Hodgkin's disease, those immunized two days prior to splenectomy had similar antibody levels when compared to those immunized on the day of surgery and those receiving pneumococcal vaccine within two days of splenectomy. During subsequent follow-up, serum antibody levels declined significantly more in those patients treated with both chemotherapy and radiation compared to the asplenic and healthy controls. A booster immunization given three months after the completion of chemotherapy in Hodgkin's disease patients resulted in no significant change in serum antibody levels.

Ruben *et al.* (1984) investigated the serum IgM and IgG antibody responses to bivalent meningococcal groups A and C polysaccharide vaccine given intramuscularly to healthy control subjects and patients who had been splenectomized for trauma, lymphoid tumor or non-lymphoid tumor. The only antibody responses which were significantly lower, in terms of the number of responding subjects, were the IgM responses to group A and group C meningococcal antigens in the patients with underlying lymphoid tumor. They also had significantly lower mean levels of both IgM and IgG antibodies in the post-vaccination serum specimens, when compared to normal controls. Those who had undergone splenectomy for trauma had a serum antibody response which was nearly the same as that of controls. The authors recommended routine administration of meningococcal vaccine to patients without a spleen or with splenic hypofunction.

The humoral antibody response to pneumococcal polysaccharide vaccine is encouraging; however, whether this humoral immunity prevents subsequent pneumococcal septicemia is not entirely clear (Brivet *et al.*, 1984; Evans, 1984; Giebink *et al.*, 1979; Sumaya *et al.*, 1981). Vaccine efficacy was evident in the study by Ammann *et al.* (1977). Two year follow-up of their patients revealed the occurrence of eight *S. pneumoniae* infections (all septicemias) in unimmunized sickle cell disease patients but no pneumococcal infection in the sickle cell disease group immunized with pneumococcal vaccine ($P < 0.025$).

Hebert *et al.* (1983) compared the cumulative mortality after challenge with aerosolized pneumococci in three groups of CD-1 mice. The first group of mice was first splenectomized and then vaccinated intraperitoneally with type 3 pneumococcal vaccine. The second group received the same pneumococcal vaccine and then seven days later was splenectomized; the third group received the vaccine followed by sham operation. When challenged with aerosolized pneumococci of the same serotype seven days later, the mice subjected to early splenectomy had a significantly higher mortality. The authors concluded that asplenic individuals may have impaired immunological responses and increased susceptibility to infection, and that pneumococcal vaccines should be given before elective splenectomy, since the group of mice given the vaccine seven days before splenectomy had a cumulative mortality which was not significantly different from the group of vaccinated normal mice.

Vaccination with polysaccharide antigen preparations should be accomplished as early as possible, and at least one to two weeks prior to planned splenectomy. However, if vaccination was not achieved before splenectomy, there will still be a humoral response with later administration. The serum antibody response will be poor if the vaccine is administered earlier than the age of two years whether or not a normal spleen is present, and if administered after chemotherapy and splenic irradiation. While it is apparent from the literature that type specific serum antibody should improve hepatic macrophage clearance of bacteremia, the literature does contain reports of cases in which pneumococcal vaccine was unsuccessful in preventing serious infection with vaccine serotypes (Brivet et al., 1984; Evans, 1984; Giebink et al., 1979; Sumaya et al., 1981).

12.9.2   ANTIBIOTIC PROPHYLAXIS

No large series or controlled study effectively demonstrates penicillin prophylaxis to be effective in the prevention of overwhelming postsplenectomy infections. However, there are several recommendations in the literature to the effect that oral penicillin should be given, at least during the first two years after splenectomy, and particularly in children. Whether amoxicillin or trimethoprim-sulfamethoxazole should be used instead for their activity against *H. influenzae*, particularly in children under the age of 5 years, has not been definitively studied. An alternative to oral penicillin prophylaxis is depot-penicillin injection on a monthly basis (Case records, 1983; Dickerman, 1979; Francke and Neu, 1981; Sherman, 1981). Trimethoprim-sulfamethoxazole or erythromycin prophylaxis have been recommended as substitutes for patients allergic to penicillin. However, in addition to the evidence that oral prophylaxis is effective, there are a number of disadvantages to prophylactic penicillin administration: these include noncompliance by patients and inadequate dosage, failure to achieve activity against all the organisms commonly responsible for overwhelming postsplenectomy infections, and induction of penicillin-resistant pneumococcal strains in patients taking this antibiotic. Cases of overwhelming pneumococcal infection have been reported in asplenic patients taking penicillin, and have led to further uncertainty regarding the efficacy of chronic penicillin prophylaxis (Brivet et al., 1984; Evans, 1984). Zarrabi and Rosner (1986) reviewed 14 reported cases of postsplenectomy sepsis in patients who regularly took penicillin prophylaxis. All but one were less than 17 years old and splenectomy had been done for various indications, including Hodgkin's disease in nine patients. In six patients, the sepsis was due to bacteria other than pneumococcus. These authors concluded that failure of penicillin prophylaxis is, in fact, rare.

However, there are additional reasons for questioning the usefulness of prolonged oral penicillin prophylaxis, of which the principal is the potential for poor compliance. Buchanan et al. (1982) studied compliance with an oral penicillin prophylactic regimen in patients splenectomized for miscellaneous conditions, and in a group with homozygous sickle cell anemia. Compliance was monitored by testing for the presence of penicillin in urine; in these two groups, 72% and 64% respectively of the urine samples collected showed the presence of penicillin. These authors felt that compliance tended to improve after reinforcement of the recommendations during follow-up clinic visits. Borgna-Pignatti *et al.* (1984) found a similar rate of compliance with penicillin prophylaxis in splenectomized thalassemics (79%).

Scher, Wroczynski and Jones (1983) investigated the effect of penicillin administered to splenectomized rats one hour prior to intraperitoneal injection of *S. pneumoniae* type 3. Sham-operated control rats, and animals which were splenectomized and given pneumococcal vaccine two weeks after splenectomy, were both protected significantly better than other groups of rats in the study. The resolution of bacteremia was significantly better in these two groups than in (1) rats in which the only intervention was splenectomy, (2) splenectomized rats given 5000 units of penicillin, and (3) splenectomized rats given 300 000 units of penicillin, one hour prior to the challenge with pneumococci. This suggests that the effectiveness of penicillin prophylaxis may be significantly less than has previously been suggested.

The use of oral penicillin prophylaxis in the splenectomized patient is controversial. Prophylaxis may be most efficacious in childhood and during the first two years following splenectomy. An alternative approach to the use of prolonged oral antibiotic prophylaxis is the institution of therapeutic antibiotics parenterally at the first sign of febrile illness. It has been recommended that any splenectomized patient should have penicillin available for oral administration at the time of onset of febrile illness, and that these patients should be promptly evaluated by a physician for any illness accompanied by a temperature greater than 102°F (Sherman, 1981).

12.9.3   GAMMA-GLOBULIN AND IMMUNOSTIMULATORS

Another suggested approach to the early treatment of severe pneumococcal infection in splenectomized individuals is the parenteral administration of human gamma-globulin. No human studies have been reported, but Offenbartl *et al.* (1986b) found that splenectomized rats receiving human gamma-globulin (Sandoglobulin^R) intravenously, after intravenous challenge with *S. pneumoniae* type 1, showed a significantly better survival than did animals receiving intravenous human albumin after the pneumococcal challenge. This suggests a new option for the treatment of overwhelming post-splenectomy infection. Offenbartl *et al.* (1986a) also demonstrated that the human gamma-globulin preparation administered to splenectomized rats 24 hours before pneumococcal challenge reduces mortality. Reduction in mortality with doses lower than 37.5 mg/kg of gamma-globulin occurred only when combined with penicillin treatment given 18 hours after pneumococcal challenge. Penicillin treatment alone did not reduce mortality. It is apparent, therefore, that a synergistic effect occurred between prophylactic gamma-globulin in a subprotective dose and penicillin treatment. This suggests that even relatively low concentrations of antibody, such as those remaining in the circulation weeks after the infusion, might be clinically relevant. A potential advantage with this preparation in humans is the avoidance of serum sickness which occurs with the administration of animal hyperimmune sera. Further trials are needed to assess the clinical implications of these animal studies in man.

Immunostimulators may eventually prove useful in protection of the splenectomized host. Almdahl *et al.* (1987) found that semisoluble aminated glucan injected intraperitoneally before or after splenectomy protected rats from experimental intraperitoneal and intravenous challenge with *E. coli*. The duration of bacteremia was also shorter than in control animals. Semisoluble aminated glucan stimulates macrophages both *in vitro* and *in vivo*, and enhances the intraperitoneal macrophage entrapment and degradation of *E. coli*. It may also stimulate bacterial clearance mechanisms at extraperitoneal sites. Browder *et al.* (1983) also reported improved survival among splenecto-mized mice given intravenous glucan and challenged with pneumococci introduced intranasally. Further studies are needed to establish the therapeutic potential of this approach to producing improved resistance to infection in splenectomized subjects.

12.9.4 PRESERVATION OF SPLENIC TISSUE

Preservation of splenic tissue by partial (instead of total) splenectomy, splenic autotransplants or ectopic splenic tissue may also preserve splenic function (see also Chapter 18). Traub *et al.* (1987) reported that reticuloendothelial function (measured by the mean percentage of pocked erythrocytes and the clearance of antibody-coated autologous erythrocytes) was better preserved after partial splenectomy and splenic repair than after splenic autotransplantation, but that autotransplantation was superior to total splenectomy in a series of 51 patients who had initially presented with abdominal trauma and suspected splenic rupture. However, there is evidence that the presence of splenic tissue is not in itself a guarantee of efficient splenic function (Sass *et al.*, 1983). Preservation of the splenic artery and normal splenic architecture appear to be of great importance to the maintenance of effective splenic function; this is shown by cases of fatal pneumococcal septicemia occurring after splenectomy for trauma in patients found at autopsy to have numerous nodules of splenic tissue present in the peritoneal cavity (Rice and James, 1980).

Animal studies have been used to test various methods of preserving splenic function. Livingston, Levine and Sirinek (1983) challenged rats with a transtracheal inoculation of *S. pneumoniae* type 3 after one of the following procedures: (1) sham operation, (2) splenectomy with splenic implants within the mesentery or portal vein splenic autotransplantation, and (3) splenectomy without transplantation of splenic tissue to other sites. Pneumococcal challenge was administered 12 weeks after the splenectomy: it was found that rats submitted to sham operation had a significantly lower mortality rate than did rats which were splenectomized, with or without subsequent portal vein splenic autotransplants. The rats with mesenteric splenic autotransplants, however, had a mortality rate similar to that of sham-operated rats, showing that this type of splenic implant may have been protective. It was therefore suggested that peritoneal implants after trauma in humans may result in a lower rate of postsplenectomy sepsis for this particular group. However, Schwartz *et al.* (1978) found that autotransplantation of macerated splenic tissue into the peritoneal cavity of splenectomized rats did not significantly protect these animals from intravenous challenge with *S. pneumoniae* type 25. The LD_{50} for the autotransplanted rats and for asplenic rats was less than 4×10^3 colony-forming units of bacteria, and all the animals in these two groups died. The LD_{50} for the control sham-operated rats was 8×10^6 colony-forming units and none of the rats receiving 4×10^5 colony-forming units in this group of controls died as a result of the intravenous pneumococcal challenge. Thus, there remains some controversy regarding the effectiveness of filtration by small peritoneal splenic implants.

Alwmark *et al.* (1983) found that rats with a two-thirds splenic resection had a lower mortality rate when challenged with *S. pneumoniae* type 1 intravenously, than did rats which were splenectomized and subsequently had splenic tissue implanted either subcutaneously or into the omentum, or had dispersed splenic tissue injected subcutaneously, intramuscularly or retroperitoneally. They found that there was a lesser degree of splenic tissue regeneration in those animals which were injected with dispersed splenic tissue than in those in which pieces of splenic tissue were implanted. This suggested that preservation of the splenic microarchitecture might be important for tissue regeneration. In addition, they found that rats with pieces of splenic tissue reimplanted had a significantly longer median survival than rats with reimplantation of dispersed splenic tissue. Steely *et al.* (1987) reported a decrease in the incidence of septic death following pneumococcal I.V. challenge in rats which underwent splenectomy and omental splenic autotransplantation, partial splenectomy, or sham operation, compared with those animals which underwent total splenectomy. Diminished mortality and the reduced incidence of *S. pneumoniae* bacteremia were dependent on the amount of splenic remnant present in the respective groups of rats. Van Wyck, Witte and Witte (1986) found that subtotal splenic resection with preservation of blood flow and the segmental anatomy of the spleen resulted in better survival in the face of pneumococcal challenge, than occurred in rats subjected to total splenectomy and splenic autografting.

In summary, it appears from this work with animal models, that preservation of a portion of the spleen, preferably with arterial structures and splenic architecture intact, would be desirable whenever practicable in the treatment of patients requiring splenic resection. Indeed, Boles, Haase and Hamoudi (1978) have reported encouraging results with respect to partial splenectomy during staging laparotomy of patients with Hodgkin's disease and found no evidence that evaluation of splenic involvement was compromised. There is still a pressing need for further data to assess the indications for partial splenectomy in this and other hematological diseases, and to partial splenectomy and repair of the spleen (splenorrhaphy) in other situations, such as splenic rupture and lacerations, commonly treated by total splenectomy (Werbin and Lodha, 1982). Further discussion of the surgical approach is given in Chapter 18.

REFERENCES

Abrams, D. I. *et al.* (1986) Antibodies to human T-lymphotropic virus type III and development of the acquired immunodeficiency syndrome in homosexual men presenting with immune thrombocytopenia. *Ann. Intern. Med.*, **104**, 47–50.

Addiego, J. E. Jr *et al.* (1980) Response to pneumococcal polysaccharide vaccine in patients with untreated Hodgkin's disease. *Lancet*, **ii**, 450–3.

Adler, S. P. (1983) Transfusion-associated cytomegalovirus infections. *Rev. Infect. Dis.*, **5**, 977–93.

Almdahl, S. *et al.* (1987) The effect of splenectomy on *Escherichia coli* sepsis and its treatment with semisoluble aminated glucan. *Scand. J. Gastroenterol.*, **22**, 261–7.

Alwmark, A. *et al.* (1983) Splenic resection or heterotopic transplantation of splenic tissue as alternatives to splenectomy. *Eur. Surg. Res.*, **15**, 217–22.

Ammann, A. J. *et al.* (1977) Polyvalent pneumococcal-polysaccharide immunization of patients with sickle-cell anemia and patients with splenectomy. *N. Engl. J. Med.*, **297**, 897–900.

Askergren, J. and Björkholm, M. (1980) Postsplenectomy septicaemia in Hodgkin's disease and other disorders. *Acta Chir. Scand.*, **146**, 569–75.

Austin, T. W., Sargeant, H. L. and Warwick, O. H. (1980) Fulminant gonococcaemia after splenectomy. *Can. Med. Assoc. J.*, **123**, 195–6.

Barbour, A. G. *et al.* (1979) Kawasaki-like disease in a young adult: association with primary Epstein–Barr virus infection. *J. Am. Med. Assoc.*, **241**, 397–8.

Barbui, T. *et al.* (1987) Does splenectomy enhance risk of AIDS in HIV-positive patients with chronic thrombocytopenia? *Lancet*, **ii**, 342–3.

Barrett-Connor, E. (1971) Bacterial infection and sickle cell anemia. An analysis of 250 infections in 166 patients and a review of the literature. *Medicine*, **50**, 97–112.

Baumgartner, J. D. *et al.* (1982) Severe cytomegalovirus infection in multiply transfused, splenectomised, trauma patients. *Lancet*, **ii**, 63–6.

Bisno, A. L. and Freeman, J. C. (1970) The syndrome of asplenia, pneumococcal sepsis, and disseminated intravascular coagulation. *Ann. Intern. Med.*, **72**, 389–93.

Boles, E. T., Jr., Haase, G. M. and Hamoudi, A.B. (1978) Partial splenectomy in staging laparotomy for Hodgkin's disease: An alternative approach. *J. Pediatr. Surg.*, **13**, 581–6.

Borgna-Pignatti, C. *et al.* (1984) Penicillin compliance in splenectomised thalassemics. *Eur. J. Pediatr.*, **142**, 83–5.

Bourgault, A. M. *et al.* (1979) Severe infection due to *Streptococcus pneumoniae* in asplenic renal transplant patients. *Mayo Clin. Proc.*, **54**, 123–6.

Brivet, F. *et al.* (1984) Fatal post-splenectomy pneumococcal sepsis despite pneumococcal vaccine and penicillin prophylaxis. *Lancet*, **ii**, 356–7.

Browder, W. *et al.* (1983) Protective effect of non-specific immunostimulation in postsplenectomy sepsis. *J. Surg. Res.*, **35**, 474–9.

Brown, E. J., Hosea, S. W. and Frank, M. M. (1983) The role of antibody and complement in the reticuloendothelial clearance of pneumococci from the bloodstream. *Rev. Infect. Dis.*, **5** (Suppl.), S797–S805.

Buchanan, G. R. *et al.* (1982) Oral penicillin prophylaxis in children with impaired splenic function: A study of compliance. *Pediatrics*, **70**, 926–30.

Buchanan, G. R. *et al.* (1983) Bacterial infection and splenic reticuloendothelial function in children with hemoglobin SC disease. *Pediatrics*, **72**, 93–8.

Case Records of the Massachusetts General Hospital, Case 20–1983. (1983) *N. Engl. J. Med.*, **308**, 1212–18.

Centers for Disease Control (1988) Recommendations of the Immunization Practices Advisory Committee (ACIP). Update: Prevention of *Haemophilus influenzae* type b disease. *Morbidity and Mortality Weekly Report (MMWR)*, **37**, 13–16.

Chaikof, E. L. and McCabe, C. J. (1985) Fatal overwhelming postsplenectomy infection. *Am. J. Surg.*, **149**, 534–9.

Chen, L. T. and Moxon, E. R. (1983) Effect of splenic congestion associated with hemolytic anemia on mortality of rats challenged with *Haemophilus influenzae* b. *Am. J. Hematol.*, **15**, 117–21.

Chilcote, R. R. *et al.* (1976) Septicemia and meningitis in children splenectomized for Hodgkin's disease. *N. Engl. J. Med.*, **295**, 798–800.

Coleman, C. N. *et al.* (1982) Functional hyposplenia after splenic irradiation for Hodgkin's disease. *Ann. Intern. Med.*, **96**, 44–7.

Coleman, R. M. *et al.* (1975) Splenic mediated erythrocyte cytotoxicity in malaria. *Immunology*, **29**, 49–54.

Curti, A. J., Lin, J. H. and Szabo, K. (1985) Overwhelming post-splenectomy infection with *Plesiomonas shigelloides* in a patient cured of Hodgkin's disease. *Am. J. Clin. Pathol.*, **83**, 522–4.

Dailey, M. O., Coleman, C. N. and Kaplan, H. S. (1980) Radiation-induced splenic atrophy in patients with Hodgkin's disease and non-Hodgkin's lymphomas. *N. Engl. J. Med.*, **302**, 215–17.

Dammin, G. J. *et al.* (1981) The rising incidence of clinical *Babesia microti* infection. *Hum. Pathol.*, **12**, 398–400.

Dickerman, J. D. (1979) Splenectomy and sepsis: A warning. *Pediatrics*, **63**, 938–41.

Eichner, E. R. (1979) Splenic function: normal, too much and too little. *Am. J. Med.*, **66**, 311–20.

Eraklis, A. J. *et al.* (1967) Hazard of overwhelming infection after splenectomy in childhood. *N. Engl. J. Med.*, **276**, 1225–9.

Evans, D. I. K. (1984) Fatal post-splenectomy sepsis despite prophylaxis with penicillin and pneumococcal vaccine. *Lancet*, **i**, 1124.

Foster, K. J. *et al.* (1982) Overwhelming pneumococcal septicaemia in a patient with ulcerative colitis and splenic atrophy. *Gut*, **23**, 630–2.

Foster, P. N., Hardy, G. J. and Losowsky, M. S. (1984) Fatal salmonella septicaemia in a patient with systemic lupus erythematosus and splenic atrophy. *Br. J. Clin. Pract.*, **38**, 434–5.

Francke, E. L. and Neu, H. C. (1981) Postsplenectomy infection. *Surg. Clin. North. Am.*, **61**, 135–55.

Giebink, G. S. *et al.* (1979) Vaccine-type pneumococcal pneumonia; occurrence after vaccination in an asplenic patient. *J. Am. Med. Assoc.*, **241**, 2736–7.

Goffinet, D. R., Glatstein, E. J. and Merigan, T. C. (1972) Herpes zoster-varicella infections and lymphoma. *Ann. Intern. Med.*, **76**, 235–40.

Granoff, D. M., Boies, E. G. and Munson, R. S., Jr (1984) Immunogenicity of *Haemophilus influenzae* type b polysaccharide-diphtheria toxoid conjugate vaccine in adults. *J. Pediatr.*, **105**, 22–7.

Green, D. M. *et al.* (1979) The incidence of postsplenectomy sepsis and herpes zoster in children and adolescents with Hodgkin disease. *Med. Pediatr. Oncol.*, **7**, 285–97.

Green, J. B. *et al.* (1986) Late septic complications in adults following splenectomy for trauma: A prospective analysis in 144 patients. *J. Trauma*, **26**, 999–1003.

Guinee, V. F. *et al.* (1985) The incidence of herpes zoster in patients with Hodgkin's disease, an analysis of prognostic factors. *Cancer*, **56**, 642–8.

Hebert, J. C. *et al.* (1983) Lack of protection by pneumococcal vaccine after splenectomy in mice challenged with aerosolized pneumococci. *J. Trauma*, **23**, 1–6.

Heier, H. E. (1980) Splenectomy and serious infections. *Scand. J. Haematol.*, **24**, 5–12.

Hicklin, H., Verghese, A. and Alvarez, S. (1987) Dysgonic fermenter 2 septicemia. *Rev. Infect. Dis.*, **9**, 884–90.

Hitzig, W. H. (1985) Immunological and hematological consequences of deficient function of the spleen. *Prog. Pediatr. Surg.*, **18**, 132–8.

Holmes, F. F. *et al.* (1981) Fulminant meningococcemia after splenectomy. *J. Am. Med. Assoc.*, **246**, 1119–20.

Horan, M. and Colebatch, F. H. (1962) Relation

between splenectomy and subsequent infection. A clinical study. *Arch. Dis. Child.*, **37**, 398–414.

Hosea, S. W. (1983) Role of the spleen in pneumococcal infection. *Lymphology*, **16**, 115–120.

Hosea, S. W. *et al.* (1981a) Opsonic requirements for intravascular clearance after splenectomy. *N. Engl. J. Med.*, **304**, 245–50.

Hosea, S. W. *et al.* (1981b) Impaired immune response of splenectomised patients to polyvalent pneumococcal vaccine. *Lancet*, **i**, 804–7.

Israeli, A., Shapiro, M. and Ephros, M. A. (1987) *Plasmodium falciparum* malaria in an asplenic man. *Trans. R. Soc. Trop. Med. Hyg.*, **81**, 233–4.

Istre, G. R. *et al.* (1987) Invasive disease due to *Streptococcus pneumoniae* in an area with a high rate of relative penicillin resistance. *J. Infect. Dis.*, **156**, 732–5.

Johnston, R. B., Jr, Newman, S. L. and Struth, A. G. (1973) An abnormality of the alternative pathway of complement activation in sickle-cell disease. *N. Engl. J. Med.*, **288**, 803–8.

Jones, J. F. *et al.* (1975) Atypical rubeola infection after splenectomy. *Lancet*, **i**, 111–12.

Jones, J. M., Amsbaugh, D. F. and Prescott, B. (1976) Kinetics of the antibody response to type III pneumococcal polysaccharide. II. Factors influencing the serum antibody levels after immunization with an optimally immunogenic dose of antigen. *J. Immunol.*, **116**, 52–64.

Kalb, R. *et al.* (1985) Cutaneous infection at dog bite wounds associated with fulminant DF-2 septicemia. *Am. J. Med.*, **78**, 687–90.

Katzenstein, D. A., Yu, G. S. M. and Jordan, M.C. (1983) Lethal infection with murine cytomegalovirus after early viral replication in the spleen. *J. Infect. Dis.*, **148**, 406–11.

King, H. and Shumacker, H. B., Jr (1952) Splenic studies I. Susceptibility to infection after splenectomy performed in infancy. *Ann. Surg.*, **136**, 239–42.

Kingston, M. E. and MacKenzie, C. R. (1979) The syndrome of pneumococcaemia, disseminated intravascular coagulation and asplenia. *Can. Med. Assoc. J.*, **121**, 57–61.

Krivit, W. (1977) Overwhelming postsplenectomy infection. *Am. J. Hematol.*, **2**, 193–201.

Langenhuijsen, M. M. A. C. and van Toorn, D. W. (1982) Splenectomy and the severity of cytomegalovirus infection. *Lancet*, **ii**, 820.

Lepow, M. L., Samuelson, J. S. and Gordon, L. K. (1984) Safety and immunogenicity of *Haemophilus influenzae* type b polysaccharide-diphtheria toxoid conjugate vaccine in adults. *J. Infect. Dis.*, **150**, 402–6.

Littman, E. (1974) Splenectomy in hereditary spherocytosis: effect on course of relapsing vivax malaria. *Am. J. Med. Sci.*, **267**, 53–6.

Livingston, C. D., Levine, B. A. and Sirinek, K. R. (1983) Improved survival rate for intraperitoneal autotransplantation of the spleen following pneumococcal pneumonia. *Surg. Gynecol Obstet.*, **156**, 761–6.

Llende, M., Santiago-Delpín, E. A. and Lavergne, J. (1986) Immunobiological consequences of splenectomy: a review. *J. Surg. Res.*, **40**, 85–94.

Loggie, B. W. and Hinchey, J. (1986) Does splenectomy predispose to meningococcal sepsis? An experimental study and clinical review. *J. Pediatr. Surg.*, **21**, 326–30.

Looareesuwan, S. *et al.* (1987) Dynamic alteration in splenic function during acute falciparum malaria. *N. Engl. J. Med.*, **317**, 675–9.

Martone, W. J. *et al.* (1980) Post-splenectomy sepsis with DF-2: Report of a case with isolation of the organism from the patient's dog. *Ann. Intern. Med.*, **93**, 457–8.

Meier, F. P., Waldvogel, F. A. and Zwahlen, A. (1985) Role of splenectomy in the pathogenesis of *Haemophilus influenzae* type f meningitis. *Eur. J. Clin. Microbiol.*, **4**, 598–600.

Miller, L. H., Usami, S. and Chien, S. (1971) Alteration in the rheologic properties of *Plasmodium knowlesi*-infected red cells: a possible mechanism for capillary obstruction. *J. Clin. Invest.*, **50**, 1451–5.

Monfardini, S. *et al.* (1975) Herpes zoster-varicella infection in malignant lymphomas. Influence of splenectomy and intensive treatment. *Eur. J. Cancer*, **11**, 51–7.

Moxon, E. R., Goldthorn, J. F. and Schwartz, A. D. (1980) *Haemophilus influenzae* b infection in rats: effect of splenectomy on blood stream and meningeal invasion after intravenous and intranasal inoculations. *Infect. Immun.*, **27**, 872–5.

Mufson, M. A. (1981) Pneumococcal infections. *J. Am. Med. Assoc.*, **246**, 1942–8.

Naraqi, S. *et al.* (1977) Prospective study of prevalence, incidence and source of herpesvirus infections in patients with renal allografts. *J. Infect. Dis.*, **136**, 531–540.

Nooruddin and Ahmed, S. S. (1967) The effects of splenectomy on parasitic infections, and the role of the spleen in filariasis – a brief appraisal of our present knowledge. *J. Trop. Med. Hyg.*, **70**, 229–32.

Offenbartl, K. S. *et al.* (1986a) Synergism between gamma-globulin prophylaxis and penicillin treatment in experimental postsplenectomy sepsis in the rat. *Int. Arch. Allergy Appl. Immunol.*, **79**, 45–8.

Offenbartl, K. *et al.* (1986b) Treatment of pneumococcal postsplenectomy sepsis in the rat with human gamma-globulin. *J. Surg. Res.*, **40**, 198–201.

Okun, D. B. and Tanaka, K. H. (1978) Profound leukemoid reaction in cytomegalovirus mononucleosis. *J. Am. Med. Assoc.*, **240**, 1888–9.

Overturf, G. D., Powars, D. and Baroff, L. J. (1977) Bacterial meningitis and septicemia in sickle cell disease. *Am. J. Dis. Child.*, **131**, 784–7.

Pearson, H. A. (1977) Sickle cell anemia and severe infection due to encapsulated bacteria. *J. Infect. Dis.*, **136** (Suppl), S25–S30.

Pearson, H. A. *et al.* (1978) The born-again spleen, return of splenic function after splenectomy for trauma. *N. Engl. J. Med.*, **298**, 1389–92.

Peterson, P. K. *et al.* (1980) Cytomegalovirus disease in renal allograft recipients: a prospective study of the clinical features, risk factors and impact on renal transplantation. *Medicine*, **59**, 283–300.

Purtilo, D. T. *et al.* (1980) Persistent tranfusion-associated infectious mononucleosis with transient acquired immunodeficiency. *Am. J. Med.*, **68**, 437–40.

Reboul, F., Donaldson, S. S. and Kaplan, H. S. (1978) Herpes zoster and varicella infections in children with Hodgkin's disease. *Cancer*, **41**, 95–9.

Rice, H. M. and James, P. D. (1980) Ectopic splenic tissue failed to prevent fatal pneumococcal septicaemia after splenectomy for trauma. *Lancet*, **i**, 565–6.

Rosner, F. and Zarrabi, M. H. (1983) Late infections following splenectomy in Hodgkin's disease. *Cancer Invest.*, **1**, 57–65.

Rosner, F. *et al.* (1984) Babesiosis in splenectomized adults. Review of 22 reported cases. *Am. J. Med.*, **76**, 696–701.

Rowley, D. A. (1950) The formation of circulating antibody in the splenectomized human being following intravenous injection of heterologous erythrocytes. *J. Immunol.*, **65**, 515–21.

Ruben, F. L. *et al.* (1984) Antibody responses to meningococcal polysaccharide vaccine in adults without a spleen. *Am. J. Med.*, **76**, 115–21.

Sass, W. *et al.* (1983) Overwhelming infection after splenectomy in spite of some spleen remaining and splenosis; a case report. *Klin. Wochenschr.*, **61**, 1075–9.

Scher, K. S., Wroczynski, A. F. and Jones, C. W. (1983) Protection from post-splenectomy sepsis: Effect of prophylactic penicillin and pneumococcal

vaccine on clearance of type 3 pneumococcus. *Surgery*, **93**, 792–7.

Schimpff, S. *et al.* (1972) Varicella-zoster infection in patients with cancer. *Ann. Intern. Med.*, **76**, 241–54.

Schoolnik, G. K., Buchanan, T. M. and Holmes, K. K. (1976) Gonococci causing disseminated gonococcal infection are resistant to the bactericidal action of normal human sera. *J. Clin. Invest.*, **58**, 1163–73.

Schwartz, A. D. and Pearson, H. A. (1972) Impaired antibody response to intravenous immunization in sickle cell anemia. *Pediatr. Res.*, **6**, 145–9.

Schwartz, A. D. *et al.* (1978) Lack of protective effect of autotransplanted splenic tissue to pneumococcal challenge. *Blood*, **51**, 475–8.

Schwartz, P. E. *et al.* (1982) Postsplenectomy sepsis and mortality in adults. *J. Am. Med. Assoc.*, **248**, 2279–83.

Sherman, R. (1981) Rationale for and methods of splenic preservation following trauma. *Surg. Clin. North Am.*, **61**, 127–34.

Shute, P. G. (1975) Splenectomy and susceptibility to malaria and babesia infection. *Br. Med. J.*, **1**, 516.

Siber, G. R. *et al.* (1978) Impaired antibody response to pneumococcal vaccine. *N. Engl. J. Med.*, **299**, 442–8.

Siber, G. R. *et al.* (1986) Antibody response to pretreatment immunization and post-treatment boosting with bacterial polysaccharide vaccines in patients with Hodgkin's disease. *Ann. Intern. Med.*, **104**, 467–75.

Singer, D. B. (1973) Postsplenectomy sepsis. *Perspect. Pediatr. Pathol.*, **1**, 285–311.

Steely, W. M. *et al.* (1987) Comparison of omental splenic autotransplant to partial splenectomy. Protective effect against septic death. *Am. Surg.*, **53**, 702–5.

Sullivan, J. L. *et al.* (1978) Immune response after splenectomy. *Lancet*, **i**, 178–81.

Sumaya, C. V. *et al.* (1981) Pneumococcal vaccine failures, two case reports and review. *Am. J. Dis. Child.*, **135**, 155–8.

Tapper, M. L. and Armstrong, D. (1976) Malaria complicating neoplastic disease. *Arch. Intern. Med.*, **136**, 807–10.

Traub, A. *et al.* (1987) Splenic reticuloendothelial function after splenectomy, spleen repair and spleen autotransplantation. *N. Engl. J. Med.*, **317**, 1559–64.

Van Wyck, D. B., Witte, M. H. and Witte, C. L. (1986) Compensatory spleen growth and protective function in rats. *Clin. Sci.*, **71**, 573–9.

Wählby, L. and Domellöf, L. (1981) Splenectomy after blunt abdominal trauma. A retrospective study of 413 children. *Acta Chir. Scand.*, **147**, 131–5.

Walzer, P. D., Gibson, J. J. and Schultz, M. G. (1974) Malaria fatalities in the United States. *Am. J. Trop. Med. Hyg.*, **23**, 328–33.

Wara, D. W. (1981) Host defense against *Streptococcus pneumoniae*: the role of the spleen. *Rev. Infect. Dis.*, **3**, 299–309.

Werbin, N. and Lodha, K. (1982) Malign effects of splenectomy – the place of conservative treatment. *Postgrad. Med. J.*, **58**, 65–9.

Winkelstein, J. A. and Lambert, G. H. with the technical assistance of Swift, A. (1975) Pneumococcal serum opsonizing activity in splenectomized children. *J. Pediatr.*, **87**, 430–3.

Wyler, D. J., Miller, L. H. and Schmidt, L. H. (1977) Spleen function in quartan malaria (due to *Plasmodium inui*): evidence for both protective and suppressive roles in host defence. *J. Infect. Dis.*, **135**, 86–93.

Wyler, D. J., Oster, C. N. and Quinn, T. C. (1978) The role of the spleen in malaria infections. *Tropical Diseases Research Series*, **1**, 183–204.

Wyler, D. J., Quinn, T. C. and Chen, L-T. (1981) Relationship of alterations in splenic clearance function and microcirculation to host defense in acute rodent malaria. *J. Clin. Invest.*, **67**, 1400–4.

Zarrabi, M. H. and Rosner, F. (1984) Serious infections in adults following splenectomy for trauma. *Arch. Intern. Med.*, **144**, 1421–4.

Zarrabi, M. H. and Rosner, F. (1986) Rarity of failure of penicillin prophylaxis to prevent postsplenectomy sepsis. *Arch. Intern. Med.*, **146**, 1207–8.

HEMOLYSIS, THROMBOCYTOPENIA AND THE SPLEEN

David R. Anderson and John G. Kelton

13.1 INTRODUCTION

Some organs of the body are uniquely associated with specific diseases resulting from disturbance or failure of their own structure or function. For example, renal failure is the consequence of disorders of the kidneys, and myocardial infarction results from structural damage to the heart. But the spleen is in many respects unique, and the disorders which are most closely associated with the spleen have their etiological origins elsewhere. For example, hereditary disorders of the red cell membrane lead to red cell destruction by the spleen. Likewise in autoantibody-mediated blood cell damage, the spleen may play both a causal and a consequential role. In these conditions, the spleen produces the autoantibodies which initiate cell damage and also provides the filtration mechanism which destroys the antibody-sensitized cells.

The recognition of the predominant role of the spleen in many autoimmune disorders is relatively recent. In this chapter, the focus will be on the clinical and experimental observations which have clarified the role of the spleen in both autoimmune and non-immune hemolytic and thrombocytopenic disorders, and in particular two common and important diseases, idiopathic thrombocytopenic purpura (ITP) and autoimmune hemolytic anemia (AIHD). The comparable and contrasting mechanisms of clearance of the red cells and platelets in these

two autoimmune disorders will be addressed.

Once a cell becomes sensitized by IgG antibody or complement, the fate of this cell is identical irrespective of whether its removal is useful for the body. Removal of an infecting microorganism, or an antigenically transformed cell such as a malignant cell, may be regarded teleologically as 'serving a useful purpose'. However, the same mechanism may place the subject at hazard when removing an otherwise autoantibody-sensitized red cell or platelet. Consequently there is an important relationship between the physiological and pathological aspects of particle clearance.

There is a unique anatomy to the spleen which allows it to function both as a generator of autoantibodies and as a clearance organ of the autoantibody-sensitized cells. (See also Chapters 3 and 4.)

13.2 ANATOMY OF THE SPLEEN

The anatomy of the spleen has been described in detail in Chapters 1 to 4 and this description is confined to aspects especially relevant to blood cell destruction. Within the spleen are large numbers of lymphocytes, monocytes and macrophages, so that there is a unique opportunity for communication between blood in the vasculature and the lymphatic and reticuloendothelial systems. The white pulp consists of periarterial lymphatic sheaths and lymphatic nodules. The red pulp contains complex vascu-

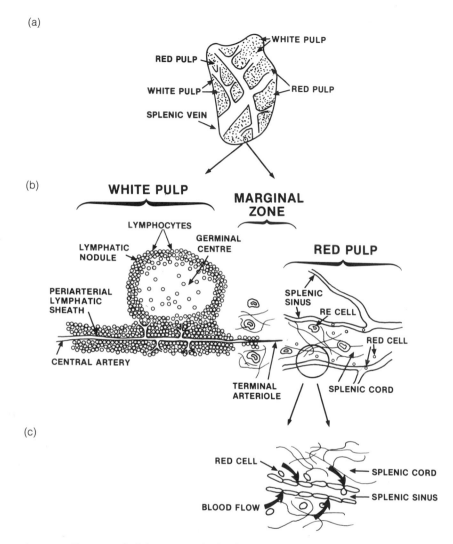

Figure 13.1 Sequentially magnified diagrams which schematically represent the splenic anatomy as it pertains to blood cell clearance. (a) A cross-section of the spleen, its venous tributaries and the red and white pulp. (b) Schematic representation of the white and red pulp. The white pulp is composed of periarterial lymphatic sheaths and lymphatic nodules. The red pulp consists of splenic cords and sinuses. Interspersed between is the marginal zone. Blood enters the white pulp through the central artery, which is enveloped by the periarterial lymphatic sheath. Arteriolar vessels leave the central artery at right angles and this results in the skimming of the plasma from the parent vessel. The remaining concentrated blood passes through the marginal zone and enters the splenic cords of the red pulp *via* the terminal arterioles. The splenic cords are a non-endothelialized reticular meshwork rich in RE cells. Blood cells pass through the cords before entering the splenic sinuses. (c) The route blood cells must follow to enter a splenic sinus. There are few direct connections between the cords and sinuses, and most blood cells enter the splenic sinuses by passing through the narrow interendothelial spaces. (Reprinted from Murphy and Kelton (1988), by courtesy of Marcel Dekker, Inc. and the editors.)

lar pathways identified as splenic cords and sinuses, and there is an abundance of RE cells (monocytes and macrophages). Between the white pulp and the red pulp is the marginal zone (Figure 13.1), which is a fine reticular area containing lymphocytes and RE cells.

The spleen receives about 5% of the total cardiac output: blood passes from the splenic artery to the trabecular arteries, and in turn to the central arteries, which enter the white pulp (Bishop and Lansing, 1982). The central arteries give off lateral branches which leave at right angles to penetrate the periarterial lymphatic sheaths (Eichner, 1979). Teleologically the peculiar anatomy of these arteries and their orientation at right angles to the parent arteries can be understood as providing for plasma skimming: rapidly flowing blood in small vessels assumes a characteristic flow pattern, with the red cells in the center of the vessel and the plasma at the periphery. The right-angled arteries of the spleen skim the plasma from the flowing blood, so that the plasma carries soluble antigens to the white pulp, where they are captured by specialized macrophages, termed dendritic or antigen-presenting cells. Second, the monomeric IgG in the plasma, which can inhibit RE cell function, is separated from the cellular elements: this increases the likelihood that IgG-sensitized cells will bind to the Fc-receptor bearing RE cells.

Concentrated blood leaves the white pulp and enters the red pulp *via* the terminal arterioles. These vessels end in the splenic cords, which form a non-endothelialized reticular meshwork consisting of fibrils and interstitial cells, with a large population of monocytes and macrophages (Chen and Weiss, 1972). Blood cells must traverse these tortuous cords in order to enter the splenic sinuses, which form the first vessels of the venous microcirculation of the red pulp. There are relatively few direct connections between the cords and the sinuses. The cords are actually spaces lying between the sinuses within the red pulp (Weiss and Tavassoli, 1972). In order for a cell to enter the sinus lumen it must pass through the three-layered wall of the sinus, which consists of an inner endothelial layer, a middle basement membrane, and an outer lining of adventitial cells. The endothelium contains filaments, which may be contractile and is potentially able to regulate the size of the interendothelial cell slits (Bishop and Lansing, 1982; see Chapter 2). Scanning and transmission electron microscopic pictures of the splenic sinus demonstrate that there are no fixed apertures in the sinus endothelium (Chen and Weiss, 1972; Weiss, 1974). However, potential spaces exist between the endothelial cells which allow the passage of blood cells into the sinuses.

Functionally the direct pathways between the terminal arterioles and the splenic sinuses are unimportant, so that most blood cells must pass through the monocyte and macrophage-rich cordal circulation during each passage through the spleen.

The red pulp plays a dual role in the removal of cells from the circulation; first, antibody-sensitized cells may be removed by the splenic RE cells. Second, cells with reduced deformability are unable to transverse the interendothelial slits of the sinus endothelium and are retained by the spleen. By these two mechanisms the red pulp plays a pivotal role in the clearance from the circulation of normal and pathologically altered cells.

13.3 THE RETICULO-ENDOTHELIAL FUNCTION OF THE SPLEEN

The monocytes and macrophages of the spleen effect the removal of infectious agents, foreign antigens, tumor antigens and antibody-sensitized cells. It is by the removal of IgG-sensitized platelets and red cells that splenic phagocytes are involved in the pathogenesis of autoimmune thrombocytopenia and hemolysis. This section will outline: (1) factors influencing splenic RE cell function; (2) the measurement of Fc-dependent RE function; (3) the mechanism of RE cell-mediated cell destruction; and (4) the importance of the splenic RE cells in the clearance of cells from the circulation.

13.3.1 FACTORS INFLUENCING RE CELL FUNCTION

(a) IgG subclass

The monocytes and macrophages of the spleen have specific binding sites (termed Fc receptors) for the gamma-2 region of the heavy chain of IgG (Lobuglio, Cotran and Jandl, 1967; Huber and Fudenberg, 1968). There are differences in affinity for the different subclasses of IgG, with IgG subclasses 1 and 3 having the highest binding affinity and IgG subclasses 2 and 4 having a low binding affinity (van der Meulen *et al.*, 1978). The IgG on sensitized cells binds to the unoccupied Fc receptors of the RE cells. There are several different types of Fc receptors on the RE cells: some have a very high binding affinity for the IgG and others have a low binding

affinity. Increasing evidence suggests that it is the low affinity Fc receptors that are the most important for antibody-mediated cell clearance, because the high affinity receptors tend to be occupied by the monomeric IgG.

(b) Plasma concentration of monomeric IgG

The monomeric IgG in the plasma can bind to the Fc receptors. When this occurs, the receptors are unavailable for interacting with IgG-sensitized cells. Indeed, it is likely that when the plasma concentration of IgG is sufficiently high, even the low affinity Fc receptors are occupied. This observation has been exploited therapeutically. Intravenous IgG can dramatically raise the concentration of IgG in the plasma and this maneuver can prevent the clearance of IgG-

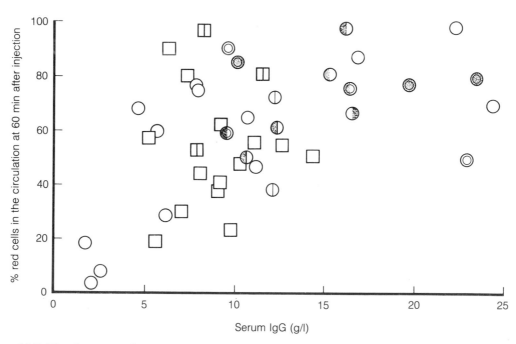

Figure 13.2 The clearance of IgG-sensitized red cells (ordinate) for 17 control subjects (□) and 27 patients (○) in relation to the serum concentration of IgG (g/l); (⊞) indicates the patient or control subject has the HLA-B8/DR3 haplotype; (◑) indicates a positive PEG assay for immune complexes; (◉) indicates a positive Raji cell assay for immune complexes; (◎) indicates a positive assay for antinuclear antibodies. (Reprinted with permission of the author and the publisher, Grune and Stratton, Inc. from Kelton *et al.* (1985) *Blood*, **66**, 492.)

sensitized platelets or red cells (Figure 13.2; Kelton *et al.*, 1985). As noted previously, the anatomy of the spleen counteracts this. As plasma is skimmed from the cellular elements of the blood, the monomeric IgG moves with the plasma. Consequently, as the cellular elements percolate through the splenic cords, there is a significant reduction in the local concentration of monomeric IgG. This monomeric IgG might otherwise occupy the Fc receptors of the RE cells. *In vitro* studies confirm that the decrease in the concentration of IgG to levels found in the red pulp of the spleen improves the efficiency of phagocytosis of sensitized red blood cells (Lobuglio, Cotran and Jandl, 1967). In addition, the slow flow in the splenic cords increases the likelihood that IgG-sensitized cells will have the opportunity of interacting with the Fc receptors on the RE cells within the spleen.

(c)   Amount of IgG and complement on the cells

IgG-sensitized cells can be cleared by splenic macrophages by two mechanisms. Macrophages and monocytes can bind to the Fc portion of the IgG and subsequently initiate the phagocytosis of the cell. Surface immunoglobulins on sensitized cells can also induce clearance by activating the complement system on the cell membrane. Several IgG molecules in close proximity can initiate the complement cascade by activating C1 (Frank, 1987). This event triggers the classical complement cascade which leads to the cleavage of C4 and C2 and the formation of the C4b2b complex, also known as the C3 cleaving enzyme. C3 is subsequently proteolysed to C3a, which is released from the cell surface, and C3b which remains surface bound. C3b is the main opsonin of the complement cascade and RE cells have C3b receptors on their cell membranes (Huber *et al.*, 1968; Lay and Nussenzweig, 1968; Ross *et al.*, 1973). Not surprisingly, the expression of C3b is under tight control: two plasma proteins, H and I, can convert C3b into its inactive form, C3dg. As will be discussed subsequently, C3b-sensitized cells

both alone and in combination with IgG play an important role in the antibody-mediated clearance of cells.

13.3.2   MEASUREMENT OF Fc-DEPENDENT RE FUNCTION

It is possible to study the Fc-dependent RE function in humans. This is accomplished by taking Rh-positive red cells from the individual to be tested, labeling the cells with ^{51}Cr and then sensitizing them with a known amount of IgG alloantibody (Kelton, 1987). Anti-D represents an ideal alloantibody for several reasons. First, its target (the Rh-positive cell) is found with high frequency in the population (85%); second, the Rh antigens are not clustered or mobile, and consequently the anti-D tends not to activate complement. Third, anti-D binds with a high affinity, which minimizes *in vivo* elution of the IgG from the red cells.

After injection of the ^{51}Cr-labeled, IgG-sensitized autologous red cells, samples of whole blood are collected at various times and the rate of clearance of these radiolabeled cells is measured. Because the amount of sensitizing alloantibody is controlled, the only variable affecting the rate of clearance of the radiolabeled red cells is the functional activity of the RE system. Studies using this technique have established the following:

1. The spleen is the dominant organ for clearance of IgG-sensitized red cells. When the red cells are moderately sensitized (2000 molecules of IgG per cell), they are rapidly cleared within hours of injection. Following splenectomy, the cells are cleared at a very reduced rate (Kelton *et al.*, 1985; Hosea *et al.*, 1981).

2. The plasma concentration of IgG is an important determinant of the rate of clearance of the IgG-sensitized cells (Kelton *et al.*, 1985). Patients with agammaglobulinemia have an enhanced rate of clearance and patients with either a naturally occurring or a pharmacologically induced hypergamma-

globulinemia have a reduced rate of clearance.

3. Splenic Fc-dependent RE clearance is governed by other as yet poorly understood factors, including certain genes, such as those for the HLA B8/DR3 alloantigens (Frank *et al.*, 1983; Lawley *et al.*, 1981), certain disease states such as systemic lupus erythematosus and HIV infections (Bender *et al.*, 1985; Frank *et al.*, 1979), and certain medications, especially methyldopa (Kelton, 1985). All these conditions impair splenic Fc-dependent RE cell clearance.

13.4 THE MECHANISM OF DESTRUCTION OF SENSITIZED CELLS

13.4.1 RED CELLS

Electron microscopic studies *in vitro* have shown that the interaction of RE cells and sensitized red cells depends upon whether IgG or complement coats their surface. IgG-sensitized red cells form rosettes with monocytes and macrophages (Lobuglio, Cotran and Jandl, 1967; Rosse, de Boisfleury and Bessis, 1975) and the red cells are either ingested completely or a portion of the red cell membrane is removed. Sensitized red cells with abnormal shapes, such as spherocytes, are engulfed completely. Light microscopic studies showed that following monocyte rosette formation, sensitized red cells become spherocytic. Sensitized red cells which are not rosetted show no such transformation.

Unlike IgG-sensitized red cells which initiate phagocytosis, complement-coated red cells adhere efficiently to RE cells but are rarely ingested (Rosse, de Boisfleury and Bessis, 1975; Ehlenberger and Nussenzweig, 1977; Bianco, Griffin and Silverstein, 1975). If the cell is ingested by the monocyte or macrophage, it often escapes from the phagocytic vacuole and is released from the cell. However, when sensitized red cells are coated with both IgG and complement, significantly fewer IgG molecules are required for ingestion to occur. The

mechanism of this synergism is now apparent. Monocyte and macrophage C3b-receptor binding leads to strong adherence of the red cell to the phagocytic cell surface. The Fc receptors for IgG on the RE cells then mediate the ingestion of the already tightly bound red cell and this results in phagocytosis.

These observations offer a probable explanation for the clinical observation that spherocytes are commonly found with warm autoimmune hemolytic anemia and are usually absent in cold agglutinin disease. Warm autoimmune hemolytic anaemia is mediated by IgG-sensitization of red cells. Microscopic studies demonstrate that RE cells are capable of removing portions of the red cell membrane from the IgG-sensitized cell, resulting in spherocyte formation. Cold agglutinin disease is mediated solely by IgM-induced complement activation. Since complement-sensitized red cells are poorly ingested by RE cells, spherocyte formation is uncommon. Studies in rats have demonstrated that IgG-mediated hemolysis leads to a loss of about 25% of the lipid-rich components of the red cell membrane within 24 hours of sensitization (Cooper, 1972).

13.4.2 PLATELETS

Histological examination of spleens from patients with ITP demonstrates that platelets are phagocytosed as whole cells, usually in the splenic cords (Tavassoli and McMillan, 1975; Luk, Musclow and Simon, 1980). It is not known whether IgG and complement-sensitized platelets are processed differently by the splenic RE cells.

13.5 THE ROLE OF SPLENIC PHAGOCYTES IN CELL CLEARANCE

Splenic monocytes and macrophages are important in cell clearance under both physiological and pathological circumstances. This section outlines their role in the clearance of senescent cell populations and antibody-mediated cell destruction.

13.5.1 THE PHYSIOLOGICAL CLEARANCE OF SENESCENT CELLS

(a) Red cells

There is increasing evidence that the clearance of senescent red cells is triggered by the binding of autoantibodies to the red cell membrane. Kay (1975) first demonstrated that when red cells aged *in vitro* were incubated with autologous or allogeneic IgG, the cells were phagocytosed by macrophages. They also found that less than 5% of young red cells were phagocytosed by macrophages whereas over 30% of the old cells were destroyed. Kay concluded that an IgG autoantibody attached to the older red cells *in vivo* and this sensitization initiated the removal of the cells by the RE system. Kay's hypothesis has been confirmed by other groups (Khansari and Fudenberg, 1983). Old red cells have elevated levels of surface IgG, bound by the Fab fragment (Lutz, Flepp and Stringaro-Wipf, 1984; Freedman, 1987). Eluates of IgG from senescent red cells rebind to red cells, causing the clearance of senescent but not young red cells (Khansari and Fudenberg, 1983; Kay *et al.*, 1982).

The target of IgG has been termed the senescent antigen. Recent work has located the antigen to band 3, which is an integral protein of the red cell membrane (Lutz, Flepp and Stringaro-Wipf, 1984; Low *et al.*, 1985; Lutz and Wipf, 1982). Although IgG binds to band 3 *in vitro*, a conformational alteration of this protein may act as the epitope for the immunoglobulin *in vivo*. This alteration occurs as a consequence of red cell aging. The precise characterization of the senescent antigen is not complete. Several groups have confirmed that it is composed of the extracellular and intramembranous portions of band 3, but not the cytoplasmic component of this protein. What also remains unknown is the mechanism of band 3 alteration that causes autoantibody sensitization. Kay *et al.* (1982) have reported that the senescent antigen forms as a result of the specific proteolytic cleavage of band 3 protein.

Low *et al.* (1985) suggest that the formation of this antigen is secondary to oligomerization of band 3 molecules in the red cell membrane. IgG capable of binding to the senescent antigen has been isolated from pooled plasma (Lutz and Wipf, 1982; Lutz, Flepp and Stringaro-Wipf, 1984); it can be absorbed by incubating plasma with senescent red cells, band 3 protein, or the senescent antigen (Kay *et al.*, 1982; Kay, 1984). Recently it has been shown *in vitro* that the senescent IgG antibody can induce complement deposition on the red cell surface (Lutz et al., 1987) and that complement may contribute to the clearance of senescent red cells. Consistent with this hypothesis is the recognition that the small number of IgG molecules bound per senescent red cell is inadequate to cause clearance of the sensitized cells solely by the Fc receptors of the RE system.

It is possible that IgG sensitization represents a general mechanism of cell clearance. For example, increased red cell IgG has also been found in patients with sickle cell anemia (Green, Rehn and Kalra, 1985; Galili, Clark and Shohet, 1986). This disorder is associated with shortened red cell survival due to other factors, but autoantibody sensitization of the red cells may represent an additional mechanism of premature cell clearance.

Senescent red cells are cleared by the cells of the macrophage system. The evidence that this clearance is mediated by IgG sensitization to a specific band 3 product suggests that the spleen is responsible for the clearance of at least a proportion of senescent red cells. However, the lifespan of red cells is apparently unaltered in asplenic individuals, and it is therefore assumed that other components of the RE system are capable of phagocytosing senescent red cells and compensating for the absence of the spleen.

(b) Platelets

The mechanism of the clearance of senescent platelets is not understood but is probably similar to that of red cells. For example, in normal individuals the small, low-density platelets, which are probably the oldest, carry large amounts of IgG on their surface (Kelton and Denomme, 1982).

13.5.2 THE CLEARANCE OF PATHOLOGICALLY SENSITIZED RED CELL POPULATIONS

(a) Red cells

Jandl and Kaplan (1960) demonstrated the effect of various levels of IgG-sensitization on red cell destruction *in vivo*. They found that low or moderate levels of IgG on the red cells resulted in splenic clearance; however, large amounts of antibody led to hepatic clearance. Subsequently it was shown that high levels of sensitization by IgG resulted in complement deposition on the red cells, which is presumed to shift the predominant clearance of red cells from the spleen to the liver. Schreiber and Frank (1972b) demonstrated that 1.4 complement molecules per cell were capable of decreasing the survival of IgG-sensitized cells. Work in both guinea pigs and humans has shown that with low levels of IgG sensitization, clearance of ^{51}Cr-labeled red cells is predominantly by the spleen (Schreiber and Frank, 1972a; Frank *et al.*, 1977). Furthermore, animals and humans with C4 deficiency or C1-esterase deficiency showed a reduced rate of clearance of IgG-sensitized red cells. However, the clearance rate does not return to normal suggesting that IgG alone can accelerate red cell clearance and the effect of complement is synergistic. With increasing levels of IgG sensitization, more C3b activation occurs and the survival of the sensitized cells is further shortened (Frank *et al.*, 1977; Mollison *et al.*, 1965).

The clearance of IgM-sensitized red cells is quite different from that of IgG-coated cells. There are no specific receptors on macrophages for IgM, and IgM can only mediate cell clearance through the activation of complement. IgM is much more efficient in activating complement than IgG and only one molecule of IgM is required to initiate the complement cascade

(Frank, 1987). With low levels of IgM sensitization, most red cells are removed from the circulation and sequestered in the liver. However, a portion of these cells returns to the circulation where they have a normal survival (Frank *et al.*, 1977). These cells have iC3d on their surface, which protects them from being subjected to further cell clearance.

If the level of IgM sensitization is increased, the initial sequestration in the liver is increased and fewer cells are returned to the circulation. Patients with C1-esterase deficiency show no significant clearance of IgM-sensitized red cells at levels that would normally lead to hemolysis.

(b) Platelets

Understanding of the importance of antibody and complement sensitization to the clearance of platelets comes principally from studying patients with idiopathic thrombocytopenic purpura (ITP). Human and animal studies have demonstrated low baseline levels of IgG on normal platelets (Winiarski and Holm, 1983). Increased levels of IgG result in rapid clearance of the platelets by the spleen. Increased platelet-associated complement has been reported in some but not all patients with immune thrombocytopenia, with some patients having marked elevations in platelet-bound complement. It is difficult to make comparisons between the various studies that have been made because of the different techniques used for measuring complement, and the use of measurements of different complement components. However, platelet-associated C3b, C3c, C3d, C4 and C9 have all been reported to be increased on ITP platelets (Winiarski and Holm, 1983; Kurata *et al.*, 1986; Cines and Schreiber, 1979; Panzer *et al.*, 1986; Lehman *et al.*, 1987; Hedge, Bowes and Roter, 1985; Myers *et al.*, 1982; Hauch and Rosse, 1977; Kayser *et al.*, 1983).

There has been speculation on how complement is bound to the platelet surface. McMillan and Martin (1981) demonstrated that purified antiplatelet autoantibody produced *in vitro* by splenic cells from patients with ITP causes the binding of C3 to the platelet surface; this suggests that complement can be activated *in vivo* with resulting augmentation of the clearance of IgG-sensitized platelets. Complement on the platelet surface has the potential for shifting the primary organ of clearance from the spleen to the liver, and this was found in one study (Panzer *et al.*, 1986). This is of more than theoretical importance as it might imply that splenectomy would be unsuccessful in such patients.

A recent case report provides evidence that complement-mediated immune platelet destruction can occur (Lehman *et al.*, 1987). A patient with a lymphoreticular disease was shown to have increased levels of platelet-associated IgG, IgM, C3c and C3d. Serum from this patient was reported to deposit complement on the platelet surface and result in platelet lysis. This mechanism of platelet destruction may account for the patient's unresponsiveness to therapy.

The relationship between platelet-associated IgG, platelet-associated IgM, and platelet-associated complement remains unclear. Some authors have reported correlations between platelet-associated IgG and platelet-associated complement (Winiarski and Holm, 1983; Kurata *et al.*, 1986; Myers *et al.*, 1982; Kayser *et al.*, 1983), while others have reported an association between platelet-associated IgM and platelet-associated complement (Lehman *et al.*, 1987; Hedge, Bowes and Roter, 1985).

13.6 SPLENIC ANTIBODY FORMATION

The spleen has an important function in forming antibodies against soluble plasma antigens. As arterial blood passes through the spleen, plasma is separated from the cellular elements and directed to the white pulp. Soluble antigens in the plasma bind to the antigen-processing cells. These cells partially digest the antigens and then present them to adjacent T-lymphocytes where the process of antibody formation begins. Following splenectomy, the levels of serum IgG and IgA do not change, although the level of IgM drops slightly. There is a significant increase in the risk of serious infection following splenectomy, especially infections caused by encapsulated organisms such as *Streptococcus pneumoniae* and *Haemophilus influenzae* (Eraklis *et al.*, 1967; see also Chapters 11 and 12).

The spleen is a major source of antiplatelet autoantibody in patients with ITP. Evidence supporting this statement is both direct and indirect. The indirect evidence comes from measuring platelet-associated IgG (PAIgG) on platelets from patients with ITP before and after splenectomy. In most patients, as the platelet count rises to normal levels, the level of PAIgG drops to normal levels (Cines and Schreiber, 1979; Karpatkin, Strick and Siskind, 1972; Dixon, Rosse and Ebbert, 1975). However, this decrease in PAIgG may also be dilutional: thus if the total amount of antiplatelet antibody is constant, the quantity of antiplatelet antibody per platelet will fall because the PAIgG will be distributed throughout a larger platelet mass. Hence, it is important to examine more direct evidence implicating the spleen as a major site for antiplatelet antibody production. McMillan *et al.* (1972, 1974) demonstrated that *in vitro* spleen cultures from patients with ITP have IgG production that is several times higher than that of controls. In most patients, the IgG has specific antiplatelet activity. These observations have been confirmed and extended by others who have shown that lymphocytes obtained from the spleens of ITP patients produce antiplatelet autoantibody both spontaneously and following stimulation with B-lymphocyte activators such as pokeweed mitogen (Karpatkin, Strick and Siskind, 1972).

13.7 THE FILTERING FUNCTION OF THE SPLEEN

The anatomy of the spleen provides the means for it to act as a fine filter. In the present context its most important function is the removal from the circulation of abnormal red cells or their inclusions, such as the physiological inclusions of reticulocytes and siderocytes; and also of red cells with pathological inclusions such as parasites. Conversely, the filtering function of the spleen appears to have a limited role in platelet pathophysiology.

13.7.1 THE REMOVAL OF INTRACELLULAR INCLUSIONS

Reticulocytes, which are the youngest circulating red blood cells, have the largest surface area to volume ratio of all red cells. During the first few passages of reticulocytes through the spleen, some of the cell membrane is lost (Come, Shohet and Robinson, 1974; Shattil and Cooper, 1972). The membrane lost is largely lipid in composition, although a specific high-molecular-weight protein is also removed (Lux and John, 1977). Simultaneously, nuclear remnants termed Howell–Jolly bodies are also removed (Crosby, 1957).

The spleen removes other red cell inclusions including iron-containing particles from sidero-

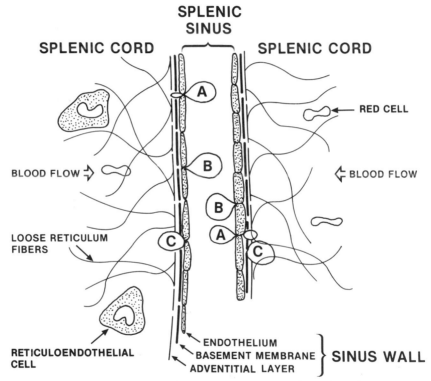

Figure 13.3 Schematic representation of the microcirculation of the red pulp. Blood flows from the splenic cords to the sinuses. The sinus endothelium is incompletely covered by a basement membrane and an adventitial cell lining. Red cells must undergo dramatic changes in shape to pass through the interendothelial cell slits. Alterations in red cell deformability may slow or prevent the passage of the cells. In the diagram the red cells labeled A contain inclusion bodies. Although the greater part of the cell may pass through the sinus endothelium, the inclusions are pinched off and remain in the splenic cord. Removal of pathological inclusions by the spleen results in the loss of small amounts of the red cell membrane. The loss of membrane further reduces the red cell deformability and increases the likelihood of subsequent splenic retention. The red cells labeled B are normal red cells, which are able to pass through the sinus endothelium unhindered. The red cells labeled C are spherocytes which, because of their reduced deformability, are unable to pass through the interendothelial slits. Red cells and inclusions unable to penetrate the sinus endothelium will be removed by the RE cells.

cytes, Heinz bodies consisting of hemoglobin denatured by oxidative stress (Chen and Weiss, 1973), and intraerythrocytic parasites (Schnitzer *et al.*, 1972), following which the red cells are returned to the circulation.

Electron microscopy studies have demonstrated that inclusion bodies are 'pitted' from red cells as they pass through the interendothelial slits of the sinus endothelium. It is probable that the inclusion is physically trapped and forced to remain within the splenic cords (Figure 13.3). Whether there is an additional 'recognition signal' which optimizes the conformation of splenic structures for the removal of an inclusion is unknown.

13.7.2 THE REMOVAL OF INDIVIDUAL CELLS

(a) Red cells

For passage through narrow apertures, such as the interendothelial slits of the splenic sinuses, the red cells depend on their high surface to volume ratio and the flexibility of the cell membrane. Factors affecting red cell deformability include the viscoelastic properties of the membrane, the geometry of the cell, and the viscosity of the intracellular hemoglobin (Mohandas, Phillips and Bessis, 1979). Congenital and acquired conditions which adversely affect these will lead to decreased red cell survival. The major obstacle to survival in most of these disorders is the inability of red cells to pass through the splenic microcirculation.

The fate of antibody-sensitized red cells depends both on the immune and the filtration functions of the spleen. Once a red cell is sensitized by IgG, there are several possible sequelae. First, the surface concentration of the autoantibody may be so low, or the functional activity of the reticuloendothelial system may be sufficiently impaired, that the cell is not cleared from the circulation. Second, IgG-sensitized red cells may be removed from the circulation by binding to the Fc or complement receptors on

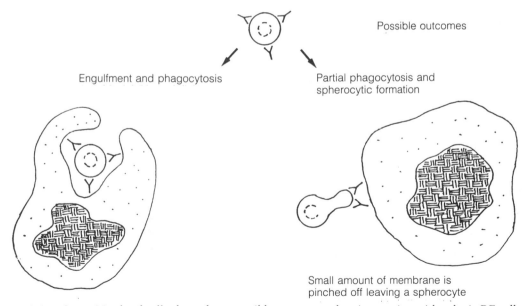

Possible outcomes

Engulfment and phagocytosis

Partial phagocytosis and spherocytic formation

Small amount of membrane is pinched off leaving a spherocyte

Figure 13.4 IgG-sensitized red cells show three possible outcomes when interacting with splenic RE cells; (1) the red cells may be engulfed and phagocytosed by the RE cells; (2) the red cells may be partially phagocytosed resulting in the formation of spherocytes; or (3) the red cells may not interact with the RE cells. Phagocytosis is most likely to occur with high levels of IgG sensitization, surface complement activation and normal RE cell function. This diagram schematically outlines the first two possibilities.

the RE cells. This outcome is most likely for those cells carrying the largest amount of IgG on the cell surface. Third, the IgG-sensitized red cells may bind to the RE cells, without being destroyed during this first interaction: the red cell escapes complete phagocytosis, but leaves a portion of its membrane behind, which in turn causes it to assume a spherical shape (Figure 13.4). The change of shape increases the risk of removal by means of the spleen's filtering function.

The filtering capacity of the spleen can be measured *in vivo* by determining the clearance of radiolabeled (usually ^{51}Cr) heat-treated autologous red cells or by measuring the clearance of radiolabeled aggregates of albumin. Heat treatment denatures spectrin and causes the red cells to become spherocytic (Palek and Lux, 1983).

(b) Platelets

The filtration function of the spleen is unimportant in platelet destruction. There is, however, indirect evidence that the spleen retains the youngest and most hemostatically active platelets. Transfusion studies have shown that platelets from asplenic donors have a 2-day longer survival than those from normal controls (Shulman *et al.*, 1968).

In a few uncommon disorders, the spleen modifies the platelets and possibly contributes to their subsequent destruction. Wiskott–Aldrich syndrome is an immunodeficiency syndrome characterized by frequent infections, eczema, and thrombocytopenia with small platelets. Splenectomy has been shown to alleviate the thrombocytopenia and bleeding symptoms in one group of 16 patients (Lum *et al.*, 1980). Interestingly, the morphology of the platelets returned to normal after removal of the spleen; the mechanism of interaction between the platelet and the spleen in this condition is unknown. Case reports have also suggested a role for the spleen in the destruction of platelets in patients with the Bernard–Soulier syndrome and the 'grey platelet syndrome' (Na-

jean *et al.*, 1963; Raccuglia, 1971). Whether the thrombocytopenia of these two conditions associated with large platelets is related to the filtration system of the spleen is unknown.

13.7.3 CELL POOLING BY THE SPLEEN (see also Chapter 8)

(a) Red cells

Despite the extensive filtering system, there is relatively little retention of normal red cells by the spleen in humans. Following the intravenous injection of radiolabeled red cells, less than 5% of the cells are retained by the spleen (Hedge *et al.*, 1973). With splenomegaly, the spenic red cell pool may increase to more than 20% of the red cell mass (Jandl and Aster, 1967). Increased red cell pooling is found with lymphoproliferative disorders, myeloproliferative disorders, and warm autoimmune hemolytic anemia (Christensen, 1973a; Lewis *et al.*, 1977; Bateman *et al.*, 1978).

The transit time of a red cell through the normal spleen is relatively brief, and usually less than one minute (Ferrant *et al.*, 1987). The splenic transit time is increased in patients with splenomegaly, and is especially increased in patients with hereditary spherocytosis and autoimmune hemolytic anemia in association with splenomegaly (Bowdler, 1962). This suggests that red cell abnormalities and splenic enlargement are additive in delaying the passage of erythrocytes through the spleen.

(b) Platelets

The relationship of platelets to the spleen differs from the interaction of red cells with the organ. First, in healthy individuals between 25 and 45% of the platelet mass is found in the spleen (Peters and Lavender, 1983; Aster, 1966; Penny, Rozenberg and Firkin, 1966). These platelets can be mobilized by stress or the infusion of adrenaline. The mechanism maintaining these platelets within the spleen is unknown but it could be age-related or antibody-dependent.

Also, the average transit time of platelets through the spleen is much longer than that of red cells, being approximately 10 minutes compared to 1 minute (Peters *et al.*, 1980). As in the case of red cells, splenomegaly leads to an increase in the splenic platelet mass, but there is no increase in the transit time of platelets through the spleen (Aster, 1966; Penny, Rozenberg and Firkin, 1966; Peters, 1983).

13.8 DISEASES ASSOCIATED WITH SPLENIC IMMUNOLOGICAL AND FILTERING ABNORMALITIES

Some diseases are associated with either enhanced or impaired splenic function; these are summarized in Table 13.1. Important examples of the role of the spleen are provided by two major autoimmune disorders, idiopathic thrombocytopenic purpura and autoimmune hemolytic anemia, and by hereditary red cell abnormalities associated with decreased cell de-

formability. These conditions will illustrate a complex but dominant role played by the spleen in blood cell destruction.

13.8.1 IDIOPATHIC THROMBOCYTOPENIC PURPURA

Idiopathic thrombocytopenic purpura (ITP) is an autoimmune disease of uncertain etiology, despite which much of the mechanism of platelet destruction is well understood. Platelet destruction is initiated by the binding of IgG antiplatelet autoantibodies to specific platelet glycoproteins and the secondary binding of IgG and other plasma proteins to the platelet membrane. The sensitized platelets are subsequently cleared by the RE cells (Kelton and Steeves, 1983; Kelton, 1983; McMillan *et al.*, 1987).

There are two basic patterns of ITP which depend on the age of the patient at presentation. Acute ITP occurs principally in young children. It usually follows a viral infection and

Table 13.1 Conditions associated with enhanced or decreased splenic RE cell and filtration activity

Splenic RE cell activity

Increased	Decreased
Chronic infection	Systemic lupus erythematosus
Agammaglobulinemia	Acquired immunodeficiency syndrome/
Idiopathic thrombocytopenic purpura	Immunodeficiency virus infection
Autoimmune hemolytic anemia	Drugs: methyldopa
Collagen-vascular diseases	Hypergammaglobulinemia
	Certain leukocyte alloantigens
	(B8/DR3)

Splenic filtering activity

Increased	Decreased*
Congenital red cell membrane abnormalities	Celiac disease
hemoglobinopathies and thalassemias	Sickle cell anemia
Autoimmune hemolytic anemia	Essential thrombocythemia
Splenomegaly with hypersplenism	Graves' disease

*See also Chapter 11.

spontaneously resolves in over 75% of cases (Karpatkin, 1985). In most, the disease lasts for less than six months. By contrast, chronic ITP is a disease which typically occurs in adults and spontaneous recovery is the exception (Difino *et al.*, 1980; McMillan, 1981). Occasionally, autoimmune thrombocytopenia is associated with a lymphoproliferative disorder such as chronic lymphocytic leukemia. Sometimes thrombocytopenia complicates a more generalized autoimmune disorder such as systemic lupus erythematosus or rheumatoid arthritis. However, for most patients there are no predisposing factors or associated diseases.

Most patients with ITP are asymptomatic, but some have evidence of hemostatic impairment which parallels the platelet count. When this is above $20 \times 10^9/l$, most patients do not bleed, and the disease is often discovered by routine laboratory testing. Once the platelet count falls below $10–20 \times 10^9/l$, petechiae and purpura often occur. Very low platelet counts are associated with evidence of generalized hemostatic impairment including mucous membrane bleeding, hematuria, melena, and menorrhagia. Life-threatening bleeding such as intracerebral hemorrhage is rare but does occur (Karpatkin, 1985; McMillan, 1981; Komrower and Watson, 1954).

Physical examination is usually normal in patients with ITP, except for the petechiae and purpura. Patients at especially high risk for serious bleeding are more likely to have 'wet purpura', with blood blisters in the mouth and evidence of mucous membrane bleeding (Crosby, 1975). Splenomegaly does not occur in ITP and its presence should lead one to search for alternative causes for the thrombocytopenia.

Laboratory investigation in the majority of adults and children with ITP is characterized by isolated thrombocytopenia. Often the platelets are increased in size, which may reflect increased platelet turnover and increased megakaryocyte ploidy. White cell and red cell changes are non-specific and can indicate an associated illness such as infectious mononucleosis or a chronic bleeding disorder that has

resulted in iron deficiency anemia. Bone marrow examination demonstrates normal to increased numbers of megakaryocytes. Other laboratory tests often performed in these patients include the rheumatoid factor, antinuclear antibody tests, and serological tests for infectious mononucleosis and, when appropriate, the human immunodeficiency virus. These tests are negative in patients with ITP. Because ITP may be associated with an abnormally functioning thyroid gland, thyroid function studies should be performed in adult ITP patients at presentation and periodically during the management of the patient.

(a)   Special tests used in the investigation of ITP

There are two special tests which may be useful in the investigation of ITP patients: these are (a) platelet antibody tests, and (b) the measurement of platelet survival using radiolabeled platelets.

(i)   *Measurement of platelet-associated IgG*

Immunoglobulins have been measured on platelets for more than 30 years and as yet an ideal assay remains to be identified. Perhaps the best evidence for this is that there are more than one hundred assays for measuring platelet-associated IgG. These can be grouped into several categories and the following briefly summarizes them in relation to the chronological order of their introduction.

Phase I assays were developed following the observation by Harrington and his associates that thrombocytopenia develops in healthy individuals after infusion of plasma from patients with ITP. All Phase I assays share the same basic principle: test serum is mixed with normal platelets, and a platelet-dependent endpoint is measured. Endpoints have included platelet aggregation, platelet release of radioactive tracers, platelet factor 3 availability, and inhibition of specific platelet functions, such as platelet migration or clot retraction. Phase I assays are no longer regarded as satisfactory because they lack both sensitivity and specificity.

Phase II assays share the general characteristic of directly measuring IgG, or other immunoglobulins, proteins or complement, on the surface of washed platelets. The test may be performed directly on platelets collected from the patient; alternatively, test serum from the patient is mixed with normal platelets and IgG adsorbed onto the platelets is measured. All Phase II assays measure IgG using an antibody or staphylococcal protein A as the probe. Staphylococcal protein A binds to IgG subclasses 1, 2 and 4 and is a very specific ligand. Phase II assays can be divided into three general groups: the first includes the direct binding assays in which the ligand is labeled directly with either fluorescein, an enzyme or a radioactive marker, then mixed with the test platelets, and after the reaction has reached equilibrium, unbound ligand is separated by washing. Direct binding assays are simple to perform but difficult to quantitate.

The second general type of phase II assay is the two-stage assay in which the ligand is incubated with the washed test platelets and after this reaction has achieved equilibrium, residual unbound ligand is measured in a second phase by measuring its interaction with IgG (or another protein of interest) bound to a solid phase. Two-stage assays are more complex than direct binding assays but are simpler to quantitate.

The final type of Phase II assay includes assays for 'total' PAIgG in which the platelet membrane is dissolved and all platelet IgG, both surface and internal, is measured.

There is now general agreement that all Phase II assays have a similar sensitivity and specificity: in ITP, positive reactions are obtained in the majority of thrombocytopenic patients. However, there is a low specificity for ITP and positive results may occur in many different thrombocytopenic disorders, some of which are usually considered not to be caused by immune mechanisms.

Phase III assays have been introduced in the past several years and there is still little information on their overall sensitivity and speci-

ficity. Phase III assays measure the binding of IgG to individual platelet glycoproteins, in the expectation that this maneuver may overcome the low specificity of phase II assays. There are three general types of phase III assays including immunoblotting in which the platelet membrane glycoproteins are separated according to size, and fixed to a solid surface (nitrocellulose); following this the binding of the test serum to the glycoproteins is measured. Radioimmunoprecipitation is performed by radiolabeling the surface platelet glycoproteins, solubilizing the membranes, and then reacting the patient's serum with this mixture. Patient IgG binding to the radiolabeled platelet glycoproteins is separated by an immunoprecipitation step, and then the radiolabeled glycoproteins are isolated according to size. The final type of phase III assay is the antigen capture assay in which a monoclonal antibody is attached to a solid phase such as a bead or a microtiter well. Solubilized platelets are incubated with this, and after a further wash, the patient's serum is allow to react. If the patient's serum carries an antibody against the particular glycoprotein, then increased binding of IgG to the monoclonal antibody-platelet glycoprotein will be detected.

(ii) The clinical usefulness of antiplatelet antibody assays in ITP

It is now generally agreed that phase I assays lack sufficient sensitivity and specificity to be used as diagnostic tests for ITP. The clinical usefulness of phase II assays in ITP remains controversial, but there is little evidence that any particular phase II assay differs significantly in overall sensitivity and specificity for ITP. It is likely that major differences among the various assays concerning sensitivity and specificity are related principally to differences in assay experience between laboratories rather than to any intrinsic advantages for a particular assay. Second, there is general agreement that PAIgG is elevated in 80−90% of ITP patients, with the increase being inversely proportional to the platelet count (Panzer *et al.*, 1986; Karpatkin, 1985; McMillan, 1981; Kernoff, Blake and Shackleton, 1980). Consequently, patients with severe thrombocytopenia almost always have elevated levels of PAIgG, whereas those with mild thrombocytopenia often have normal levels of PAIgG. Finally, there is general agreement that these assays are relatively non-specific and positive results are observed in many different thrombocytopenic disorders (Kelton, Powers and Carter, 1982) and in patients who are not thrombocytopenic (Kelton *et al.*, 1984). We believe that increased PAIgG characterizes a variety of thrombocytopenic disorders, including some which traditionally have not been considered to be caused by immune mechanisms.

In summary, PAIgG assays are positive in most thrombocytopenic patients with ITP. A positive test is consistent with ITP, but not diagnostic of it. As previously discussed, platelet-associated complement components have been found in elevated quantities in many patients with ITP. The pathological significance of this finding is still unclear.

(iii)   Platelet survival studies using radionuclides

Platelet kinetic studies can be performed in patients with ITP using sodium ^{51}chromate (^{51}Cr) or ^{111}indium oxime (^{111}In). These studies have provided important information concerning the mechanism of platelet destruction in ITP. Before summarizing these studies, the advantages and disadvantages of each label will be described. Both ^{51}Cr and ^{111}In are taken up by platelets and both are gamma emitters. However, the platelet labeling efficiency of ^{111}In is far higher (over 80%) than ^{51}Cr (less than 10%). This has a major impact on labeling procedures especially when using autologous platelets. The low labeling efficiency of ^{51}Cr means that far more platelets are required to provide a sufficiently high level of radioactive emissions to be counted. Consequently, auto-

logous platelet survival studies cannot be accurately performed in severely thrombocytopenic patients using ^{51}Cr. In contrast, the high labeling efficiency of ^{111}In allows the performance of autologous platelet survivals even in thrombocytopenic patients. The pattern of gamma emission for ^{111}In is also better than ^{51}Cr for counting and organ visualization. Finally there is evidence that ^{51}Cr can be released from platelets by several stimuli including certain antiplatelet autoantibodies (Nagasawa, Kim and Baldini, 1977; Baldini, 1978; Joist and Baker, 1981), whereas ^{111}In binds to a large-molecular-weight protein within the platelets and is not released unless the platelets are destroyed. The major disadvantages of ^{111}In are its expense and its much shorter decay half-life (2.8 days) by comparison with ^{51}Cr.

(iv)   Application of platelet life-span studies in ITP

As with many aspects of ITP, there is at present no complete agreement concerning typical platelet survival in an ITP patient, the dominant organ of clearance, and whether platelet survival studies or measurement of organ clearance predict response to therapy. (See also Chapter 8.) Virtually all thrombocytopenic ITP patients show shortening of platelet life-span, whether this is measured by ^{51}Cr or ^{111}In (Peters and Lavender, 1983; Peters *et al.*, 1980; Kernoff, Blake and Shackleton, 1980; Aster, 1972; Branehog, Kutti and Weinfeld, 1974). However, the reported degree of shortening of the platelet lifespan differs dramatically between the various studies. In some patients, there is a correlation between the level of platelet-associated IgG and the platelet survival (Kernoff, Blake and Shackleton, 1980; Mueller-Eckhardt *et al.*, 1980, 1982), whereas in other patients this relationship is not observed (Ballem *et al.*, 1987).

The results of platelet survival studies have been used to elucidate the pathophysiology of thrombocytopenia in ITP. Two major platelet kinetic studies in the 1970s using ^{51}Cr-labeled platelets supported the view that the thrombocytopenia was secondary to a marked increase in platelet destruction (Harker, 1970; Branehog et al., 1975). In these studies the mean platelet count was $21 \times 10^9/l$ and $27 \times 10^9/l$ and the average platelet survival was 0.34 and 0.57 days. Both studies showed increases in megakaryocytic size and number and elevated platelet turnover values in comparison to controls. These results strongly suggested that the major mechanism of the thrombocytopenia was peripheral destruction and that there was a compensatory increase in platelet production.

Recently these observations have been questioned: Ballem et al. (1987) reported that the majority of their patients with chronic ITP had only moderate shortening of platelet survival and normal rates of platelet turnover. They used ^{111}In-labeled autologous platelets in their study. The platelet lifespans ranged from 1 to 7 days. These investigators suggested that the discrepancy between their data and previous studies was due to the use of autologous rather than homologous labeled platelets. They also reported a three-fold increase in DNA synthetic activity by megakaryocytic stem cells in nonsplenectomized ITP patients. Despite this finding most of these patients had normal platelet turnover rates. These results suggest that although there is a stimulus for increased platelet production at the level of the stem cells and early megakaryocytic forms, the platelet precursors are not reaching full maturation or are not releasing platelets into the circulation. An observation consistent with this is the finding that some patients with ITP have cytotoxic antibodies directed against megakaryocytes (Hoffman et al., 1985).

(v)   Correlation of the level of platelet-associated IgG with platelet survival, organ clearance and response to therapy

It might be expected that the platelets with the most IgG on their surface would be destroyed not only in the spleen, but also in the liver. Some investigators have reported just that: patients with moderately increased levels of platelet-associated IgG show principally splenic destruction, whereas those with the largest amount of PAIgG have mainly hepatic destruction (Kernoff, Blake and Shackleton, 1980). However, other investigators have not confirmed this correlation between the level of platelet-associated IgG and the pattern of sequestration (Panzer et al., 1986; Mueller-Eckhardt et al., 1982). Furthermore, there is no evidence that the pattern of platelet clearance predicts the response to splenectomy in individual patients.

(vi)   Splenic pathology and ITP

The pathology of the spleen in ITP is nonspecific. The organ is normal in size (Tavassoli and McMillan, 1975; Hayes et al., 1985), and an enlarged spleen suggests that the patient does not have ITP. It has been reported that the white pulp has increased numbers of germinal centers, and that they contain increased numbers of activated lymphocytes (Luk, Musclow and Simon, 1980). More recently, others have observed these findings in only about half of all cases of ITP. However, even those who do not report an increase in germinal centers have observed increased numbers of plasma cells within the germinal centers of such spleens (Kristensen and Jensen, 1985).

The splenic red pulp of ITP patients contains increased numbers of RE cells and neutrophils. Many of the monocytes and macrophages have a lipid-laden cytoplasm and are termed foamy histiocytes. Some investigators have described partially degraded platelets within these macrophages, which may account for the cytoplasmic lipids (Tavassoli and McMillan, 1975). Although foamy histiocytes are not observed by light microscopy in every ITP patient, they can be observed in most when the histiocytes are examined using electron microscopy (Hayes et al., 1985; Kristensen and Jensen, 1985).

13.8.2 AUTOIMMUNE HEMOLYTIC ANEMIA

Warm-antibody autoimmune hemolytic anemia (AIHD) is an uncommon acquired disorder caused by the development of IgG anti-red cell autoantibodies. Additionally, the autoantibody sometimes deposits complement on the red cell surface. Hemolysis is almost exclusively extravascular with RE cells phagocytosing the IgG-sensitized red cells. The IgG is referred to as a warm antibody because it is preferentially active at 37°C. In a majority of patients with warm-antibody AIHD the disease is idiopathic, although this depends in part on the rigor with which associated disorders are distinguished from 'primary' in the various series. However, in about one-third the anemia is clearly associated with a lymphoproliferative disorder, other autoimmune disease, or a collagen–vascular disorder, most commonly systemic lupus erythematosus (Chaplin and Avioli, 1977). There is a wide range of age at presentation, with three-quarters of patients being over the age of 40 years (Petz and Garratty, 1980). In patients under 50 years of age, the idiopathic form is much more common. The principal symptoms on presentation are highly variable and are usually related to the severity of the patient's anemia; physical examination is often remarkable only for the patient's pallor, and sometimes slight icterus, and most (57%) have a palpable spleen (Allgood and Chaplin, 1967), which is usually only slightly or moderately enlarged.

Warm-antibody autoimmune hemolytic anemia is usually a chronic disease. Patients have periodic exacerbations and the response to different therapeutic agents varies appreciably. Prognosis is difficult to estimate on an individual basis, but earlier series suggested an overall mortality of 30–50% (Crosby and Rappaport, 1957; Dacie, 1962; Allgood and Chaplin, 1967). More recent studies have suggested a lower mortality, possibly as the result of improved management (Worlledge, Hughes Jones and Bain, 1982; Silverstein et al., 1972).

Laboratory investigations show that most patients are anemic at presentation and 40% have an initial hemoglobin of less than 70 g/l. The red cells may show spherocytosis with increased osmotic fragility. The reticulocyte count is usually elevated, but exceptionally cases with reticulocytopenia can occur (Liesveld, Rowe and Lichtman, 1987; Conley et al., 1982). The indirect bilirubin and LDH levels are elevated with moderate hemolysis. The direct antiglobulin test for surface immunoglobulin or complement is positive in more than 95% of the cases. Bone marrow examination usually shows erythroid hyperplasia.

[51]Cr-labeled red cell survival studies demonstrate a shortened survival in patients with warm-antibody AIHD. The site of red cell destruction is usually the spleen. [51]Cr red cell studies have a limited value in predicting the efficacy of splenectomy in patients with this disorder, and this depends critically on the positioning of the external counter, the frequency of observations, and the mathematical analysis of the pattern of spleen-related uptake.

Pathology of the spleen in warm-antibody autoimmune hemolytic anemia

In contrast to its normal size in ITP, the spleen is usually enlarged in patients with warm-antibody AIHD (Jensen and Kristensen, 1986; Schwartz, Bernard and Adams, 1970). Histological examination of splenic tissue from patients with autoimmune hemolytic anemia demonstrates that the enlargement is principally within the red pulp, and in particular the cords, where there is a striking increase in the number of trapped red cells and spherocytes. In addition, there are also increased numbers of monocytes and macrophages.

Splenomegaly also characterizes other extravascular hemolytic disorders (Jandl et al., 1965; Molnar and Rappaport, 1972). Histologically, the red pulp in such cases also contains many red cells, which emphasizes the lack of specificity of this appearance in hemolytic anemias, and also the importance of the filtration func-

Table 13.2 The participation of the spleen in the pathogenesis of ITP and AIHD

	ITP	AIHD
Antibody production	+ +	+
IgG-dependent RE cell clearance	+ + +	+ +
Filtration capacity	– – –	+ +
Response to splenectomy	+ + +	+ +

tion of the spleen in these disorders. The difficulty with which spherocytic red cells pass through the splenic sinus wall obstructs the passage of red cells through the spleen: this enhances the interaction of RE cells with sensitized red cells within the splenic cords as well as causing the cords to enlarge. The combination of macrophage activity and passive filtration by the spleen are additive in producing increased destruction of sensitized red cells (Table 13.2). The interactions of the microvasculature of the spleen and blood cells in passage are discussed in detail in Chapters 3 and 4.

13.8.3 TREATMENT OF ITP AND AUTOIMMUNE HEMOLYTIC ANEMIA

The various approaches to therapy for both ITP and warm-antibody AIHD will be discussed in parallel, in view of their similarity with respect to the role of the spleen in their pathophysiology, predisposing causes, and response to therapy. The modalities of treatment will be summarized according to the probable mechanism of effect. It is well recognized that a treatment often acts by more than one mechanism, and in these instances we will discuss the effects under the response most likely to be predominant.

(a) Impairment of reticuloendothelial function and suppression of autoantibody formation

The spleen is the dominant organ of autoantibody formation in both warm-antibody AIHD and ITP. In addition, the spleen removes the IgG-sensitized red cells and platelets from the circulation. However, it is not the only organ that can serve both functions; this poses a problem for clinicians because the relative importance of the spleen compared to other lymphocyte-rich macrophage-rich organs in autoantibody generation and cell clearance cannot be unequivocally determined in individual patients.

(i) Corticosteroids

Corticosteroids are the first choice of treatment for both ITP and AIHD. A typical dose is 1–2 mg/kg body weight of prednisone per day, although a recent study suggests much lower doses can be equally efficacious in ITP (Bellucci et al., 1988). A positive response with a rise in the platelet count (ITP) or a rise in the hemoglobin level (AIHD) can be anticipated in at least two-thirds of patients (Karpatkin, 1985; Difino et al., 1980; Allgood and Chaplin, 1967; Bellucci et al., 1988; Christensen, 1973b).

The mechanism of the effect of corticosteroids in these diseases has been studied in detail: the major mechanism is probably the impairment of reticuloendothelial cell function. In vitro studies have shown that corticosteroids inhibit RE receptors for IgG and C3 and cause a dose-dependent decrease in the numbers of RE cell Fc-receptors (Schreiber et al., 1975; Fries, Brickman and Frank, 1983). Consequently steroids inhibit the adhesion, ingestion and subsequent destruction of platelets and red cells by mononuclear cells (Verp and Karpatkin, 1975), and also inhibit chemotaxis and the migration of monocytes (Rinehart et al., 1974).

There is indirect evidence to suggest that corticosteroids decrease autoantibody production in patients with AIHD and ITP (Rosse, 1971). This is largely based on the observation that the amount of cell-specific antibody is decreased in those patients with AIHD or ITP who respond to corticosteroid therapy. Finally, corticosteroids may have a unique action in ITP, which could account for the rapid reduction of bleeding, even before there is a rise in platelet count. Corticosteroids have been reported to decrease capillary fragility, and thus decrease the local risk of bleeding by a mechanism which involves the impairment of prostaglandin I_2 biosynthesis (Faloon, Greene and Lozner, 1952; Stefanini and Martino, 1956; Kitchens, 1977; Blajchman et al., 1979).

Because of the serious long-term side effects of corticosteroids, once a patient has achieved an optimal clinical response, which is usually 1–2 weeks, the dose of corticosteroids should be reduced, with tapering from high to low doses over one to two months. Frequently, the patient shows evidence of relapse during this time, with a decrease in the platelet count (ITP), or the hemoglobin level (AIHD). In these patients, it is appropriate to resume high-dosage corticosteroids, and after a response is achieved to taper them for a second time. However, in the majority of adult patients, ITP and AIHD are chronic illnesses and to continue long-term corticosteroid therapy in the hope of ultimate remission may represent an undue hazard for a patient with little chance of long-lasting remission (Difino et al., 1980; Allgood and Chaplin, 1967; Thompson et al., 1972; Doan, Bouroncle and Wiseman, 1960).

(ii) Splenectomy

Splenectomy is the definitive treatment for both ITP and warm-antibody AIHD, because the spleen is both a major site of autoantibody formation and an important site for red cell and platelet destruction. Evidence confirming its role in autoantibody formation comes from the *in vitro* studies discussed previously in which splenic lymphocytes produce antiplatelet autoantibodies. The levels of antiplatelet autoantibody (Myers et al., 1982) and anti-red cell autoantibody (Allgood and Chaplin, 1967) fall dramatically in the majority of patients following splenectomy. Evidence implicating the role of the spleen in IgG-mediated cell clearance is also strong. IgG-sensitized red cells are rapidly removed from the circulation in healthy individuals, but are cleared at a very slow rate in patients following splenectomy (Hosea et al., 1981). A fourfold increase in the IgG sensitization of red cells is required for the clearance rate in splenectomized subjects to be comparable to that in non-splenectomized subjects. Similar results have been found for IgG-mediated platelet clearance. The amount of antiplatelet antibody must be increased at least sixfold to produce a similar degree of thrombocytopenia in individuals who have undergone splenectomy, by comparison with individuals with a normal spleen (Shulman, Marder and Weinrach, 1965).

In both ITP and AIHD attempts have been made to predict which patients are more likely to respond to splenectomy, but at present it is not possible to state with certainty which prognostic factors are important. Both very high and very low levels of PAIgG have been associated with a poor response to splenectomy (Dixon, Rosse and Ebbert, 1975; Court et al., 1987). Patients with cold agglutinin disease, with only complement on the red cells, are unlikely to respond to splenectomy, and this procedure is generally avoided in those patients.

Measurement of platelet life-span, and splenic-hepatic sequestration patterns, have not in general been predictive of response to splenectomy (Nagasawa, Kim and Baldini, 1977; Najean and Ardaillou, 1971; Ries and Price, 1974; Gugliotta et al., 1981; Najean et al., 1967). Indeed potential pitfalls in using the pattern of platelet destruction in deciding on therapy are illustrated by one patient, whose pattern of sequestration varied throughout the illness (Aster and Keene, 1969).

There is better agreement concerning the predictive nature of a previous response to therapy. Patients with ITP who have had a good response to corticosteroids, defined as a dramatic rise in platelet count, or who respond to a lower than expected dose of corticosteroids, are more likely to respond to splenectomy (Brennan et al., 1975; Difino et al., 1980; Karpatkin, 1985). Unfortunately, such correlates do not necessarily hold for the individual patient.

Following splenectomy about 20% of patients with ITP will show clinical relapse. Unfortunately, the results with AIHD are not as good and more than one-third of complete responders will relapse within one year of therapy. When a late relapse in ITP occurs, the possibility of an accessory spleen should be considered. The presence of Howell–Jolly bodies, siderocytes, and other evidence of hyposplenism in the peripheral blood film does not exclude the possibility of an accessory spleen (Verheyden et al., 1978; Gibson et al., 1986) because the filtering capacity of the spleen differs from its antibody-based Fc-dependent clearing function. Accessory spleens can be observed using technetium scanning (Gibson et al., 1986), but it appears that more sensitive techniques are radionuclide scanning following ^{111}In-labeled platelet lifespan measurements, and CT scans of the abdomen (Verheyden et al., 1978; Hansen and Jarhult, 1986. See also Chapter 17).

The acute mortality of splenectomy in patients with ITP and AIHD is very low. There exists a low but real long-term risk of septicemia, which is, however, not as pronounced as in children under 4 years of age and in patients with otherwise impaired immunity. Postsplenectomy septicemia can occur in otherwise healthy individuals (Eraklis et al., 1967; Whitaker, 1969); therefore any patient not previously immunized should receive multivalent pneumococcal vaccine 1 to 2 weeks before surgery. Occasionally pneumococcal vaccine has been found to exacerbate immune thrombocytopenia (Kelton, 1981). The infectious sequelae of splenectomy are also addressed in Chapters 11 and 12.

(b) Agents acting by reticuloendothelial cell blockade

Most agents effective in ITP and AIHD have more than one mechanism of action. However, in several instances the mechanism of action appears to be highly focused and acts by preventing the clearance of IgG-sensitized cells. The first to be described is still experimental whereas the second is already widely used.

(i) Reticuloendothelial blockade using monoclonal antibodies

A recent report described the use of a monoclonal antibody in a patient with refractory ITP (Clarkson et al., 1986). The monoclonal antibody had activity against the low affinity Fc receptors on macrophages. The patient was treated with this monoclonal antibody on two separate occasions and on both there was an increase in the platelet count. The mechanism was presumed to be one of specific RE blockade, and this was supported by demonstration of impaired clearance of ^{51}Cr-labeled, IgG-sensitized autologous red cells. This study appears to be important not only because it offers the promise of a new approach to clinical management, but also because of its importance to understanding the pathophysiology of this and related diseases.

(ii) High dose intravenous IgG (IV-IgG)

Several years ago it was observed that treatment of children with large doses of IV-IgG for agammaglobulinemia might result in resolution of associated autoimmune thrombocytopenia. This observation was soon confirmed and now IV-IgG represents an important therapy for children with acute immune thrombocytopenia and patients with chronic ITP of all ages (Bussel et al., 1983a,b, 1985; Mori et al., 1983; Newland et al., 1983; Oral et al., 1984; Imbach et al., 1981). Clinical trials have shown that the administration of IV-IgG in doses of 2 g/kg body weight to children with acute ITP produces in many patients a significantly more rapid rise in the platelet count than corticosteroids (Imbach et al., 1985).

In both children and adults with chronic ITP, IV-IgG raises the platelet count in about 75% of patients. Although the rise tends to be less dramatic in chronic than in acute ITP, in most patients the increase results in the patient achieving safe platelet levels. Unfortunately, for most patients with chronic ITP the response is relatively short lived and the platelets return to their original levels within about a month. Rarely a patient will have a long-term remission following the administration of high doses of IV-IgG (Mori et al., 1983; Oral et al., 1984).

IV-IgG significantly impairs Fc-dependent macrophage function while the plasma concentration of IgG remains at high levels. Consequently, it is likely that the mechanism of action of IV-IgG is mediated by preventing the clearance of IgG-sensitized platelets. In patients with acute ITP, the platelet count is kept at safe levels by the RE blockade. Simultaneously, the antiplatelet autoantibody in the plasma slowly declines in amount and the patient has an apparently spontaneous cure of the illness. In patients with chronic ITP, the platelet count rises because of RE blockade, but as the plasma concentration of IgG declines, and normal RE function returns, the continued formation of autoantibodies causes the patient to relapse.

Although high-dose IV-IgG has been used in small numbers of patients with AIHD, experience is not sufficiently large to allow one to comment upon the efficacy of this therapy. The early pessimistic reports were followed by more hopeful descriptions of IV-IgG in AIHD (Stiehm et al., 1987; Besa, 1988). Consequently, the usefulness of IV-IgG in AIHD still remains to be defined.

The mechanism of action of IV-IgG in ITP and AIHD may be more complex than simple Fc-dependent RE blockade. Some patients have a long-term remission following treatment with IV-IgG. In these patients it has been postulated that an anti-idiotypic interaction interrupts the formation of autoantibody and alters the basic pathophysiology of the disease. This possibility implies that in these patients a small fraction of the IV-IgG is responsible for the long-term benefit.

(iii) Treatment with anti-D

Salama and his associates (1984, 1986) have reported that the administration of 1 to 2 mg of anti-D to Rh-positive individuals with ITP resulted in a rise in the platelet count in many of the these patients. We have observed similar benefit from anti-D in ITP patients. Presumably, the mechanism of action is by a temporary RE blockade. Anti-D is much less expensive than IV-IgG and can rapidly be given subcutaneously or intravenously depending upon the preparation. This may prove useful in the ambulatory management of patients with chronic ITP.

(iv) Danazol

Danazol is an attenuated androgen with limited virilizing effects. It was first reported to be effective in ITP by Ahn et al. (1983) using relatively high doses (400–800 mg daily). Subsequent reports by the original investigators have found that danazol may also be used successfully in the treatment of autoimmune hemolytic anemia, and that doses as low as 50 mg per day could be effective in some patients with ITP (Ahn et al., 1985, 1987). Initially it was felt that the medication suppressed autoantibody formation, as shown by a decrease in the level of antiplatelet autoantibody. A more recent study has suggested that the mechanism of action is principally by RE blockade: in a longitudinal study of six patients with ITP, Schreiber et al. (1987) demonstrated that the level of PAIgG did not change in patients responding to danazol. However, there was a reduction in the number of Fc receptors on monocytes.

Danazol is generally well tolerated. Side effects include myalgias, headaches, occasional nausea and weight gain (Ahn et al., 1983); it should not be used during pregnancy as it may be teratogenic (Wentz, 1982).

(c) Agents acting by suppression of autoantibody formation

Azathiaprine and cyclophosphamide have been used successfully in patients with chronic ITP (Finch et al., 1974) and autoimmune hemolytic anemia. These agents act by decreasing the formation of antiplatelet and anti-red cell autoantibodies. Evidence for this is given by the reduction in the level of antiplatelet and anti-red cell autoantibodies and the delay in response, which often does not occur for several months following the initiation of therapy. Because secondary malignancies have been associated with these medications, their use is limited essentially to cases in which other therapies have failed.

13.8.4   CONDITIONS ASSOCIATED WITH DECREASED RED CELL DEFORMABILITY

Reduced red cell deformability is the consequence of alterations in the red cell membrane, an increase in intracellular viscosity, or a decrease in the surface area to volume ratio of the cells. Subtle alterations in deformability can lead to splenic sequestration; with more marked changes in red cell properties, an increasing proportion of red cell destruction occurs in other RE rich organs such as the liver. Intravascular red cell destruction may also occur under these circumstances. This pattern of clearance of abnormal red cells has been confirmed by experimental, red cell survival, and pathological studies.

(a)   Experimental studies

Much has been learned about the patterns of red cell destruction by using phenylhydrazine as an oxidizing agent to induce Heinz body formation. Rifkind (1965) showed that when phenylhydrazine is injected into rabbits, about 50% of the circulating blood cells contain Heinz bodies within 24 hours. Histological examination of the liver reveals little or no red cell ingestion by the Kupffer cells. However, the spleen shows a marked increase in the numbers of red cells within the cords: almost all these red cells contain Heinz bodies and many of the cells are being ingested by monocytes and macrophages. Fewer red cells are seen in the splenic sinuses.

When high doses of phenylhydrazine are administered, the red cells are ingested by the hepatic Kupffer cells and there is evidence of intravascular hemolysis. Microscopic examina-

tion of the liver shows red cell ingestion by the RE cells but there is no extracellular sequestration such as occurs in the splenic cords. This study emphasizes the importance of the microcirculation of the spleen in the clearance of red cells with mild to moderate impairment in deformability. The interendothelial slits between the cords and sinusoids act as an important barrier to the passage of deformed red cells. This obstruction promotes increasing contact between abnormal red cells and cordal RE cells, and subsequently leads to erythrophagocytosis. However, when damage to the red cell is severe, the major site of clearance becomes the liver. (See also Chapters 3 and 4.)

(b)   Clinical data

(i)   Thalassemia

The pathogenesis of the anemia of thalassemia is multifactorial. Inclusion bodies are rarely found in the peripheral blood of thalassemic patients with a normally functioning spleen. However, splenectomized patients with thalassemia major show inclusion bodies within their red cells indicating that the spleen is important for the clearance of globin chain precipitates (Rigas and Koler, 1961; Slater, Muir and Weed, 1968; Wennberg and Weiss, 1968). ^{51}Cr-labeled red cell studies showed increased uptake of the thalassemic cells by the spleen.

Light-microscopic examination of splenic tissue from patients with thalassemia major shows an accumulation of red cells within the splenic cords. The interendothelial slits are the most important barrier to red cell passage: electron microscopic studies demonstrate a marked distortion of the thalassemic cells as they pass through these apertures, and red cells containing inclusion bodies are disrupted during their passage through them (Figure 13.3). The red cells become teardrop in shape and pass into the splenic sinuses; however, the inclusion bodies remain in the splenic cords where phagocytosis occurs. The formation of teardrop cells and red cell fragments by the microcirculation of the spleen accounts for the finding of these cells in the peripheral blood of patients with thalassemia major. However, after splenectomy these abnormal cells are not as commonly seen (Wennberg and Weiss, 1968; Slater, Muir and Weed, 1968; Nathan and Gunn, 1966).

Splenomegaly is a common sequela of thalassemia major. This can result in hypersplenism and increased red cell transfusion requirements. Hypertransfusion programs designed to maintain the patient's hemoglobin within the normal range have decreased the spleen size in some patients (Beard, Necheles and Allen, 1969; O'Brien, Pearson and Spencer, 1977), which may be due to diminished red cell pooling, or possibly a reduction in extramedullary hematopoiesis within the spleen.

Some thalassemia patients benefit from splenectomy performed to alleviate the hypersplenism and decrease red cell transfusion requirements. Several studies have attempted to define factors capable of predicting the optimal time for splenectomy in these patients. Some would recommend splenectomy when transfusion requirements progressively rise above their previous baseline (Modell, 1977). In a study analyzing the transfusion requirements and hemoglobin levels of a group of thalassemic patients before and after splenectomy, it was found that the mean transfusion requirements were significantly higher in the presplenectomy group (Cohen, Markenson and Schwartz, 1980).

There is some disagreement about the long-term benefit of splenectomy in patients with thalassemia: opinion is at present divided between those who believe that most patients with increasing transfusion requirements have a long-term benefit from splenectomy (Modell, 1977), and others who feel that the improvement is at best temporary (Engelhard, Cividalli and Rachmilewitz, 1975).

(ii) Hemoglobinopathies

Sickle cell anemia In young patients with homozygous sickle cell anemia, splenomegaly is common although splenic function is usually impaired (Pearson *et al.*, 1979). By the age of 8 about 50% of affected children will develop splenic fibrosis and functional asplenia, probably caused by recurrent splenic thromboses. However, patients with splenomegaly who develop increasing transfusion requirements or thrombocytopenia may be helped by splenectomy. In these cases the splenectomy will usually lead to resolution of thrombocytopenia, reduce the transfusion requirements and increase the red cell life-span (Sprague and Paterson, 1958; Szwed, Yum and Hogan, 1980; Emond *et al.*, 1984. See also Chapter 16).

Patients with functioning spleens are also susceptible to the development of acute splenic red cell sequestration, characterized by a sudden decrease in the hemoglobin concentration, hypovolemia and evidence of rapid splenic enlargement. This condition usually occurs in children although it is known to occur in adults (Solanki, Kletter and Castro, 1986). In some patients, the splenic sequestration crisis is triggered by acute splenic venous occlusion. Treatment involves red cell transfusions, and exchange transfusion may need to be considered. This complication may be fatal and splenectomy is indicated for recurrent cases (Seelder and Shwiaki, 1972). For further consideration of the significance of the spleen in sickle cell disease, see Chapter 16.

Unstable hemoglobins Unstable hemoglobins result in hemoglobinopathies in which a structural abnormality of hemoglobin leads to the formation in red cells of insoluble hemoglobin inclusions known as Heinz bodies. The disorder is diagnosed by showing that hemolysates containing these hemoglobins denature when heated in iso-osmotic phosphate buffer to 50°C. The spectrum of clinical disease associated with unstable hemoglobins varies from mild hemolysis to severe life-threatening red cell destruction; splenomegaly may be present. Patients with mild to moderate disease principally show spleen-mediated red cell destruction, and will respond to splenectomy. More severe unstable hemoglobinopathies are less likely to benefit from splenectomy (Miller *et al.*, 1971; White and Dacie, 1971).

(iii)   Red cell membrane abnormalities

Hereditary spherocytosis Hereditary spherocytosis is an inherited hemolytic disorder, with extravascular hemolysis caused by structural red cell membrane abnormalities (Weed and Bowdler, 1966; Becker and Lux, 1985). Inheritance is usually as an autosomal dominant. Patients with this disorder have laboratory evidence of chronic but low-grade hemolysis, spherocytic red cell morphology and commonly splenomegaly.

^{51}Cr red cell survival studies demonstrate that the red cells have a shortened lifespan with destruction occurring predominantly in the spleen. Splenectomy cures the expression of the disorder, although it does not alter the abnormality of the red cell membrane or the increased osmotic fragility.

Investigation of the role of the spleen in the pathogenesis of the hemolysis of hereditary spherocytosis has provided a unique insight into the manner in which the spleen is capable of conditioning red cells to premature destruction. The filtration system of the splenic microcirculation delays or prevents the passage of the poorly deformable spherocytic cells, and this results in loss of cell membrane ('fragmentation') during the slow passage through the red pulp and the interendothelial slits of the sinus wall. This progressively decreases the surface area to volume ratio of the cell. The conditions in the splenic pulp may create a metabolic competition which aggravates the loss of integrity of the membrane (*vide infra*). The RE cells of the splenic cords are exceptionally active and phagocytose many of the trapped spherocytic cells; however, it is clear that this accounts for only part of the total cells destroyed. A significant fraction is conditioned by the spleen and destroyed at other sites (Ferrant, 1983).

One characteristic abnormality of red cells in hereditary spherocytosis is their high sodium flux, which requires a highly active sodium–potassium pump to maintain normal intracellular electrolytes. This is not, however, the cause of the spherocytosis. When the red cells are trapped in the splenic cords cellular ATP levels remain normal, but there is a decrease in intracellular glucose and pH which could impair activity of the sodium–potassium pump and lead to further cell membrane damage (Becker and Lux, 1985; Emerson *et al.*, 1956; Prankerd, 1963; Murphy, 1967).

Hereditary elliptocytosis is also due to a congenital defect of the red cell membrane and is morphologically characterized by elliptical red cells. Inheritance is as an autosomal dominant, and the homozygous form is associated with a severe hemolytic disorder in affected infants. However, in most instances the heterozygous form is found to be a clinical epiphenomenon, without significant anemia or hemolysis. Occasional cases show severe hemolysis and splenomegaly and the severity of the anemia is usually improved by splenectomy. As with hereditary spherocytosis, the morphological abnormality of the red cells continues after splenectomy (Palek, 1985).

Hereditary pyropoikilocytosis is a rare condition, related to hereditary elliptocytosis in that both have an inherent instability in the cytoskeleton, expressed by heat-induced cell fragmentation at temperatures lower than for normal red cell membranes. The red cell morphology shows microspherocytes and a wide variety of bizarre red cell shapes. Splenectomy lessens the hemolysis, and the spleen is probably a major site of cell destruction.

13.8.5   HYPERSPLENISM

Hypersplenism is essentially a clinical syndrome rather than a process, and it can be defined as the condition present when (a) there are decreased numbers of one or more blood cell lines in the peripheral blood; (b) there is at least a normal, and sometimes increased production of that cell line present on bone marrow examination; (c) splenomegaly is present; and (d) splenectomy corrects the cytopenia. Anemia, leukopenia and thrombocytopenia occur to differing degrees in association with splenomegaly and 'hypersplenism', and it is difficult to define any predictable relationship between splenomegaly and the degree of cytopenia induced by the wide variety of primary and secondary disorders that can cause splenic enlargement.

(a) Anemia

Splenomegaly from many causes tends to increase the mass of red cells pooled in the spleen, and this may lead to a moderate shortening of the red cell lifespan. In itself this is seldom sufficient in degree to exceed the compensatory reserve of the bone marrow, but the volume of pooled red cells, and slight shortening of red cell survival, may diminish the sustainable population of red cells in the extrasplenic circulation. Of more importance is the dilutional effect of expansion of blood volume in the presence of limited red cell production capacity (see Chapter 9).

(b) Thrombocytopenia

The thrombocytopenia of hypersplenism is principally caused by the increased pooling of platelets in the spleen with a normal (or only slightly shortened) platelet survival (Najean et al., 1967; Cooney and Smith, 1968; Toghill, Green and Ferguson, 1977; Heyns et al., 1985). Karpatkin and Freedman (1978) studied platelet size as a means of differentiating the thrombocytopenia of ITP from that of hypersplenism, and showed that the mean platelet volume was significantly greater in patients with ITP than those with hypersplenism. Karpatkin (1978, 1983) hypothesized that the spleen is enriched with young and large platelets, termed megathrombocytes, and speculated that these platelets could be released into the circulation at times of stress. This would explain the low degree of hemostatic impairment in patients with thrombocytopenia secondary to hypersplenism.

REFERENCES

Ahn, Y. S. et al. (1983) Danazol for the treatment of idiopathic thrombocytopenic purpura. N. Engl. J. Med., 308, 1396–9.

Ahn, Y. S. et al. (1985) Danazol therapy for autoimmune hemolytic anemia. Ann. Intern. Med., 102, 298–301.

Ahn, Y. S. et al. (1987) Low dose danazol therapy in idiopathic thrombocytopenic purpura. Ann. Intern. Med., 107, 177–81.

Allgood, J. W. and Chaplin H. Jr (1967) Idiopathic acquired autoimmune hemolytic anemia: a review of 47 cases treated from 1955 through 1965. Am. J. Med., 43, 254–73.

Aster, R. H. (1966) Pooling of platelets in the spleen: role in the pathogenesis of 'hypersplenic' thrombocytopenia. J. Clin. Invest., 45, 645–57.

Aster, R. H. (1972) Platelet sequestration studies in man. Br. J. Haematol., 22, 259–63.

Aster, R. H. and Keene, W. R. (1969) Sites of platelet destruction in idiopathic thrombocytopenic purpura. Br. J. Haematol., 16, 61–73.

Baldini, M. G. (1978) Platelet production and destruction in idiopathic thrombocytopenic purpura: a controversial issue. J. Am. Med. Assoc., 239, 2477–9.

Ballem, P. J. et al. (1987) Mechanisms of thrombocytopenia in chronic autoimmune thrombocytopenic purpura: evidence of both impaired platelet production and increased platelet clearance. J. Clin. Invest., 80, 33–40.

Bateman, S. et al. (1978) Splenic red cell pooling: a diagnostic feature in polycythaemia. Br. J. Haematol., 40, 389–96.

Beard, M. E. J., Necheles, T. F. and Allen, D. M. (1969) Clinical experience with intensive transfusion therapy in Cooley's anemia. Ann. NY Acad. Sci., 165, 415–22.

Becker, P. S. and Lux, S. E. (1985) Hereditary spherocytosis and related disorders. Clin. Haematol., 14, 15–43.

Bellucci, S. et al. (1988) Low doses vs conventional doses of corticoids in immune thrombocytopenic purpura (ITP): results of a randomized clinical trial in 160 children, 223 adults. Blood, 71, 1165–9.

Bender, B. S. et al. (1985) Defective reticuloendothelial system Fc-receptor function in patients with Acquired Immunodeficiency Syndrome. J. Infect. Dis., 152, 409–12.

Besa, E. C. (1988) Rapid transient reversal of anemia and long-term effects of maintenance intravenous immunoglobulin for autoimmune hemolytic anemia in patients with lymphoproliferative disorders. *Am. J. Med.*, **84**, 691–7.

Bianco, C., Griffin, F. M. and Silverstein, S.C. (1975) Studies of the macrophage complement receptor: alteration of receptor function upon macrophage activation. *J. Exp. Med.*, **141**, 1278–90.

Bishop, M. D. and Lansing, L. S. (1982) The spleen: a correlative overview of normal and pathologic anatomy. *Hum. Pathol.* **13**, 334–42.

Blajchman, M. A. *et al.* (1979) Shortening of the bleeding time in rabbits by hydrocortisone caused by inhibition of prostacyclin generation by the vessel wall. *J. Clin. Invest.*, **63**, 1026–35.

Bowdler, A. J. (1962) Theoretical considerations concerning measurement of the splenic red cell pool. *Clin. Sci.*, **23**, 181–95.

Branehog, I., Kutti, J. and Weinfeld, A. (1974) Platelet survival and platelet production in idiopathic thrombocytopenic purpura. *Br. J. Haematol.*, **27**, 127–43.

Branehog, I. *et al.* (1975) The relation of thrombo-kinetics to bone marrow megakaryocytes in idiopathic thrombocytopenic purpura. *Blood*, **45**, 551–62.

Brennan, M. F. *et al.* (1975) Correlation between response to corticosteroids and splenectomy for adult idiopathic thrombocytopenic purpura. *Am. J. Surg.*, **129**, 490–2.

Bussel, J. B. *et al.* (1983a) Intravenous use of gam-maglobulin in the treatment of chronic immune thrombocytopenic purpura as a means to defer splenectomy. *J. Pediatr.*, **103**, 651–4.

Bussel, J.B. *et al.* (1983b) Intravenous gammaglobulin treatment of chronic idiopathic thrombocytopenic purpura. *Blood*, **62**, 480–6.

Bussel, J. B. *et al.* (1985) Treatment of acute idiopathic thrombocytopenia of childhood with intravenous infusions of gammaglobulin. *J. Pediatr.*, **106**, 886–90.

Chaplin, H. and Avioli, L. V. (1977) Autoimmune hemolytic anemia. *Arch. Intern. Med.*, **137**, 346–51.

Chen, L. and Weiss, L. (1972) Electron microscopy of the red pulp of human spleen. *Am. J. Anat.*, **134**, 425–58.

Chen, L. and Weiss, L. (1973) The role of the sinus wall in the passage of erythrocytes through the spleen. *Blood*, **41**, 529–37.

Christensen, B. E. (1973a) Erythrocyte pooling and sequestration in enlarged spleens. Estimations of splenic erythrocyte and plasma volume in spleno-megalic patients. *Scand. J. Haematol.*, **10**, 106–19.

Christensen, B. E. (1973b) The pattern of erythrocyte sequestration in immunohaemolysis: effects of prednisone treatment and splenectomy. *Scand. J. Haematol.*, **10**, 120–9.

Cines, D. B. and Schreiber, A. D. (1979) Immune thrombocytopenia: use of a Coombs' antiglobulin test to detect IgG and C3 on platelets. *N. Engl. J. Med.*, **300**, 106–11.

Clarkson, S. B. *et al.* (1986) Treatment of refractory immune thrombocytopenic purpura with an anti-Fc γ-receptor antibody. *N. Engl. J. Med.*, **314**, 1236–9.

Cohen, A., Markenson, A. L. and Schwartz, E. (1980) Transfusion requirements and splenectomy in thalassemia major. *J. Pediatr.*, **97**, 100–2.

Come, S. E., Shohet, S. B. and Robinson, S.H. (1974) Surface remodeling *vs* whole-cell hemolysis of reti-culocytes produced with erythroid stimulation or iron deficiency anemia. *Blood*, **44**, 817–29.

Conley, C. L. *et al.* (1982) Autoimmune hemolytic anemia with reticulocytopenia and erythroid mar-row. *N. Engl. J. Med.*, **306**, 281–6.

Cooney, D. P. and Smith, B. A. (1968) The pathophysiology of hypersplenic thrombocy-topenia. *Arch. Intern. Med.*, **121**, 332–7.

Cooper, R. A. (1972) Loss of membrane components in the pathogenesis of antibody-induced sphero-cytosis. *J. Clin. Invest.*, **51**, 16–21.

Court, W. S. *et al.* (1987) Platelet surface-bound IgG in patients with immune and nonimmune throm-bocytopenia. *Blood*, **69**, 278–83.

Crosby, W. H. (1957) Siderocytes and the spleen. *Blood*, **12**, 165–70.

Crosby, W. H. (1975) Wet purpura, dry purpura. *J. Am. Med. Assoc.*, **232**, 7441–45.

Crosby, W. H. and Rappaport, H. (1957) Autoim-mune hemolytic anemia. I. Analysis of hemato-logic observations with particular reference to their prognostic value. A survey of 57 cases. *Blood*, **12**, 42–9.

Dacie, J. F. (1962) *The Haemolytic Anaemias, Con-genital and Acquired.* 2nd edn. Churchill, London.

Difino, S. M. *et al.* (1980) Adult idiopathic thrombo-cytopenic purpura: clinical findings and response to therapy. *Am. J. Med.*, **69**, 430–42.

Dixon, R., Rosse, W. and Ebbert, L. (1975) Quan-titative determination of antibody in idiopathic thrombocytopenic purpura: correlation of serum and platelet-bound antibody with clinical re-sponse. *N. Engl. J. Med.*, **292**, 230–6.

Doan, C. A., Bouroncle, B. A. and Wiseman, B. K. (1960) Idiopathic and secondary thrombocyto-penic purpura: clinical study and evaluation of 381 cases over a period of 28 years. *Ann. Intern. Med.*, **53**, 861–76.

Ehlenberger, A. G. and Nussenzweig, V. (1977) The role of membrane receptors for C3b and C3d in phagocytosis. *J. Exp. Med.*, **145**, 357–71.

Eichner, E. R. (1979) Splenic function: normal, too much and too little. *Am. J. Med.*, **66**, 311–20.

Emerson, C. P. *et al.* (1956) Studies on the destruction of red blood cells. *Arch. Intern. Med.*, **97**, 1–38.

Emond, A. M. *et al.* (1984) Role of the splenectomy in homozygous sickle cell disease in childhood. *Lancet*, i, 88–91.

Engelhard, D., Cividalli, G. and Rachmilewitz, E. A. (1975) Splenectomy in homozygous beta-thalassaemia: a retrospective study of 30 patients. *Br. J. Haematol.*, **31**, 391–403.

Eraklis, A. J. *et al.* (1967) Hazard of overwhelming infection after splenectomy in childhood. *N. Engl. J. Med.*, **276**, 1225–9.

Faloon, W. W., Green, R. W. and Lozner, E. L. (1952) The hemostatic defect in thrombocytopenia as studied by the use of ACTH and cortisone. *Am. J. Med.*, **13**, 12–20.

Ferrant, A. (1983) The role of the spleen in haemolysis. *Clin. Haematol.*, **12**, 489–504.

Ferrant, A. *et al.* (1987) The spleen and haemolysis: evaluation of the intrasplenic transit time. *Br. J. Haematol.*, **65**, 31–4.

Finch, S. C. *et al.* (1974) Immunosuppressive therapy of chronic idiopathic thrombocytopenic purpura. *Am. J. Med.*, **56**, 4–12.

Frank, M. M. (1987) Complement in the pathophysiology of human disease. *N. Engl. J. Med.*, **316**, 1525–30.

Frank, M. M. *et al.* (1977) Pathophysiology of immune hemolytic anemia. *Ann. Intern. Med.*, **87**, 210–22.

Frank, M. M. *et al.* (1979) Defective reticuloendothelial system Fc-receptor function in systemic lupus erythematosis. *N. Engl. J. Med.*, **300**, 518–23.

Frank, M. M. *et al.* (1983) Immunoglobulin G Fc-receptor-mediated clearance in autoimmune diseases. *Ann. Intern. Med.*, **98**, 206–18.

Freedman, J. (1987) The significance of complement on the red cell surface. *Transfusion Med. Rev.*, **1**, 58–70.

Fries, L.F., Brickman, C.M. and Frank, M.M. (1983) Monocyte receptors for the Fc portion of IgG increase in number in autoimmune hemolytic anemia and other hemolytic states and are decreased by corticosteroid therapy. *J. Immunol.*, **131**, 1240–5.

Galili, U., Clark, M.R. and Shohet, S.B. (1986) Excessive binding of natural anti-alpha-galactosyl immunoglobin G to sickle erythrocytes may contribute to extravascular cell destruction. *J. Clin. Invest.*, **77**, 27–33.

Gibson, J. *et al.* (1986) Management of splenectomy failures in chronic immune thrombocytopenic purpura: role of accessory splenectomy. *Aust. NZ J. Med.*, **16**, 695–8.

Green, G.A., Rehn, M.M. and Kalra, V.K. (1985) Cell-bound autologous immunoglobulin in erythrocyte subpopulations from patients with sickle cell disease. *Blood*, **65**, 1127–33.

Gugliotta, L. *et al.* (1981) Chronic idiopathic thrombocytopenic purpura: site of platelet sequestration and results of splenectomy. *Scand. J. Haematol.*, **26**, 407–12.

Hansen, S. and Jarhult, J. (1986) Accessory spleen imaging: radionuclide, ultrasound and CT investigations in a patient with thrombocytopenia 25 years after splenectomy for ITP. *Scand. J. Haematol.*, **37**, 74–7.

Harker, L.A. (1970) Thrombokinetics in idiopathic thrombocytopenic purpura. *Br. J. Haematol.*, **19**, 95–104.

Hauch, T.W. and Rosse, W.F. (1977) Platelet-bound complement (C3) in immune thrombocytopenia. *Blood*, **50**, 1129–36.

Hayes, M.M. *et al.* (1985) Splenic pathology in immune thrombocytopenia. *J. Clin. Pathol.*, **38**, 985–8.

Hedge, U.M., Bowes, A. and Roter, B.L.T. (1985) Platelet associated complement components (PAC_{3c} and PAC_{3d}) in patients with autoimmune thrombocytopenia. *Br. J. Haematol.*, **60**, 49–55.

Hedge, U.M. *et al.* (1973) Measurement of splenic red cell volume and visualization of the spleen with ^{99m}Tc. *J. Nucl. Med.*, **14**, 769–71.

Heyns, A. duP. *et al.* (1985) Kinetics and mobilization from the spleen of indium-111-labelled platelets during plateletpheresis. *Transfusion*, **25**, 215–18.

Hoffman, R. *et al.* (1985) An antibody cytotoxic to megakaryocyte progenitor cells in a patient with immune thrombocytopenic purpura. *N. Engl. J. Med.*, **312**, 1170–4.

Hosea, S.W. *et al.* (1981) Opsonic requirements for intravascular clearance after splenectomy. *N. Engl. J. Med.*, **304**, 245–50.

Huber, H. and Fudenberg, H.H. (1968) Receptor sites of human monocytes for IgG. *Int. Arch. Allergy*, **34**, 18–31.

Huber, H. *et al.* (1968) Human monocytes: distinct receptor sites for the third component of complement and for immunoglobulin G. *Science*, **162**, 1281–3.

Imbach, P. *et al.* (1981) High-dose intravenous gammaglobulin for idiopathic thrombocytopenic purpura in childhood. *Lancet*, i, 1228–31.

Imbach, P. *et al.* (1985) Intravenous immunoglobulin versus oral corticosteroids in acute immune thrombocytopenic purpura in childhood. *Lancet*, ii, 464–8.

Jandl, J.H. and Aster, R.H. (1967) Increased splenic pooling and the pathogenesis of hypersplenism. *Am. J. Med. Sci.*, 253, 383–98.

Jandl, J.H. and Kaplan, M.E. (1960) The destruction of red cells by antibodies in man. III. Qualitative factors influencing the patterns of hemolysis *in vivo*. *J. Clin. Invest.*, 39, 1145–56.

Jandl, J.H. *et al.* (1965) Proliferative response of the spleen and liver to hemolysis. *J. Exp. Med.*, 122, 299–325.

Jensen, O.M. and Kristensen, J. (1986) Red pulp of the spleen in autoimmune haemolytic anemia and hereditary spherocytosis: morphometric light and electron microscopic studies. *Scand. J. Haematol.*, 36, 263–6.

Joist, J.H. and Baker, R.K. (1981) Loss of [111]Indium as indicator of platelet injury. *Blood*, 58, 350–3.

Karpatkin, S. (1978) Heterogeneity of human platelets. VI. Correlation of platelet function with platelet volume. *Blood*, 51, 307–16.

Karpatkin, S. (1983) The spleen and thrombocytopenia. *Clin. Haematol.*, 12, 591–604.

Karpatkin, S. (1985) Autoimmune thrombocytopenic purpura. *Semin. Hematol.*, 22, 260–88.

Karpatkin, S. and Freedman, M.L. (1978) Hypersplenic thrombocytopenia differentiated from increased peripheral destruction by platelet volume. *Ann. Intern. Med.*, 89, 200–3.

Karpatkin, S., Strick, N. and Siskind, G.W. (1972) Detection of splenic antiplatelet antibody synthesis in autoimmune thrombocytopenic purpura. *Br. J. Haematol.*, 23, 167–76.

Kay, M.M.B. (1975) Mechanism of removal of senescent cells by human macrophages *in situ*. *Proc. Natl. Acad, Sci. USA*, 72, 3521–5.

Kay, M.M.B. (1984) Localization of senescent cell antigen on band 3. *Proc. Natl. Acad. Sci. USA*, 81, 5753–7.

Kay, M.M.B. *et al.* (1982) Antigenicity, storage, and aging: physiologic autoantibodies to cell membrane and serum proteins and the senescent cell antigen. *Mol. Cell. Biochem.*, 49, 65–85.

Kayser, W. *et al.* (1983) Platelet associated complement C3 in thrombocytopenic states. *Br. J. Haematol.*, 54, 353–63.

Kelton, J.G. (1981) Vaccination-associated relapse of immune thrombocytopenia. *J. Am. Med. Assoc.*, 245, 369–71.

Kelton, J.G. (1983) The measurement of platelet-bound immunoglobulins: An overview of the methods and the biological relevance of platelet-associated IgG. in *Progress in Hematology*. Vol. XIII (ed. E.B. Brown), Grune and Stratton, NY, pp. 163–99.

Kelton, J.G. (1985) Impaired reticuloendothelial function in patients treated with methyldopa. *N. Engl. J. Med.*, 313, 596–600.

Kelton, J.G. (1987) Platelet and red cell clearance is determined by the interaction of the IgG and complement on the cells and the activity of the reticuloendothelial system. *Transfusion Med. Rev.*, 1, 75–84.

Kelton, J.G. and Denomme, G. (1982) The quantitation of platelet-associated IgG on cohorts of platelets separated from healthy individuals by buoyant density centrifugation. *Blood*, 60, 136–9.

Kelton, J.G., Powers, P.J. and Carter, C.J. (1982) A prospective study of the usefulness of the measurement of platelet-associated IgG for the diagnosis of idiopathic thrombocytopenic purpura. *Blood*, 60, 1050–3.

Kelton, J.G. and Steeves, K. (1983) The amount of platelet-bound albumin parallels the amount of IgG on washed platelets from patients with immune thrombocytopenia. *Blood*, 62, 924–7.

Kelton, J.G. *et al.* (1984) The relationship among platelet-associated IgG, platelet lifespan, and reticuloendothelial cell function. *Blood*, 63, 1434–8.

Kelton, J.G. *et al.* (1985) The concentration of IgG in the serum is a major determinant of Fc-dependent reticuloendothelial function. *Blood*, 66, 490–5.

Kernoff, L.M., Blake, K.C.H. and Shackleton, D. (1980) Influence of the amount of platelet-bound IgG on platelet survival and site of sequestration in autoimmune thrombocytopenia. *Blood*, 55, 730–3.

Khansari, N. and Fudenberg, H.H. (1983) Phagocytosis of senescent erythrocytes by autologous monocytes: requirement of membrane-specific autologous IgG for immune elimination of aging red blood cells. *Cell. Immunol.*, 78, 114–121.

Kitchens, C.S. (1977) Amelioration of endothelial abnormalities by prednisone in experimental thrombocytopenia in the rabbit. *J. Clin. Invest.*, 60, 1129–34.

Komrower, G.M. and Watson, G.H. (1954) Prognosis of idiopathic thrombocytopenic purpura of childhood. *Arch. Dis. Childh.*, 29, 502–6.

Kristensen, J. and Jensen, O.M. (1985) Splenic pulp, plasma cells and foamy histiocytes in immune thrombocytopenia: combined morphometric, immunohistochemical and ultrastructural studies. *Scand. J. Haematol.*, **34**, 340–4.

Kurata, Y. *et al.* (1986) Platelet-associated complement in chronic ITP. *Br. J. Haematol.*, **60**, 723–33.

Lawley, T.J. *et al.* (1981) Defective Fc-receptor functions associated with the HLA-B8/DRw3 haplotype. *N. Engl. J. Med.*, **304**, 185–92.

Lay, W.H. and Nussenzweig, V. (1968) Receptors for complement on leukocytes. *J. Exp. Med.*, **128**, 991–1009.

Lehman, H.A. *et al.* (1987) Complement-mediated autoimmune thrombocytopenia. Monoclonal IgM antiplatelet antibody associated with lymphoreticular malignant disease. *N. Engl. J. Med.*, **316**, 194–8.

Lewis, S.M. *et al.* (1977) Splenic red cell pooling in hairy cell leukaemia. *Br. J. Haematol.*, **35**, 351–7.

Liesveld, J.L., Rowe, J.M. and Lichtman, M.A. (1987) Variability of the erythropoietic response in autoimmune hemolytic anemia: analysis of 109 cases. *Blood*, **69**, 820–6.

Lobuglio, A.F., Cotran, R.S. and Jandl, J.H. (1967) Red cells coated with immunoglobulin G: binding and sphering by mononuclear cells in man. *Science*, **158**, 1582–5.

Low, P.S. *et al.* (1985) The role of hemoglobin denaturation and band 3 clustering in red blood cell aging. *Science*, **227**, 531–3.

Luk, S.C., Musclow, E. and Simon, G.T. (1980) Platelet phagocytosis in the spleen of patients with idiopathic thrombocytopenic purpura. *Histopathology*, **4**, 127–36.

Lum, L.G. *et al.* (1980) Splenectomy in the management of the thrombocytopenia of the Wiskott–Aldrich syndrome. *N. Engl. J. Med.*, **302**, 892–6.

Lutz, H.U., Flepp, R. and Stringaro-Wipf, G. (1984) Naturally occurring autoantibodies to exoplasmic and cryptic regions of band 3 protein, the major integral membrane protein of human red blood cells. *J. Immunol.*, **133**, 2610–18.

Lutz, H.U. and Wipf, G. (1982) Naturally occurring autoantibodies to skeletal proteins from human red blood cells. *J. Immunol.*, **128**, 1695–9.

Lutz, H.U. *et al.* (1987) Naturally occurring anti-band-3 antibodies and complement together mediate phagocytosis of oxidatively stressed human erythrocytes. *Proc. Natl. Acad. Sci. USA*, **84**, 7368–72.

Lux, S.E. and John, K.M. (1977) Isolation and partial characterization of a high molecular weight red cell membrane protein complex normally removed by the spleen. *Blood*, **50**, 625–41.

McMillan, R. (1981) Chronic idiopathic thrombocytopenic purpura. *N. Engl. J. Med.*, **304**, 1135–47.

McMillan, R. and Martin, M. (1981) Fixation of C3 to platelets *in vitro* by antiplatelet antibody from patients with immune thrombocytopenic purpura. *Br. J. Haematol.*, **47**, 251–6.

McMillan, R. *et al.* (1972) Immunoglobulin synthesis *in vitro* by splenic tissue in idiopathic thrombocytopenic purpura. *N. Engl. J. Med.*, **286**, 681–4.

McMillan, R. *et al.* (1974) Quantitation of platelet-binding IgG produced *in vitro* by spleens from patients with idiopathic thrombocytopenic purpura. *N. Engl. J. Med.*, **291**, 812–17.

McMillan, R. *et al.* (1987) Platelet-associated and plasma anti-glycoprotein autoantibodies in chronic ITP. *Blood*, **70**, 1040–5.

van der Meulen, F.W. *et al.* (1978) The role of adherence to human mononuclear phagocytes in the destruction of red cells sensitised with non-complement binding IgG antibodies. *Br. J. Haematol.*, **38**, 541–9.

Miller, D.R. *et al.* (1971) Hemoglobin Köln disease occurring as a fresh mutation: erythrocyte metabolism and survival. *Blood*, **38**, 715–29.

Modell, B. (1977) Total management of thalassemia major. *Arch. Dis. Child.*, **52**, 489–500.

Mohandas, N., Phillips, W.M. and Bessis, M. (1979) Red blood cell deformability and hemolytic anemias. *Semin. Hematol.*, **16**, 95–114.

Mollison, P.L. *et al.* (1965) Rate of removal from the circulation of red cells sensitised with different amounts of antibody. *Br. J. Haematol.*, **11**, 461–70.

Molnar, Z. and Rappaport, H. (1972) Fine structure of the red pulp of the spleen in hereditary spherocytosis. *Blood*, **39**, 81–98.

Mori, P.G. *et al.* (1983) Chronic idiopathic thrombocytopenia treated with immunoglobulin. *Arch. Dis. Child.*, **58**, 851–5.

Mueller-Eckhardt, C. *et al.* (1980) The clinical significance of platelet-associated IgG: a study on 298 patients with various disorders. *Br. J. Haematol.*, **46**, 123–31.

Mueller-Eckhardt, C. *et al.* (1982) Platelet associated IgG, platelet survival, and platelet sequestration in thrombocytopenic states. *Br. J. Haematol.*, **52**, 49–58.

Murphy, J.R. (1967) The influence of pH and temperature on some physical properties of normal erythrocytes and erythrocytes from patients with hereditary spherocytosis. *J. Lab. Clin. Med.*, **69**, 758–75.

Murphy, W.G. and Kelton, J.G. (1988) Role of the

spleen in autoimmune disorders. In *Disorders of the Spleen: Pathophysiology and Management* (eds C. Pochedly, R.H. Sills and A.D. Schwartz), Marcel Dekker Inc., New York and Basel.

Myers, T.J. *et al.* (1982) Platelet-associated complement C3 in immune thrombocytopenic purpura. *Blood*, **59**, 1023–8.

Nagasawa, T., Kim, B.K. and Baldini, M.G. (1977) In vivo elution of ^{51}Cr from labelled platelets induced by antibody. *Fed. Proc.*, **36**, 380.

Najean, Y. and Ardaillou, N. (1971) The sequestration site of platelets in idiopathic thrombocytopenic purpura: its correlation with the results of splenectomy. *Br. J. Haematol.*, **21**, 153–64.

Najean, Y. *et al.* (1963) Survival of radiochromium-labelled platelets in thrombocytopenia. *Blood*, **22**, 718–32.

Najean, Y. *et al.* (1967) The platelet destruction site in thrombocytopenic purpura. *Br. J. Haematol.*, **13**, 409–26.

Nathan, D.G. and Gunn, R.B. (1966) Thalassemia: the consequences of unbalanced hemoglobin synthesis. *Am. J. Med.*, **41**, 815–30.

Newland, A.C. *et al.* (1983) High-dose intravenous IgG in adults with autoimmune thrombocytopenia. *Lancet*, **i**, 84–7.

O'Brien, R.T., Pearson, H.A. and Spencer, R.P. (1977) Transfusion induced decrease in spleen size in thalassemia major: documentation by radioisotopic scan. *J. Pediatr.*, **81**, 105–7.

Oral, A. *et al.* (1984) Intravenous gammaglobulin in the treatment of chronic idiopathic thrombocytopenic purpura in adults. *Am. J. Med.*, **76**(3A), 187–92.

Palek, J. (1985) Hereditary elliptocytosis and related disorders. *Clin. Haematol.*, **14**, 45–87.

Palek, J. and Lux, S.E. (1983) Red cell membrane skeletal defects in hereditary and acquired hemolytic anemias. *Sem. Hematol.*, **20**, 189–224.

Panzer, S. *et al.* (1986) Platelet-associated immunoglobulins IgG, IgM, IgA and complement C3c in chronic idiopathic autoimmune thrombocytopenia: relation to the sequestration pattern of ^{111}Indium labelled platelets. *Scand. J. Haematol.*, **37**, 97–102.

Pearson, H. A. *et al.* (1979) Developmental aspects of splenic function in sickle cell diseases. *Blood*, **53**, 358–65.

Penny, R., Rozenberg, M. C. and Firkin, B. G. (1966) The splenic platelet pool. *Blood*, **27**, 1–16.

Peters, A. M. (1983) Splenic blood flow and blood cell kinetics. *Clin. Haematol.*, **12**, 421–47.

Peters, A. M. and Lavender, J. P. (1983) Platelet kinetics with indium-111 platelets: comparison with chromium-51 platelets. *Semin. Thromb.*

Hemostas., **9**, 100–14.

Peters, A. M. *et al.* (1980) Use of ^{111}Indium-labelled platelets to measure splenic function. *Br. J. Haematol.*, **46**, 587–93.

Petz, L. D. and Garratty, G. (1980) *Acquired Immune Hemolytic Anemias*, Churchill Livingstone, New York and London, Chapter 2, pp. 22–37.

Prankerd, T. A. J. (1963) The spleen and anaemia. *Br. Med. J.*, **2**, 517–24.

Raccuglia, G. (1971) Gray platelet syndrome: a variety of qualitative platelet disorder. *Am. J. Med.*, **51**, 818–28.

Ries, C. A. and Price, D. C. (1974) [^{51}Cr]Platelet kinetics in thrombocytopenia: correlation between splenic sequestration of platelets and response to splenectomy. *Ann. Intern. Med.*, **80**, 702–7.

Rifkind, R. A. (1965) Heinz body anemia: an ultrastructural study. II. Red cell sequestration and destruction. *Blood*, **26**, 433–48.

Rigas, D. A. and Koler, R. D. (1961) Decreased erythrocyte survival in hemoglobin H disease as a result of the abnormal properties of hemoglobin H: the benefit of splenectomy. *Blood*, **18**, 1–17.

Rinehart, J. J. *et al.* (1974) Effect of corticosteroids on human monocyte function. *J. Clin. Invest.*, **54**, 1337–43.

Ross, G. D. *et al.* (1973) Two different complement receptors on human lymphocytes. *J. Exp. Med.*, **138**, 798–811.

Rosse, W. F. (1971) Quantitative immunology of immune hemolytic anemia. II. The relationship of cell-bound antibody to hemolysis and the effect of treatment. *J. Clin. Invest.*, **50**, 734–43.

Rosse, W. F., de Boisfleury, A. and Bessis, M. (1975) The interaction of phagocytic cells and red cells modified by immune reactions. Comparison of antibody and complement coated red cells. *Blood Cells*, **1**, 345–58.

Salama, A. *et al.* (1984) Treatment of autoimmune thrombocytopenic purpura with rhesus antibodies (anti-Rh$_0$(D)). *Blut*, **49**, 29–35.

Salama, A., Kiefel, V. and Mueller-Eckhardt, C. (1986) Effect of IgG anti-Rh$_0$(D) in adult patients with chronic autoimmune thrombocytopenia. *Am. J. Hematol.*, **22**, 241–50.

Schnitzer, B. *et al.* (1972) Pitting function of the spleen in malaria: ultrastructural observations. *Science*, **177**, 175–7.

Schreiber, A. D. and Frank, M. M. (1972a) Role of antibody and complement in the immune clearance and destruction of erythrocytes. I. *In vivo* effects of IgG and IgM complement-fixing sites. *J. Clin. Invest.*, **51**, 575–82.

Schreiber, A. D. and Frank, M. M. (1972b) Role of antibody and complement in the immune clearance and destruction of erythrocytes. II. Molecular nature of IgG and IgM complement-fixing sites and effects of their interactions with serum. *J. Clin. Invest.*, **51**, 583–9.

Schreiber, A. D. *et al.* (1975) Effect of corticosteroids on the human monocyte IgG and complement receptors. *J. Clin. Invest.*, **56**, 1189–97.

Schreiber, A. D. *et al.* (1987) Effect of danazol in immune thrombocytopenic purpura. *N. Engl. J. Med.*, **316**, 503–8.

Schwartz, S. I., Bernard, R. P. and Adams, J. T. (1970) Splenectomy for hematologic disorders. *Arch. Surg.*, **101**, 338–47.

Seelder, R. A. and Shwiaki, M. Z. (1972) Acute splenic sequestration crisis (ASSC) in young children with sickle cell anemia: clinical observations in 20 episodes in 14 children. *Clin. Pediatr.*, **11**, 701–4.

Shattil, S. J. and Cooper, R. A. (1972) Maturation of macroreticulocyte membrane *in vivo*. *J. Lab. Clin. Med.*, **79**, 215–27.

Shulman, N. R., Marder, V. J. and Weinrach, R. S. (1965) Similarities between known antiplatelet antibodies and the factor responsible for thrombocytopenia in idiopathic purpura. Physiologic, serologic, and isotopic studies. *Ann. NY Acad. Sci.*, **124**, 499–542.

Shulman, N. R. *et al.* (1968) Evidence that the spleen retains the youngest and hemostatically most effective platelets. *Trans. Assoc. Am. Physicans*, **81**, 302–13.

Silverstein, M. N. *et al.* (1972) Idiopathic acquired hemolytic anemia. Survival in 117 cases. *Arch. Intern. Med.*, **129**, 85–93.

Slater, L. M., Muir, W. A. and Weed, R. I. (1968) Influence of splenectomy on insoluble hemoglobin inclusion bodies in β-thalassemic erythrocytes. *Blood*, **31**, 766–77.

Solanki, D. L., Kletter, G. G. and Castro, O. (1986) Acute splenic sequestration crisis in adults with sickle cell disease. *Am. J. Med.*, **80**, 985–90.

Sprague, C. C. and Paterson, J. C. S. (1958) Role of the spleen and effect of splenectomy in sickle cell disease. *Blood*, **13**, 569–81.

Stefanini, M. and Martino, N. B. (1956) Use of prednisone in the management of some hemorrhagic states. *N. Engl. J. Med.*, **254**, 313–17.

Stiehm, E. R. *et al.* (1987) Intravenous immunoglobulins as therapeutic agents. *Ann. Intern. Med.*, **107**, 367–82.

Szwed, J. J., Yum, M. and Hogan, R. (1980) A beneficial effect of splenectomy in sickle cell anemia and chronic renal failure. *Am. J. Med. Sci.*, **279**, 169–172.

Tavassoli, M. and McMillan, R. (1975) Structure of the spleen in idiopathic thrombocytopenic purpura. *Am. J. Clin. Pathol.*, **64**, 180–91.

Thompson, R. L. *et al.* (1972) Idiopathic thrombocytopenic purpura: long-term results of treatment and the prognostic significance of response to corticosteroids. *Arch. Intern. Med.*, **130**, 730–4.

Toghill, P. J., Green, S. and Ferguson, R. (1977) Platelet dynamics in chronic liver disease with special reference to the role of the spleen. *J. Clin. Pathol.*, **30**, 367–71.

Verheyden, C. N. *et al.* (1978) Accessory splenectomy in management of recurrent idiopathic thrombocytopenic purpura. *Mayo Clin. Proc.*, **53**, 442–6.

Verp, M. and Karpatkin, S. (1975) Effect of plasma, steroids or steroid products on the adhesion of human opsonized thrombocytes to human leukocytes. *J. Lab. Clin. Med.*, **85**, 478–86.

Weed, R. I. and Bowdler, A. J. (1966) Metabolic dependence of the critical hemolytic volume of human erythrocytes: relationship to osmotic fragility and autohemolysis in hereditary spherocytosis and normal red cells. *J. Clin. Invest.*, **45**, 1137–49.

Weiss, L. (1974) A scanning electron microscopic study of the spleen. *Blood*, **43**, 665–91.

Weiss, L. (1983) The red pulp of the spleen: structural basis of blood flow. *Clin. Haematol.*, **12**, 375–93.

Weiss, L. and Tavassoli, M. (1972) Anatomic hazards to the passage of erythrocytes through the spleen. *Sem. Hematol.*, **7**, 372–80.

Wennberg, E. and Weiss, L. (1968) Splenic erythroclasia: an electron microscopic study of hemoglobin H disease. *Blood*, **31**, 778–90.

Wentz, A. C. (1982) Adverse effects of danazol in pregnancy. *Ann. Intern. Med.*, **96**, 672–3.

Whitaker, A. N. (1969) Infection and the spleen: association between hyposplenism, pneumococcal sepsis and disseminated intravascular coagulation. *Med. J. Aust.*, **1**, 1213–19.

White, J. M. and Dacie, J. V. (1971) The unstable hemoglobins: molecular and clinical features. *Progr. Hematol.*, **7**, 69–109.

Winiarski, J. and Holm, G. (1983) Platelet associated immunoglobulins and complement in idiopathic thrombocytopenic purpura. *Clin. Exp. Immunol.*, **53**, 201–7.

Worlledge, S., Hughes Jones, N. C. and Bain, B. (1982) in *Blood and Its Disorders* (eds R. M. Hardisty and D. J. Weatherall), Chapter 11, Blackwell Scientific, Oxford and Boston, pp. 485–93.

THE SPLEEN IN THE MYELOPROLIFERATIVE DISORDERS

Michael T. Shaw

14.1   INTRODUCTION

The term 'myeloproliferative syndrome' was coined by Dameshek (1951) and most hematologists today would regard the myeloproliferative disorders as comprising polycythemia vera, essential thrombocythemia, agnogenic (primary) myeloid metaplasia, and chronic granulocytic leukemia. With the possible exception of essential thrombocythemia, they are considered to be panmyeloses, and are clonal hemopathies which arise from a pluripotent stem cell (Adamson and Fialkow, 1978). Each disease appears to show a characteristic emphasis on the proliferation of one cell line. Thus in polycythemia vera erythropoiesis predominates, whereas in essential thrombocythemia and chronic granulocytic leukemia thrombopoiesis and granulopoiesis are emphasized respectively. In agnogenic myeloid metaplasia there is fibrosis of the bone marrow which does not seem to be part of the underlying myeloid proliferative process, but is probably a reaction to the abnormal myeloid cell development.

The only consistent chromosomal abnormality in this group of disorders is the Philadelphia chromosome (Ph[1]) found in all the hemopoietic cell precursors in patients with chronic granulocytic leukemia. The Ph[1] is known to represent reciprocal translocation of sections of the long arms of chromosomes 9 and 22. This important molecular event involves translocation of the Abelson proto-oncogene (c-abl) from chromo-some 9 to within the breakpoint cluster region (bcr) on chromosome 22, with the formation of a chimeric bcr/c-abl gene (Champlin *et al.*, 1986).

The spleen is an organ which is intimately associated with the hemopoietic system. Physiologically it is responsible for trapping effete circulating blood cells, and pathologically this removal of cells may become excessive, as in patients with immune thrombocytopenic purpura, various hemolytic anemias and some myeloproliferative disorders. In many mammals, the spleen plays a role in the development of hemopoiesis during embryonic life, and it is therefore not unexpected that it is involved in the hematopathology of the myeloproliferative disorders. In this chapter, the pathophysiological processes which occur in the spleen in these diseases will be reviewed, together with the clinical implications of splenomegaly, and finally the indications for and results of splenectomy and splenic radiotherapy.

14.2   SPLENIC HEMATOPOIESIS AND MYELOID METAPLASIA

Extramedullary hematopoiesis in man occurs in the spleen to a variable extent during embryonic life from the twelfth week to birth (Wintrobe *et al.*, 1976; Lewis, 1983). Embryologically, the spleen originates as a thickening of the mesenchyme of the gastric mesentery. Large basophilic stem cells differentiate into erythroblasts and megakaryocytes within the sinusoids, and into granulocytes adjacent to the arterioles. Stromal cells in mice have been found to proliferate in the embryonic spleen prior to the appearance of splenic hematopoiesis, and to decrease when splenic hematopoiesis becomes established (van den Heuvel *et al.*, 1987). The hematopoietic tissue completely fills the spleen prior to the development of lymphatic tissue (Thiel and Downey, 1921; Block, 1964; Ward and Block, 1971). In most mammals, myeloid tissue persists in the red pulp after embryonic life, but in man only a few granulocytes, erythroblasts and megakaryocytes are found here at birth, and these totally disappear soon afterwards.

It is claimed by Ward and Block (1971) that as far as embryonic hematopoiesis is concerned, ontogeny recapitulates phylogeny, and that mature fishes, amphibia, and reptiles normally have splenic hematopoiesis. Because extramedullary hematopoiesis in man occurs in sites of normal hematopoiesis in lower vertebrates, these areas, including the spleen, must either retain mesenchymal cells capable of differentiating into hematopoietic stem cells, or alternatively, the microenvironment is suitable for recolonization by hematopoietic stem cells. The potential for splenic hematopoiesis remains after birth, and when there is hematological stress, as in megaloblastic or hemolytic anemias, extramedullary erythropoiesis and megakaryopoiesis may be found in the spleen. It is further postulated that in these conditions injury to the endothelial cells of the bone marrow sinuses occurs, allowing immature cells to escape into the blood and become trapped in the splenic red pulp. Further mitotic divisions result in the formation of 'nests' of erythroid and megakaryocytic cells (Lewis, 1983).

In contrast, Keleman, Calvo and Fliedner (1979) claim that the spleen is not a significant organ of hematopoiesis in the human fetus, and that most previous observations have been made in non-human mammals. Wolf, Luevano and Neiman (1983) studied spleens from 65 aborted human fetuses and stillborn infants, with a gestational age varying from 12 to 40 weeks. They used immunohistochemical and cytochemical methods to study hematopoiesis and found surprisingly few hematological precursor cells. What few erythroid precursors were seen, were scattered within the red pulp, and not in clusters. They were mainly late normoblasts; there were even fewer granulocytic precursors and only very rare mature megakaryocytes. Similar findings were obtained when monoclonal antibodies prepared against transferrin receptors were used to demonstrate erythroid and myeloid precursors. These investigators believe that hematopoietic cells found in embryonic spleens merely reflect splenic trapping of these cells from the peripheral blood.

Some workers claim, however, that pluripotential stem cells (CFUs) occur normally in the spleen as well as in the bone marrow of mature man (Schofield, 1979). Murphy (1983) suggested that erythroid-committed stem cells (BFUe and CFUe) migrate from the bone marrow into the spleen. In the context of pathological myeloproliferation, Lutton and Levere (1979) obtained a peripheral blood mononuclear cell fraction by density gradient centrifugation from patients with polycythemia vera and myelofibrosis with myeloid metaplasia, which contained erythroid precursor cells of high proliferative capacity. The erythroid precursor cells formed erythroid colonies which appeared in culture in 5 to 7 days in the absence of exogenous erythropoietin, in contrast to normal

---

Figure 14.1 Number of granulocyte colonies (CFU-C) per ml of blood and neutrophil count per μl of blood assayed 1 hour after irradiation. Solid line represents mean CFU-C $\pm$ SE per ml of blood. The mean represents triplicate cultures plated at 0.5, 1.0 and 2 × 10^5 peripheral blood cells per dish. Dotted line shows neutrophil concentration per μl and arrows indicate time of irradiation. Patients 1 (a) and 2 (b) had myelofibrosis and received splenic irradiation. (c) Astrocytoma control patients 3 (×) and 4 (●) had malignant gliomas and received brain irradiation. (Reproduced from Koeffler *et al.* (1979) *Br. J. Haematol.*, with permission.)

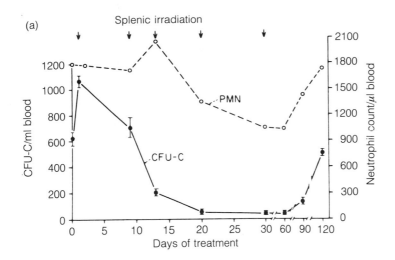

(a)

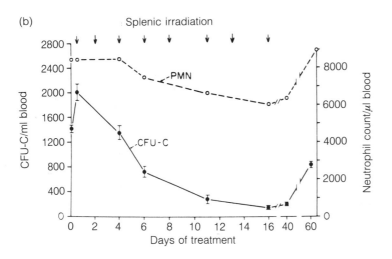

(b)

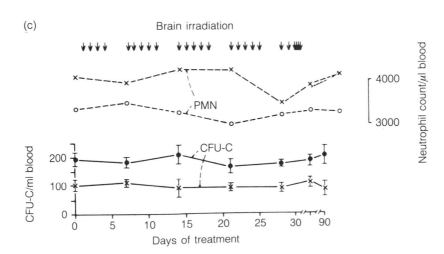

(c)

peripheral blood cells in which erythroid colonies appear later (10–14 days), and only in the presence of exogenous erythropoietin. Spleen cells from a patient with myelofibrosis behaved like spleen cells in polycythemia vera. Furthermore, patients with agnogenic myeloid metaplasia and chronic granulocytic leukemia have increased numbers of circulating myeloid precursors capable of producing colony forming units (CFU-C) *in vitro*. Splenic irradiation in patients with agnogenic myeloid metaplasia and chronic granulocytic leukemia produces a marked fall in circulating CFU-C, which remains depressed for several weeks (Barret *et al.*, 1977; Koeffler, Cline and Golde, 1979; Figure 14.1) suggesting that radiation therapy destroys splenic proliferating precursor cells. One patient with probable chronic granulocytic leukemia was found to have higher numbers of granulocyte–monocyte committed stem cells (CFU-GM) in the splenic vein than in the peripheral blood (Bagby, 1978). CFU-GM numbers rapidly fell after splenectomy. Greenberg and Steed (1981) found a hundred-fold increase in CFU-GM in spleens removed from chronic granulocytic leukemic patients compared to normal spleens. In patients with agnogenic myeloid metaplasia the splenic vein has also been found to have more CFU-GM than the peripheral venous blood. The number of CFU-GM in the splenic vein of two patients with agnogenic myeloid metaplasia were shown to be much higher than in other peripheral veins, suggesting granulocyte production by the spleen (Kirschner, Goldberg and Landaw, 1980).

It thus appears that in patients with myeloproliferative disorders, especially chronic granulocytic leukemia and agnogenic myeloid metaplasia, a very high proportion of total hematopoietic stem cell proliferation is shifted from the bone marrow to the spleen (Adler, 1976). In a few cases, there is evidence that virtually the entire hematopoietic stem cell population may have shifted to the spleen. An analogous situation may be demonstrated experimentally in mice, in which a few CFUs are always present in the spleen. When the bone marrow has been ablated with ^{89}Sr, there is a marked increase of splenic CFUs. If these mice are splenectomized 2 to 3 weeks after ^{89}Sr has been administered, they die from the complications of pancytopenia (Adler, 1976). It is postulated that in agnogenic myeloid metaplasia and chronic granulocytic leukemia, the site in which the hematopoietic cells proliferate depends first on the character of the hematopoietic population itself (Moore, 1975) and second on the characteristics of the microenvironment of the supporting organs (Wolf and Trentin, 1968). It is possible that the cells acquire 'fetal characteristics' resulting in a predilection for growth in sites of fetal hemopoietic tissue. In agnogenic myeloid metaplasia, alteration of the microenvironment may be caused by myeloid fibrosis. In chronic granulocytic leukemia, infiltration of the microenvironment with myeloid elements could result in suppression of local stem cell proliferation.

In summary, extramedullary hematopoiesis in the spleen occurs in those conditions which result in a stressed bone marrow producing normal or megaloblastic myeloid elements. Myeloid metaplasia, on the other hand, is a specific form of extramedullary hematopoiesis in which the myeloid cells, found in both the bone marrow and the spleen, are dysplastic or neoplastic. In the latter situation, the spleen shares in this pathological process.

14.3 PATHOLOGY OF THE SPLEEN IN MYELOPROLIFERATIVE SYNDROMES

14.3.1 POLYCYTHEMIA VERA

Slight to moderate splenomegaly is the rule in this disease (Westin *et al.*, 1972). The spleen often shows vascular thromboses and infarcts. Histologically, the sinuses are engorged with blood, the splenic cords may show histiocytic hyperplasia, and hemosiderin is scant or absent. Extramedullary hematopoiesis is usually absent, but when present, is limited to a few foci of erythropoiesis. If extramedullary hematopoiesis is more than scant, it usually signifies conversion to myelofibrosis (Rappaport, 1966; Pettit, Lewis and Nicholas, 1979).

14.3.2   ESSENTIAL THROMBOCYTHEMIA

The spleen in this disorder is either enlarged, weighing from 400 to more than 2000 g or it is found to be atrophic, weighing less than 15 g (Rappaport, 1966). The most prominent microscopic feature is the large number of clumped platelets in the sinuses. Very few megakaryocytes are seen, but when found, they are occasionally atypical. No other extramedullary hematopoiesis is present. It is suggested (Rappaport, 1966; Waweru and Lewis, 1985) that the spleen traps some of the excess platelets and that patients with splenic atrophy reveal the hematological and clinical manifestations of thrombocythemia before those with splenomegaly. In addition, the spleen often shows widening of the pulp cords, probably due to reticulin fibrosis.

14.3.3   AGNOGENIC MYELOID METAPLASIA

The spleen is always enlarged in this disease, weighing between 700 and 4000 g. The splenic capsule is often thickened with scars from previous infarcts, although infarcts are said by some to be fewer than in chronic granulocytic leukemia (Jackson, Parker and Lemon, 1940; Rappaport, 1966). However, others have denied this claim, and have found no significant difference (Ward and Block, 1971). Microscopically, extramedullary hematopoiesis is always found in the red pulp (Figure 14.2). The trabeculae and Malpighian corpuscles are widely separated; hematopoietic islands are found in the cords and sinuses, with nucleated red cells and granulocytes in varying proportions. Megakaryocytes are prominent and sometimes they predominate and are dysplastic (Wolf and Neiman, 1985). The degree of splenic hematopoiesis is not correlated with the degree of bone marrow fibrosis (Ward and Block, 1971; Wolf

and Neiman, 1985). Splenic cords show increased cellularity or fibrosis or both; increased reticulin can be seen when specimens are treated with silver stains (Rappaport, 1966). However, Ward and Block (1971) claim that fibrosis occurs in mild to moderate amounts in only a few progressive cases. Many histiocytes have been observed in the splenic cords, and in some cases, hemosiderin abounds in macrophages. On electron microscopy, the hemopoietic cells demonstrate loops and blebs in the nucleus. There is also cytoplasmic degeneration, suggesting that splenic hematopoiesis may, to a great extent, be ineffective (Tavassoli and Weiss, 1973). In the white pulp, the Malphigian corpuscles are atrophic. Ultrastructural studies by Tavassoli (1973) have shown focal cytoplasmic degeneration involving mitochondria and elements of endoplasmic reticulum in the lymphocytes and reticulum cells.

14.3.4   CHRONIC GRANULOCYTIC LEUKEMIA

The spleen is often very large, weighing between 1500 and 4000 g. The capsule reveals adhesions. Obliteration of normal architecture can be seen on the cut section, and ischemic and hemorrhagic infarcts may be present. Histologically, myeloid metaplasia, predominantly granulocytic, is the most notable feature. The pulp cords are infiltrated with granulocytes at all stages of maturation. Neutrophil and eosinophil myelocytes predominate, and basophils may be conspicuous. Myeloid foci are seen in the splenic sinuses together with nucleated red cells, granulocytes and megakaryocytes (Figure 14.3). In long-standing cases or after splenic radiation therapy, fibrosis of the splenic cords may be observed. In the white pulp, the Malphigian corpuscles become atrophic and widely separated as the disease progresses (Rappaport, 1966).

The similarities and differences in the pathological processes which occur in the spleen in the myeloproliferative disorders are summarized in Table 14.1.

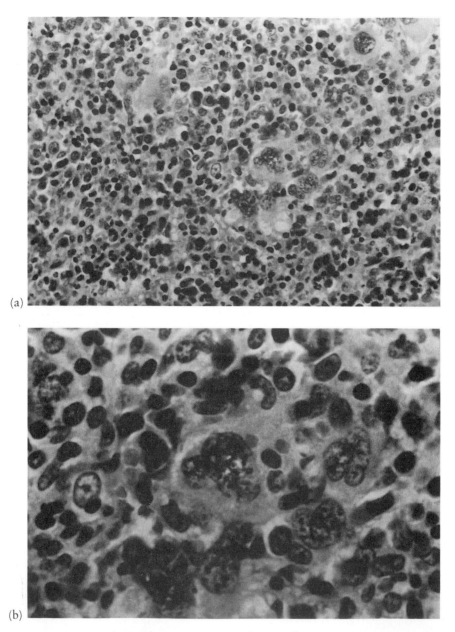

Figure 14.2 (a) Section of spleen from a patient with agnogenic myeloid metaplasia showing complete replacement of normal architecture with myeloid metaplasia. (H & E ×200). (b) Same showing megakaryocytic hyperplasia with atypical features. (H & E ×200).

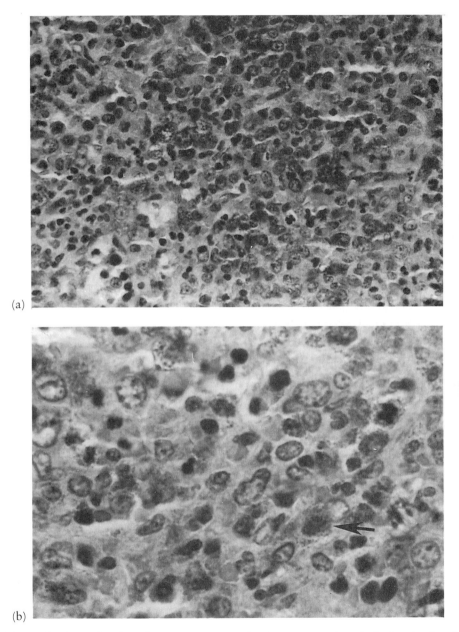

Figure 14.3 (a) Section of spleen from a patient with chronic granulocytic leukemia showing myeloid infiltration. (H & E ×200). (b) Same. Note eosinophil myelocyte shown with arrow. (H & E ×500).

Table 14.1 Splenic pathology in the myeloproliferative disorders

	P. vera	E. thromb.	AMM	CGL
Splenomegaly	+	+/−	++	++
Splenic infarct	+	?	++	++
Myeloid metaplasia	−	−	+	+
Reticulin fibrosis of cords	−	+	+	+/−

Abbreviations; P. vera, polycythemia vera; E. thromb; essential thrombocythemia; AMM, agnogenic myeloid metaplasia; CGL, chronic granulocytic leukemia.

14.4 CLINICAL IMPLICATIONS OF SPLENOMEGALY IN THE MYELOPROLIFERATIVE DISORDERS

14.4.1 POLYCYTHEMIA VERA

Splenomegaly is clinically detectable in about 60% of patients with polycythemia vera. When the spleen is scanned by means of radioisotopic techniques, splenomegaly can be found in 90% of patients. The spleen size is variable but modest. Increasing size of the spleen or massive splenomegaly in a patient with a diagnosis of polycythemia vera usually means progression to myelofibrosis. In some cases, the spleen remains impalpable during the whole course of the disease. Splenic vein thrombosis is a rare complication leading to portal hypertension and bleeding from esophageal varices. Splenic pain may occasionally occur and is more likely to be due to splenic enlargement than to splenic infarct (Wetherley-Mein and Pearson, 1982). Phlebotomy sufficient to produce a normal packed cell volume produces no evident change in the size of the spleen, but it does shrink after treatment with myelosuppressive agents (Westin *et al.*, 1972). Splenic rupture occurs very rarely (Fernandez *et al.*, 1983).

Ferrokinetic studies indicate minimal or no extramedullary erythropoiesis; however, a few patients present with features of both polycythemia vera and myelofibrosis. In these patients, ^{52}Fe uptake in the spleen resembles that seen in myelofibrosis rather than in polycythemia vera. Clinically and hematologically, patients may remain in a relatively stable steady state for several years, and this syndrome has been called 'transitional myeloproliferative disorder' (Pettit, Lewis and Nicholas, 1979).

A 'spent' phase of polycythemia vera has been described by Najean *et al.* (1984) in which there is persistent splenomegaly in spite of treatment, frequent cytopenias of one or more lines, persistent red cell hypervolemia, persistence of myeloid hyperplasia with no collagen myelofibrosis, and no hepatosplenic erythroblastic metaplasia as measured by radioiron studies or ^{111}In-transferrin scintigraphy. This phase is significantly more common in patients treated by phlebotomy than in those treated with myelosuppressive agents.

14.4.2 ESSENTIAL THROMBOCYTHEMIA

As outlined earlier, patients with essential thrombocythemia may show either splenomegaly or splenic atrophy, or the spleen size may be normal. In one series of 94 patients, splenomegaly occurred in 48% (Belucci *et al.*, 1986). Splenomegaly was always moderate, with the splenic tip not exceeding 4 cm below the costal margin in any case. In another series, 30% of patients had detectable splenomegaly (Murphy *et al.*, 1982).

The spleen enlarges when the complications of portal vein or hepatic vein thrombosis occur and also in those few cases progressing to myelofibrosis (Waweru and Lewis, 1985). Marsh, Lewis and Szur (1966) used ^{51}Cr-labeled heat-damaged red cells to study splenic function, and described splenic atrophy in a subset of patients with essential thrombocythemia. It has been proposed that the etiology of splenic atrophy is extensive infarction due to multiple splenic arterial thrombi, comparable to the 'autosplenectomy' of adults with sickle cell disease, but there may well be other unrelated causes. Patients with splenic atrophy tend to have higher platelet counts, probably due to the absence of platelet pooling by the spleen. Ferrokinetic studies with [52]Fe have also been used to demonstrate absence of extramedullary hematopoiesis (Waweru and Lewis, 1985).

14.4.3   AGNOGENIC MYELOID METAPLASIA

Moderate to massive splenomegaly is found in this disease and is progressive. The duration of the disease can be roughly correlated with the degree of splenomegaly (Hickling, 1937; Ward and Block, 1971), although others have denied the correlation (Wolf and Neiman, 1985). Patients in whom the spleen extends into the iliac fossa probably have had the disease for between 13 and 27 years. Rarely, rapid enlargement of the spleen occurs over 1 to 2 years (Chevalier, 1949; Skinner and Sophean, 1951). In a few cases, the spleen is not palpable at presentation, but in all cases enlargement later develops, and is always apparent at some period in the course of the disease (Silverstein, Wollaeger and Baggentoss, 1973).

Portal hypertension is a well-documented complication of agnogenic myeloid metaplasia and may compound the degree of splenomegaly. The cause is somewhat obscure, but it has been suggested that cirrhosis from hepatitis following frequent blood transfusions, hemosiderosis in the liver from iron storage and buildup, and portal and splenic vein thromboses, may be contributing factors (Ward and Block, 1971). In addition, liver biopsies performed in patients with agnogenic myeloid metaplasia have demonstrated myeloid metaplasia (Silverstein, Wollaeger and Baggentoss, 1973; Ligumski, Polliack and Benbassat, 1978), the presence of which may lead to atrophy or necrosis of the liver parenchyma followed by reparative fibrosis. Increased portal blood flow is also thought to be important in the pathogenesis of portal hypertension (Garnett et al., 1969; Hess et al., 1971, 1976), which may play a role in the causation of dilutional anemia (see Chapter 9).

As the spleen progressively enlarges, the effects on the formed elements of the blood become more pronounced. Anemia may be caused by various factors including splenic pooling of red cells, hemolysis and the dilutional effects on hemoglobin concentration of the increased plasma volume (Bowdler, 1983). One classical theory of the cause of anemia was that erythropoiesis in the bone marrow was depressed by the activity of a humoral substance produced by the enlarged spleen; however, this has never been convincingly supported by experimental studies (Goldman and Nolasco, 1983). The 'hypersplenic' effect often involves platelets, and in the patient with a markedly enlarged spleen, more than 90% of the circulating platelets may be intrasplenic (Bowdler, 1983). This results in profound thrombocytopenia due to maldistribution of the platelets. Neutropenia may be due to increased polymorphonuclear leukocyte margination in the splenic blood vessels depleting the circulating cells (Fieschi and Sacchetti, 1964; Scott et al., 1971).

Laboratory evidence that splenic erythropoiesis makes a useful contribution to red cell production is inconclusive. [52]Fe and ^{59}Fe studies often show uptake and release of the isotope in a pattern similar to that seen in the normal marrow, confirming the presence of splenic erythropoiesis, but there is not a quantitatively effective production of red cells (Bowdler, 1961; Wetherley-Mein and Pearson, 1982).

14.4.4   CHRONIC GRANULOCYTIC LEUKEMIA

As in agnogenic myeloid metaplasia, the spleen size tends to correlate with the duration of the disease, and the spleen is nearly always palpably enlarged at presentation. In six cases in which the spleen was not palpably enlarged, the peripheral blood leukocyte count was less than $100 \times 10^9/l$ (Thompson and Stainsby, 1982). It is generally agreed that splenic size in the chronic phase of the disease at the time of diagnosis is an important prognostic indicator, a small spleen being associated with longer survival and conversely a large spleen being associated with short survival (Medical Research Council, 1983). During treatment of the chronic phase, rapid shrinkage occurs when adequate control is achieved. Often a previously easily palpable or massively enlarged spleen become impalpable; in others, however, a palpable spleen remains the only clinical hint of the presence of the disease.

The spleen is not usually tender to palpation during the chronic phase of chronic granulocytic leukemia. Abdominal discomfort or vague digestive complaints such as early satiety may be noticed by the patient. During the accelerated phase, the spleen enlarges rapidly and splenic pain, either felt locally or referred to the shoulder tip, is common. Likewise pain in this disorder is often associated with splenic infarction. The pain is exacerbated by breathing or movement and a splenic rub may be evident on auscultation. Portal hypertension has occasionally been described, as previously noted in agnogenic myeloid metaplasia, and the cause may be similar (Thompson and Stainsby, 1982). Increased plasma volume and red cell pooling play a part in the production of anemia. Splenic rupture has occasionally been described (Bauer, Haskins and Armitage, 1981).

The spleen is certainly important as an organ of hematopoiesis in this disease, being secondary only to the bone marrow and considerable traffic of granulocytes takes place between the marrow and the spleen (Pederson, 1979). Some-times, however, a falling myeloid and rising splenic contribution to granulopoiesis occurs, coincident with the development of relapse. Indeed it has been suggested that the spleen may be the initial site of evolution of cytogenetic changes leading to the terminal phase of the disease, as aneuploidy has been seen in cells in the spleen before the bone marrow has shown any chromosomal change (Shaw, 1982). However, a case has been described in which chromosomal changes associated with the accelerated phase occurred in the bone marrow but not in the spleen (Brandt, 1975). Splenectomy has not been successful in delaying the terminal phase, so that at the present time evidence for the splenic origin of this phase is inconclusive.

14.5   SPLENECTOMY AND ITS EFFECTS IN THE MYELOPROLIFERATIVE DISORDERS

The two myeloproliferative disorders in which splenectomy has been performed most frequently are agnogenic myeloid metaplasia and chronic granulocytic leukemia. Of historical interest is an early study by Hickling (1937), who reviewed 27 patients with agnogenic myeloid metaplasia who had had splenectomy. He noted that 15 died in the immediate postoperative period and six others died within the first year. He therefore believed that this operation was contraindicated in patients with agnogenic myeloid metaplasia, and inferred that the spleen was an important and perhaps indispensable source of hematopoiesis in this disorder. Green *et al.* (1953) also reviewed splenectomy in agnogenic myeloid metaplasia, and found that only 6 of their 29 patients had died within 6 months of splenectomy. They concluded that death following the operation had previously been related to a high rate of postoperative complications, and not to an indispensable spleen. The pendulum of thought on this procedure, however, then swung in the opposite direction until Crosby (1972) subsequently recommended splenectomy in all cases of agnogenic myeloid metaplasia as soon as the diagnosis of the condition had been made.

In agnogenic myeloid metaplasia the principal indications for splenectomy are hypersplenism and symptomatic splenomegaly (Garrison et al., 1984). With hypersplenism, thrombocytopenia and anemia progressively worsen and result in increasing transfusion requirements. Studies in some patients have shown increased splenic sequestration of ^{51}Cr-labeled red cells (Cabot et al., 1978). To sustain a diagnosis of hypersplenism, a formal demonstration of adequate bone marrow function is needed, using such means as ferrokinetic studies and ^{59}Fe or ^{52}Fe sacral uptake or ^{111}indium scanning. Results have been far from conclusive in predicting the outcome of splenectomy, however, and are currently performed much less frequently than in the past (Wilson et al., 1985). It is interesting to note that ferrokinetic studies before and after splenectomy in two series of patients with agnogenic myeloid metaplasia showed increased myeloid erythropoiesis as measured by the ^{59}Fe sacral uptake following splenectomy (Wetherley-Mein and Pearson, 1982; Barosi et al., 1984). It has been suggested that after splenectomy, there is a reorganization of erythropoiesis. The long-standing theory of a splenic humoral substance acting as an inhibitor of erythropoiesis in the marrow could possibly be relevant in this context, but no satisfactory supporting evidence has yet been proposed.

Less common indications for splenectomy in agnogenic myeloid metaplasia are portal hypertension, if there is adequate liver function (Sullivan, Rheinlander and Weintraub, 1974; Silverstein and ReMime, 1979), and rupture of the spleen. A contraindication to splenectomy is the presence of thrombocytosis, because of the very real danger of postsplenectomy thromboses (Ward and Block, 1971). Conversely, the most pressing indication for splenectomy remains thrombocytopenia.

The operative details of splenectomy vary, but the operation is now usually performed through a midline or left paramedian incision (Goldstone, 1978; Cabot et al., 1978). To decrease the risk of massive bleeding, most surgeons mobilize the spleen and divide the short gastric vessels and lienogastric and lienocolic ligaments, before approaching the markedly enlarged splenic artery and vein (Goldstone, 1978; Coon and Liepman, 1982). Postoperative complications include subphrenic abscess and other intra-abdominal infections, postoperative bleeding, pleural effusion, pneumonia, deep venous thrombosis and pulmonary embolism, hepatic failure and, very occasionally, pericardial effusion (Nagler et al., 1986). The postoperative survival is also said to be shortened in males as opposed to females (Silverstein and ReMime, 1974) and in patients with anemia, massive splenomegaly, and elevated serum alkaline phosphatase levels (Penchas et al., 1982).

Splenectomy in agnogenic myeloid metaplasia results in hematological and clinical changes. The most profound hematological change is seen in the platelet count, which often rises dramatically (Heaton et al., 1976; Cabot et al., 1978; Coon, 1985; Wilson et al., 1985). The hemoglobin and hematocrit values often rise also. In one study, polycythemia occurred following splenectomy in three cases (Barosi et al., 1984). The peripheral white cell count also tends to rise (Mulder, Steenbergen and Haanen, 1977; Cabot et al., 1978). In another study, the number of teardrop poikilocytes in the peripheral blood fell (DiBella, Silverstein and Hoagland, 1977). An interesting observation by Aviram et al. (1986) was that the spleen plays an important role in cholesterol metabolism: they showed that after splenectomy in patients with myeloproliferative disorders, cholesterol, apolipoprotein B and low density lipoproteins were significantly increased. In general, the quality of life may be considerably improved in those patients who may have needed frequent red cell or platelet transfusions. However, the natural history of the disease is not altered and there is probably no demonstrable survival benefit from the operation.

Long-term complications include thromboses, including mesenteric venous and arterial thrombosis, portal vein thrombosis, deep vein thrombosis and pulmonary embolism, related to the rapid rise in platelet count (Heaton *et al.*, 1976; Mulder, Steenbergen and Haanen, 1977; Cabot *et al.*, 1978; Goldstone, 1978; Wobbes, van der Sluis and Lubbers, 1984; Wilson *et al.*, 1985). The long-term risk of bacterial infection is present, as with other splenectomized patients, and is due to the impaired removal of microorganisms by phagocytosis from the blood (see also Chapters 11 and 12). Serum concentration of IgM, tuftsin and properdin decrease (*Lancet*, 1985). Slow enlargement of the liver is an inevitable consequence of splenectomy, but previously reported cases of explosive hepatomegaly have not been confirmed (Ward and Block, 1971).

Splenectomy in chronic granulocytic leukemia was, for many years, rejected as not being a useful form of treatment. However, in 1968, Baikie suggested that elective splenectomy early in the course of the disease, might prolong survival by deferring the terminal phase. This proposal was made because of the cytogenetic evidence, referred to earlier in this chapter, that in some cases, the spleen may be the initial site of evolution of the terminal phase. Spiers *et al.* (1975) reviewed 26 patients in whom splenectomy had been performed, and found that the number who entered the terminal phase was significantly fewer than in a comparable retrospective group of non-splenectomized patients. Two further retrospective studies (Ihde *et al.*, 1976; McBride and Hester, 1977) showed no evidence of prolonged survival in splenectomized patients. A controlled trial from Italy of early splenectomy in the chronic phase showed no benefit in the splenectomized group (Baccarani, Corbelli and Tura, 1981), and a similar Medical Research Council trial (1983) also reported negative findings.

One benefit of splenectomy in the chronic phase of the disease is the reduction of morbidity during the terminal phase, and symptoms from a rapidly enlarging spleen may be prevented (Coon, 1985). An uncomplicated chronic phase is not now generally believed to be an indication for splenectomy. In symptomatic chronic granulocytic leukemia and in the terminal phase, splenectomy may produce some beneficial effects. Canellos, Nordland and Carbone (1972) reported benefit in patients made thrombocytopenic after treatment with busulphan. In the terminal phase in some patients splenectomy has produced short-term improvement in the severe pain of splenic infarction, or of splenomegaly without infarction. Likewise there may be improvement in thrombocytopenia or anemia which may be requiring frequent transfusions (Gomez *et al.*, 1976).

It should be emphasized that in polycythemia vera and essential thrombocythemia, a high proportion of the total red cell mass and platelets is sequestered in the spleen (Aster, 1966). If splenectomy is performed, the subsequent severe thrombocytosis is very likely to result in thrombotic or hemorrhagic disorders (Murphy, 1983). Bensinger, Logue and Rundles (1970) described the effectiveness of melphalan in four patients with postsplenectomy thrombocytosis in such cases, but splenectomy is considered to be contraindicated in both polycythemia vera and essential thrombocythemia.

14.6 SPLENIC RADIATION THERAPY

In the myeloproliferative disorders, the use of radiation therapy to the spleen as a treatment modality has been recognized in chronic granulocytic leukemia in the chronic phase, since the beginning of the twentieth century (Pusey, 1902; Senn, 1903). This form of therapy remained the standard for chronic granulocytic leukemia for many years and was found to produce alleviation of symptoms, with shrinkage of the spleen and marked improvement of the blood counts in total doses of 600–1000 cGy (Hotchkiss and Block, 1962; Schoen and Baur, 1968).

In 1968, the Medical Research Council published the results of a randomized trial using busulphan *versus* radiation therapy in the treatment of chronic granulocytic leukemia. Those patients treated with radiation therapy had a median survival time of 2.5 years as opposed to

3.5 years in those treated with busulphan. This trial has been criticized for the lack of adequate standardization of radiation therapy. However, the results were supported by others (Gollerkeri and Shah, 1971; Conrad, 1973), and radiation therapy has now been superseded by chemotherapy and bone marrow transplantation. Splenic radiation therapy is still used for symptomatic splenomegaly unresponsive to chemotherapy, in patients unable to tolerate chemotherapy, and in pregnant females (Richards and Spiers, 1975).

In agnogenic myeloid metaplasia, radiation therapy has been used much less than in chronic granulocytic leukemia. In 1953, Hickling described splenic radiation therapy as an effective method of reducing the white cell count in agnogenic myeloid metaplasia. In 1971, Ward and Block concluded that radiation therapy was seldom indicated, and suggested that only an occasional patient might obtain transient relief of abdominal symptoms. The general opinion today concedes that the use of low-dose radiation therapy to the spleen is an acceptable method of alleviating splenic pain and of reducing the size of a massive spleen (Szur et al., 1973; Parmentier et al., 1977; Greenberger et al., 1977; Wagner et al., 1986). Doses vary from 100 to 1500 cGy delivered over 9 to 15 days. Radiation therapy is also indicated in patients in whom splenectomy is contraindicated. It results in a moderate to marked decrease in the peripheral blood granulocyte count. The mechanism of this seems to be destruction of proliferating precursor cells in the splenic tissue and sinuses (Koeffler, Cline and Golde, 1979). Effects on bone marrow erythropoiesis as shown by ferrokinetic studies have been variable (Szur et al., 1973; Parmentier et al., 1977).

14.7 OTHER METHODS OF TREATING SPLENOMEGALY

Canellos et al. (1979) treated five patients in the blastic phase of chronic granulocytic leukemia, who had symptomatic splenomegaly, with splenic artery infusions of cytosine arabinoside. All of them had reduction in the size of the spleen with symptomatic relief. In another study, Hocking, Machleder and Golde (1980) advocated splenic embolization with inert materials prior to splenectomy to alleviate the complications of removing a massively enlarged spleen. Neither of these procedures has yet achieved wide clinical acceptance.

REFERENCES

Adamson, J. W. and Fialkow, P. J. (1978) The pathogenesis of myeloproliferative syndromes. *Br. J. Haematol.*, **38**, 299–303.

Adler, S. S. (1976) The pathogenesis of spleen mediated phenomena in chronic myeloid leukaemia and agnogenic myeloid metaplasia: a non-abscopal mechanism. *Scand. J. Haematol.*, **17**, 153–9.

Aster, R. H. (1966) Pooling of platelets in the spleen: role in the pathogenesis of 'hypersplenic' thrombocytopenia. *J. Clin. Invest.*, **45**, 645–57.

Aviram, M. et al. (1986) Increased low-density lipoprotein levels after splenectomy: a role for the spleen in cholesterol metabolism in myeloproliferative disorders. *Am. J. Med. Sci..*, **291**. 25–8.

Baccarani, M., Corbelli, G. and Tura, S. (1981) Early splenectomy and polychemotherapy versus polychemotherapy alone in chronic myeloid leukaemia. *Leukemia Res.*, **5**, 149–57.

Bagby, G. C. (1978) Stem cell (CFU-C) proliferation and emergence in a case of chronic granulocytic leukaemia. *Scand. J. Haematol.*, **20**, 193–9.

Baikie, A. G. (1968) The place of splenectomy in the treatment of chronic granulocytic leukaemia: some random observations, a review of the earlier literature and a plea for its proper study in a cooperative therapeutic trial. *Aust. Ann. Med.*, **17**, 175–6 (Abstract).

Barosi, G. et al. (1984) Polycythaemia following splenectomy in myelofibrosis with myeloid metaplasia. *Scand. J. Haematol.*, **32**, 12–18.

Barret, A. J. et al. (1977) Effect of splenic irradiation on colony-forming cells in chronic granulocytic leukaemia. *Br. Med. J.*, **1**, 1259.

Bauer, T. W., Haskins, G. E. and Armitage, J. O. (1981) Splenic rupture in patients with hematologic malignancies. *Cancer*, **48**, 2729–33.

Belucci, S. et al. (1986) Essential thrombocythemia: clinical, evolutionary and biological data. *Cancer*, **58**, 2440–7.

Bensinger, T. A., Logue, G. L. and Rundles, R. W. (1970) Hemorrhagic thrombocythemia; control of postsplenectomy thrombocytosis with melphalan. *Blood*, **36**, 61–8.

Block, M. (1964) Studies on the blood and blood-forming tissues of the newborn opossum. I. Normal development. *Ergeb. Anat. Entw. Gesch.*, **37**, 237.

Bowdler, A. J. (1961) Radioisotope investigations in primary myeloid metaplasia. *J. Clin. Pathol.*, **14**, 595–602.

Bowdler, A. J. (1983) Splenomegaly and hypersplenism. *Clin. Haematol.*, **12**, 467–88.

Brandt, L. (1975) Comparative studies of bone marrow and extramedullary haemopoietic tissue in chronic myeloid leukemia. *Ser. Hematol.*, **8** (4), 75–80.

Cabot, E. B. *et al.* (1978) Splenectomy in myeloid metaplasia. *Ann. Surg.*, **187**, 24–30.

Canellos, G. P., Nordland, J. and Carbone, P. P. (1972) Splenectomy for thrombocytopenia in chronic granulocytic leukemia. *Cancer*, **29**, 660–5.

Canellos, G. P. *et al.* (1979) Treatment of refractory splenomegaly in myeloproliferative disease by splenic artery infusion. *Blood*, **53**, 1014–17.

Champlin, R. E. *et al.* (1986) Chronic leukemias: oncogenes, chromosomes and advances in therapy. *Ann. Intern. Med.*, **104**, 671–88.

Chevalier, P. (1949) Les splenomegalies myeloides et leurs formes complexes. *Sang*, **20**, 112.

Conrad, R. G. (1973) Survival in chronic granulocytic leukemia. *Arch. Intern. Med.*, **131**, 684–5.

Coon, W. W. (1985) The limited role of splenectomy in patients with leukemia. *Surg. Gynecol. Obstet.*, **160**, 291–4.

Coon, W. W. and Liepman, M. K. (1982) Splenectomy for agnogenic myeloid metaplasia. *Surg. Gynecol. Obstet.*, **154**, 561–3.

Crosby, W. H. (1972) Splenectomy in hematologic disorders. *N. Engl. J. Med.*, **286**, 1252–4.

Dameshek, W. (1951) Some speculations on the myeloproliferative syndromes. *Blood*, **6**, 372–5.

DiBella, N. J., Silverstein, M. N. and Hoagland, H. (1977) Effect of splenectomy on teardrop-shaped erythrocytes in agnogenic myeloid metaplasia. *Arch. Intern. Med.*, **137**, 380–1.

Fernandez, S. F. *et al.* (1983) Rotura pathologica del bazo secundaria a policitema vera. *Rev. Clin. Esp.*, **168**, 139–41.

Fieschi, A. and Saccheti, C. (1964) Clinical assessment of granulopoiesis. *Acta Haematol.*, **31**, 150–62.

Garnett, E. S. *et al.* (1969) The spleen as an arteriovenous shunt. *Lancet*, **i**, 386–8.

Garrison, R. N. *et al.* (1984) Splenectomy in hematologic malignancy. *Am. Surg*, **50**, 428–32.

Goldman, J. M. and Nolasco, I. (1983) The spleen in myeloproliferative disorders. *Clin. Haematol.*, **12**, 505–16.

Goldstone, J. (1978) Splenectomy for massive splenomegaly. *Am. J. Surg.*, **135**, 385–8.

Gollerkeri, M. P. and Shah, G. B. (1971) Management of chronic myeloid leukemia: a five-year survey with a comparison with oral busulfan and splenic irradiation. *Cancer*, **21**, 596–601.

Gomez, G. A. *et al.* (1976) Splenectomy for palliation of chronic myelocytic leukemia. *Am. J. Med.*, **61**, 14–22.

Green, T. W. *et al.* (1953) Splenectomy for myeloid metaplasia of the spleen. *N. Engl. J. Med.*, **248**, 211–19.

Greenberg, P. L. and Steed, S. M. (1981) Splenic granulocytopoiesis and production of colony-stimulating activity in lymphoma and leukemia. *Blood*, **57**, 119–29.

Greenberger, J. S. *et al.* (1977) Irradiation for control of hypersplenism and painful splenomegaly in myeloid metaplasia. *Int. J. Radiat. Oncol. Biol. Phys.*, **2**, 1083–90.

Heaton, A. *et al.* (1976) Experience with splenectomy in autoimmune thrombocytopenia and agnogenic myeloid metaplasia. *S. Afr. Med. J.*, **50**, 1506–12.

Hess, C. E. *et al.* (1971) Dilutional anemia of splenomegaly: an indication for splenectomy. *Ann. Surg.*, **173**, 693–9.

Hess, C. E. *et al.* (1976) Mechanism of dilutional anemia in massive splenomegaly. *Blood.* **47**, 629–44.

Hickling, R. A. (1937) Chronic non-leukaemic myelosis. *Q. J. Med.*, **6**, 253–75.

Hickling, R. A. (1953) Treatment of patients with myelosclerosis. *Br. Med. J.*, **2**, 411–13.

Hocking, W. G., Machleder, H. I. and Golde, D. W. (1980) Splenic artery embolisation prior to splenectomy in end-stage polycythemia vera. *Am. J. Haematol.*, **8**, 123–7.

Hotchkiss, D. R. and Block, M. A. (1962) Effect of splenic irradiation on systemic hematopoiesis. *Ann. Intern. Med.*, **109**, 697–711.

Ihde, D. C. *et al.* (1976) Splenectomy in the chronic phase of chronic granulocytic leukemia. *Ann. Intern. Med.*, **84**, 17–21.

Jackson, H. Jr, Parker, F. Jr and Lemon, H. M. (1940) Agnogenic myeloid metaplasia of the spleen. *N. Engl. J. Med.*, **222**, 985.

Keleman, E., Calvo, W. and Fliedner, T. M. (1979) *Atlas of Hematopoietic Development*, Springer-Verlag, New York, pp. 156–71.

Kirschner, J. J., Goldberg, J. and Landaw, S. A. (1980) The spleen as a site of colony-forming cell production in myelofibrosis. *Proc. Soc. Exp. Biol. Med.*, **165**, 279–82.

Koeffler, H. P., Cline, M. J. and Golde, D. W. (1979) Splenic irradiation in myelofibrosis: effect on circulating myeloid progenitor cells. *Br. J. Haematol.*, **43**, 69–77.

Lancet (1985) Splenectomy: long-term risk of infection. Leading Article, *Lancet*, ii, 928–9.

Lewis, S. M. (1983) The spleen–mysteries solved and unresolved. *Clin. Haematol.*, **12**, 363–73.

Ligumski, M., Polliack, A. and Benbassat, J. (1978) Nature and incidence of liver involvement in agnogenic myeloid metaplasia. *Scand. J. Haematol.*, **21**, 81–93.

Lutton, J. D. and Levere, R. D. (1979) Endogenous erythroid colony formation by peripheral blood mononuclear cells from patients with myelofibrosis and polycythemia vera. *Acta Haematol.*, **62**, 94–9.

McBride, C. M. and Hester, J. P. (1977) Chronic myelogenous leukemia: management of splenectomy in a high risk population. *Cancer*, **39**, 653–8.

Marsh, G. W., Lewis, S. M. and Szur, L. (1966) The use of ^{51}Cr-labeled heat-damaged red cells to study splenic function. *Br. J. Haematol.*, **12**, 167–71,

Medical Research Council's Working Party for Therapeutic Trials in Leukaemia (1968) Chronic granulocytic leukemia: comparison of radiotherapy and busulphan therapy. *Br. Med. J.*, **1**, 201–8.

Medical Research Council (1983) Randomised trial of splenectomy in Phl-positive chronic granulocytic leukaemia including an analysis of prognostic features. *Br. J. Haematol.*, **54**, 415–30.

Moore, M. A. S. (1975) Embryologic and phylogenetic development of the hematopoietic systems. *Adv. Biosci.*, **16**, 87–101, Pergamon Press, Vieweg, Germany.

Mulder, H., Steenbergen, J. and Haanen, C. (1977) Clinical course and survival after elective splenectomy in 19 patients with primary myelofibrosis. *Br. J. Haematol.*, **35**, 419–27.

Murphy, S. (1983) Thrombocytosis and thrombocythemia. *Clin. Haematol.*, **12**, 89–106.

Murphy, S. *et al.* (1982) Essential thrombocythemia: response during first year of therapy with melphalan and radioactive phosphorus: a Polycythemia Vera Study Group report. *Cancer Treat. Rep.*, **66**, 35–40.

Nagler, A. *et al.* (1986) Postsplenectomy pericardial effusion in two patients with myeloid metaplasia. *Ann. Intern. Med.*, **146**, 600–1.

Najean, Y. *et al.* (1984) The 'spent' phase of polycythaemia vera: hypersplenism in the absence of myelofibrosis. *Br. J. Haematol.*, **56**, 163–70.

Parmentier, C. *et al.* (1977) Splenic irradiation in myelofibrosis. Clinical findings and ferrokinetics. *Int. J. Radiat. Oncol. Biol. Phys.*, **2**, 1075–81.

Pederson, B. (1979) Spleen and relapse in chronic myeloid leukaemia. *Scand. J. Haematol.*, **22**, 369–74.

Penchas, S. *et al.* (1982) Splenectomy in agnogenic myeloid metaplasia: factors of possible prognostic significance. *Postgrad. Med. J.*, **58**, 212–15.

Pettit, J. E., Lewis, S. M. and Nicholas, A. W. (1979) Transitional myeloproliferative disorder. *Br. J. Haematol.*, **43**, 167–84.

Pusey, W. A. (1902) Report of cases treated with Roentgen rays. *J. Am. Med. Assoc.*, **38**, 911–19.

Rappaport, H. (1966) Tumors of the hematopoietic system. *An Atlas of Tumor Pathology.* Section, fascicle 8. Armed Forces Institute of Pathology, Washington, DC, pp. 237–336.

Richards, H. G. H. and Spiers, A. S. D. (1975) Chronic granulocytic leukaemia in pregnancy. *Br. J. Radiol.*, **48**, 261–4.

Schoen, D. and Bauer, R. (1968) Ergebnisse mit der Milzbestralung bei 175 fallen mit chronischer myelischer Leukämie. *Strahlentherapie*, **135**, 1–10.

Schofield, R. (1979) The pluripotent stem cell. *Clin. Haematol.*, **8**, 221–37.

Scott, J. L. *et al.* (1971) Leukocyte labelling with 51-chromium. II. Leukocyte kinetics in chronic myelocytic leukemia. *Blood*, **38**, 162–73.

Senn, N. (1903) Case of splenomedullary leukemia successfully treated by the use of Roentgen ray. *Medical Rec.*, **64**, 281–2.

Shaw, M. T (1982) Clinical and haematological manifestations of the terminal phase. In *Chronic Granulocytic Leukaemia* (ed. M. T. Shaw), Praeger, Eastbourne, pp. 169–88.

Silverstein, M. N. and ReMime, W. H. (1974) Sex, splenectomy, and myeloid metaplasia. *J. Am. Med. Assoc.*, **227**, 424–5.

Silverstein, M. N. and ReMime, W. H. (1979) Splenectomy in myeloid metaplasia. *Blood.* **53**, 515–18.

Silverstein, M. N., Wollaeger, E. E. and Baggentoss, A. H. (1973) Gastrointestinal and abdominal manifestations of agnogenic myeloid metaplasia. *Arch. Intern. Med.*, **131**, 532–7.

Skinner, H. C. and Sophean, L. S. (1951) Agnogenic myeloid metaplasia in the spleen: follow-up after splenectomy. *J. Int. Coll. Surg.*, **15**, 343–6.

Spiers, A. S. D. *et al.* (1975) Chronic granulocytic leukaemia: effect of elective splenectomy on the course of the disease. *Br. Med. J.*, **1**, 175–9.

Sullivan, A., Rheinlander, H. and Weintraub, L. R.

(1974) Esophageal varices in agnogenic myeloid metaplasia: disappearance after splenectomy. A case report. *Gastroenterology*, **66**, 429–32.

Szur, L. *et al.* (1973) The effect of radiation on splenic function in myelosclerosis: studies with ^{52}Fe and ^{99}Tc. *Br. J. Radiol.*, **46**, 295–301.

Tavassoli, M. (1973) Splenic white pulp in myeloid metaplasia. *Arch. Pathol.*, **95**, 419–21.

Tavassoli, M. and Weiss, L. (1973) An electron microscopic study of spleen in myelofibrosis with myeloid metaplasia. *Blood*, **42**, 267–79.

Thiel, G. and Downey, H. (1921) The development of the mammalian spleen, with special reference to its hemopoietic activity. *Am. J. Anat.*, **28**, 279.

Thompson, R. B. and Stainsby, D. (1982) The clinical and haematological features of chronic granulocytic leukaemia in the chronic phase. In *Chronic Granulocytic Leukaemia* (ed. M. T. Shaw), Praeger, Eastbourne, pp. 137–68.

Van den Heuvel, R. L. *et al.* (1987) Stromal stem cells (CFU-f) in yolk sac, liver, spleen, and bone marrow of pre- and postnatal mice. *Br. J. Haematol.*, **66**, 15–20.

Wagner, H. *et al.* (1986) Splenic irradiation in the treatment of patients with chronic myelogenous leukemia or myelofibrosis with myeloid metaplasia. *Cancer*, **58**, 1204–7.

Ward, H. P. and Block, M. H. (1971) The natural history of agnogenic myeloid metaplasia (AMM) and a critical evaluation of its relationship with the myeloproliferative syndrome. *Medicine*, **50**, 357–421.

Waweru, F. and Lewis, S. M. (1985) Blood volume, erythrokinetics and spleen function in thrombocythemia. *Acta Haematol.*, **73**, 219–23.

Westin, J. *et al.* (1972) Spleen size in polycythemia. *Acta Med. Scand.*, **181**, 431–6.

Wetherley-Mein, G. and Pearson, T. C. (1982) The myeloproliferative disorders. in *Blood and Its Disorders* (eds. R. M. Hardisty and D. J. Weatherall), 2nd edn, Chapter 32, Blackwell Scientific Publications, Oxford, pp. 1269–316.

Wilson, R. E. *et al.* (1985) Splenectomy for myeloproliferative disorders. *World J. Surg.*, **9**, 431–6.

Wintrobe, M. M. *et al.* (1976) *Clinical Hematology*, 7th edn, Lee and Febiger, Philadelphia.

Wobbes, T., van der Sluis, R. F. and Lubbers, E. C. (1984) Removal of the massive spleen: a surgical risk? *Am. J. Surg.*, **147**, 800–2.

Wolf, B. C., Luevano, E. and Neiman, R. S. (1983) Evidence to suggest that the human fetal spleen is not a hematopoietic organ. *Am. J. Clin. Pathol.*, **80**, 140–4.

Wolf, B. and Neiman, R. S. (1985) Myelofibrosis with myeloid metaplasia: pathophysiologic implications of the correlation between bone marrow changes and progression of splenomegaly. *Blood*, **65**, 803–9.

Wolf, N. S. and Trentin, J. J. (1968) Hemopoietic colony studies. V. Effect of hemopoietic stroma on differentiation of pluripotent stem cells. *J. Exp. Med.*, **127**, 205–14.

Peter C. Raich

15.1 SPLENIC INVOLVEMENT IN LYMPHOPROLIFERATIVE DISORDERS

'The viola is like the spleen. We have one but no one knows why or what it's doing there.' Harry Rumpler, violist.

15.1.1 INTRODUCTION

Lymphoproliferative disorders include both malignant and benign conditions, with lymphoid hyperplasia as the common feature. Since the spleen is the largest lymphoid organ in the body it is not surprising that it is frequently involved in the lymphoproliferative disorders (see Table 15.1). In malignant lymphoma, splenic involvement, manifested by splenomegaly and at times the associated features of hypersplenism, may be a presenting feature together with lymph node enlargement, or it may appear later in the course of the disease, on relapse or with disease resistant to therapy. Occasionally lymphomas present with involvement limited to the spleen. In chronic lymphocytic leukemia splenomegaly may be one of the earliest findings, but this appears to have little influence on the outcome of the disease. In hairy cell leukemia splenomegaly may be the major finding alerting the physician to the possibility of that diagnosis, and subsequent removal of the spleen will frequently be associated with lasting remission.

In this section, the extent of splenic involvement observed in the malignant lymphoproliferative disorders (MLPDs) will be discussed, as well as how this involvement pertains to the diagnosis, staging, prognosis and treatment of each disorder.

15.1.2 LYMPHOCYTE FUNCTION, DIFFERENTIATION AND KINETICS

In man the spleen serves principally as a large lymphoid organ, in addition to its specialized blood filtering function. Hematopoiesis in the spleen, other than lymphopoiesis, takes place only during fetal life, and as extramedullary hematopoiesis in certain disorders characterized by impaired immune function.

MLPDs initially and primarily involve the lymphoid system. The malignant cells represent a monoclonal population of cells characterized by surface markers as having predominantly B- or T-lymphocyte features (Greaves, 1975; Seligman, Preud'Homme and Brouet, 1973). The marked pleomorphism observed in Hodgkin's disease has been attributed to the host's reaction to the malignant cells, while the cells in non-Hodgkin's lymphomas have been shown to be expanded clones of specific lymphocyte precursors and functional cell types. The increased availability and application of cell surface markers has led to the identification of malignant lymphoma cells corresponding to various stages of differentiation of B- and T-cells, as well as of antigenically stimulated, activated

Table 15.1 Splenic involvement in the lymphoproliferative malignancies

Disease	Splenomegaly	White pulp	Red pulp
Hodgkin's disease	late	early	late
Non-Hodgkin's lymphomas			
small, cleaved cell	common	early	late
large cell	variable	+	
small, non-cleaved	common	+	
ALL	in children	early	late
CLL	common	early	late
Hairy cell leukemia	common	late	early
T-cell lymphoproliferative			
disorders	variable	+	+
Waldenström's			
macroglobulinemia	common	early	late

Source: Adapted from Maurer (1985).

cell types (see Table 15.2). Several classification systems of these 'immunoproliferative' diseases based on functional and immunological studies have been proposed, including those by Lukes, Butler and Hicks (1966), Lennert (1967), Lukes and Collins (1974), the Kiel classification (Lennert, 1978; Meuge, Hoerni and De Mascarel, 1978) and most recently the 'Working Formulation' (Rosenberg et al., 1982; see Table 15.3).

Since these immunoproliferative cells retain many of the characteristics of normal B- and T-cells, it is probable that they will retain other traits, such as recirculation through the lymphatic (immune) system, as well as the predilection to accumulate and proliferate in certain compartments of the immune system. Malignancies arising from cells corresponding to the primary differentiation pathway, such as ALL, involve the bone marrow but less often the spleen, while those linked to the secondary differentiation pathway, including most of the lymphomas, frequently involve the lymph nodes and spleen.

An orderly recirculation of B- and T-lymphocytes has been demonstrated in normal animals and in man (Wagstaff et al., 1981; Crowther and Wagstaff, 1983). These are predominantly small lymphocytes and are thought to become antigenically stimulated during their travels.

The lymphocyte pools in the human spleen have been shown to comprise more than one-third of the total recirculating lymphocyte mass (Christensen et al., 1978), and a brisk exchange, especially of T-cells, occurs between these and the circulating lymphocytes. Their specific location within the spleen may be determined by their surface antigenic pattern. Malignant lymphocytes may be expected to follow similar pathways to areas of sequestration and proliferation. Such 'homing in' may be facilitated by specific leukocyte-related antigens in splenic sinusoidal endothelial cells (Giorno, 1984).

Since there appears to be a certain degree of organ specificity for the different MLPDs, it has been postulated that surface phenotype and cell maturation may determine the degree and pattern of spread. Small cell MLPDs, such as CLL, are frequently widespread at presentation and invariably show bone marrow involvement (Spivak and Perry, 1970; Bazerbashi, Reeve and Chanarin, 1978). Lymphomas of follicular center cells (poorly differentiated or small cell, cleaved) produce a nodular pattern of infiltration in lymph nodes and marrow. Large cell lymphomas can be expected to have less bone marrow involvement, since normal immunoblasts do not circulate freely and are removed rapidly from the blood, possibly by the spleen.

Table 15.2 B-lymphocyte differentiation and origins of B-cell lymphomas

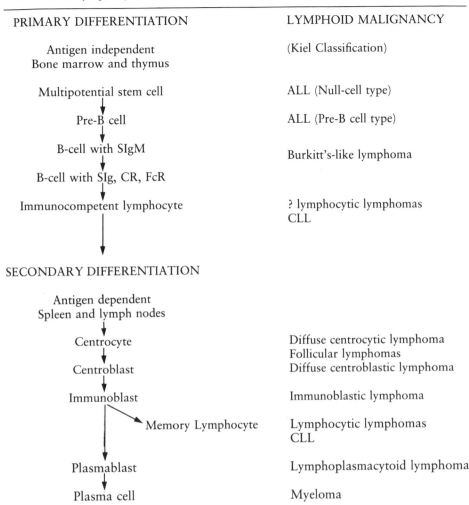

PRIMARY DIFFERENTIATION	LYMPHOID MALIGNANCY
Antigen independent Bone marrow and thymus	(Kiel Classification)
Multipotential stem cell	ALL (Null-cell type)
Pre-B cell	ALL (Pre-B cell type)
B-cell with SIgM	Burkitt's-like lymphoma
B-cell with SIg, CR, FcR	
Immunocompetent lymphocyte	? lymphocytic lymphomas CLL

SECONDARY DIFFERENTIATION	
Antigen dependent Spleen and lymph nodes	
Centrocyte	Diffuse centrocytic lymphoma Follicular lymphomas
Centroblast	Diffuse centroblastic lymphoma
Immunoblast	Immunoblastic lymphoma
Memory Lymphocyte	Lymphocytic lymphomas CLL
Plasmablast	Lymphoplasmacytoid lymphoma
Plasma cell	Myeloma

SIg — Surface immunoglobulin-bearing cells
CR — Complement receptors
FcR — Receptors for Fc portion of Ig
Source: After Magrath (1981).

It is, however, quite common to observe circulating lymphoma cells ('clonal excess') in the more well-differentiated lymphomas, even in those with no demonstrable microscopic bone marrow involvement (Ault, 1979; Ligler et al., 1980).

Other phenomena characteristic of certain lymphomas can also be explained by these recirculation features. Fluctuations in the size of lymph nodes, and even spontaneous regression, occur in the small cell (low grade) lymphomas. In CLL extracorporeal irradiation of blood and irradiation of local lymphoid organs, such as the spleen, is often followed by a marked decrease in blood lymphocytosis as well as reduction in generalized lymphadenopathy (the

Table 15.3 A comparison of working formulation with Rappaport and Kiel classifications of non-Hodgkin's lymphomas

Working formulation	Rappaport equivalents	Keil classification
Low grade		
Small lymphocytic	Diffuse lymphocytic, well differentiated	Lymphocytic, B- and T-types
Follicular small cleaved cell	Nodular, poorly differentiated, lymphocytic	Centroblastic centrocytic (small centrocytes) follicular or diffuse
Follicular mixed small cleaved and large cell	Nodular, mixed lymphocytic–histiocytic	
Intermediate grade		
Follicular large cell	Nodular histiocytic	Centroblastic (large centrocytes)
Diffuse small cleaved cell	Diffuse poorly differentiated, lymphocytic	Centrocytic (small centrocytes)
Diffuse mixed small and large cell	Diffuse mixed lymphocytic–histiocytic	Centroblastic–centrocytic diffuse
Diffuse large cell	Diffuse histiocytic	Centrocytic (large cells) Centroblastic
High grade		
Diffuse large cell immunoblastic	Diffuse histiocytic	Immunoblastic
Lymphoblastic	Lymphoblastic	Lymphoblastic
Small non-cleaved cell/ Burkitt's and non-Burkitt's	Diffuse undifferentiated/ Burkitt's	Lymphoblastic Burkitt's type and others

abscopal effect: Parmentier *et al.*, 1974; Byhardt, Brace and Wiernick, 1975; Singh, Bates and Wetherley-Mein, 1986). The progressive invasion and destruction of lymphoid organs by these malignant cells compromises the function of normal lymphocytes, leading to unexpected avenues of spread as well as to immunological abnormalities and other defects observed in the MLPDs.

15.1.3   HODGKIN'S DISEASE

In contrast to most of the other MLPDs, Hodgkin's disease (HD) has been thought to begin locally in a lymphoid organ and then to spread in an orderly centripetal fashion to adjacent lymphoid structures and, at times, adjacent non-lymphoid structures. This concept of spread 'by contiguity' was favored by Kaplan and coworkers (Rosenberg and Kaplan, 1966), after careful assessment of a large number of patients with Hodgkin's disease. This approach, when applied to the design of radiation therapy to include the adjacent uninvolved lymphoid areas ('extended field'), resulted in high cure rates (Kaplan, 1980).

It is, however, difficult to accept that spread into the abdomen occurs frequently in retrograde fashion via the thoracic duct, or that it spreads from one side of the neck to the other or to the axillae. Staging laparotomy studies in Hodgkin's disease patients have shown that the spleen is the most frequently involved intra-abdominal site. Rates of 36–44% splenic involvement, compared to 6–28% for para-aortic lymph node involvement, have been reported (Aisenberg and Qazi, 1974; Glees et al., 1982). Splenic involvement as the only site of intra-abdominal disease has been reported in 3–14% (Mann, Hafez and Longo, 1986), while intra-abdominal lymph node disease without splenic involvement occurs in less than 10% (Mauch et al., 1983; Krikorian, Portlock and Mauch, 1986). In a recent review by Leibenhaut et al. (1987) patients with CS (clinical stage) I-A subdiaphragmatic disease with negative lymphoangiograms had only a 10% probability of splenic involvement, contrasting with the 30% probability in patients with supradiaphragmatic disease and negative lymphoangiograms.

The 'susceptibility' theory developed by Smithers (Smithers, 1970; Smithers, Lillicrap and Barnes, 1974) presents a more plausible concept to explain intra-abdominal spread. According to this concept, malignant cells migrate via the lymph to the blood stream, and then localize preferentially at certain sites. Initial spread to the spleen is thought to be by hematogenous routes, independently of other intra-abdominal disease. From there Hodgkin's disease can spread to other intra-abdominal sites, such as lymph nodes and liver, as well as to the bone marrow. That Hodgkin's disease can spread through the blood is supported by the finding of characteristic Reed–Sternberg cells circulating in peripheral blood in some Hodgkin's disease patients (Bouroncle, 1966; Schiffer, Levi and Wiernick, 1975).

In an evaluation of staging laparotomy data for 76 patients, Stein et al. (1982) showed a correlation between anatomical substaging and splenic involvement in patients with pathological stage III Hodgkin's disease. Patients with substage III-1 more often had 'minimal' involvement of the spleen (1 to 4 nodules) as compared to 'extensive' involvement (more

than 4 nodules), the proportions being 56% and 44% respectively. 'Extensive' involvement of the spleen was seen in 76% of patients with substage III-2. Thus, involvement of the spleen per se does not necessarily imply a bad prognosis or a high probability of hematogenous spread to liver, bone marrow and other extra-lymphatic organs. Patients with stage III-1 disease have experienced generally good results with a treatment program of total nodal irradiation only (Stein et al., 1982). Splenic vascular invasion, however, has been associated with systemic involvement and a poor prognosis (Strum, Allen and Rappaport, 1971; Kirschner et al., 1974; Haskell, 1981).

Splenomegaly is rarely present at the initial presentation of Hodgkin's disease. In late stages of the disease, however, it may become massive. In a series reported by Glatstein et al. (1969), spleen weights ranged from 100 to 1300 g, with those weighing more than 400 g invariably being affected by Hodgkin's disease. The difficulty of establishing splenic involvement by means short of splenectomy, is borne out by data presented by Kaplan (1970). In a series of 340 consecutive untreated patients with biopsy-proven Hodgkin's disease, and evaluated principally by thorough clinical staging, 44 (13%) were felt to have splenic involvement. In a second series of untreated patients, evaluated by clinical staging and laparotomy with splenectomy, 58 of 160 (36%) patients had documented splenic disease. Spleen involvement becomes progressively greater with advancing disease. In three large series with autopsy evaluation of 335 Hodgkin's disease patients, 59–69% had documented splenic involvement (Uddstroemer, 1934; Westling, 1965; Jackson and Parker, 1947).

Hodgkin's disease nodules in the spleen range from a few millimeters in diameter to multiple large masses almost completely replacing the normal parenchyma. It is, therefore, crucial that the spleen be carefully examined following staging laparotomy. This includes slicing the entire spleen at less than 5 mm intervals, and sampling all suspicious areas for microscopic examination (Farrer-Brown *et al.*, 1972). Since small nodules of Hodgkin's disease may be scattered randomly throughout the spleen, it would appear that partial splenectomy, at times recommended in children with Hodgkin's disease, would not be as accurate for staging (Boles, Haase and Hamoudi, 1978).

Early lesions of Hodgkin's disease in the spleen are usually found near the central artery in the periarterial lymphatic sheaths of the white pulp or in adjacent lymphoid follicles (Yam and Li, 1976; Halie *et al.*, 1978; Butler, 1983). As these initially small nodules grow and expand, they tend to compress the red pulp rather than invade it. This may be due to characteristics of the special splenic environment. Such small Hodgkin's disease nodules frequently show a halo or corona of small lymphocytes surrounding the nodule. The prominence of this lymphocyte layer tends to decrease in larger nodules and in spleens involved by lymphocyte-depletion Hodgkin's disease. This finding, and the observation that the splenic follicles nearest to the Hodgkin's nodule are larger, with centers nearly devoid of small lymphocytes but with prominent large cells, implies an immune reaction to the malignant nodule (Halie *et al.*, 1978).

The histological criteria applied to foci of Hodgkin's disease in the spleen are the same as those for involved lymph nodes (Lukes, 1971). The presence of typical Reed–Sternberg and Hodgkin's cells, in a background of a mixed cell population of lymphocytes, plasma cells and eosinophils, leads to the diagnosis of involvement by Hodgkin's disease. It is, however, important not to overinterpret such findings, since multinucleated giant cells, closely resembling Reed–Sternberg cells, have been found in other malignant and non-malignant disorders (Lukes, Tindle and Parker, 1969; Strum, Park and Rappaport, 1970). Furthermore, epithelioid granulomas are commonly seen in the spleens of Hodgkin's disease patients; they are observed in 9% of otherwise uninvolved spleens. The presence of these granulomas without splenic involvement is considered a favorable prognostic sign (O'Connell *et al.*, 1975; Sacks *et al.*, 1978).

15.1.4   NON-HODGKIN'S MALIGNANT LYMPHOMAS

The malignant cells in the great majority of these disorders are B-lymphocytes in varying degrees of differentiation. In contrast to Hodgkin's disease, the non-Hodgkin's lymphomas (NHL) most often present in more disseminated fashion. While malignant lymphoma presenting in the spleen as the only area of involvement is rare (see below, section 15.1.5), involvement of the spleen during the course of lymphoma presenting at another site is common (Ahmann, Kiely and Harrison, 1966). In an extensive review by Rosenberg *et al.* (1961) of 1269 patients with NHL, 0.8% presented with a palpable spleen, 35.9% developed a palpable spleen during the course of the disease, and 53.7% showed splenic involvement at autopsy. This is comparable to previously reported series, which observed palpable spleens during the patients' lifetime in 21–56% of cases (Sugarbaker and Craver, 1940; Gall and Mallory, 1942; Wetherley-Mein *et al.*, 1952). Nodular lymphomas involve the spleen in 50–60% of cases, whereas the diffuse types show this in about 30% (Heifetz, Fuller and Rodgers, 1980).

Initial splenic involvement in malignant lymphoma typically involves the white pulp, and therefore presents in nodular fashion in both the nodular and diffuse types of lymphomas. 'Small cell' lymphomas usually form small uniform nodules, representing infiltration and enlargement of the Malpighian corpuscles, evenly distributed throughout the spleen, while the 'large cell' lymphomas form bulky and irregular nodules (Maurer, 1985; Kim and Dorfman, 1974; Galton *et al.*, 1978). In the follicular lymphomas, it is not unusual to observe lymphoma cells in the red pulp. This would seem to correspond to the relatively high percentage of 'lymphosarcoma cell leukemia' presentations in patients with follicular lymphomas (Spiro *et al.*, 1975).

As in Hodgkin's disease, splenic size is not a reliable indicator of lymphoma involvement. Although large spleens are commonly involved, splenic lymphoma may also be found in spleens of normal weight (Kim and Dorfman, 1974). Involved spleens weighed from 75 to 4500 g in lymphoma patients (Skarin, Davey and Moloney, 1971), whereas uninvolved spleens weighed less than 270 g (Lotz, Chabner and DeVita, 1976). Rosenberg *et al.* (1961) showed that 59% of spleens involved with lymphoma at autopsy were palpable premortem, whereas 29% of palpable spleens showed no lymphoma in the spleen post-mortem. Although it is difficult to assess splenic involvement by non-invasive methods, definite documentation of disease in the spleen is much less important than in Hodgkin's disease: because of the more generalized presentation of the non-Hodgkin's lymphomas, the question of splenic involvement seldom influences treatment.

Splenic involvement is also seen in the less-common histological types of non-Hodgkin's lymphoma. Lennert and Mestdagh (1968) described a lymphoma characterized by a high content of epithelioid histiocytes. In a subsequent series reported by Kim *et al.* (1978), splenomegaly was present in 10 of 19 patients. On staging laparotomy and splenectomy, all 7 patients with splenomegaly had splenic disease, with splenic weights ranging from 225 to 1350 g. The undifferentiated lymphomas, including Burkitt's lymphoma, typically present with disease outside the lymphatic system (Burkitt and O'Connor, 1961). Splenomegaly may be found occasionally; however, in the abdomen other abdominal tumor masses usually predominate (Wright, 1970).

Although of B-cell lineage, the non-Hodgkin's lymphomas associated with HIV infection and AIDS demonstrate several striking differences. The majority are of high-grade histological type, either small non-cleaved lymphoma (undifferentiated, Burkitt's or Burkitt's-like), or immunoblastic lymphoma (Ziegler, 1981; Ziegler, Beckstead and Volberding, 1984; Levine *et al.*, 1984; Kalter *et al.*, 1985; Ioachim, Cooper and Hellman, 1985; Levine and Gill, 1987; Knowles *et al.*, 1988). Most patients present with 'B' symptoms, and with a high proportion of extranodal involvement, especially of the gastrointestinal tract, central

nervous system, bone marrow, and myocardium. In this respect they are very similar to the malignant lymphomas associated with other immunosuppressive states, such as accompany cardiac and renal allotransplantation (Weintraub and Warnke, 1982; Matas *et al.*, 1976) and in primary immunodeficiency syndromes. Splenomegaly was present in 2 of 21 patients with AIDS (Ioachim, Cooper and Hellman, 1985). T-cell leukemia-lymphoma, which has been linked to infection with HTLV-I, and has been described in some AIDS patients, will be discussed in more detail in section 15.1.9(b).

15.1.5 PRIMARY LYMPHOMA OF THE SPLEEN

Malignant lymphoma presenting in the spleen as the only manifestation is rare. In a series from the Memorial Sloan-Kettering Institute 2.6% of stage I cases showed localization to the spleen (Straus, Filippa and Lieberman, 1983). Primary lymphoma of the spleen may develop after chronic immune stimulation, including infection and idiopathic splenomegaly (Dacie *et al.*, 1969; Stahel, Maurer and Cavalli, 1982). Skarin, Davey and Moloney (1971) described 11 patients with primary lymphosarcoma of the spleen confirmed by splenectomy. All presented with palpably enlarged spleens, and eight with features of hypersplenism, in addition to absence of blood lymphocytosis and palpable lymph nodes, and only mild lymphocytosis in the bone marrow. A blood picture of chronic lymphocytic leukemia subsequently developed in 6 of the 11 patients. The latter cases may well represent the so-called 'splenomegalic aleukemic CLL' as identified by Videbaek, Christensen and Jonsson (1982). Although in most cases unexplained splenomegaly is the presenting feature of primary splenic lymphoma, chronic hemorrhagic ascites was the main presenting feature in one case (Hacker *et al.*, 1982).

15.1.6 ACUTE LYMPHOCYTIC LEUKEMIA (ALL)

Splenomegaly, lymphadenopathy and hepatomegaly are common in childhood ALL.

However, such organomegaly is seldom prominent and may be absent. In adults with ALL, extramedullary manifestations such as splenomegaly and adenopathy are rare. Splenomegaly appearing in children who have achieved hematological remission, does not necessarily indicate a relapse. Manoharan et al. (1980) described five children in whom an isolated finding of splenomegaly was evaluated. Splenectomy was performed in three: none of the spleens was involved with leukemia. However, all three died in leukemic recurrence within 28 months, while the two non-splenectomized children remained in complete remission, 2 and 6 years after the appearance of splenomegaly.

15.1.7 CHRONIC LYMPHOCYTIC LEUKEMIA AND ITS VARIANTS

Chronic lymphocytic leukemia (CLL) is a generalized lymphoproliferative disease affecting the small lymphocyte (Dameshek and Gunz, 1964). A variety of cell markers and clinical features delineate several subtypes.

(a) B-cell chronic lymphocytic leukemia (B-cell CLL)

In approximately 95% of cases cell surface membrane immunoglobulin markers will identify the small abnormal lymphocytes of CLL as B-cells. They proliferate slowly, and circulate through the blood, the spleen, bone marrow and lymph nodes. The spleen is often involved, and may occasionally present as an isolated initial manifestation (Dighiero et al., 1979; see section 15.1.5). The spleen is palpably enlarged in 50% of patients at diagnosis (Hansen, 1973); splenomegaly progresses with advancing disease (Videbaek, Christensen and Jonsson, 1982). Total body tumor mass, as reflected by areas of involvement and symptoms, is related to prognosis. To assist in making treatment decisions in CLL patients, a clinical staging system was proposed by Rai et al. (1975) as shown in Table 15.4. More recently, a simpler staging scheme has been adopted by an international study group (Binet et al., 1981; see Table 15.5).

The commonest pattern of splenic involvement in CLL is expansion of the white pulp and infiltration of the red pulp (Lampert et al., 1980a). The white pulp may be infiltrated in either a nodular or diffuse fashion. The degree of red pulp infiltration will usually parallel the degree of peripheral blood lymphocytosis. T-cells are displaced from their usual periarterial location, and appear more often in the red pulp (Lampert, 1983).

Praz et al. (1984) have demonstrated that CLL cells can activate the alternative complement pathway in vitro and that C3 molecules

Table 15.4 Rai clinical staging system for CLL

Stage	Findings at diagnosis
O	Lymphocytes in blood 15 000 per microliter or higher, and 40% marrow lymphocytosis.
I	Above, plus enlarged lymph nodes.
II	Above, plus splenomegaly, hepatomegaly, or both.
III	Above, plus anemia (hemoglobin less than 11 g/dl).
IV	Above, plus thrombocytopenia (platelets less than 100 000 per microliter).

From Rai et al. (1975).

Table 15.5 International clinical staging system for CLL

Stage	Findings at diagnosis
Stage A	Lymphocytosis in blood 15 000 per microliter or higher, 40% marrow lymphocytosis. No anemia or thrombocytopenia, and less than three areas of nodal involvement.
Stage B	Above with three or more areas of lymphoid involvement, including lymph nodes, spleen or liver. No anemia or thrombocytopenia.
Stage C	Above with anemia (hemoglobin less than 11 g/dl in men and less than 10 g/dl in women) or thrombocytopenia (less than 100 000 per microliter) regardless of the number of lymphoid areas involved.

Note: Each cervical, axillary and inguinal area, whether unilateral or bilateral, as well as spleen and liver, count as one area each. From Binet *et al.* (1981).

are detectable on CLL cells *in vivo*. The authors postulate that these CLL cells could interact with splenic and hepatic macrophages, thereby sequestering preferentially in these organs.

(b) T-cell chronic lymphocytic leukemia (T-CLL)

T-cell CLL is rare in the Western world, but is the most common type of CLL in Japan (Hanaoka *et al.*, 1979). It is frequently associated with splenomegaly, skin infiltration and early neurologic manifestations (Brouet *et al.*, 1975). The involved spleen shows enlargement of both the red and white pulp, with, however, prominent residual germinal centers (Lampert, 1983). Cell typing has shown these cells phenotypically and functionally to be suppressor T-cells, which may explain the hypogammaglobulinemia observed in a number of cases.

T-cells from patients with the syndrome of chronic T-8 hyperlymphocytosis and neutropenia have been shown to express natural killer (NK)-related antigens (Grillot-Courvalin *et al.*, 1986). The relationship of this entity to chronic T-cell leukemia is presently unclear (Newland *et al.*, 1984; Pandolfi *et al.*, 1984; McKenna *et al.*, 1985; Loughran *et al.*, 1985).

See section 15.1.9(b) for discussion of adult T-cell leukemia-lymphoma associated with HTLV-I infection.

(c) Prolymphocytic leukemia

Prolymphocytic leukemia is a more aggressive disease than CLL, with a poor response to chemotherapy. It typically presents with massive splenomegaly and marked leukocytosis but no lymphadenopathy (Galton *et al.*, 1974). Prolymphocytes are of intermediate size, with a characteristic nucleus showing well-condensed chromatin and a prominent nucleolus (Catovsky, 1977). Splenectomy and leukapheresis have led to temporary therapeutic responses (Buskard *et al.*, 1976).

The majority of spleens in this condition have shown enlargement of the white pulp and infiltration of the red pulp (Lampert, 1983). A nodular pattern is often seen, with the larger, abnormal cells at the periphery of the 'nodules' (Lampert *et al.*, 1980b).

(d) Heavy chain disease

Six of seven patients with mu heavy-chain disease reported by Franklin (1975) presented clinically as CLL, often with marked splenomegaly but infrequently with peripheral lymphadenopathy (Jonsson *et al.*, 1976). Associated findings are kappa light-chains in the urine and vacuolated plasma cells in the marrow (Franklin, 1975).

Gamma heavy-chain disease frequently presents as a lymphoma, with lymphadenopathy, hepatosplenomegaly and systemic symptoms (Franklin *et al.*, 1964). Alpha heavy-chain disease may present with enteric manifestations and abdominal masses ('Mediterranean lymphoma') or with respiratory tract infiltration (Seligmann *et al.*, 1968). Spleen and liver are usually not involved, but such involvement has been described (Plesnicar, Sumi-Kriznik and Golouh, 1975).

(e) Waldenström's macroglobulinemia

Clinically this condition mimics 'aleukemic' CLL, with manifestations of hyperviscosity due to the IgM monoclonal gammopathy (Kyle and Garton, 1987). Moderate hepatosplenomegaly and lymph node enlargement are also part of the clinical presentation. Splenomegaly was reported in 37% of patients reported by McCallister *et al.* (1967) and MacKenzie and Fudenberg (1972).

(f) Multiple myeloma and plasma cell leukemia

Only rarely has splenomegaly been observed in multiple myeloma. In a review of plasma cell leukemia by Kosmo and Gale (1987) a 5% incidence of splenomegaly was derived from a combined analysis of 1045 cases of multiple myeloma. By contrast, a 60% frequency of splenomegaly was noted in 30 patients with primary (*de novo*) plasma cell leukemia, and in three of eight patients with the secondary form, in the late leukemic phase of multiple myeloma.

15.1.8 HAIRY CELL LEUKEMIA

Hairy cell leukemia (HCL) or leukemic reticuloendotheliosis accounts for 2–5% of all leukemias (Katayama and Finkel, 1974; Golomb, Catovsky and Golde, 1978; Bouroncle, 1979). Present evidence points to a B-lymphocyte as the malignant cell, which, however, possesses certain monocyte characteristics (Catovsky, 1977; Meijer *et al.*, 1984). The 'hairy cell' can be shown to have numerous cytoplasmic filamentous projections when observed by phase microscopy of the peripheral blood, the bone marrow, and the spleen. The malignant cells usually demonstrate typical acid phosphatase positivity resistant to tartrate, or TRAP (Yam, Li and Finkel, 1972); however, cases with negative TRAP reactivity have been described (Schaefer *et al.*, 1975). The typical appearance of the marrow infiltrated with a loose network of mononuclear cells is more diagnostic, especially when associated with prominent splenomegaly and pancytopenia (Catovsky, 1977).

Splenomegaly is present in 80–90% of cases (see Table 15.6). In a review by Maurer (1985) of three reported series (Burke, Byrne and Rappaport, 1974; Mintz and Golomb, 1979), the

Table 15.6 Hepatosplenomegaly in hairy cell leukemia

	Splenomegaly(%)	Hepatomegaly (%)
Catovsky (1977)	85	35
Golomb, Catovsky and Golde (1978)	82	19
Bouroncle (1979)	93	40
Cawley, Burns and Hayhoe (1980)	84	40
Flandrin *et al.* (1984)	72	20

average spleen weight was 1500 g with a range of 250–4650 g. At surgery, involved spleens typically have a homogeneous, red, fleshy appearance without nodularity (Maurer, 1985; Breitfeld and Lee, 1975). It is the only lymphoproliferative disorder which involves primarily the red pulp of the spleen (see Table 15.1). The microscopic picture is distinctive and diagnostic: the white pulp is atrophic and may be partially obliterated in massively enlarged spleens (Burke, 1981). The hairy cells diffusely infiltrate the cords of the red pulp, and the sinusoids are filled with similar cells. This obliteration of red pulp architecture differs from other MLPDs, and is considered pathognomic for HCL. Subendothelial infiltration of the trabecular veins by hairy cells has also been described as characteristic (Burke and Rappaport, 1984). This finding, and a monoclonal antibody phenotype characteristic of HCL, led to the confirmation of splenic involvement in a 140 g spleen (Burke *et al.*, 1987).

'Pseudosinuses' and 'red cell pools' are located within the splenic cords of patients with HCL (Nanba, Soban and Bowling, 1977). The hairy cells tend to attach to endothelial cells and to each other, as well as to red blood cells, leading to plugging of sinus pores, increased intrasinusal pressure and dilatation of the cord structures to form blood-lakes (Burke, Mackay and Rappaport, 1976; Pilon, Davey and Gordon, 1981, 1982). These structural abnormalities of the spleen would explain the prominent functional hypersplenism and the cases of splenic rupture observed in patients with HCL (see sections 15.3.1 and 15.3.2). The splenic blood pool in HCL is especially prominent (Maurer, 1985). The increased splenic blood pool, and the congestion and decreased blood flow of the cords, leads to increased exposure of blood cells to the cordal macrophages, and results in removal of these cells from the circulation and contributes to the peripheral cytopenia.

Elkon *et al.* (1979) described four men in whom polyarteritis nodosa developed after the diagnosis of HCL. The onset of vasculitis was attributed to the impaired clearance of circulating antigens and immune complexes in these patients. More recently, the case of a woman who developed HCL in splenic implants secondary to splenectomy for splenic rupture was reported (Goedert *et al.*, 1981). Evidence for limited vasculitis was present prior to the diagnosis of HCL, with florid systemic expression of the vasculitis following diagnosis of the hematological disorder. It would appear more likely, however, that the reticuloendothelial impairment in hairy cell leukemia may allow for a more clinically obvious expression of the vasculitis than that it should be a primary cause of the HCL.

15.1.9 T-CELL LYMPHOPROLIFERATIVE DISORDERS

(a) Cutaneous T-cell lymphomas (mycosis fungoides and Sézary syndrome)

Mycosis fungoides and the Sézary syndrome are closely related and are commonly grouped as part of the spectrum of malignant T-cell lymphomas with a predilection for skin infiltration (Crossen *et al.*, 1971; Edelson *et al.*, 1974). The malignant cells in both disorders are mature T-lymphocytes, often with helper-inducer phenotypes (Brouet, Flandrin and Seligmann, 1973; Braylan, Variakojis and Yachnin, 1975; Broder *et al.*, 1976; Kung *et al.*, 1981). A number of patients tested had peripheral blood neoplastic T-cells which showed helper cell activity *in vitro* (Broder, Uchiyama and Waldmann, 1979). These cells also demonstrate the same striking convoluted and cerebriform nuclear pattern (Zucker-Franklin, 1974) and frequently have non-specific chromosomal abnormalities (Whang-Peng *et al.*, 1979). These cutaneous T-cell lymphoma cells have been shown to have active T-cell growth factor (TCGF) receptors on their surface (Gootenberg *et al.*, 1981).

Individuals with these disorders usually progress through stages from the initial premycotic, to infiltrating plaque, to cutaneous tumor, and finally to the generalized erythro-

Table 15.7 Clinical staging system for cutaneous T-cell lymphoma

Stage		Description
O		Premalignant lesions
I		Erythematous plaque or generalized erythema
II		Indurated plaque or exfoliative erythroderma, or both
III		Tumors with or without papules, plaques, or generalized erythroderma
IV		Visceral involvement
	A	Without a leukemic phase
	B	With a leukemic phase

From Zucker-Franklin (1974).

dermia stage associated with the presence of abnormal T-lymphocytes in the blood (Lutzner et al., 1975). In the leukemic phase, lymphadenopathy and hepatosplenomegaly are not uncommon. Although the earlier, cutaneous stages may remain indolent for some time, visceral involvement has been described in up to 81% (Long and Mihm, 1974). The clinical features heralding the onset of extracutaneous dissemination of mycosis fungoides include fever, weight loss, widespread lymphadenopathy, and often hepatosplenomegaly. In the series by Long and Mihm (1974), 6 of 15 patients presented with splenomegaly at the time of dissemination. At autopsy, 12 of 15 had splenic involvement, with a mean spleen weight of 310 g, and a range of 110–2050 g.

Staging laparotomy may be of some value in assessing extracutaneous spread and for the definition of treatment options (Variakojis,

Table 15.8 National cutaneous T-cell lymphoma workshop staging classification*

T Skin	N Lymph nodes	M Visceral organs
T_1 Limited plaques (10% BSA)	N_0 No adenopathy, histology negative	M_0 No involvement
T_2 Generalized plaques	N_1 Adenopathy, histology negative	M_1 Visceral involvement
T_3 Cutaneous tumors	N_2 No adenopathy, histology positive	
T_4 Generalized erythroderma	N_3 Adenopathy, histology positive	

Stage I	Limited (IA) or generalized plaques (IB) without adenopathy or histological involvement of lymph nodes or viscera (T_1, N_0, M_0, or T_2, N_0, M_0)
Stage II	Limited or generalized plaques with adenopathy (IIA) or cutaneous tumors with or without adenopathy (IIB); without histologic involvement of lymph nodes or viscera (T_{1-2}, N_1, M_0 or T_3, N_{0-1}, M_0)
Stage III	Generalized erythroderma with or without adenopathy; without histological involvement of lymph nodes or viscera (T_4, N_{0-1}, M_0)
Stage IV	Histological involvement of lymph nodes (IVA) or viscera (IVB) with any skin lesion and with or without adenopathy (T_{1-4}, N_{2-3}, M_0 for IVA; T_{1-4}, N_{0-3}, M_1 for IVB)

*Blood involvement should be recorded as absent ($\widehat{B}_0$) or present (B_1) but is not currently used to determine final stage.
BSA – body surface area
From Bunn and Lamberg (1979).

Rosas-Uribe and Rappaport, 1974). Staging evaluation employing non-invasive methods, including cytological and chromosomal evaluation of blood and lymph node cells, shows a high percentage of cases with extracutaneous dissemination (Bunn *et al.*, 1980).

Several clinical and histological staging systems have been proposed (Griem *et al.*, 1975; see Table 15.7). More recently, the National Workshop on Cutaneous T-Cell Lymphoma has adopted a clinical staging system which is presently being evaluated (Bunn and Lamberg, 1979; see Table 15.8).

(b) Adult T-cell leukemia-lymphoma (ATL)

Uchiyama *et al.* (1977) have reported a distinct T-cell lymphoproliferative disorder affecting adults in the southwestern part of Japan, especially in Kyushu. Subsequently, clusters of an aggressive T-cell malignancy were described in Caribbean black immigrants in London (Catovsky *et al.*, 1982), and in blacks from the southeastern part of the United States (Blayney *et al.*, 1983a). The clinical features of this adult T-cell leukemia-lymphoma (ATL) have been described in over 100 cases from Japan, but in only a few from other endemic areas, including the Caribbean basin and the southeastern United States (Bunn *et al.*, 1983; Swerdlow *et al.*, 1984; Urba and Longo, 1985; Takatsuki *et al.*, 1985; Gibbs, Loffers and Campbell, 1987). The syndrome presents with nearly identical features in these different geographic areas, and includes peripheral lymph node enlargement (86%), hepatomegaly (72%), splenomegaly (51%), and skin lesions (49%). In other series, splenomegaly was present in 63% of Japanese cases (Uchiyama *et al.*, 1977), in 25% of Jamaican cases (Gibbs, Loffers and Campbell, 1987) and in none of the US patients with ATL (Blayney *et al.*, 1983a).

Lytic bone lesions have been described in about 50% of patients, and hypercalcemia has been present in 24% of Japanese patients and in 40–90% of cases outside Japan. The bone marrow has been found to be involved in all cases.

A high incidence of CNS involvement and of opportunistic infections has been noted. All patients experience an aggressive clinical course.

The peripheral white blood cell count is moderately elevated, with pleomorphic neoplastic cells showing irregular nuclear contours and characteristic lobulation, and which are difficult to distinguish from Sézary cells. Cell surface marker analysis has identified the malignant cells in ATL as mature T-lymphocytes of helper-inducer phenotype, with T1, T3, T4 and T11 positivity and T8 negativity (Hattori *et al.*, 1981; Catovsky *et al.*, 1982; Takatsuki *et al.*, 1982). ATL may originate from suppressor cells: in approximately 50% of cases the leukemic T-cells appeared to act as suppressor cells (Uchiyama *et al.*, 1978). These cells have been shown to display IL-2 receptors, and to release biologically active IL-1 (Wano *et al.*, 1987), which possibly explains the osteoclast activation and fever observed in such patients. In 1980 Poiesz *et al.* isolated a retrovirus, termed HTLV-I, from a cell line from a black patient with what was thought to be mycosis fungoides. This virus could be definitely linked to ATL when seroepidemiological studies showed that more than 90% of cases from the endemic areas were HTLV-1 antibody positive (Gallo, 1984; Gallo *et al.*, 1981, 1983; Essex *et al.*, 1984; Gallo and Wong-Staal, 1982; Wong-Staal and Gallo, 1985). Although some patients who present with typical ATL do not show the presence of HTLV-1 infection (Shimoyama *et al.*, 1983), they still demonstrate the typical chromosomal changes of HTLV-1 associated ATL (Shimoyama, Abe and Miyamoto, 1987). The presence of TCGF receptors (Tac) on ATL cells, as measured by reactivity with anti-Tac antibody, can help to distinguish HTLV-1 associated ATL from other T-cell malignancies (Broder *et al.*, 1984).

A second transforming retrovirus (HTLV-II) has been found to be associated with a T-cell hairy cell leukemia (Kalyanaraman *et al.*, 1982), but this virus has only been isolated from four individuals worldwide.

The spread of these two retroviruses is not

yet clearly defined. Drug abusers in the United States have been shown to have a high rate of exposure. Positive serology to HTLV-I/II was found in up to 61% of drug abusers, especially in older blacks in New Orleans and in Newark. Antibody prevalence in white drug abusers over 40 years old was 17.5–36.4% (Weiss *et al.*, 1987). However, these high prevalence rates have recently been challenged: Manns *et al.* (1988) claim that the test used in these studies lacked specificity. They found an HTLV-1 seroprevalence of 0.8 per 1000 in US homosexual males.

Thus far the majority of cases of ATL in the United States have been seen in migrants from Caribbean islands and southern US-born blacks who have moved to northern cities. The full implications of seropositivity to HTLV-I/II, its interaction with HIV-I, and the possibilities of a similar epidemic of an aggressive lymphoid malignancy in the future remain to be determined.

15.2   DIAGNOSIS OF SPLENIC INVOLVEMENT

15.2.1   LABORATORY EVALUATION

Hematological abnormalities may be pronounced in the lymphoproliferative diseases. Often these can be directly attributed to the enlarged or involved spleen. In such cases, the hematological changes are part of the wider array of symptoms and signs ascribed to hypersplenism (Dameshek and Estren, 1947), big spleen disease (Hamilton *et al.*, 1967) or splenomegaly syndrome (Videbaek, Christensen and Jonsson, 1982). The pathophysiological mechanisms observed in the hypersplenism associated with MLPDs will be discussed in more detail in section 15.3.1.

The presence of pancytopenia with a normocellular or hyperplastic bone marrow is usually attributed to hypersplenism, no matter what its cause. Anemia has been attributed to erythrocyte pooling in the spleen, hemodilution anemia (Bowdler, 1967), and excessive destruction of

red cells due to the increased time spent in the unfavorable splenic environment (Videbaek, Christensen and Jonsson, 1982). In hairy cell leukemia, the splenic erythrocyte pool is especially large, possibly because of the prominent red pulp involvement (Lewis *et al.*, 1977).

Autoimmune hemolytic anemia (AIHD) is common in the MLPDs, especially in CLL and the lymphocytic lymphomas. In CLL approximately 30% of patients will develop a positive Coombs' test at some stage of their disease (Hansen, 1973). The onset of this hemolytic anemia may precede the diagnosis of CLL or lymphoma by several years (Bowdler and Glick, 1966). In a series of 234 patients with autoimmune hemolytic anemia reported by Pirofsky (1969), 48% were found to be due to an associated MLPD. In 113 cases of secondary AIHD, 60% were seen in patients with MLPDs. Especially in those patients with warm-reacting antibody type AIHD, the spleen plays a major role in red cell destruction, and splenectomy or corticosteroids often effectively improve the anemia (Christensen, 1973b).

At times, despite the absence of a positive Coombs' test, immune hemolysis may still exist. This has been attributed to a relatively small number of antibody molecules per red cell (Gilliland, Baxter and Evans, 1971; Videbaek, Christensen and Jonsson, 1982). Because of the high number of Fc receptors on the splenic phagocytes, even sensitized red cells with few surface antibody molecules attach to monocytes and are partially or entirely phagocytosed (LoBuglio, Cotran and Jandl, 1967).

Thrombocytopenia in lymphoproliferative splenomegaly has been ascribed to intensified pooling of platelets in the enlarged spleen (Aster, 1966), while platelet survival is usually normal. Neutropenia has been ascribed to both splenic sequestration and increased destruction.

Wedelin *et al.* (1981) correlated the results of a number of routine laboratory tests in 39 untreated patients with Hodgkin's disease with the size and degree of splenic involvement. They found that large spleens, irrespective of tumor involvement, were correlated with lower hemoglobin, decreased lymphocyte counts, elevated reticulocyte counts, and lower IgG and IgM levels. No such correlations were found when involved spleens weighed less than 500 g. Other laboratory tests showed no differences, and the authors concluded that other routine laboratory tests yield no specific information with respect to spleen size or involvement in Hodgkin's disease.

The erythrocyte sedimentation rate (ESR) is elevated in approximately half of Hodgkin's disease patients at presentation, and is increased in almost all patients with large body tumor burden, B symptoms and extensive prior treatment (Le Bourgeois and Tubiana, 1977; Jaffe, Paed and Bishop, 1970). There appears to be no specific correlation between splenic involvement or enlargement and elevation of the ESR. This also seems true for other non-specific laboratory abnormalities, including the levels of serum copper, zinc, uric acid, lactic dehydrogenase, alkaline phosphatase, haptoglobin and acute phase reactants (Ray, Wolf and Kaplan, 1973). Serum iron and iron binding capacity are decreased in Hodgkin's disease, presenting a picture of 'anemia of chronic disease'. This does not represent an iron deficiency state, since tissue iron stores, including those in the spleen, are increased (Britten et al., 1986). This is reflected in elevated serum ferritin levels, which are often as high as ten times the normal level, especially in extensive and advanced disease (Jaffe, Paed and Bishop, 1970; Jones et al., 1972; Bieber and Bieber, 1973).

Anemia, neutropenia and thrombocytopenia are commonly observed in patients with hairy cell leukemia. In a series of 211 patients reported by Flandrin et al. (1984), the mean hemoglobin was 10.2 g/dl, the mean platelet count 92 000/mm^3, the mean WBC 5000/mm^3, and the mean neutrophil count 949/mm^3. Pancytopenia was present in 59% of patients. They found no significant correlation between hemoglobin or WBC and spleen size. A weak inverse relationship was found between spleen size and platelet counts, and between spleen size and neutrophil counts. In a comparison of patients presenting with and without splenomegaly, the authors found no statistically significant difference between the two groups with regard to clinical features and survival, or with laboratory findings, such as anemia, thrombocytopenia and neutropenia. Jansen and Hermans (1981), in a series of 391 patients with HCL, did demonstrate a negative prognostic effect of decreased hemoglobin, neutrophils and platelets on presentation. They concluded that the larger the spleen and the lower the hemoglobin level, the poorer the prognosis. Catovsky (1977) also linked low levels of hemoglobin, neutropenia and thrombocytopenia with survival. Reed–Sternberg cells are only very occasionally encountered in the peripheral blood of patients with Hodgkin's disease (Bouroncle, 1966), whereas in the NHLs, abnormal and presumably malignant lymphocytes are observed in approximately 10%. Such abnormal cells are especially common in patients with the follicular small cleaved cell and the diffuse large cell types of NHL (Come et al., 1980). By using cytofluorometric methods with monoclonal surface immunoglobulins to identify such abnormal lymphocyte clones, 'clonal excess' has been detected in 30–40% of NHL patients without morphological blood involvement (Ault, 1979; Ligler et al., 1980).

15.2.2 PHYSICAL EXAMINATION

The frequent finding of Hodgkin's disease in spleens of normal size and weight at routine staging laparotomy including splenectomy, became apparent at an early stage (Glatstein et al., 1969, 1970; Enright, Trueblood and Nelsen, 1970). Between one-third and one-half of spleens removed from patients without clinically or radiographically detectable splenomegaly were found to have gross or microscopic involvement. In addition to this 'false negative' error, 'false positive' findings of splenomegaly prior to laparotomy could not be attributed to splenic Hodgkin's disease in 35–40% of cases (Glatstein et al., 1969, 1970; Rosenberg and Kaplan, 1970). In a series reported by Askergren *et al.* (1981), 17 of 48 non-palpable spleens showed tumor involvement, while palpable spleens, all of which weighed over 600 g, were all involved. In one patient with Hodgkin's disease, cyclical splenomegaly was associated with cyclical fever and hemolysis (McKenna *et al.*, 1979).

The spleen has to be enlarged from 1.5 to 3 times its normal size for it to become palpable. In addition, a palpable spleen is not necessarily enlarged, while a moderately enlarged spleen may not be palpable on the most skilled examination. Radiographical methods, especially CT scanning, are considerably more reliable as indicators of splenic enlargement.

In contrast to Hodgkin's disease, clinically detectable splenomegaly in the non-Hodgkin's lymphomas, CLL and hairy cell leukemia usually does reflect splenic involvement. At autopsy, 40–50% of patients with non-Hodgkin's lymphoma have documented splenic disease (Rosenberg *et al.*, 1961; Risdall, Hoppe and Warnke, 1979). Patients with earlier stages of NHL, who underwent staging laparotomy and splenectomy, showed involvement in 30–40% of cases (Goffinet, Castellino and Kim, 1973; Moran *et al.*, 1975).

15.2.3   RADIONUCLIDE SCANNING

Since physical examination and customary x-rays of the abdomen have been unreliable in assessing splenic involvement in malignancy, a number of special, non-invasive techniques have been applied to the spleen in an effort to provide such information prior to, or instead of, splenectomy. (See also Chapter 17.) This is especially important in Hodgkin's disease, where the extent of disease and specific organ involvement frequently determine the best treatment for individual patients. In the early days of organ scanning with radionuclides, [^{51}Cr]-chromate attached to heat-damaged red blood cells was employed to measure microvascular function of the spleen. In a series of 68 patients with Hodgkin's disease reported by Ell *et al.* (1975), this method was found to be an unreliable technique for staging. Splenic contraction in response to adrenaline following the administration of ^{51}Cr-labeled red blood cells, was found by spleen scanning to be less in those patients with Hodgkin's disease involving the spleen (Osadchaya, Vasilo and Baisogolov, 1980). This has been confirmed with ^{99m}Tc-labeled heat-treated red blood cells (Rosen *et al.*, 1982). ^{67}Ga-labeled citrate scanning is also unreliable in detecting splenic disease (Kay and McCready, 1972; Johnston *et al.*, 1974; Levi *et al.*, 1975; Seabold *et al.*, 1976; Horn, Ray and Kriss, 1976), and has been found to be more useful in detecting disease above the diaphragm than abdominal involvement.

The splenic scintigram with [^{99m}Tc]-sulfur colloid has been the most commonly employed radionuclide scanning method for the spleen. When the results of such scanning are compared to the findings at laparotomy and splenectomy, this method is found to lack sensitivity with respect to borderline splenic enlargement, especially for Hodgkin's disease involvement (Askergren *et al.*, 1981). In a study from the Walter Reed Army Hospital, Washington, 15 of 66 spleens judged normal by spleen scan were found to be positive for tumor, whereas 13 of 23 spleens considered to be enlarged on scan contained no disease (Harris, Tang and Weltz, 1978). Similar results have been reported by others (Silverman *et al.*, 1972; Milder *et al.*, 1973; Hermreck, Kofender and Bell, 1975; see Table 15.9).

Even the finding of definite large filling defects on the scan of an enlarged spleen is not always evidence for active or persistent disease. A patient with Stage IV-A, nodular sclerosing Hodgkin's disease, with a large filling defect seen on spleen scan prior to treatment, showed a persistent defect following six months of MOPP chemotherapy. Subsequent laparotomy showed the spleen to be disease-free and histologically normal (Dickerman and Clements, 1975). With the advent of CT and MRI technology, splenic scintiscans may remain useful as a secondary method to assess splenic function and blood flow, and to differentiate between

Table 15.9 Comparison of non-invasive imaging methods of the spleen

	No. of patients	Sensitivity[a]	Specificity[a]	Accuracy[a]
Computed tomography				
Alcorn *et al.* (1977)	16	–	–	0.78
Redman *et al.* (1977)	22	0.50	–	0.80
Breiman *et al.* (1978)	16	0.90	1.00	0.94
Frick *et al.* (1981)	18	0.75	1.00	0.89
Castellino *et al.* (1984)	121	0.33	0.76	0.58
Strijk *et al.* (1985)	35	0.57	1.00	0.77
Ultrasound				
Glees *et al.* (1977)	20	0.77	0.72	0.75
Frick *et al.* (1981)	22	0.35	0.82	0.68
King *et al.* (1985)	22	0.60	0.88	0.82
Radionuclide scan (^{99m}Tc-sulfur colloid)				
Alcorn *et al.* (1977)	15	–	–	0.66
Glees *et al.* (1977)	19	0.61	0.66	0.55
Frick *et al.* (1981)	39	0.75	0.88	0.86
Hermreck *et al.* (1975)	28	0.36	0.65	0.53
Milder *et al.* (1973)	50	0.74	0.63	0.70
Silverman *et al.* (1972)	42	0.40	0.82	0.62
Harris *et al.* (1978)	87	0.40	0.79	0.67

[a]See text for definition.

enlarged splenic hilar nodes and accessory spleens (Frick, Feinberg and Loken, 1981). The presence of an ectopic or 'wandering' spleen may be suspected when no splenic image is seen in its usual location, and definite uptake is noted elsewhere in the abdomen or pelvis (Waldman and Suissa, 1978).

In the non-Hodgkin's lymphomas, the finding of focal splenic defects usually correlates with splenic disease (Lindfors *et al.*, 1984). Large cell lymphomas with splenic involvement are especially prone to show this pattern, which usually improves or disappears with effective chemotherapy (Sagar, DelDuca and Mecklenburg, 1979). A case of splenic accumulation of ^{99m}Tc-diphosphonate, a radionuclide employed for bone scanning, has been reported in a patient with extensive lymphomatous involvement in the absence of increased iron deposition (Birch, Garvie and Ackery, 1980). Immunoscin-

tography utilizing radionuclide-labeled monoclonal antibodies may offer increased specificity in scanning for areas of lymphomatous involvement in the near future (Carde *et al.*, 1988).

15.2.4 ULTRASONIC SCANNING

The usefulness of ultrasound examination lies primarily in detecting borderline enlargement of the spleen, which may not be palpable on physical examination, but which, because of its size, has a greater likelihood of being diseased (Koga and Morikawa, 1975; Glees *et al.*, 1977; Frick, Feinberg and Loken, 1981; King, Dawson and Bayliss, 1985). Both decreased and increased splenic echogenicity have been associated with malignant involvement (Siler *et al.*, 1980). The calculated sensitivity, specificity and accuracy of ultrasound in detecting splenic lymphoma from three series of patients are listed in

Table 15.9 and are compared to other imaging methods. Sonography has also been employed as an adjunct to splenic aspiration and biopsy (Lindgren *et al.*, 1985; Solbiati *et al.*, 1983).

15.2.5 COMPUTED TOMOGRAPHY

Computed tomography (CT) has revolutionized the non-invasive staging of patients with malignancies, especially the assessment of the intra-abdominal extent of the malignant lymphomas. Lymphoma nodules of 1 cm or greater can usually be well identified in the spleen as single or multiple low-density lesions (Piekarski *et al.*, 1980; Earl *et al.*, 1980). Early studies indicated that this would prove to be a much more sensitive non-invasive method than others in assessing spleen size and tumor involvement (Jones, Tobias and Waldman, 1978; Redman *et al.*, 1977). However, small miliary deposits of lymphoma remain elusive.

Many reports have appeared in the literature, assessing the usefulness and accuracy of CT of the spleen in detecting lymphoma involvement. Several are summarized in Table 15.9, and compared to a similar assessment for ultrasound and radionuclide scanning (Alcorn *et al.*, 1977; Redman *et al.*, 1977; Breiman *et al.*, 1978; Frick, Feinberg and Loken, 1981; Castellino *et al.*, 1984; Strijk *et al.*, 1985). In Table 15.9, sensitivity refers to the percentage of patients with histologically proven disease in the spleen whose imaging studies were correctly interpreted as positive. Specificity refers to the percentage of patients with no histological disease in the spleen whose imaging studies were correctly interpreted as negative. Overall accuracy is the percentage of patients whose imaging studies were correctly interpreted as either positive or negative.

Although CT has been shown to be the most useful and reliable non-invasive test to detect splenic disease, a number of problems and weaknesses remain. In approximately two-thirds of the cases of splenic involvement with Hodgkin's disease, the tumor nodules measure less than 1 cm in diameter (Castellino *et al.*, 1984), a size usually not detectable by CT. Although CT is excellent for assessing spleen size, not all large spleens are involved by lymphoma and many normal-sized spleens have been shown to contain lymphoma nodules. Calculation of total splenic volume by deriving a 'splenic index' from the CT, has been proposed as a means for improving diagnostic accuracy (Strijk *et al.*, 1985). Splenic hilar nodes and accessory spleens are well detected by CT (Frick, Feinberg and Loken, 1981), although at times ^{99m}Tc-sulfur colloid scanning may provide additional useful information. The use of dynamic CT scans following bolus administration of iodinated contrast material, does not add to the accuracy of detecting splenic disease, but will distinguish accessory spleens from enlarged lymph nodes or splenic varices (Glazer *et al.*, 1981).

Magnetic resonance imaging (MRI) has two major applications to the monitoring of malignancy: it can produce high-resolution images without the use of ionizing radiation, and it can chemically characterize the tumor and tissues *in vivo* and yield biochemical information on metabolic differences (Smith, 1984). It remains to be seen if and when MRI will replace CT as the definitive, non-invasive procedure of choice for the imaging of splenic disease.*

15.2.6 SPLENIC ASPIRATION AND BIOPSY

Splenic aspiration or biopsy is seldom if ever performed in the United States or Britain at this time, primarily because of its perceived limited usefulness and the possibility of hemorrhage. However, in the earlier hematological literature there is considerable evidence that this is a safe procedure. During the 1950s and 60s splenic puncture results were described in over 1600 patients with very few minor complications

---

*'This kind of stone [the magnet] restores husbands to wives and increases elegance and charm in speech. Moreover, along with honey, it cures dropsy, spleen, fox mange, and burns . . .' Bartholomew the Englishman. (Encyclopedist, thirteenth century, AD)

(Moeschlin, 1957; Dameshek and Gunz, 1964; Soederstroem, 1970, 1979). In other parts of the world, splenic aspiration and biopsy continue to be used in the diagnosis of infectious and malignant diseases involving the spleen. In a series of 608 splenic aspirations reported from Kenya (Kager *et al.*, 1983), rapid aspiration with a small caliber needle yielded useful information, mainly for the diagnosis of kala azar and other parasitic infections. However, in four patients with splenomegaly, lymphoma was diagnosed by splenic aspirate. The patients experienced little discomfort, and preferred it over bone marrow aspiration and biopsy. One serious complication was reported in one of the lymphoma patients, with bleeding and death within one hour following the procedure.

In a report from Sweden, TrueCut needle biopsies were performed in 32 patients with a variety of malignant and non-malignant disorders (Lindgren *et al.*, 1985). Of eight patients with focally abnormal ultrasound evaluation seven had lymphoma documented on splenic biopsy. Four of the 32 patients experienced bleeding requiring transfusions; two of these occurred in patients with hairy cell leukemia, and splenectomy had to be performed in one of the hairy cell leukemia patients.

These reports point to some risk from this procedure in patients with hematological malignancies, especially those with hairy cell leukemia. Although splenic aspiration or biopsy has been recommended as an alternative to diagnostic splenectomy, especially in children who appear most susceptible to serious postsplenectomy sepsis, the incomplete information obtained from such a procedure seriously limits its usefulness (Lampert, 1983).

15.2.7 LAPAROTOMY AND SPLENECTOMY

The feasibility of an operation is not the best indication for its performance. Lord Cohen.

From the discussion so far, it is apparent that none of the non-invasive methods of evaluating splenic disease is sufficiently accurate to replace direct examination of the spleen. This is especially crucial in those patients where the presence of splenic disease would modify the pattern of treatment. Aside from diagnostic laparotomy and splenectomy in previously undiagnosed patients, this situation exists today principally in the pretreatment evaluation of patients with Hodgkin's disease.

(a)   Diagnostic splenectomy

The removal of an enlarged spleen for histological examination is often required when noninvasive investigations fail to elicit a definite diagnosis. This may include a small number of patients with protracted fever of undetermined origin (Greenall, Gough and Kettlewell, 1983). The spleen, however, should not be removed simply because it is enlarged: the diagnostic and therapeutic benefits should be carefully weighed against the potential morbidity and mortality. Exploratory laparotomy has been associated with a mortality rate of 0·5−1·0%, and a surgical complication rate of 9−15%, even in experienced hands (Kawarada *et al.*, 1976; Goffinet *et al.*, 1977; Klaue, Eckert and Kern, 1979; Traetow, Fabri and Carey, 1980; Mitchell and Morris, 1983; Larson and Ultmann, 1982).

Where diagnostic and staging laparotomies are performed frequently, about 12% are for undiagnosed splenomegaly (Long and Aisenberg, 1974; Goonewardene *et al.*, 1979; Mitchell and Morris, 1983). Of these, 90% have yielded a definite diagnosis, usually one of the lymphoproliferative disorders. One group of patients with splenomegaly which remains undiagnosed following splenectomy is that with non-tropical splenomegaly (Dacie *et al.*, 1969). In up to 20% of these patients, malignant lymphoma has occurred after several years (Dacie *et al.*, 1978).

(b)   Staging laparotomy and splenectomy

Laparotomy with splenectomy and biopsy of the liver and para-aortic lymph nodes was initially performed on selected patients with Hodgkin's disease presenting special diagnostic problems (Glatstein *et al.*, 1969). Because of an unexpectedly high frequency of Hodgkin's disease involvement of the resected spleens (61%), the value of routine laparotomy and splenectomy in unselected, previously untreated patients was evaluated (Glatstein *et al.*, 1970; Rosenberg and Kaplan, 1970; Kadin, Glatstein and Dorfman, 1971). In 100 consecutive, untreated patients reported by Rosenberg and Kaplan (1970), 50% of the clinically involved spleens, and 24% of the clinically negative spleens contained histologically documented disease. A later review of 160 cases gave an overall frequency of splenic involvement of 36% (Kaplan, 1980).

The primary purpose of the staging laparotomy is to determine as accurately as possible the extent of intra-abdominal disease. It is not considered a therapeutic procedure, although it does diminish the development of hypersplenism which may decrease tolerance to chemotherapy. By placing metal clips at the splenic hilum, future radiation therapy fields can be designed more precisely, although more recently the presence of metal clips is less desirable as it interferes with subsequent CT evaluation of the abdomen. Absence of the spleen also avoids the need for radiation involving a field including the left kidney and the base of the left lung (Greenberger, Come and Weichselbaum, 1979). It is now well established that the noninvasive methods of CT and radionuclide scanning cannot replace splenectomy as a staging procedure (Aisenberg, 1978).

Staging laparotomy and splenectomy for Hodgkin's disease and the lymphomas is indicated only if the findings may lead to a change in treatment from that planned from clinical staging (see Table 15.10). In several series assessing changes in stage pre- and postoperatively, the findings at laparotomy led to changes in stage in 30–43% of patients (Kaplan, 1972; Gill, Souter and Morris, 1980; Sterchi and Myers, 1980; Glees *et al.*, 1982). Patients with stage III disease who had splenic involvement were found to have a shorter disease-free interval than those who did not (Worthy, 1981). Several authors have suggested that patients with stage IIIA disease, whose abdominal disease is limited to the spleen and the upper abdominal nodes (anatomical substage III-1), respond well to radiotherapy alone, whereas those with lower abdominal disease (anatomical substage III-2) respond poorly and require primary treatment with chemotherapy (Desser, Moran and Ultmann, 1973; Stein *et al.*, 1978, 1982). Assessment of data from Stanford University, however, found no prognostic advan-

---

Table 15.10 Indications for staging laparotomy in lymphoma patients

---

Hodgkin's disease:
1. Clinical stage IA and IIA
   except: (a) isolated high cervical nodes only
   (b) bulky mediastinal disease

2. Clinical stage IIIA (without involvement of lower abdominal nodes)

3. Presence of splenomegaly when RT main therapy

4. Equivocal lymphangiogram/abdominal CT

5. Preservation of ovarian function prior to RT

Non-Hodgkin's lymphomas:
1. Clinical stage I (diffuse large cell lymphomas)

---

tage to such substaging, and identified a group of PS* IIIA patients with extensive splenic disease, which they defined as more than four nodules, who benefited from chemotherapy in addition to radiation therapy (Hoppe *et al.*, 1982). Data from the University of Chicago did show a correlation between anatomical substaging and splenic involvement in 76 patients with PS IIIA Hodgkin's disease (Larson and Ultmann, 1982). Patients with stage III-2 disease tended to have extensive involvement with more than four splenic nodules, whereas stage III-1 patients more often had minimal splenic disease, and were therefore felt to be at lower risk for occult liver involvement.

The likelihood of splenic involvement has been shown to be strongly dependent on the histological subtype of Hodgkin's disease (Kaplan, 1972). The spleen was found to be involved in 16% of lymphocyte predominant (LP), in 35% of nodular sclerosing (NS), in 59% of mixed cellularity (MC), and in 83% of lymphocyte depletion cases. The probability of change in stage following laparotomy could also be correlated with histological subtype; a change in stage was seen in 13% of LP, in 19% of NS, and in 37% of MC types.

With the development of more effective combination chemotherapy regimens and the judicious combination of radiation and chemotherapy, laparotomy has become less important as a routine staging procedure (Rosenberg, 1988). Its present indications are outlined in Table 15.10. For Hodgkin's disease, staging laparotomy is recommended for CS† IA and IIA, except for those with nodal disease limited to one high cervical area, and those with bulky mediastinal adenopathy, who should receive chemotherapy with or without radiation. Patients presenting with subdiaphragmatic CS IIB disease may not require laparotomy, because of an extremely high probability of splenic involvement (89%), which is best treated with chemotherapy (Leibenhaut *et al.*,

*Pathological stage.
†Clinical stage.

1987). Laparotomy is also indicated in CS IIIA, where evidence for lower abdominal disease is absent or equivocal, and in those with splenomegaly where radiation therapy is planned as the initial treatment. Women who wish to preserve ovarian function may benefit from the surgical relocation of the ovaries at laparotomy.

The role of staging laparotomy with splenectomy in non-Hodgkin's lymphomas (NHL) is much less clearly defined. The great majority of these patients present with advanced, stage III and IV disease, and in only relatively few will surgical staging affect treatment decisions (Come and Chabner, 1979). Although splenic involvement was noted in 32% of a series of unselected and untreated lymphoma patients who underwent staging laparotomy (Goffinet, Castellino and Kim, 1973), 60–75% of NHL patients are stage IV by virtue of bone marrow, liver or other extranodal involvement (Come and Chabner, 1979). Splenic evaluation in such cases is superfluous. On the other hand, splenic involvement is relatively uncommon in diffuse large cell (histiocytic) lymphoma (Goffinet, Castellino and Kim, 1973; Heifetz, Fuller and Rodgers, 1980). This type of NHL also presents more often as stage I and II when compared with the nodular lymphomas (Rosenberg, Ribas-Mundo and Goffinet, 1978). Therefore in patients presenting as CS I diffuse large cell lymphoma, staging laparotomy may be an important aspect of their overall evaluation to exclude intra-abdominal and splenic disease.

Truly localized NHL can be successfully treated by radiation therapy alone, if either subtotal or total lymphoid irradiation is employed (Kaminski *et al.*, 1986), with results similar to limited field radiation plus adjuvant chemotherapy. However, excellent results have recently been reported in clinically staged I and II patients with histologically aggressive lymphomas treated with 3 cycles of CHOP chemotherapy (cyclophosphamide, doxorubicin, vincristine and prednisone) followed by 3000 cGy of involved field radiation therapy to the original site of disease (Connors *et al.*, 1987).

Restaging or 'second look' laparotomy for

Hodgkin's disease patients in apparently complete remission following treatment, has been studied by several groups (Sutcliffe *et al.*, 1978, 1982; Goodman *et al.*, 1982), in order to document complete remission. These studies showed that residual disease is only rarely found in patients with normal clinical restaging following completion of therapy. Of 46 Hodgkin's disease patients who underwent posttreatment laparotomy, four patients with a normal clinical evaluation showed splenic involvement only, whereas of 14 patients with clinically suspicious findings, only two had evidence of active disease on laparotomy (Sutcliffe *et al.*, 1982). At this time, restaging laparotomy is not recommended as a routine procedure, especially in patients who have undergone pretreatment laparotomy with removal of the spleen.

Because of the high risk of postsplenectomy sepsis, especially in children with Hodgkin's disease (Singer, 1973; Chilcote *et al.*, 1976; Lanzkowsky *et al.*, 1976; Dickerman, 1979), which has been estimated at about 10% with a 50% mortality rate, partial splenectomy has been recommended and performed at a number of institutions (Boles, Haase and Hamoudi, 1978; Pearson, 1980; Katz and Schiller, 1980). The use of an ultrasonic scalpel has been proposed for this procedure for better hemostasis (Hodgson and McElhinney, 1982). Boles, Haase and Hamoudi (1978) estimated only a 2–3% understaging of patients with Hodgkin's disease when partial splenectomy was performed. However data from other authors point to a larger error: Dearth *et al.* (1978) reported that 11.6% of splenic disease would have been missed with partial splenectomy, whereas Sterchi, Buss and Bayer (1984) found a 6.2% understaging of splenic involvement. A plea has been made to preserve accessory spleens at time of initial staging laparotomy and splenectomy in patients with Hodgkin's disease (Strauch, 1979), although accessory spleens do not always protect from postsplenectomy sepsis, and a critical mass of functioning splenic tissue may be required to provide adequate protection (Goldthorn and Schwartz, 1978;

Moore *et al.*, 1983). Splenic autotransplantation has also been proposed to provide some degree of splenic function after splenectomy (Traub *et al.*, 1987).

(c)   Laparoscopy

Laparoscopy has also been proposed as an alternative to staging laparotomy and splenectomy, because of the risk of postsplenectomy infections, the avoidance of operative risk and the fact that chemotherapy is being employed more frequently, with or without radiation therapy, whether the spleen is involved or not (DeVita *et al.*, 1971, 1973; Bagley *et al.*, 1973; Beretta *et al.*, 1976). In a series of 121 unselected and previously untreated patients with Hodgkin's disease reported by Beretta *et al.* (1976), findings on laparoscopy were compared with subsequent laparotomy and splenectomy. Needle biopsy of the liver during laparoscopy was helpful in detecting extranodal disease. While needle biopsies of the spleen were positive in 13%, subsequent laparotomy and splenectomy demonstrated disease in an additional 26 spleens. The authors concluded that, although laparoscopy appears to be a useful staging procedure in Hodgkin's disease patients, especially for the detection of liver involvement, it is not recommended in patients where splenic evaluation is an important part of the staging.

In NHL, laparoscopy may be useful in localized disease, where combined radiotherapy and chemotherapy is indicated, to detect stage IV disease by virtue of hepatic involvement. This procedure has also been employed to reevaluate NHL patients for completeness of response and to detect sites of relapse (Anderson *et al.*, 1976).

15.3   COMPLICATIONS OF SPLENIC INVOLVEMENT AND SPLENECTOMY

The problems encountered in patients with enlarged spleens, designated as the 'splenomegaly syndrome' by Videbaek, Christensen and Jonsson (1982), center principally on the pancytopenia of hypersplenism, although other compli-cations, such as hypermetabolic symptoms, in-cluding fever (McKenna *et al.*, 1979), and mechanical problems of pain and rupture, should also be included. This section will address those complications specifically en-countered in patients with splenomegaly associ-ated with the MLPDs, as well as problems which follow splenectomy.

15.3.1   HYPERSPLENISM

Anemia, thrombocytopenia and leukopenia in the presence of a normocellular or hypercellular bone marrow are the presenting features of hypersplenism (Dameshek and Estren, 1947; Hamilton *et al.*, 1967). Anemia is especially common in the MLPDs, which, however, may not reflect a true reduction in total red cell volume. In patients with enlarged spleens, no matter what the cause, expansion of plasma volume leads to a hemodilutional anemia (Bowdler, 1970), which is sometimes exagger-ated by the diversion of red cells into a large splenic pool. As discussed in section 15.1, splenic involvement by the MLPDs leads to expansion of the extrasinusal space by lymphocytes (Har-ris, McAlister and Prankerd, 1958), while the red pulp remains relatively intact, allowing for increased blood flow and for accumulation of red cells (Videbaek, Christensen and Jonsson, 1982). In patients with CLL, Christensen (1973a) has shown a direct correlation between the degree of splenomegaly and size of the splenic erythrocyte pool. For spleens weighing about 1000 g the erythrocyte pool was 10% of the total red cell mass, increasing to 40% for spleens weighing 4000 g. (See also Chapter 8).

In hairy cell leukemia, because of the es-pecially prominent parenchymal changes de-scribed in section 15.1.8, the splenic erythro-cyte pool is unusually large (Lewis *et al.*, 1977), and contributes to the prominent anemia of this disorder (Flandrin *et al.*, 1984). In this disease also, expansion of plasma volume and dilu-tional anemia are related to the degree of splen-omegaly and contribute to the reduced hemo-globin levels (Castro-Malaspina, Najean and Flandrin, 1979).

There appears to be a similar relationship between spleen size and splenic pooling of pla-telets as with red cell pooling. Normally, about 30% of the circulating platelet mass is pooled in the spleen (Aster, 1966). As the size of the spleen increases, the platelet pool expands, reaching values up to 90% of the total circulat-ing platelet mass. On the other hand, despite significant splenic enlargement, platelet survival usually remains normal (Aster and Jandl, 1964).

There is some evidence for splenic pooling of granulocytes, which increases with spleno-megaly (Vincent, 1977). There also appears to be increased margination of granulocytes in the splenic vessels, thereby reducing the peripheral neutrophil count (Fieschi and Sacchetti, 1964; Scott *et al.*, 1971).

Hypermetabolic manifestations are at times a prominent feature of the hypersplenism observed in the MLPDs. These include weight loss, fever, hyperhydrosis, and increased basal metabolic rate, which are often reversed by splenectomy (Christensen, Hansen and Vide-baek, 1977; McKenna *et al.*, 1979).

15.3.2   SPLENIC PAIN AND RUPTURE

The discomfort experienced by MLPD patients with splenomegaly is usually vague and undra-matic, except when due to splenic infarction. In general, splenic infarction is more common in the chronic leukemias than in acute leukemia or lymphoma, and is often associated with the sudden onset of left flank, back or shoulder pain, at times pleuritic in nature, or sometimes mimicking an acute abdomen.

Splenic infarction may predispose to splenic rupture, although acute rupture of the spleen occurs more often in the acute than the chronic MLPDs. Bauer, Haskins and Armitage (1981) have reviewed the diagnoses in 53 cases of splenic rupture; the following numbers of cases were observed: AML 11, ALL 10, unclassified acute leukemia 9, NHL 9, CML 6, HD 5, CLL

3. A report by Johnson, Rosen and Sheehan (1979) notes that 1% of patients with acute leukemia experience splenic rupture. In 34% of ruptured spleens in cases of acute leukemia, this was the presenting event of the leukemia (Bauer, Haskins and Armitage, 1981). It is possible that the leukemic infiltration of the spleen contributes to spontaneous rupture, either by causing capsular invasion or ischemic infarction.

Splenic rupture has also been observed in hairy cell leukemia. Eleven cases have been described in the literature (Rosier and Lefer, 1977; Yam and Crosby, 1979; Schmitt et al., 1981). Again a major correlation appears to be with the frequency of splenic infarction (Yam and Crosby, 1979), which in turn is most probably related to the vascular changes observed in such spleens (see section 15.1.8).

Two cases of splenic rupture in plasma cell leukemia have been described (Stephens and Hudson, 1969; Rogers and Shah, 1980). Infarction, followed by subcapsular hematoma, was postulated as the possible mechanism for the splenic rupture.

15.3.3   IMMUNE DEFICIENCIES

'Then a sentimental passion of a vegetable fashion must excite your languid spleen.' Sir William Gilbert (1836–1911) in *Patience*.

Most patients with Hodgkin's disease, including those presenting with limited disease, demonstrate an impairment of cell-mediated immunity. Clinically, this deficit is expressed by an increased susceptibility to certain unusual, 'opportunistic' infections, including fungi and viruses (Casazza, Duvall and Carbone, 1966; Goffinet, Glatstein and Merigan, 1972). Anergy is expressed by impaired delayed hypersensitivity responses (Sokol and Primikiros, 1961; Aisenberg, 1962; Young et al., 1972; Chang, Stutzman and Sokal, 1975). Numerous *in vitro* studies have shed additional light on the cellular immune defects observed in Hodgkin's disease: these include depression of lymphocyte prolifer-

ative responses to mitogens and alloantigens (Faguet, 1975; Han and Sokal, 1970; Levy and Kaplan, 1974; Sibbit, Bankhurst and Williams, 1978; Schulof, Lacher and Gupta, 1981), a serum factor which affects T-lymphocyte E-rosette formation (Fuks, Strober and Kaplan, 1976), lymphopenia and reduction in circulating T-cells (Posner, Reinherz and Brerad, 1981), and excess suppressor cells (Twomey et al., 1975; Hillinger and Herzig, 1977).

The suppressor cells observed in patients with Hodgkin's disease have been characterized as either monocytes (Goodwin et al., 1977; Schechter and Soehnlen, 1978; Han, 1980; Vanhaelen and Fisher, 1981), or T-lymphocytes (Zarling, Berman and Raich, 1980; Lauria et al., 1983). In the study by Zarling, Berman and Raich (1980) the cytotoxic responses of patients' lymphocytes could be enhanced by removing suppressor lymphocytes by passing them through columns containing histamine-coated Sepharose beads. The presence of suppressor cells has been shown to persist following treatment and long-lasting remission (Yanes et al., 1975). The extent to which the spleen contributes to these defects in cellular immunity has been examined by numerous investigators.

The depression of cell-mediated immunity observed in Hodgkin's disease may reflect a reduction in a specific T-cell subset by sequestration in the spleen and other lymphoid organs. Several authors have demonstrated elevated T-cell numbers in the spleen in Hodgkin's disease, and these show relatively normal PHA reactivity (Payne et al., 1976; Kaur et al., 1974; DeSousa et al., 1977; Matchett, Huang and Kremer, 1973; Han et al., 1980; Minassian, 1986). Some workers have indicated that involved splenic tissue tends to have somewhat fewer T-lymphocytes than uninvolved spleens (Stathopoulos et al., 1977; Han et al., 1980; Dorreen, Habeshaw and Wrigley, 1982), while others found elevated numbers in involved spleens (Baroni et al., 1982), or no differences between involved and uninvolved spleens (Posner, Reinherz and Brerad, 1981). Splenectomy in Hodgkin's disease patients led to a normalization of peripheral blood T-cell numbers and PHA responses within 18 months of splenectomy (DeSousa et al., 1977; Wagener et al., 1976; Wagener, Geestman and Wessels, 1975; Gupta and Tan, 1980; Bjoerkholm, Askergren and Holm, 1980). In trauma-related splenectomies, peripheral blood suppressor cell activity drops within 2 weeks and remains stable thereafter (Robertson et al., 1982), although Posner, Reinherz and Brerad (1981) found that circulating T-cell subsets were not changed 5–14 days following splenectomy.

There is additional evidence that at least some of the blood lymphocyte abnormalities observed in Hodgkin's disease are due to the removal of functionally active lymphocytes by the spleen (Posner, Reinherz and Brerad, 1981). Whether this is related to splenic involvement, B-symptoms, splenomegaly, or perhaps all of these, has not been definitely established (Bjoerkholm, Askergren and Wederlin, 1980). By studying lymphocyte counts and function in arterial and venous blood in patients undergoing splenectomy, Bjoerkholm et al. (1983) found that spontaneous lymphocyte DNA synthesis, as well as that induced by pokeweed mitogen and concanavalin A, was significantly lower in venous than arterial blood in most of the patients studied.

The possibility that specific subpopulations of lymphocytes may be removed by the spleen is reinforced by the finding of increased suppressor lymphocyte numbers and activity in the peripheral blood of Hodgkin's disease patients (Hillinger and Herzig, 1978; Twomey et al., 1980; Zarling, Berman and Raich, 1980). Increased suppressor cell activity, of either the T-lymphocytic or the monocytic type, has not been found in the spleen cell population of Hodgkin's disease patients (Han, 1980; Toge et al., 1983; Minassian, 1986), although several authors have also demonstrated increased proportions of T-helper/inducer cells relative to T-suppressor cells in the spleens of Hodgkin's disease patients (Hunter et al., 1977; Gupta, 1980; Poppema et al., 1982; Borowitz, Croker

and Metzgar, 1982). Ruco et al. (1982) observed increased natural killer cell activity in Hodgkin's disease spleens.

The cause for this selective sequestration of specific T-cell subsets in the spleen is not clear. Antilymphocyte antibodies have been suggested to be involved, since antibody-coated blood cells of various types are removed from the circulation by the spleen (Siegal, 1976). Fuks, Strober and Kaplan (1976) described a serum factor in patients with Hodgkin's disease which inhibited sheep-erythrocyte-rosetting capacity of their lymphocytes. The lymphocytes of normal individuals could not be inhibited by this serum factor. Bieber, Fuks and Kaplan (1977) were able to demonstrate an E-rosette inhibiting factor in extracts of Hodgkin's disease spleens. A lymphocytotoxic substance was also noted by Bjoerkholm, Wedelin and Holm (1982) in approximately 30% of patients. This factor was found more frequently in large, tumor-involved spleens, and persisted following treatment. The increased ferritin found associated with macrophages from spleens of Hodgkin's disease patients has also been held responsible for selective lymphocyte sequestration (Britten et al., 1986).

Hodgkin's disease patients with large involved spleens, usually reflecting advanced disease, may show decreased levels of IgG and IgM in their blood (Wedelin et al., 1981). Specific antibodies against Haemophilus influenzae were significantly reduced in Hodgkin's disease patients receiving specific treatment, but were normal in untreated patients (Weitzman et al., 1977). Splenectomy had no effect on these antibodies, although chemotherapy in splenectomized patients had a greater effect in reducing IgM levels.

Suppressor cells have also been demonstrated in the peripheral blood of patients with non-Hodgkin's lymphoma (Zarling, Berman and Raich, 1980), CLL (Faguet, 1979), and a variety of solid tumors (Bean et al., 1977; Yu et al., 1977). Whether the mechanisms are similar to those described in patients with Hodgkin's disease has not been determined.

15.3.4   OVERWHELMING POSTSPLENECTOMY INFECTION (OPSI)

The immunological functions of the spleen are described in detail in Chapter 5. The most important mechanisms by which the spleen protects the body from infections are outlined in Table 15.11 (Baesl and Filler, 1985; Lockwood, 1983). Although as early as 1919, Morris and Bullock (1919) suggested that splenectomy would result in an increased susceptibility to infection, it was not until King and Schumacker (1952) described five infants who developed fulminant sepsis 3 months to 3 years following splenectomy for hereditary spherocytosis, that this connection was made. In a survey of 2795 cases collected by Singer (1973), it was estimated that the early mortality from severe infections in the asplenic population was at least 50 times greater than in a normal population. More recent reviews provide additional information regarding the concern that splenectomy performed in patients with Hodgkin's disease and NHL carries with it a greater risk of severe infections than splenectomy performed for other hematological disorders or trauma (Ravry et al., 1972; Krivit, 1977; Trigg, 1979; Mitchell and Morris, 1983; Baesl and Filler, 1985. See also Chapter 12).

Most cases of overwhelming postsplenectomy infection (OPSI) reported in the literature occur within three years of surgery, and children are clearly more susceptible than adults (Winkelstein and Lambert, 1975). Chilcote et al. (1976) have reviewed 200 children splenectomized for the staging of Hodgkin's disease, and found the incidence of OPSI to be 10%, with a 50% mortality of the infected cases. In contrast, a review of OPSI following splenectomy for trauma in children revealed a 2.5% incidence and a 25% fatality rate (Sherman, 1980). Reports in adult patients have also suggested a higher infection rate in patients splenectomized for causes other than trauma (Weitzman and Aisenberg, 1977; O'Neal and McDonald, 1981; Francke and Neu, 1981).

Conversely, other studies have reported that the occurrence of OPSI in adults following splenectomy did not differ between patients with and without lymphoma (Donaldson et al., 1972; Cormia and Campos, 1973; Schimpff et al., 1975; Carlstedt and Tholin, 1984). A review of a number of reports of postsplenectomy infections in lymphoma patients up to 1972 by Desser and Ultmann (1972), demonstrated a morbidity of 1.4% and an overall mortality of 0.5%. These figures are substantially less than those reported at that time for infection following splenectomy for other causes. The report by Donaldson et al. (1972) contrasted a rate for severe infection of 4.5% in lymphomas to a rate of 9.3% in non-lymphoma patients.

In summary then, the available literature points to a definitely increased risk of OPSI in children following splenectomy for any cause other than trauma. This increased risk can be essentially eliminated by prophylactic antibiotic administration (Krivit, Giebink and Leonard,

---

Table 15.11 Immune functions of the spleen

1.   Removal of circulating particulate antigen.
2.   Primary IgM antibody response to intravenous antigen.
3.   Secondary IgG antibody response to intravenous antigen.
4.   Maintenance of IgM serum levels.
5.   Alternative pathway of complement activation.
6.   Production of tuftsin (stimulates phagocytes).

Adapted from Baesl and Filler (1985).

1979). In adult patients, the risk for developing OPSI appears no greater, and may even be less, than in patients undergoing splenectomy for causes other than trauma. One explanation for this observed difference is that of 'splenosis', or the seeding of spleen cells from the traumatized spleen to produce multiple nodules of splenic tissue within the peritoneal cavity. This has been documented by reappearance of radiocolloid uptake following splenectomy for splenic trauma (Pearson et al., 1978), the loss of those features of blood morphology characteristic of the asplenic state, and normal levels of serum tuftsin (Orda et al., 1981).

Functional hyposplenia and splenic atrophy have been described following radiation therapy to the spleen for Hodgkin's disease (Coleman et al., 1982). This appears to be associated with an increased risk of developing overwhelming pneumococcal sepsis. Functional asplenia has also been reported in patients with immunoblastic lymphoma who had extensive splenic involvement and replacement (Gross et al., 1982).

Following splenectomy, there are increased opsonization requirements for the clearance of organisms from the circulation (Hosea et al., 1981). The bacterial organisms responsible for OPSI include principally the encapsulated organism Streptococcus pneumoniae, although Haemophilus influenzae, Neisseria meningitidis, Escherichia coli and Listeria monocytogenes (Jacobson et al., 1972) have also contributed to sepsis and meningitis in such patients. Schimpff et al. (1975) observed that infections with S. pneumoniae and H. influenzae were distinctly uncommon in splenectomized Hodgkin's disease patients during remission, whereas such infections were more commonly observed in patients undergoing radiation and/or intensive chemotherapy, especially when associated with severe granulocytopenia. Recent intensive treatment also appears to have been a factor in the 21% incidence of fulminant sepsis observed in the series reported by Weitzman and Aisenberg (1977). Weitzmann et al. (1977) also observed that prior splenectomy significantly

potentiated the decrease in IgM levels caused by intensive chemotherapy, which may predispose to postsplenectomy septicemia in patients with Hodgkin's disease. Neutrophil function has been shown to be impaired in Hodgkin's disease, with improvement following splenectomy (von Fliedner et al., 1980).

Schimpff et al. (1975) also commented on the more frequent occurrence of other infections in splenectomized patients in remission. They reported a 24% incidence of herpes zoster, which was also related to prior radiation and/or chemotherapy. Cormia and Campos (1973) relate a 9.4% rate of herpes zoster in splenectomized Hodgkin's disease patients, in contrast to a 1.6% rate observed in patients splenectomized for other conditions. Cytomegalovirus (CMV) has become more frequent because of transfusion-transmitted infection in immunosuppressed patients, especially in premature infants and transplant recipients (Yeager et al., 1981; Bove, 1986; Hersman et al., 1982; Menitove, 1987). Several authors have reported that presumptive seronegative patients transfused during or after splenectomy appear to have an increased risk of severe transfusion-associated CMV infection (Baumgartner et al., 1982; Drew and Miner, 1982).

Prophylaxis against OPSI is indicated in splenectomized children up to the age of 18 or for at least 5 years following the splenectomy (Mitchell and Morris, 1983; Baesl and Filler, 1985). For elective splenectomy, patients should be vaccinated with polyvalent pneumococcal vaccine (Pneumovax) at least 2 to 3 weeks prior to splenectomy. In children under 10 years of age, H. Influenzae type b vaccine is also advised at the same time (Baesl and Filler, 1985). If such immunization cannot be planned before surgery, it should be given as soon as possible postoperatively. No booster injections of pneumococcal vaccine are recommended at this time.

Antibiotic prophylaxis should consist of trimethoprim-sulfamethoxazole (Septra or Bactrim) 2.5 mg/kg body weight twice daily for children under the age of 10 (since H. influen-

zae is more common in this age group), while penicillin 250 mg twice daily is recommended for those 10 years of age and older (Horan and Colebatch, 1962). For patients allergic to sulfonamides or penicillin, amoxicillin may be substituted. In light of the present low rate of OPSI in adults (Schwartz *et al.*, 1982), antibiotic prophylaxis is not recommended for patients over the age of 18, although the administration of pneumococcal vaccine prior to splenectomy is advised. Prompt medical attention should be given to acute febrile illnesses in both children and adults with a history of prior splenectomy.

15.3.5 SECOND MALIGNANCIES

The greater than expected incidence of second malignancies, especially acute leukemia, in patients treated for Hodgkin's disease has been known for some time (Arsenau *et al.*, 1972; Raich *et al.*, 1975; Cadman, Capizzi and Bertino, 1977). Those patients treated with sequential radiation and intensive chemotherapy, including alkylating agents, were felt to be especially at risk.

There is now recent evidence that splenectomy may be associated with the subsequent appearance of acute non-lymphocytic leukemia in Hodgkin's disease patients who have received MOPP chemotherapy, consisting of mustine, vincristine, procarbazine, and prednisone (van Leeuwen, Somers and Hart, 1987; Rosenberg, 1988). The data from Stanford implies that this is an especially high risk in patients over the age of 40 years. It will be of interest to see if other chemotherapy combinations containing non-alkylating agents will show a lesser risk of leukemia, even in the face of splenectomy (Hoppe, Horning and Rosenberg, 1985).

15.4 THE TREATMENT OF SPLENIC INVOLVEMENT

15.4.1 SPLENECTOMY

'Splenectomy should be done when the patient does not need it. If one waits until the patient needs the operation he may not be able to tolerate it.' William H. Crosby (1972).

During the past 75 years splenectomy has become a relatively common procedure in the treatment of hypersplenism. This generalization includes the lymphoproliferative disorders which are often complicated by symptomatic splenomegaly. The first successful splenectomies employed in the treatment of MLPDs were reported by Giffin (1921). A number of more recent studies have confirmed the therapeutic value of splenectomy in this setting (Strumia, Strumia and Bassert, 1966; Christensen *et al.*, 1970; Crosby, 1972).

As defined by Dameshek and Estren (1947), hypersplenism is characterized by the tetralogy of peripheral blood cytopenias, bone marrow hyperplasia, splenomegaly, and correction of the cytopenias following splenectomy. In the MLPDs, blood cytopenias most often reflect the combined effects of splenic sequestration, splenic pooling, increased plasma volume, bone marrow infiltration and replacement, and possibly marrow suppression due to therapy. Correction of the hematological abnormalities following splenectomy is commonly observed in hypersplenism associated with malignant lymphomas and CLL. Morris, Cooper and Madigan (1975) and later Gill, Souter and Morris (1981), reported nearly identical results following splenectomy in such patients. Of the patients with Hodgkin's disease 53% obtained a hematological remission of the hypersplenism, as did 55% of non-Hodgkin's lymphoma patients (Mitchell and Morris, 1983). Approximately 50% of the patients were able to return to full chemotherapy dosages.

Clinically significant hypersplenism develops in 5–10% of patients with Hodgkin's disease (Crosby, 1972), and splenectomy may allow more effective therapy and a reduction of complications (Cooper *et al.*, 1974). The great majority of splenectomies performed in Hodgkin's disease patients are for the purpose of accurate surgical staging early in the course of the disease, as discussed in section 15.2.7(b).

In CLL, splenectomy has a limited role and is associated with a high operative mortality (Christensen et al., 1970). This is due to the fact that the standard approach to treatment of CLL usually consists of chemotherapy and possibly radiotherapy, and only late in the course of the disease, when the patient is refractory and presents with massive splenomegaly, is splenectomy considered. Yam and Crosby (1974) showed that early splenectomy for hypersplenism was well tolerated in patients with CLL, well-differentiated lymphomas and hairy cell leukemia, in contrast to the poor results observed in large cell lymphomas. In a series reported by Christensen, Hansen and Videbaek (1977), a group of CLL patients was splenectomized electively at a relatively early stage in the course of their disease, and compared with a non-splenectomized control group. Generally, splenectomy was performed for progressive splenomegaly and hypersplenism. The mean survival for the splenectomized group was 54 months, compared to 30 months for the control group. The median hemoglobin values rose from 100 g/l to 130 g/l within 3 months of operation, and platelet counts rose from a median of 90 000/mm^3 to 270 000/mm^3. The need for transfusion was considerably reduced, and hypermetabolic symptoms associated with hypersplenism were frequently improved. No cases of fulminant postsplenectomy septicemia were observed. Other investigators have also reported dramatic improvements in platelet counts in CLL patients with refractory thrombocytopenia (Merl et al., 1983).

Splenectomy has been beneficial in patients with prolymphocytic leukemia, where chemotherapy is frequently ineffective (Buskard et al., 1976). On the other hand, in patients presenting with non-tropical idiopathic splenomegaly (Dacie et al., 1969, 1978; Manoharan, Bader and Pitney, 1982; Rowbotham, Brearley and Collins, 1986), primary lymphosarcoma of the spleen (Skarin, Davey and Moloney, 1971), or as splenomegalic aleukemic CLL (Videbaek, Christensen and Jonsson, 1982), splenectomy may lead to the clinical expression of a CLL-like disorder, which at times follows an aggressive course.

Hairy cell leukemia (HCL) is now known to have a quite variable natural history. There is a subset of approximately 10% of patients who remain clinically stable without treatment for several years (Champlin et al., 1986). For those patients who present with an enlarged spleen and peripheral blood cytopenias, splenectomy remains the initial treatment of choice. The usual indications for such treatment include progressive cytopenias, massive splenomegaly, and recurrent infections. Although most patients with enlarged spleens will present more frequently with significant pancytopenia, it is not possible to predict, by spleen size, which patient will respond to splenectomy (Flandrin et al., 1984; Golomb, 1987). The degree of response tends to be greater in patients with massive splenomegaly (Mintz and Golomb, 1979). However, Golomb and Vardiman (1983) reported that patients with pancytopenia, but without a palpable spleen, may respond to splenectomy, whereas Jansen and Hermans (1981) found such treatment unsuccessful. It should be borne in mind that in patients with HCL, the spleen may be found to be enlarged to two to three times normal at surgery but has escaped detection by clinical examination (Golomb, 1987).

In most series a good hematological response is observed in more than 50% of HCL patients undergoing splenectomy (Bouroncle, Wiseman and Doan, 1958; Rubin et al., 1969; Schrek and Donnelly, 1966; Yam, Li and Finkel, 1972; Flandrin et al., 1973, 1984; Burke, Byrne and Rappaport, 1974; Catovsky et al., 1974; Naeim and Smith, 1974; Golde, 1982; Golomb, Ratain and Vardiman, 1986). In 28 splenectomized patients with HCL followed by Catovsky (1977), 61% achieved complete remission and 39% partial remission within 2 weeks of splenectomy. Complete remission was defined as a rise in hemoglobin above 110 g/l, neutrophils above 1000/mm^3 and platelets greater than 100 000/mm^3. In 85 splenectomized patients reported by Flandrin et al.

(1981) 61% achieved a complete remission of HCL, as defined by Catovsky (1977). In 170 patients reviewed by Golomb, Ratain and Vardiman (1986) the mean pre- and postsplenectomy values changed as follows, with hemoglobin rising from 104 to 115 g/l, granulocytes from 552 to 1754/mm^3, and platelets from 87 000 to 211 000/mm^3.

In the series reported by Catovsky (1977) and Flandrin et al. (1984) the survival for splenectomized patients was better than for non-splenectomized patients. Although both were non-randomized studies, a clear advantage is evident for the splenectomized patients. The median survival time was more than five times that of the non-splenectomized patients in Catovsky's series, while Flandrin et al. (1984) reported a median survival time of more than 200 months in splenectomized patients and 37 months in non-splenectomized patients. There was no significant difference in survival in those patients whose spleens were palpable at 4 cm or less below the costal margin: their survival rate was, in fact, similar to those with larger spleens who underwent splenectomy.

Golomb, Ratain and Vardiman (1986) reported that approximately one-third of their patients required further therapy after splenectomy with a median interval to additional treatment of 8.3 months. In the Catovsky (1977) series, relapse of pancytopenia occurred in all patients who achieved partial responses, and in one-half of those who showed a complete response. However, the median time to relapse was 16 months in the complete responders as compared to 2.5 months in the remaining patients.

Most reported cases of HCL with prolonged remissions and survival have been in splenectomized patients. Catovsky (1977) describes three long-term complete responders, continuing between 37 and 180 months following splenectomy, and Mycrs et al. (1981) describe a case continuing in complete remission 21 years after removal of the spleen. We have seen a similar survival in a patient with HCL, diagnosed initially as lymphosarcoma of the spleen, who remains in peripheral remission 22 years following splenectomy (Flink, 1988).

The precise mechanism by which excellent responses occur following splenectomy is not clear. The spleen is a preferred area of infiltration and growth for the neoplastic hairy cells. As discussed in section 15.3.1, hypersplenism is the major mechanism for the pancytopenia in these patients. In addition to improvement in absolute blood counts, improvement in platelet function has also been observed following splenectomy (Champlin et al., 1986). Rosove et al. (1980) describe degranulation of platelets circulating through the HCL spleen, leading to an acquired 'storage pool' functional defect.

Because of the strong susceptibility of the pancytopenic HCL patient to infections, including opportunistic infections such as those due to atypical mycobacteria, extreme care must be taken before and after surgery to investigate and treat all sources of infection.

Among the splenectomized patients reported by Catovsky (1977), one patient died of bronchopneumonia two and a half weeks following surgery, and six other patients died during the first six months, all from infections. Four of these patients had received chemotherapy just prior to the infections, and Catovsky warns that cytotoxic drugs are contraindicated in the pre- and immediately postoperative periods. The usefulness of protective measures, such as prophylactic antibiotics, remains to be evaluated in such patients.

15.4.2   RADIATION THERAPY

Although a splenic irradiation port is included in patients with Hodgkin's disease receiving total nodal radiation therapy, this is associated with radiation damage to the left kidney and the base of the left lung (Greenberger, Come and Weichselbaum, 1979; Le Bourgeois et al., 1979). Staging laparotomy with splenectomy removes the need to irradiate the spleen, and the increased effectiveness of combination chemotherapy programs in achieving prolonged complete remissions in patients with more advanced stages of Hodgkin's disease, has also decreased the need to add radiation treatment to the spleen.

In early stage Hodgkin's disease, patients with a supradiaphragmatic presentation may be considered for radiation to the upper abdomen in place of staging laparotomy and splenectomy. In a controlled clinical trial by the European Organisation for the Research and Treatment of Cancer (EORTC) reported by Tubiana *et al.* (1981) 300 patients with clinical stages I and II Hodgkin's disease were randomized to receive either splenic irradiation or splenectomy. All patients received mantle field irradiation as well as para-aortic lymph node irradiation. Both the survival rates and relapse-free survival rates were almost identical in the two groups. However, the authors state that the prognostic significance of the finding of splenic involvement is valuable in selecting patients who benefit from 'prophylactic' para-aortic node irradiation, even in those patients with otherwise good prognostic indicators, such as young age, absence of symptoms and favorable histology.

In the non-Hodgkin's lymphomas, radiation of the spleen may be included as part of abdominal radiation fields, or as part of total abdominal irradiation (Goffinet *et al.*, 1976). Radiation to an enlarged spleen may also be beneficial later in the course of the disease to relieve pain not responding to chemotherapy, or for hypersplenism in patients who are not candidates for surgery or chemotherapy (Newell, 1963; Comas, Andrews and Nelson, 1968). Transient decreases in blood counts may be encountered during and following such radiation.

Patients with Hodgkin's disease and NHL who have undergone radiation therapy including the spleen have experienced atrophy and functional hyposplenism, occasionally leading to fatal pneumococcal sepsis (Dailey, Coleman and Kaplan, 1980). When irradiated spleens obtained at autopsy from patients with Hodgkin's disease and other lymphomas are compared to non-irradiated spleens, major differences are observed (Dailey, Coleman and Fajardo, 1981). After an interval of 1 to 8 years, and following an average radiation dose of 3900 cGy, most of the irradiated spleens were found to be small, with an average weight of 75 g, with a thickened capsule and diffuse fibrosis of the red pulp. Intimal thickening of the arteries, and at times the veins, was also observed. It is of interest that in one study ^{99m}Tc-sulfur colloid scans did not reveal splenic atrophy or decrease in reticuloendothelial function following radiation (Spencer and Knowlton, 1975).

Splenic irradiation in CLL dates back to the early therapeutic use of radiation (Senn, 1903). More extensive lymphoid irradiation, including total body irradiation (Del Regato, 1974), has been explored during the past quarter century. These techniques do not appear to be consistently superior to chemotherapy, and are often associated with excessive marrow suppression. In a review of the role of radiotherapy in CLL by Paule, Cosset and Le Bourgeois (1985), only fractional low-dose splenic irradiation was found to lead to a long-lasting decrease in the lymphocyte count, and improvement in anemia and thrombocytopenia. Most patients treated show relief of painful splenomegaly as well as improvement in blood counts (Parmentier *et al.*, 1974; Byhardt, Brace and Wiernik, 1975; Singh, Bates and Wetherley-Mein, 1986). These studies have shown a reduction of lymphocytic bone marrow infiltration by 20–50% with total doses of 600–800 cGy to the spleen.

Splenic irradiation in CLL leads to the destruction of a large portion of the malignant B-cell clone with low doses, and potentially the somewhat more resistant subset of T-suppressor cells present in the spleen is affected by higher doses of radiation (Paule, Cosset and Le Bourgeois, 1985). T-suppressor cells have been shown to contribute to bone marrow stem cell inhibition, resulting in anemia and thrombocytopenia in some patients with CLL (Mangan, Chikkappa and Farley, 1982; Nagasawa, Abe and Nakagawa, 1981). Normalization of helper/suppressor T-cell ratios have been observed following splenic irradiation (McCann *et al.*, 1982; Paule and Cossett, 1984). An additional mechanism for improvement of anemia in these patients is suggested by Awwad *et al.* (1967), who showed decreased red cell destruction and increased red cell survival after splenic irradiation.

Splenic irradiation in patients with CLL is generally well tolerated with little hematological toxicity. A transient decrease in neutrophils and platelets occurs, but is seldom severe (Singh, Bates and Wetherley-Mein, 1986). Occasionally hyperkalemia (Kurlander, Stein and Roth, 1975) and a transient increase in liver size have been described following splenic irradiation. Apart from these occasional problems, splenic irradiation is a useful mode of treatment in CLL, especially in patients refractory to chemotherapy, and a safer alternative than total body irradiation. Prolymphocytic leukemia appears more resistant to splenic radiation: only one of three patients reported by Singh, Bates and Wetherley-Mein (1986) responded.

Several reports have demonstrated complete and partial remissions of HCL with splenic irradiation (Bouroncle, 1979; Sharp and Mac-Walter, 1983; Jansen and Hermans, 1981; Gosselin, Hanlon and Pease, 1956; Schrek and Donelly, 1966; Plenderleith, 1970). Yam, Li and Finkel (1972), however, found splenic irradiation ineffective. In those patients with HCL where splenectomy is inadvisable, or is refused, and other modalities such as interferon or pentostatin are not available, splenic irradiation should be considered as a valid alternative treatment.

15.4.3 CHEMOTHERAPY

In patients with Hodgkin's and non-Hodgkin's lymphomas, combination chemotherapy has been quite effective in advanced stages, including those with splenic involvement. Long-term disease-free remissions are common. Splenic involvement and enlargement may be associated with lower blood counts and a decreased ability to tolerate full chemotherapy doses. Splenectomy has been proposed as a means for improving tolerance to chemotherapy in such patients.

When progressive disease occurs in HCL following splenectomy, this usually expresses itself by a worsening of pancytopenia due to bone marrow replacement by the hairy cells, or by a leukemic manifestation with increasing peripheral blood hairy cells. In these patients a variety of chemotherapy programs have been tried, ranging from single agents such as chlorambucil (Golomb, Schmidt and Vardiman, 1984), and rubidazone (Stewart *et al.*, 1979), to intensive combination programs (Calvo *et al.*, 1985; Joosten *et al.*, 1985). The latter were often associated with severe toxicity.

A much more promising agent for the treatment of HCL was reported by Spiers, Parekh and Bishop (1984); pentostatin (2-deoxycoformycin) acts as an inhibitor of adenosine deaminase, an enzyme of purine metabolism. Since then a number of additional reports have attested to the effectiveness of pentostatin (Spiers *et al.*, 1985; Johnston *et al.*, 1986; Kraut, Bouroncle and Grever, 1986). Prolonged, unmaintained remissions were achieved in 50–90% of patients, including regression of splenomegaly, clearing of bone marrow infiltration, and normalization of blood counts. Studies are presently under way by several cooperative groups to evaluate the relative effectiveness of pentostatin and alpha-interferon in both previously splenectomized and non-splenectomized patients with HCL.

15.4.4 BIOLOGICAL RESPONSE MODIFIERS

'New medicines, and new methods of cure, always work miracles for a while.' William Heberden.

The effective use of alpha-interferon (α-IFN) in HCL was first reported by Quesada *et al.* (1984), and additional reports since that time have established that HCL thus far is the malignancy most responsive to α-IFN (Foon *et al.*, 1984, 1986a; Ratain *et al.*, 1985; Thompson *et al.*, 1985, Jacobs, Champlin and Golde, 1985; Golomb *et al.*, 1986; Golomb, Ratain and Vardiman, 1986; Ehman and Silber, 1986). Durable objective responses, mostly partial, are seen in 75% of patients, and improvement in blood count is achieved in 90% (Thompson and Fefer, 1987; Spiegel, 1987; Fahey *et al.*, 1987; Golomb, 1987). Responses are obtained in both previously splenectomized and non-splenectomized patients (Ehman and Silber, 1986). Although in most cases hairy cells clear dramatically from the bone marrow, complete disappearance from the marrow has not been documented (Bardawil *et al.*, 1986). Because of a tendency to relapse once the α-IFN is stopped, long-term continuous or intermittent maintenance therapy may be required (Ratain *et al.*, 1987).

When α-IFN is not effective in patients with HCL, pentostatin has been tried in several cases. Foon *et al.* (1986b) reported two patients who were refractory to α-IFN but responded well to pentostatin, with a decrease in spleen size and improvement of pancytopenia. Golomb (1987) reports a patient who progressed on α-IFN and gamma-IFN, but achieved clearing of marrow hairy cells and normalization of peripheral blood counts with pentostatin.

Patients with non-Hodgkin's lymphomas, who have failed prior chemotherapy, have shown responses to α-IFN, especially in the low-grade lymphomas and the cutaneous T-cell lymphomas, where response rates of 40–50% have been reported (Louie *et al.*, 1981; Foon *et al.*, 1984; Leavitt *et al.*, 1984; Bunn *et al.*, 1984; Wagstaff and Crowther, 1984; Roth and Foon, 1986; O'Connell *et al.*, 1986; Foon, Roth and Bunn, 1986, 1987; Ochs *et al.*, 1986). In intermediate and high-grade lymphomas, α-IFN has shown less activity. The use of α-IFN in combination with conventional chemotherapy during induction, and as a single agent in maintenance therapy, is presently being explored (Hawkins *et al.*, 1985).

Patients with multiple myeloma have shown moderate response rates with α-IFN, usually in the 15–25% range (Costanzi, Cooper and Scarffe, 1985; Costanzi *et al.*, 1985; Quesada *et al.*, 1986; Cooper *et al.*, 1986; Cooper and Welander, 1987). Its activity in CLL has been disappointing (Foon, Roth and Bunn, 1986; O'Connell *et al.*, 1986). Some responses have been observed in childhood ALL (Ochs *et al.*, 1986).

At this time there is evidence that monoclonal antibodies when used alone have some limited therapeutic effect in patients with lymphomas and CLL. CLL patients treated with murine-derived monoclonal antibodies showed only a transient decrease in circulating leukemia cells (Foon *et al.*, 1983; Dillman *et al.*, 1984). Patients with cutaneous T-cell lymphoma did at times show transient reduction in size of lymph nodes and skin lesions (Foon *et al.*, 1983; Dillman *et al.*, 1984; Miller *et al.*, 1983). Anti-idiotype monoclonal antibodies have been evaluated primarily in the non-Hodgkin's lymphomas (Nadler *et al.*, 1980; Hatsubai, Maloney and Levy, 1981; Miller *et al.*, 1982; Meeker *et al.*, 1985; Giardina *et al.*, 1985). Only one patient has been reported to have had a complete and durable remission with this therapy. In order to overcome the difficulties encountered when monoclonal antibodies are used by themselves, current research is evaluating the linking of antibodies to cytotoxic drugs, toxins and radionuclides.

15.5   CONCLUSION

The spleen has been implicated in diseases afflicting mankind for the duration of recorded medical history. Since it represents the largest concentration of lymphocytes in the body and is continuously perfused by blood, it is not surprising that the spleen is involved in many diseases initiated by the immune system, and in the majority of malignancies involving the immune system. Although the spleen is seldom the only organ involved in such disorders, they do afford us a window to observe the disease mechanisms operative in the spleen.

The onset and extension of splenic involvement by the malignant lymphoproliferative disorders is determined by cell kinetics and circulation patterns, cell surface markers and stromal cell receptors, as well as local factors within the spleen. For many disorders we are now beginning to learn the reasons for the degree and timing of splenic involvement.

In addition to exploring these specific pathogenic factors, we have made extensive use of a wealth of clinical observations regarding the role of the spleen in these disorders. Staging laparotomy and splenectomy, for example, have added much information about the natural history of Hodgkin's disease, and have allowed for the development of more rational and effective treatment. Splenectomy remains one of the most effective treatments for hairy cell leukemia, although in other disorders, altered or absent splenic function is associated with immediate and long-term problems, which may need clinical attention in depth.

In continuing to provide us with new knowledge concerning the malignant lymphoproliferative disorders, the spleen deserves our continued interest and enquiry.

ACKNOWLEDGEMENTS

This work was supported by an American Cancer Society Professorship of Clinical Oncology awarded to the author.

REFERENCES

Ahmann, D. L., Kiely, J. M. and Harrison, E. G., Jr (1966) Malignant lymphoma of the spleen. A review of 49 cases in which the diagnosis was made at splenectomy. *Cancer*, **19**, 461–9.

Aisenberg, A. C. (1962) Studies on delayed hypersensitivity in Hodgkin's disease. *J. Clin. Invest.*, **41**, 1964–70.

Aisenberg, A. C. (1978) The staging and treatment of Hodgkin's disease. *N. Engl. J. Med.*, **299**, 1228–32.

Aisenberg, A. C. and Qazi, R. (1974) Abdominal involvement at the onset of Hodgkin's disease. *Am. J. Med.*, **57**, 870–4.

Alcorn, F. S. *et al.* (1977) Contributions of computed tomography in the staging and management of malignant lymphomas. *Radiology*, **125**, 717–23.

Anderson, T. *et al.* (1976) Peritoneoscopy: a useful tool in restaging lymphoma patients. *Proc. AACR and ASCO*, **17**, 268.

Arseneau, J. C. *et al.* (1972) Non-lymphomatous malignant tumors complicating Hodgkin's disease. *N. Engl. J. Med.*, **42**, 1119.

Askergren, J. *et al.*, (1981) On the size and tumour involvement of the spleen in Hodgkin's disease. *Acta Med. Scand.*, **209**, 217–20.

Aster, R. H. (1966) Pooling of platelets in the spleen: role in the pathogenesis of 'hypersplenic' thrombocytopenia. *J. Clin. Invest.*, **45**, 645–57.

Aster, R. H. and Jandl, J. H. (1964) Platelet sequestration in man. II. Immunological and clinical studies. *J. Clin. Invest.*, **43**, 856–69.

Ault, K. A. (1979) Detection of small numbers of monoclonal B lymphocytes in the blood of patients with lymphoma. *N. Engl. J. Med.*, **300**, 1401–5.

Awwad, H. *et al.* (1967) The effect of splenic X-irradiation on the ferrokinetics of chronic leukemia with a clinical study. *Blood*, **29**, 242–56.

Baesl, T. J. and Filler, R. M. (1985) Surgical diseases of the spleen. Symposium on pediatric surgery, Part I. *Surg. Clin. N. Am.*, **65**, 1260–86.

Bagley, C. M., Jr *et al.* (1973) Diagnosis of liver involvement by lymphoma: results in 96 consecutive peritoneoscopies. *Cancer*, **31**, 840-7.

Bardawil, R. G. *et al.* (1986) Changes in peripheral blood and bone marrow specimens following therapy with recombinant alpha-2-interferon for hairy cell leukemia. *Am. J. Clin. Pathol.*, **85**, 194-201.

Baroni, C. D. *et al.* (1982) Tissue T-lymphocytes in untreated Hodgkin's disease. Morphologic and functional correlations in spleens and lymph nodes. *Cancer*, **50**, 259–68.

Bauer, T. W., Haskins, G. E. and Armitage, J. O. (1981) Splenic rupture in patients with hematologic malignancies. *Cancer*, **48**, 2729–33.

Baumgartner, J. D. *et al.* (1982) Severe cytomegalovirus infection in multiply-transfused, splenectomised trauma patients. *Lancet*, i, 63–5.

Bazerbashi, M. B., Reeve, J. and Chanarin, I. (1978) Studies in chronic lymphocytic leukaemia. The kinetics of Cr-labelled lymphocytes. *Scand. J. Haematol.*, **20**, 37–51.

Bean, M. A. *et al.* (1977) Occurrence of restricted suppressor T-cell activity in man. *J. Exp. Med.*, **146**, 1455–60.

Beretta, G. *et al.* (1976) Sequential laparoscopy and laparotomy combined with bone marrow biopsy in staging Hodgkin's disease. *Cancer Treat. Rep.*, 60, 1231–7.

Bieber, C. P. and Bieber, M. M. (1973) Detection of ferritin as a circulating tumor associated antigen in Hodgkin's disease. *Nat. Cancer Inst. Monogr.*, 36, 147–53.

Bieber, M. M., Fuks, Z. and Kaplan, H. S. (1977) E-rosette inhibiting substance in Hodgkin's disease spleen extracts. *Clin. Exp. Immunol.*, 29, 369–75.

Binet, J. L. *et al.* (1981) A new prognostic classification of chronic lymphocytic leukemia derived from multivariate survival analysis. *Cancer*, 48, 198–206.

Birch, S. J., Garvie, N. W. and Ackery, D. M. (1980) Splenic accumulation of technetium 99m methyldiphosphonate in non-Hodgkin's lymphoma. *Br. J. Radiol.*, 53, 161–3.

Bjoerkholm, M., Askergren, J. and Holm, G. (1980) Long-term influence of splenectomy on immune functions in patients with Hodgkin's disease. *Scand. J. Haematol.*, 24, 87–94.

Bjoerkholm, M., Askergren, J. and Wedelin, C. (1980) Blood lymphocyte functions in relation to splenic weight and tumor involvement in untreated Hodgkin's disease. *Scand. J. Haematol.*, 25, 51–7.

Bjoerkholm, J., Wedelin, C. and Holm G. (1982) Lymphocytotoxic serum factors and lymphocyte functions in untreated Hodgkin's disease. *Cancer*, 50, 2044–8.

Bjoerkholm, M. *et al.* (1983) Lymphocyte counts and functions in arterial and venous splenic blood of patients with Hodgkin's disease. *Clin. Exp. Immunol.*, 52, 485–92.

Blayney, D. W. *et al.* (1983a) The human T-cell leukemia/lymphoma virus associated with American adult T-cell leukemia/lymphoma. *Blood*, 62, 401–5.

Blayney, D. W. *et al.* (1983b) The human T-cell leukemia/lymphoma virus, lymphoma, lytic bone lesions, and hypercalcemia. *Ann. Intern. Med.*, 98, 144–51.

Boles, E. T. Jr, Haase, G. M. and Hamoudi, A. B. (1978) Partial splenectomy in staging laparotomy for Hodgkin's disease: an alternative approach. *J. Pediatr. Surg.*, 13, 581–6.

Borowitz, M. J., Croker, B. P. and Metzgar, R. S. (1982) Immunohistochemical analysis of the distribution of lymphocyte subpopulations in Hodgkin's disease. *Cancer Treat. Rep.*, 66, 667–74.

Bouroncle, B. A. (1966) Sternberg-Reed cells in the peripheral blood of patients with Hodgkin's disease. *Blood*, 27, 544–56.

Bouroncle, B. A. (1979) Leukemic reticuloendotheliosis (hairy cell leukemia). *Blood*, 53, 412–36.

Bouroncle, B. A., Wiseman, B. K. and Doan, C. A. (1958) Leukemic reticuloendotheliosis. *Blood*, 13, 609–30.

Bove, J. R. (1986) Transfusion-transmitted diseases: current problems and challenges. *Progr. Hematol.*, 14, 123–47.

Bowdler, A. J. (1967) Dilution anaemia associated with enlargement of the spleen. *Proc. R. Soc. Med.*, 60, 44–7.

Bowdler, A. J. (1970) Blood volume studies in patients with splenomegaly. *Transfusion*, 10, 171–81.

Bowdler, A. J. and Glick, I. W. (1966) Autoimmune hemolytic anemia as the herald state of Hodgkin's disease. *Ann. Intern. Med.*, 65, 761–7.

Braylan, R., Variakojis, D. and Yachnin, S. (1975) The Sezary syndrome lymphoid cell: abnormal surface properties and mitogen responsiveness. *Br. J. Haematol.*, 31, 553–64.

Breiman, R. S. *et al.* (1978) CT-pathologic correlations in Hodgkin's disease and non-Hodgkin's lymphoma. *Radiology*, 126, 159–66.

Breitfeld, V. and Lee, R. E. (1975) Pathology of the spleen in hematologic disease. *Surg. Clin. North Am.*, 55, 233–51.

Britten, K. J. M. *et al.* (1986) The distribution of iron and iron binding proteins in spleen with reference to Hodgkin's disease. *Br. J. Cancer*, 54, 277–86.

Broder, S., Uchiyama, T. and Waldmann, T. A. (1979) Current concepts in immunoregulatory T-cell neoplasms. *Cancer Treat. Rep.*, 63, 607–12.

Broder, S. *et al.* (1976) The Sezary syndrome: A malignant proliferation of helper T-cells. *J. Clin. Invest.*, 58, 1297–306.

Broder, S. *et al.* (1984) T-cell lymphoproliferative syndrome associated with human T-cell leukemia/lymphoma virus. *Ann. Intern. Med.*, 100, 543–57.

Brouet, J. C., Flandrin, G. and Seligmann, M. (1973) Indications of the thymus-derived nature of the proliferating cells in six patients with Sezary's syndrome. *N. Engl. J. Med.*, 289, 341–4.

Brouet, J. C. *et al.* (1975) Chronic lymphocytic leukaemia of T-cell origin. Immunological and clinical evaluation in eleven patients. *Lancet*, ii, 890–3.

Bunn, P. A. and Lamberg, S. I. (1979) Report of the Committee on Staging and Classification of Cutaneous T-cell Lymphomas. *Cancer Treat. Rep.*, 63, 725–36.

Bunn, P. A., Jr *et al.* (1980) Prospective staging evaluation of patients with cutaneous T-cell lymphomas. *Ann. Intern. Med.*, 93, 223–30.

Bunn, P. A., Jr *et al.* (1983) Clinical course of

retrovirus-associated adult T-cell lymphoma in the United States. *N. Engl. J. Med.*, **309**, 257–64.

Bunn, P. A., Jr *et al.* (1984) Recombinant leukocyte A interferon: an active agent in advanced cutaneous T-cell lymphomas. *Ann. Intern. Med.*, **101**, 484–7.

Burke, J. S. (1981) Surgical pathology of the spleen: an approach to the differential diagnosis of splenic lymphomas and leukemias. Diseases of the white pulp. Diseases of the red pulp. *Am. J. Surg. Pathol.*, **5**, 681–94.

Burke, J. S., Byrne, G. E., Jr and Rappaport, H. (1974) Hairy cell leukemia (leukemic reticuloendotheliosis). A clinical pathologic study of 21 patients. *Cancer*, **33**, 1399–410.

Burke, J. S., Mackay, B. and Rappaport, H. (1976) Hairy cell leukemia (leukemic reticuloendotheliosis). Ultrastructure of the spleen. *Cancer*, **37**, 2267–74.

Burke, J. S. and Rappaport, H. (1984) The diagnosis and differential diagnosis of hairy cell leukemia in bone marrow and spleen. *Semin. Oncol.*, **11**, 334–46.

Burke, J. S. *et al.* (1987) Recognition of hairy cell leukemia in a spleen of normal weight. *J. Clin. Pathol.*, **87**, 276–81.

Burkitt, D. and O'Connor, G. T. (1961) Malignant lymphoma in African children. I. A clinical syndrome. *Cancer*, **14**, 258–69.

Buskard, N. A. *et al.* (1976) Prolymphocytic leukemia. *Hämatol. Bluttransfus.*, **18**, 237–53.

Butler, J. J. (1983) Pathology of the spleen in benign and malignant conditions. *Histopathology*, **7**, 453–74.

Byhardt, R. W., Brace, K. C. and Wiernik, P. H. (1975) The role of splenic irradiation in chronic lymphocytic leukemia. *Cancer*, **35**, 1621–5.

Cadman, E. C., Capizzi, R. L. and Bertino, J. R. (1977) Acute non-lymphocytic leukemia. A delayed complication of Hodgkin's disease therapy: analysis of 109 cases. *Cancer*, **40**, 1280–96.

Calvo, F. *et al.* (1985) Intensive chemotherapy of hairy cell leukemia in patients with aggressive disease. *Blood*, **65**, 115–19.

Carde, P. *et al.* (1988) Hodgkin's disease (HD) and immunoscintigraphy (IS): use of anti-Reed-Sternberg cells H-RS-1 monoclonal antibody (Mab) in 9 patients (pts). *Proc. ASCO*, **7**, 227.

Carlstedt, A. and Tholin, B. (1984) Infectious complications after splenectomy. *Acta Chir. Scand.*, **150**, 607–10.

Casazza, A. R., Duvall, C. P. and Carbone, P. P. (1966) Summary of infectious complications occurring in patients with Hodgkin's disease. *Cancer Res.*, **26**, 1290–6.

Castellino, R. A. *et al.* (1984) Computed tomography, lymphography, and staging laparotomy: correlations in initial staging of Hodgkin's disease. *Am. J. Roentgen.*, **143**, 37–41.

Castro-Malaspina, H., Najean, Y. and Flandrin, G. (1979) Erythrokinetic studies in hairy-cell leukaemia. *Br. J. Haematol.*, **42**, 189–97.

Catovsky, D. (1977) Hairy-cell leukaemia and prolymphocytic leukaemia. *Clin. Haematol.*, **6**, 245–68.

Catovsky, D. *et al.* (1974) Leukaemic reticuloendotheliosis ('hairy' cell leukaemia), a distinct clinico-pathological entity. *Br. J. Haematol.*, **26**, 9–27.

Catovsky, D. *et al.* (1982) Adult T-cell lymphoma-leukaemia in blacks from the West Indies. *Lancet*, **i**, 639–42.

Cawley, J. C., Burns, G. F. and Hayhoe, F. G. J. (1980) *Hairy Cell Leukaemia*, Springer-Verlag, Berlin.

Champlin, R. *et al.* (1986) Chronic leukemias: oncogenes, chromosomes, and advances in therapy. *Ann. Intern. Med.*, **104**, 671–88.

Chang, T., Stutzman, L. and Sokal, J. E. (1975) Correlation of delayed hypersensitivity responses with chemotherapeutic results in advanced Hodgkin's disease. *Cancer*, **36**, 950–5.

Chilcote, R. R. *et al.* (1976) Septicemia and meningitis in children splenectomized for Hodgkin's disease. Investigators and special studies committee of the Childrens Cancer Study Group. *N. Engl. J. Med.*, **295**, 798–800.

Christensen, B. E. (1973a) Erythrocyte pooling and sequestration in enlarged spleens. Estimations of splenic erythrocyte and plasma volume in splenomegalic patients. *Scand. J. Haematol.*, **10**, 106–19.

Christensen, B. E. (1973b) The pattern of erythrocyte sequestration in immunohaemolysis. Effects of prednisone treatment and splenectomy. *Scand. J. Haematol.*, **10**, 120–9.

Christensen, B. E., Hansen, M. M. and Videbaek, A. A. (1977) Splenectomy in chronic lymphocytic leukaemia. *Scand. J. Haematol.*, **18**, 279-87.

Christensen, B. E. *et al.* (1970) Splenectomy in haematology. Indications, results and complications in 41 cases. *Scand. J. Haematol.*, **7**, 247–60.

Christensen, B. E. *et al.* (1978) Traffic of T and B lymphocytes in the normal spleen. *Scand. J. Haematol.*, **20**, 246–57.

Coleman, C. N. *et al.* (1982) Functional hyposplenia after splenic irradiation for Hodgkin's disease. *Ann. Intern. Med.*, **96**, 44–7.

Comas, F. V., Andrews, G. A. and Nelson, B. (1968) Spleen irradiation in secondary hypersplenism.

Am. J. Roentgenol. Rad. Ther. Nucl. Med., **104**, 668–73.

Come, S. E. and Chabner, B. A. (1979) Staging in non-Hodgkin's lymphoma: approach, results and relationship to histopathology. *Clin. Haematol.*, **8**, 645–56.

Come, S. E. *et al.* (1980) Non-Hodgkin's lymphomas in leukemic phase: Clinicopathologic correlations. *Am. J. Med.*, **69**, 667–74.

Connors, J. M. *et al.* (1987) Brief chemotherapy and involved field radiation therapy for limited-stage, histologically aggressive lymphoma. *Ann. Intern. Med.*, **107**, 25–30.

Cooper, I. A. *et al.* (1974) The role of splenectomy in the management of advanced Hodgkin's disease. *Cancer*, **34**, 408–17.

Cooper, M. R. *et al.* (1986) Alpha-2 interferon, melphalan and prednisone in previously untreated patients with multiple myeloma: a phase I-II trial. *Cancer Treat. Rep.*, **70**, 473–6.

Cooper, M. R. and Welander, C. E. (1987) Interferons in the treatment of multiple myeloma. *Cancer*, Suppl. 1, **59**, 594–600.

Cormia, F. E., Jr and Campos, L. T. (1973) Infections after splenectomy. Letter to the editor. *Ann. Intern. Med.*, **78**, 149–50.

Costanzi, J., Cooper, M. R. and Scarffe, J. H. (1985) Interferon Alpha-2: use in patients with resistant and relapsing multiple myeloma. A phase II study. *Dev. Oncol.*, **27**, 75–85.

Costanzi, J. J. *et al.* (1985) Phase II study of recombinant alpha-2 interferon in resistant multiple myeloma. *J. Clin. Oncol.*, **3**, 654–9.

Crosby, W. H. (1972) Splenectomy in hematologic disorders. *N. Engl. J. Med.*, **286**, 1252–4.

Crossen, P. E. *et al.* (1971) The Sezary syndrome. *Am. J. Med.*, **50**, 24–34.

Crowther, D. and Wagstaff, J. (1983) Lymphocyte migration in malignant disease. *Clin. Exp. Immunol.*, **51**, 413–20.

Dacie, J. V. *et al.* (1969) Non-tropical idiopathic splenomegaly (primary hypersplenism): a review of ten cases and their relationship to malignant lymphomas. *Br. J. Haematol.*, **17**, 317–33.

Dacie, J. V. *et al.* (1978) Non-tropical 'idiopathic splenomegaly': a follow-up study of ten patients described in 1969. *Br. J. Haematol.*, **38**, 185–93.

Dailey, M. O., Coleman, C. N. and Fajardo, L. F. (1981) Splenic injury caused by therapeutic irradiation. *Am. J. Surg. Pathol.*, **5**, 325–31.

Dailey, M. O., Coleman, C. N. and Kaplan, H. S. (1980) Radiation-induced splenic atrophy in patients with Hodgkin's disease and non-Hodgkin's lymphomas. *N. Engl. J. Med.*, **302**, 215–17.

Dameshek, W. S. and Estren, S. (1947) *The Spleen and Hypersplenism*. Grune and Stratton, New York.

Dameshek, W. and Gunz, I. (1964) *Leukemia*, 2nd edn. Grune and Stratton, New York and London.

Das Gapta, F., Coombes, B. and Brasfield, R. D. (1965) Primary malignant neoplasm of the spleen. *Surg. Gynecol. Obstet.*, **120**, 947–60.

Dearth, J. C. *et al.* (1978) Partial splenectomy for staging Hodgkin's disease: risk of false-negative results. *N. Engl. J. Med.*, **299**, 345–6.

Del Regato, J. A. (1974) Total body irradiation in the treatment of chronic lymphogenous leukemia. *Am. J. Roentgenol. Rad. Ther. Nucl. Med.*, **120**, 504–20.

DeSousa, M. *et al.* (1977) Exotaxis: the principle and its application to the study of Hodgkin's disease. *Clin. Exp. Immunol.*, **27**, 143–51.

Desser, R. K. and Ultmann, J. E. (1972) Risk of severe infection in patients with Hodgkin's disease or lymphoma after diagnostic laparotomy and splenectomy. Editorial. *Ann. Intern. Med.*, **77**, 143–6.

Desser, R. K., Moran, E. M. and Ultmann, J. E. (1973) Staging of Hodgkin's disease and lymphoma. *Med. Clin. North Am.*, **57**, 479–98.

DeVita, V. T., Jr *et al.* (1971) Peritoneoscopy in the staging of Hodgkin's disease. *Cancer Res.*, **31**, 1746–50.

DeVita, V. T., Jr *et al.* (1973) Diagnosis of liver involvement by lymphoma: results in 96 consecutive peritoneoscopies. *Cancer*, **31**, 840–7.

Dickerman, J. D. (1979) Splenectomy and sepsis: a warning. *Pediatrics*, **63**, 938–41.

Dickerman, J. D. and Clements, J. P. (1975) Abnormal spleen scan following MOPP therapy in a patient with Hodgkin's disease: case report. *J. Nucl. Med.*, **16**, 457–8.

Dighiero, G. *et al.* (1979) Identification of a pure splenic form of chronic lymphocytic leukaemia. *Br. J. Haematol.*, **41**, 169–76.

Dillman, R. O. *et al.* (1984) Therapy of chronic lymphocytic leukemia and cutaneous T-cell lymphoma with T101 monoclonal antibody. *J. Clin. Oncol.*, **2**, 881–91.

Donaldson, S. S. *et al.* (1972) Characterization of postsplenectomy bacteremia among patients with and without lymphoma. *N. Engl. J. Med.*, **287**, 69–71.

Dorreen, M. S., Habeshaw, J. A. and Wrigley, P. F. M. (1982) Distribution of T-lymphocyte subsets in Hodgkin's disease characterised by monoclonal antibodies. *Br. J. Cancer*, **45**, 491–9.

Drew, W. L. and Miner, R. C. (1982) Transfusion-related cytomegalovirus infection following non-cardiac surgery. *J. Am. Med. Assoc.*, **247**, 2389–91.

Earl, H. M. *et al.* (1980) Computerized tomographic (CT) abdominal scanning in Hodgkin's disease. *Clin. Radiol.*, **31**, 149–53.

Edelson, R. L. *et al.* (1974) Preferential cutaneous infiltration by neoplastic thymus-derived lymphocytes. *Ann. Intern. Med.*, **80**, 685–92.

Ehman, W. C. and Silber, R. (1986) Recombinant alpha-2 interferon treatment of hairy cell leukemia without prior splenectomy. *Am. J. Med.*, **80**, 1111–14.

Elkon, K. B. *et al.* (1979) Hairy-cell leukaemia with polyarteritis nodosa. *Lancet*, **ii**, 280–2.

Ell, P. J. *et al.* (1975) An assessment of the value of spleen scanning in the staging of Hodgkin's disease. *Br. J. Radiol.*, **48**, 590–3.

Enright, L. P., Trueblood, H. W. and Nelsen, T. S. (1970) The surgical diagnosis of abdominal Hodgkin's disease. *Surg. Gynecol. Obstet.*, **130**, 853–8.

Essex, M. E. *et al.* (1984) Seroepidemiology of human T-cell leukemia virus in relation to immunosuppression and the acquired immunodeficiency syndrome. in *Human T-cell Leukemia/Lymphoma Virus* (eds R. C. Gallo and D. J. Gross), Cold Spring Harbor Laboratory, New York.

Faguet, G. B. (1975) Quantitation of immunocompetence in Hodgkin's disease. *J. Clin. Invest.*, **56**, 951–7.

Faguet, G. B. (1979) Mechanisms of lymphocyte activation. The role of suppressor cells in the proliferative responses of chronic lymphatic leukemia lymphocytes. *J. Clin. Invest.*, **63**, 67–74.

Fahey, J. L. *et al.* (1987) Immune interventions in disease. *Ann. Intern. Med.*, **106**, 257–74.

Farrer-Brown, G. *et al.* (1972) The diagnosis of Hodgkin's disease in surgically excised spleens. *J. Clin. Pathol.*, **25**, 294–300.

Fieschi, A. and Sacchetti, C. (1964) Clinical assessment of granulopoiesis. *Acta Haematol.*, **31**, 150–62.

Flandrin, G. *et al.* (1973) Leucemie à 'tricholeucocyte' (hairy cell leukemia). Etude clinique et cytologique de 55 observations. *Nouv. Rev. Fr. Hematol.*, **13**, 609–40.

Flandrin, G. *et al.* (1984) Hairy cell leukemia: clinical presentation and follow-up of 211 patients. *Semin. Oncol.*, **11**, 458–71.

Flink, E. (1988) Personal communication.

Foon, K. A., Roth, M. S. and Bunn, P. A., Jr (1986) Alpha interferon treatment of low-grade B-cell non-Hodgkin's lymphomas, cutaneous T-cell lymphomas, and chronic lymphocytic leukemia. *Semin. Oncol.*, Suppl. 2, **13**, 35–42.

Foon, K. A., Roth, M. S. and Bunn, P. A. (1987) Interferon therapy of non-Hodgkin's lymphoma. *Cancer*, Suppl. 1, **59**, 601–4.

Foon, K. A. *et al.* (1983) Monoclonal antibody therapy of chronic lymphocytic leukemia and T cell lymphoma: preliminary observations. in *Monoclonal Antibodies and Cancer*, Academic Press, Orlando, pp. 39–52.

Foon, K. A. *et al.* (1984) Treatment of advanced non-Hodgkin's lymphoma with recombinant leukocyte A interferon. *N. Engl. J. Med.*, **311**, 1148–52.

Foon, K. A. *et al.* (1986a) Recombinant leukocyte A interferon therapy for advanced hairy cell leukemia: therapeutic and immunologic results. *Am. J. Med.*, **80**, 351–6.

Foon, K. A. *et al.* (1986b) Response to 2-deoxycoformycin after failure of interferon-alpha in non-splenectomized patients with hairy cell leukemia. *Blood*, **68**, 297–300.

Francke, E. L. and Neu, H. C. (1981) Postsplenectomy infection. *Surg. Clin. North Am.*, **61**, 135–55.

Franklin, E. C. (1975) μ-chain disease. *Arch. Intern. Med.*, **135**, 71–2.

Franklin, E. C. *et al.* (1964) Heavy chain disease: A new disorder of serum γ-globulins. *Am. J. Med.*, **37**, 332–50.

Frick, M. P., Feinberg, S. B. and Loken, M. K. (1981) Noninvasive spleen scanning in Hodgkin's disease and non-Hodgkin's lymphoma. *Comput. Tomogr.*, **5**, 73–80.

Fuks, Z., Strober, S. and Kaplan, H. S. (1976) Interaction between serum factors and T-lymphocytes in Hodgkin's disease. Use as a diagnostic test. *N. Engl. J. Med.*, **295**, 1273–8.

Gall, E. A. and Mallory, T. B. (1942) Malignant lymphoma: a clinicopathologic survey of 618 cases. *Am. J. Pathol.*, **18**, 381–415.

Gallo, R. C. (1984) Human T-cell leukemia-lymphoma virus and T-cell malignancies in adults. *Cancer Surv.*, **3**, 113–59.

Gallo, R. C. and Wong-Staal, F. (1982) Retroviruses as etiologic agents of some animal and human leukemias and lymphomas and as tools for elucidating the molecular mechanisms of leukemogenesis. *Blood*, **60**, 545–57.

Gallo, R. C. *et al.* (1981) Kyoto workshop on some specific recent advances in human tumor virology (meeting report). *Cancer Res.*, **41**, 4738–9.

Gallo, R. C. *et al.* (1983) Association of the human type C retrovirus with a subset of adult T-cell cancers. *Cancer Res.*, **43**, 3892–9.

Galton, D. A. G. *et al.* (1978) Clinical spectrum of lymphoproliferative diseases. *Cancer*, **42**, 901–10.

Galton, D. A. G. *et al.* (1974) Prolymphocytic leukaemia. *Br. J. Haematol.*, **27**, 7–23.

Giardina, S. L. *et al.* (1985) The generation of monoclonal anti-idiotype antibodies to human B-cell-derived leukemias and lymphomas. *J. Immunol.*, **135**, 653–8.

Gibbs, W. N., Loffers, W. S. and Campbell, M. (1987) Non-Hodgkin lymphoma in Jamaica and its relation to adult T-cell leukemia-lymphoma. *Ann. Intern. Med.*, **106**, 361–8.

Giffin, H. Z. (1921) Present status of splenectomy as a therapeutic measure. *Minn. Med.*, **4**, 132–8.

Gill, P. G., Souter, R. G. and Morris, P. J. (1980) Results of surgical staging in Hodgkin's disease. *Br. J. Surg.*, **67**, 478–81.

Gill, P. G., Souter, R. G. and Morris, P. J. (1981) Splenectomy for hypersplenism in malignant lymphomas. *Br. J. Surg.*, **68**, 29–33.

Gilliland, B. C., Baxter, E. and Evans, R. S. (1971) Red-cell antibodies in Coombs'-negative hemolytic anemia. *N. Engl. J. Med.*, **285**, 252–6.

Giorno, R. (1984) Unusual structure of human splenic sinusoids revealed by monoclonal antibodies. *Histochemistry*, **81**, 505–7.

Glatstein, E. *et al.* (1969) The value of laparotomy and splenectomy in the staging of Hodgkin's disease. *Cancer*, **24**, 709–18.

Glatstein, E. *et al.* (1970) Surgical staging of abdominal involvement in unselected patients with Hodgkin's disease. *Radiology*, **97**, 425–32.

Glazer, G. M. *et al.* (1981) Dynamic CT of the normal spleen. *Am. J. Roentgenol.*, **137**, 343–6.

Glees, J. P. *et al.* (1977) Accuracy of grey-scale ultrasonography of liver and spleen in Hodgkin's disease and the other lymphomas compared with isotope scans. *Clin. Radiol.*, **28**, 233–8.

Glees, J. P. *et al.* (1982) The changing role of staging laparotomy in Hodgkin's disease: a personal series of 310 patients. *Br. J. Surg.*, **69**, 181–7.

Goedert, J. J. *et al.* (1981) Polyarteritis nodosa, hairy cell leukemia and splenosis. *Am. J. Med.*, **71**, 323–6.

Goffinet, D. R., Castellino, R. A. and Kim, H. (1973) Staging laparotomies in unselected previously untreated patients with non-Hodgkin's lymphomas. *Cancer*, **32**, 672–81.

Goffinet, D. R., Glatstein, E. J. and Merigan, T. C. (1972) Herpes zoster-varicella infections and lymphoma. *Ann. Intern. Med.*, **76**, 235–41.

Goffinet, D. R. *et al.* (1976) Abdominal irradiation in non-Hodgkin's lymphomas. *Cancer*, **37**, 2797–806.

Goffinet, D. R. *et al.* (1977) Clinical and surgical (laparotomy) evaluation of patients with non-Hodgkin's lymphomas. *Cancer Treat. Rep.*, **61**, 981–92.

Golde, D. W. (1982) Therapy of hairy-cell leukemia. Editorial. (1982) *N. Engl. J. Med.*, **307**, 495–6.

Goldthorn, J. F. and Schwartz, A. D. (1978) Poor protective effect of unregenerated splenic tissue to pneumococcal challenge after subtotal splenectomy. *Surg. Forum*, **29**, 469–70.

Golomb, H. M. (1987) The treatment of hairy cell leukemia. *Blood*, **69**, 979–83.

Golomb, H. M., Catovsky, D. and Golde, D. W. (1978) Hairy cell leukemia. A clinical review based on 71 cases. *Ann. Intern. Med.*, **89**, 677–83.

Golomb, H. M., Ratain, M. J. and Vardiman, J. W. (1986) Sequential treatment of hairy cell leukemia: a new role for interferon. in *Important Advances in Oncology 1986*, (ed. V. T. DeVita), Lippincott, Philadelphia.

Golomb, H. M., Schmidt, K. and Vardiman, J. W. (1984) Chlorambucil therapy of 24 post-splenectomy patients with progressive hairy cell leukemia. *Semin. Oncol.*, **11**, 502–6.

Golomb, H. M. and Vardiman, J. W. (1983) Response to splenectomy in 65 patients with hairy cell leukemia: an evaluation of spleen weight and bone marrow involvement. *Blood*, **61**, 349–52.

Golomb, H. M. *et al.* (1986) Alpha-2 interferon therapy of hairy cell leukemia: a multi-center study of 64 patients. *J. Clin. Oncol.*, **4**, 900–5.

Goodman, G. E. *et al.* (1982) Surgical restaging of Hodgkin's disease. *Cancer Treat. Rep.*, **66**, 751–7.

Goodwin, J. S. *et al.* (1977) Prostaglandin-producing suppressor cells in Hodgkin's disease. *N. Engl. J. Med.*, **297**, 963–8.

Goonewardene, A. *et al.* (1979) Splenectomy for undiagnosed splenomegaly. *Br. J. Surg.*, **66**, 62–5.

Gootenberg, J. E. *et al.* (1981) Human cutaneous T-cell lymphoma and leukemia cell lines produce and respond to T-cell growth factor. *J. Exp. Med.*, **154**, 1403–18.

Gosselin, G. R., Hanlon, D. G. and Pease, G. L. (1956) Leukaemic reticuloendotheliosis. *Can. Med. Assoc. J.*, **74**, 886–91.

Greaves, M. F. (1975) Clinical applications of cell surface markers. in *Progress in Hematology* (ed. E. B. Brown), Grune and Stratton, New York, pp. 255–303.

Greenall, M. J., Gough, M. H. and Kettlewell, M. G. (1983) Laparotomy in the investigation of patients with pyrexia of unknown origin. *Br. J. Surg.*, **70**, 356–7.

Greenberger, J. S., Come, S. E. and Weichselbaum,

R. R. (1979) Issues of controversy in radiation therapy and combined modality approaches to Hodgkin's disease. *Clin. Haematol.*, **8**, 611–24.

Griem, M. L. *et al.* (1975) Staging procedures in mycosis fungoides. *Br. J. Cancer*, **31**, (Suppl. II), 362–7.

Grillot-Courvalin, C. *et al.* (1986) The syndrome of T8 hyperlymphocytosis: variation in phenotype and cytotoxic activities of granular cells and evaluation of their role in associated neutropenia. *Blood*, **69**, 1204–10.

Gross, D. J. *et al.* (1982) Functional asplenia in immunoblastic lymphoma. *Arch. Intern. Med.*, **142**, 2213–15.

Gupta, S. (1980) Subpopulations of human T lymphocytes: XVI. Maldistribution of T cell subsets associated with abnormal locomotion of T cells in untreated adult patients with Hodgkin's disease. *Clin. Exp. Immunol.*, **42**, 186–95.

Gupta, S. and Tan, C. (1980) Abnormality of T cell locomotion and of distribution of subpopulations of T and B lymphocytes in the peripheral blood and spleen from children with untreated Hodgkin's disease. *Clin. Immunol. Immunpathol.*, **15**, 133–43.

Hacker, J. F. III, *et al.* (1982) Hemorrhagic ascites: an unusual presentation of primary splenic lymphoma. *Gastroenterology.*, **83**, 470–3.

Halie, M. R. *et al.* (1978) Hodgkin's disease in the spleen. *Virchows Arch.*, **27**, 39–48.

Hamilton, P. J. S. *et al.* (1967) Splenectomy in 'big spleen disease'. *Br. Med. J.*, **iii**, 823–5.

Han, T. (1980) Role of suppressor cells in depression of T-lymphocyte proliferative response in untreated and treated Hodgkin's disease. *Cancer*, **45**, 2102–8.

Han, T. and Sokal, J. E. (1970) Lymphocyte response to phytohemagglutinin in Hodgkin's disease. *Am. J. Med.*, **48**, 728–34.

Han, T. *et al.* (1980) Splenic T and B lymphocytes and their mitogenic response in untreated Hodgkin's disease. *Cancer*, **45**, 767–74.

Hanaoka, M. *et al.* (1979) Adult T-cell leukemia. Histological classification and characteristics. *Acta Pathol. Jpn.*, **29**, 723–38.

Hansen, M. M. (1973) Chronic lymphocytic leukaemia. Clinical studies based on 189 cases followed for a long time. *Scand. J. Haematol.*, (Suppl. 18).

Harris, I. M., McAlister, J. M. and Prankerd, T. A. J. (1958) Splenomegaly and the circulating red cell. *Br. J. Haematol.*, **4**, 97–102.

Harris, J. M., Jr, Tang, D. B. and Weltz, M. D. (1978) Diagnostic tests and Hodgkin's disease. *Cancer*, **41**, 2388–92.

Haskell, C. M. (1981) Significance of splenic vascular invasion in Hodgkin's disease. Letter to the editor. *Lancet*, **i**, 195–6.

Hattori, T. *et al.* (1981) Surface phenotype of Japanese adult T-cell leukemia cells characterized by monoclonal antibodies. *Blood*, **58**, 645.

Hatsubai, A., Maloney, D. G. and Levy, R. (1981) The use of a monoclonal anti-idiotype antibody to study the biology of a human B cell lymphoma. *J. Immunol.*, **126**, 2397–402.

Hawkins, M. J. *et al.* (1985) Phase I evaluation of recombinant A interferon alpha (rIFN-(Alpha)A) in combination with COPA chemotherapy (I-COPA). Abstract. *Proc. Ann. Meet. ASCO*, **4**, 229.

Heifetz, L. J., Fuller, L. M. and Rodgers, R. W. (1980) Laparotomy findings in lymphangiogram-staged I and II non-Hodgkin's lymphomas. *Cancer*, **45**, 2778–86.

Hermreck, A. S., Kofender, V. S. and Bell, C. (1975) The staging of Hodgkin's disease: preoperative clinical assessment versus operative evaluation. *Am. J. Surg.*, **130**, 639–42.

Hersman, J. *et al.* (1982) The effect of granulocyte transfusions on the incidence of cytomegalovirus infection after allogeneic marrow transplantation. *Ann. Intern. Med.*, **96**, 149–52.

Hillinger, S. M. and Herzig, G. P. (1977) Increased suppressor cell activity in Hodgkin's disease. *Proc. Am. Assoc. Cancer Res.*, **18**, 152.

Hillinger, S. M. and Herzig, G. P. (1978) Impaired cell-mediated immunity in Hodgkin's disease mediated by suppressor lymphocytes and monocytes. *J. Clin. Invest.*, **61**, 1620–7.

Hodgson, W. J. B. and McElhinney, A. J. (1982) Ultrasonic partial splenectomy. *Surgery*, **91**, 346–8.

Hoppe, R. T., Horning, S. J. and Rosenberg, S. A. (1985) The concept, evolution and preliminary results of the current Stanford clinical trials for Hodgkin's disease. *Cancer Surv.*, **4**, 459–75.

Hoppe, R. T. *et al.* (1982) Prognostic factors in pathologic stage III Hodgkin's disease. *Cancer Treat. Rep.*, **66**, 743–9.

Horan, M. and Colebatch, J. H. (1962) Relation between splenectomy and subsequent infection: a clinical study. *Arch. Dis. Child.*, **37**, 398–414.

Horn, N. L., Ray, G. R. and Kriss, J. P. (1976) Gallium-67 citrate scanning in Hodgkin's disease and non-Hodgkin's lymphoma. *Cancer*, **37**, 250–7.

Hosea, S. W. *et al.* (1981) Opsonic requirements for intravascular clearance after splenectomy. *N. Engl. J. Med.*, **304**, 245.

Hunter, C. P. *et al.* (1977) Increased T lymphocytes

and IgMEA-receptor lymphocytes in Hodgkin's disease spleens. *Cell Immunol.*, **31**, 193–8.

Ioachim, H. L., Cooper, M. C. and Hellman, G. C. (1985) Lymphomas in men at high risk for acquired immune deficiency syndrome (AIDS). *Cancer*, **56**, 2831–42.

Jackson, H., Jr and Parker, F., Jr (1947) *Hodgkin's Disease and Allied Disorders*. Oxford University Press, New York.

Jacobs, A. D., Champlin, R. E. and Golde, D. W. (1985) Recombinant alpha-2 interferon for hairy cell leukemia. *Blood*, **65**, 1017–20.

Jacobson, R. J. *et al.* (1972) Listeria infections after splenectomy. *N. Engl. J. Med.*, **287**, 721.

Jaffe, N., Paed, D. and Bishop, Y. M. M. (1970) The serum iron level, haematocrit, sedimentation rate and leucocyte alkaline phosphatase level in paediatric patients with Hodgkin's disease. *Cancer*, **26**, 332–7.

Jansen, J. and Hermans, J. (1981) Splenectomy in hairy cell leukaemia: a retrospective multicenter analysis. *Cancer*, **47**, 2066–76.

Johnson, C. S., Rosen, P. J. and Sheehan, W. W. (1979) Acute lymphocytic leukemia manifesting as splenic rupture. *Am. J. Clin. Pathol.*, **72**, 118–21.

Johnston, G. *et al.* (1974) Ga-citrate imaging in untreated Hodgkin's disease: preliminary report of cooperative group. *J. Nucl. Med.*, **15**, 399–403.

Johnston, J. B. *et al.* (1986) The treatment of hairy-cell leukemia with 2-deoxycoformycin. *Br. J. Haematol.*, **63**, 525–34.

Jones, P. A. E. *et al.* (1972) Ferritinaemia in leukaemia and Hodgkin's disease. *Br. J. Cancer*, **27**, 212–17.

Jones, S. E., Tobias, D. A. and Waldman, R. S. (1978) Computed tomographic scanning in patients with lymphoma. *Cancer*, **41**, 480–6.

Jonsson, V. *et al.* (1976) Mu chain disease in a case of chronic lymphocytic leukaemia and malignant histiocytoma. *Scand. J. Haematol.*, **16**, 209–17.

Joosten, P. *et al.* (1985) High-dose methotrexate with leucovorin rescue: effectiveness in relapsed hairy cell leukemia. *Blood*, **66**, 241–2.

Kadin, M. E., Glatstein, E. and Dorfman, R. F. (1971) Clinicopathologic studies of 117 untreated patients subjected to laparotomy for the staging of Hodgkin's disease. *Cancer*, **27**, 1277–94.

Kager, P. A. *et al.* (1983) Splenic aspiration: experience in Kenya. *Trop. Geogr. Med.*, **35**, 125–31.

Kalter, S. P. *et al.* (1985) Aggressive non-Hodgkin's lymphomas in immunocompromised homosexual males. *Blood*, **66**, 655–9.

Kalyanaraman, V. S. *et al.* (1982) A new subtype of human T-cell leukemia virus (HTLV-II) associated with a T-cell variant of hairy cell leukemia. *Science*, **218**, 571–3.

Kaminski, M. S. *et al.* (1986) Factors predicting survival in adults with stage I and II large-cell lymphoma treated with primary radiation therapy. *Ann. Intern. Med.*, **104**, 747–56.

Kaplan, H. S. (1970) On the natural history, treatment, and prognosis of Hodgkin's disease. *Harvey Lectures, 1968–9*. Academic Press, New York, pp. 215–59.

Kaplan, H. S. (1972) *Hodgkin's Disease*, Harvard University Press, Cambridge, Mass.

Kaplan, H. S. (1980) Hodgkin's disease: unfolding concepts concerning its nature, management and prognosis. *Cancer*, **45**, 2439–74.

Katayama, I. and Finkel, H. E. (1974) Leukemic reticuloendotheliosis. A clinicopathologic study with review of the literature. *Am. J. Med.*, **57**, 115–26.

Katz, S. and Schiller, M. (1980) Partial splenectomy in staging laparotomy for Hodgkin's disease. *Is. J. Med. Sci.*, **16**, 669–71.

Kaur, J. *et al.* (1974) Increase of T lymphocytes in the spleen in Hodgkin's disease. *Lancet*, **ii**, 800–2.

Kawarada, Y. *et al.* (1976) Staging laparotomy for Hodgkin's disease. *Am. Surg.*, **42**, 332–45.

Kay, D. N. and McCready, V. R. (1972) Clinical isotope scanning using Ga citrate in the management of Hodgkin's disease. *Br. J. Radiol.*, **45**, 437–43.

Kim, H. and Dorfman, R. F. (1974) Morphological studies of 84 untreated patients subjected to laparotomy for the staging of the non-Hodgkin's lymphomas. *Cancer*, **33**, 657–74.

Kim, H. *et al.* (1978) Malignant lymphoma with a high content of epithelioid histiocytes. *Cancer*, **41**, 620–35.

King, D. J., Dawson, A. A. and Bayliss, A. P. (1985) The value of ultrasonic scanning of the spleen in lymphoma. *Clin. Radiol.*, **36**, 473–4.

King, H. and Schumacker, H. B., Jr (1952) Splenic studies: I. Susceptibility to infection after splenectomy performed in infancy. *Ann. Surg.*, **136**, 239–42.

Kirschner, R. H. *et al.* (1974) Vascular invasion and hematogenous dissemination of Hodgkin's disease. *Cancer*, **34**, 1159–62.

Klaue, P., Eckert, P. and Kern, E. (1979) Incidental splenectomy: early and late postoperative complications. *Am. J. Surg.*, **138**, 296–300.

Knowles, D. M. *et al.* (1988) Lymphoid neoplasia associated with the Acquired Immunodeficiency Syndrome (AIDS). *Ann. Intern. Med.*, **108**, 744–53.

Koga, T. and Morikawa, Y. (1975) Ultrasonographic

determination of the splenic size and its clinical usefulness in various liver diseases. *Radiology*, **115**, 157–61.

Kosmo, M. A. and Gale, R. P. (1987) Plasma cell leukemia. *Semin. Hematol.*, **24**, 202–8.

Kraut, E. H., Bouroncle, B. A. and Grever, M. R. (1986) Low-dose deoxycoformycin in the treatment of hairy cell leukemia. *Blood*, **68**, 1119–22.

Krikorian, J. G., Portlock, C. S. and Mauch, P. M. (1986) Hodgkin's disease presenting below the diaphragm: a review. *J. Clin. Oncol.*, **4**, 1551–62.

Krivit, W. (1977) Overwhelming postsplenectomy infection. *Am. J. Hematol.*, **2**, 193–201.

Krivit, W., Giebink, G. S. and Leonard, A. (1979) Overwhelming postsplenectomy infection. *Surg. Clin. North Am.*, **59**, 223–33.

Kung, P. C. *et al.* (1981) Cutaneous T-cell lymphomas: characterization by monoclonal antibodies. *Blood*, **57**, 261–6.

Kurlander, R., Stein, R. S. and Roth, D. (1975) Hyperkalemia complicating splenic irradiation of chronic lymphocytic leukemia. *Cancer*, **36**, 926–30.

Kyle, R. A. and Garton, J. P. (1987) The spectrum of IgM monoclonal gammopathy in 430 cases. *Mayo Clin. Proc.*, **62**, 719–31.

Lampert, I. A. (1983) Splenectomy as a diagnostic technique. *Clin. Haematol.*, **12**, 535–63.

Lampert, I. *et al.* (1980a) The histopathology of prolymphocytic leukemia with particular reference to the spleen. A comparison with chronic lymphocytic leukemia. *Histopathology*, **4**, 3–19.

Lampert, I. A. *et al.* (1980b) Immunohistochemical characterization of cells involved in dermatopathic lymphadenopathy. *J. Pathol.*, **131**, 145–56.

Lanzkowsky, P. *et al.* (1976) Staging laparotomy and splenectomy: treatment and complications of Hodgkin's disease in children. *Am. J. Hematol.*, **1**, 393–404.

Larson, R. A. and Ultmann, J. E. (1982) The strategic role of laparotomy in staging Hodgkin's disease. *Cancer Treat. Rep.*, **66**, 767–74.

Lauria, F. *et al.* (1983) Increased proportion of suppressor/cytotoxic (OKT8+) cells in patients with Hodgkin's disease in long-lasting remission. *Cancer*, **52**, 1385–8.

Leavitt, R. D. *et al.* (1984) High and low dose treatment for high and low grade non-Hodgkin's lymphoma. *Proceedings of the Second International Conference on Malignant Lymphoma*, Lugano, Switzerland.

Le Bourgeois, J. P. and Tubiana, M. (1977) The erythrocyte sedimentation rate as a monitor for relapse in patients with previously treated Hodgkin's disease. *Int. J. Radiat. Oncol. Biol. Phys.*, **2**, 241–7.

Le Bourgeois, J. P. *et al.* (1979) Renal consequences of irradiation of the spleen in lymphoma patients. *Br. J. Radiol.*, **52**, 56–60.

Leibenhaut, M. H. *et al.* (1987) Sub-diaphragmatic Hodgkin's disease: laparotomy and treatment results in 49 patients. *J. Clin. Oncol.*, **5**, 1050–5.

Lennert, K. (1967) Classification of malignant lymphomas (European concept). in *Progress in Lymphology* (ed. A. Ruttimann), Thieme, Stuttgart. pp. 103–9.

Lennert, K. (1978) *Malignant Lymphomas Other Than Hodgkin's Disease: Histology, Cytology, Ultrastructure, Immunology* (eds. K. Lennert *et al.*), Springer-Verlag, New York.

Lennert, K. and Mestdagh, J. (1968) Lymphogranulomatosen mit konstant hohem Epitheloidzellgehalt. *Virchows Arch. (Pathol. Anat.)*, **344**, 1–20.

Levi, J. A. *et al.* (1975) Role of gallium citrate scanning in the management of non-Hodgkin's lymphoma. *Cancer*, **36**, 1690–701.

Levine, A. M. and Gill, P. S. (1987) AIDS-related malignant lymphoma: clinical presentation and treatment approaches. *Oncology*, **1**, 41–6.

Levine, A. M. *et al.* (1984) Development of B-cell lymphoma in homosexual men. *Ann. Intern. Med.*, **100**, 7–13.

Levy, R. and Kaplan, H. S. (1974) Impaired lymphocyte function in untreated Hodgkin's disease. *N. Engl. J. Med.*, **290**, 181–6.

Lewis, S. M. *et al.* (1977) Splenic red cell pooling in hairy cell leukaemia. *Br. J. Haematol.*, **35**, 351–7.

Ligler, F. S. *et al.* (1980) Detection of tumor cells in the peripheral blood of nonleukemic patients with B cell lymphoma. Analysis of 'clonal excess'. *Blood*, **55**, 792–801.

Lindfors, K. K. *et al.* (1984) Scintigraphic findings in large-cell lymphoma of the spleen: concise communication. *J. Nucl. Med.*, **25**, 969–71.

Lindgren, P. G. *et al.* (1985) Excision biopsy of the spleen by ultrasonic guidance. *Br. J. Radiol.*, **58**, 853–7.

LoBuglio, A. F., Cotran, R. S. and Jandl, J. H. (1967) Red cells coated with immunoglobulin G: binding and sphering by mononuclear cells in man. *Science*, **158**, 1582–5.

Lockwood, C. M. (1983) Immunological functions of the spleen. *Clin. Haematol.*, **12**, 449–65.

Long, J. C. and Aisenberg, A. C. (1974) Malignant lymphoma diagnosed at splenectomy and idiopathic splenomegaly. A clinicopathological comparison. *Cancer*, **33**, 1054–61.

Long, J. C. and Mihm, M. C. (1974) Mycosis fungoides with extracutaneous dissemination: a distinct clinicopathologic entity. *Cancer*, 34, 1745–55.

Lotz, M. J., Chabner, B. and DeVita, V. T. Jr (1976) Pathological staging of 100 consecutive untreated patients with non-Hodgkin's lymphomas. *Cancer*, 37, 266–70.

Loughran, T. P., Jr *et al.* (1985) Leukemia of large granular lymphocytes: association with clonal chromosomal abnormalities and autoimmune neutropenia, thrombocytopenia and hemolytic anemia. *Ann. Intern. Med.*, 102, 169–75.

Louie, A. C. *et al.* (1981) Follow-up observations on the effect of human leukocyte interferon in non-Hodgkin's lymphoma. *Blood*, 58, 712–18.

Lukes, R. J. (1971) Criteria for involvement of lymph node, bone marrow, spleen and liver in Hodgkin's disease. *Cancer Res.*, 31, 1755–67.

Lukes, R. J., Butler, J. J. and Hicks, E. B. (1966) Natural history of Hodgkin's disease as related to its pathologic picture. *Cancer*, 19, 317–44.

Lukes, R. J. and Collins, R. D. (1974) Immunologic characterization of human malignant lymphomas. *Cancer*, 34, 1488–503.

Lukes, R. J., Tindle, B. H. and Parker, J. W. (1969) Reed–Sternberg-like cells in infectious mononucleosis. Letter to the editor. *Lancet*, ii, 1003–4.

Lutzner, M. *et al.* (1975) Cutaneous T-cell lymphomas: the Sezary syndrome, mycosis fungoides, and related disorders. Edited transcript of 1974 NIH conference. *Ann. Intern. Med.*, 83, 534–52.

MacKenzie, M. R. and Fudenberg, H. H. (1972) Macroglobulinemia: an analysis for forty patients. *Blood*, 39, 874–89.

Magrath, I. T. (1981) Lymphocyte differentiation: an essential basis for the comprehension of lymphoid neoplasia. *J. Nat. Cancer Inst.*, 67, 501–14.

Mangan, K. F., Chikkappa, G. and Farley, P. C. (1982) T gamma cells suppress growth of erythroid colony-forming units in vitro in the pure red cell aplasia of B cell chronic lymphocytic leukemia. *J. Clin. Invest.*, 70, 1148–56.

Mann, J. L., Hafez, G. R. and Longo, W. L. (1986) Role of the spleen in the transdiaphragmatic spread of Hodgkin's disease. *Am. J. Med.*, 81, 959–61.

Manns, A. *et al.* (1988) Seroprevalence of human T-cell lymphotropic virus Type I among homosexual men in the United States. Letter to the editor. *N. Engl. J. Med.*, 318, 516–17.

Manoharan, A., Bader, L. V. and Pitney, W. R. (1982) Non-tropical idiopathic splenomegaly (Dacie's syndrome). Report of 5 cases. *Scand. J. Haematol.*, 28, 175–9.

Manoharan, A. *et al.* (1980) Significance of splenomegaly in childhood acute lymphoblastic leukaemia in remission. *Lancet*, i, 449–52.

Matas, A. J. *et al.* (1976) Post-transplant malignant lymphoma: distinctive morphologic features related to pathogenesis. *Am. J. Med.*, 61, 716–20.

Matchett, K. M., Huang, A. T. and Kremer, W. B. (1973) Impaired lymphocyte transformation in Hodgkin's disease: evidence for depletion of circulating T-lymphocytes. *J. Clin. Invest.*, 52, 1908–17.

Mauch, P. *et al.* (1983) Prognostic factors in patients with subdiaphragmatic Hodgkin's disease. *Hematol. Oncol.*, 1, 205–14.

Maurer, R. (1985) The role of the spleen in leukemias and lymphomas including Hodgkin's disease. *Experientia*, 41, 215–22.

McCallister, B. D. *et al.* (1967) Primary macroglobulinemia: review with a report on thirty-one cases and notes on the value of continuous chlorambucil therapy. *Am. J. Med.*, 43, 394–434.

McCann, S. R. *et al.* (1982) Lymphocyte subpopulations following splenic irradiation in patients with chronic lymphocytic leukaemia. *Br. J. Haematol.*, 50, 225–9.

McKenna, R. W. *et al.* (1985) Granulated T cell lymphocytosis with neutropenia: malignant or benign chronic lymphoproliferative disorder. *Blood*, 66, 259–66.

McKenna, W. *et al.* (1979) Pel-Ebstein fever coinciding with cyclical haemolytic anaemia and splenomegaly in a patient with Hodgkin's disease. *Scand. J. Haematol.*, 23, 378–80.

Meeker, T. C. *et al.* (1985) A clinical trial of anti-idiotype therapy for B cell malignancy. *Blood*, 65, 1349–63.

Meijer, J. L. M. *et al.* (1984) Immunohistochemical studies of the spleen in hairy-cell leukemia. *Am. J. Pathol.*, 115, 266–74.

Menitove, J. E. (1987) Current issues in blood component therapy: transmission of infectious diseases. *Oncology*, 1, 21–8.

Merl, S. A. *et al.* (1983) Splenectomy for thrombocytopenia in chronic lymphocytic leukemia. *Am. J. Hematol.*, 15, 253–9.

Meuge, C., Hoerni, B. and DeMascarel, A. (1978) Non-Hodgkin malignant lymphomas. Clinico-pathologic correlations with the Kiel classification. Retrospective analysis of a series of 274 cases. *Eur. J. Cancer*, 14, 587–92.

Milder, M. S. *et al.* (1973) Liver–spleen scan in Hodgkin's disease. *Cancer*, 31, 826–34.

Miller, R. A. *et al.* (1982) Treatment of B-cell lymphoma with monoclonal antiidiotype antibody. *N. Engl. J. Med.*, **306**, 517–22.

Miller, R. A. *et al.* (1983) Monoclonal antibody therapeutic trials in seven patients with T-cell lymphoma. *Blood*, **62**, 988–95.

Minassian, A. A. (1986) Suppressor cells in the peripheral blood and spleen of patients with Hodgkin's disease. *Cancer*, **57**, 1756–61.

Mintz, U. and Golomb, H. M. (1979) Splenectomy as initial therapy in 26 patients with leukemic reticuloendotheliosis (hairy cell leukemia). *Cancer Res.*, **39**, 2366–70.

Mitchell, A. and Morris, P. J. (1983) Surgery of the spleen. *Clin. Haematol.*, **12**, 565–90.

Moeschlin, S. (1957) *Spleen Puncture.* Heinemann, London.

Moore, G. E. *et al.* (1983) Failure of splenic implants to protect against fatal postsplenectomy infection. *Am. J. Surg.*, **146**, 413–14.

Moran, E. M. *et al.* (1975) Staging laparotomy in non-Hodgkin's lymphoma. *Br. J. Cancer*, (Suppl. II), **31**, 228.

Morris, D. H. and Bullock, F. D. (1919) The importance of the spleen in resistance to infection. *Ann. Surg.*, **70**, 513–21.

Morris, P. J., Cooper, I. A. and Madigan, J. P. (1975) Splenectomy for haematological cytopenias in patients with malignant lymphomas. *Lancet*, **ii**, 250–3.

Myers, T. J. *et al.* (1981) Primary splenic hairy cell leukemia: remission for 21 years following splenectomy. *Am. J. Hematol.*, **11**, 299–303.

Nadler, L. M. *et al.* (1980) Serotherapy of a patient with a monoclonal antibody directed against a human lymphoma-associated antigen. *Cancer Res.*, **40**, 3147–54.

Naeim, F. and Smith, G. S. (1974) Leukemic reticuloendotheliosis. *Cancer*, **34**, 1813–21.

Nagasawa, A., Abe, T. and Nakagawa, T. (1981) Pure red cell aplasia and hypogammaglobulinemia associated with T cell chronic lymphocytic leukemia. *Blood*, **57**, 1025–31.

Nanba, K., Soban, E. J. and Bowling, M. C. (1977) Splenic pseudosinuses and hepatic angiomatous lesions. *Am. J. Clin. Pathol.*, **67**, 415–26.

Newell, J. (1963) Splenic irradiation. *Clin. Radiol.*, **14**, 20–7.

Newland, A. C. *et al.* (1984) Chronic T cell lymphocytosis: a review of 21 cases. *Br. J. Haematol.*, **58**, 433–46.

Ochs, J. *et al.* (1986) Phase I/II study of recombinant alpha-2 interferon against advanced leukemia and lymphoma in children. *J. Clin. Oncol.*, **4**, 883–7.

O'Connell, M. J. *et al.* (1975) Epithelioid granulomas in Hodgkin disease. *J. Am. Med. Assoc.*, **233**, 886–90.

O'Connell, M. J. *et al.* (1986) Clinical trial of recombinant leukocyte A interferon as initial therapy for favorable histology non-Hodgkin's lymphomas and chronic lymphocytic leukemia: an Eastern Cooperative Oncology Group pilot study. *J. Clin. Oncol.*, **4**, 128–36.

O'Neal, B. J. and McDonald, J. C. (1981) The risk of sepsis in the asplenic adult. *Ann. Surg.*, **194**, 775–8.

Orda, R. *et al.* (1981) Postsplenectomy splenic activity. *Ann. Surg.*, **194**, 771–4.

Osadchaya, T. I., Vasilo, N. I. and Baisogolov, G. D. (1980) Diagnosis of splenic involvement in Hodgkin's disease by radionuclide evaluation of splenic contraction in response to adrenaline. *J. Nucl. Med.*, **21**, 384–6.

Pandolfi, F. *et al.* (1984) Classification of patients with T-cell chronic lymphocytic leukemia and expansions of granular lymphocytes: heterogeneity of Italian cases by a multiparameter analysis. *J. Clin. Immunol.*, **4**, 174.

Parmentier, C. *et al.* (1974) La radiothérapie dans la leucémie lymphoïde chronique: l'irradiation splénique. *Nouv. Rev. Fr. Hématol.*, **14**, 735–54.

Paule, B. and Cosset, J. M. (1984) La radiothérapie splénique comme alternative thérapeutique dans la leucémie lymphoïde chronique. *Bull. Cancer*, **71**, 72–3.

Paule, B., Cosset, J. M. and Le Bourgeois, J. P. (1985) The possible role of radiotherapy in chronic lymphocytic leukaemia. A critical review. *Radiother. Oncol.*, **4**, 45–54.

Payne, S. V. *et al.* (1976) T and B lymphocytes and Reed-Sternberg cells in Hodgkin's disease lymph nodes and spleens. *Clin. Exp. Immunol.*, **24**, 280–6.

Pearson, H. A. (1980) Splenectomy: its risks and its roles. *Hosp. Pract.*, **15**, 85–94.

Pearson, H. A. *et al.* (1978) The born-again spleen. Return of splenic function after splenectomy for trauma. *N. Engl. J. Med.*, **298**, 1389–92.

Piekarski, J. *et al.* (1980) Computed tomography of the spleen. *Radiology*, **135**, 683–9.

Pilon, V. A., Davey, F. R. and Gordon, G. B. (1981) Splenic alterations in hairy cell leukemia. *Arch. Pathol. Lab. Med.*, **105**, 577–81.

Pilon, V. A., Davey, F. R. and Gordon, G. B. (1982) Splenic alterations in hairy-cell leukemia: an electron microscopic study. *Cancer*, **49**, 1617–23.

Pirofsky, B. (1969) in *Autoimmunization and the Autoimmune Hemolytic Anemias*, Williams and Wilkins, Baltimore, p. 37.

Plenderleith, I. H. (1970) Hairy cell leukaemia. *Can. Med. Assoc. J.*, **102**, 1056–60.

Plesnicar, S., Sumi-Kriznik, T. and Golouh, R. (1975) Abdominal lymphoma with alpha heavy chain disease. *Isr. J. Med. Sci.*, **11**, 832–7.

Poiesz, B. J. *et al.* (1980) Detection and isolation of type C retrovirus particles from fresh and cultured lymphocytes of a patient with cutaneous T-cell lymphoma. *Proc. Natl. Acad. Sci. USA*, **77**, 7415–19.

Poppema, S. *et al.* (1982) In situ immunologic characterization of cellular constituents in lymph nodes and spleens involved by Hodgkin's disease. *Blood*, **59**, 226–32.

Posner, M. R., Reinherz, E. L. and Brerad, J. (1981) Lymphoid subpopulations of peripheral blood and spleen in untreated Hodgkin's disease. *Cancer*, **48**, 1170–6.

Praz, F. *et al.* (1984) Complement alternative pathway activation by chronic lymphocytic leukemia cells: its role in their hepatosplenic localization. *Blood*, **63**, 463–7.

Quesada, J. R. *et al.* (1984) Alpha interferon for induction of remission in hairy-cell leukemia. *N. Engl. J. Med.*, **310**, 15–18.

Quesada, J. R. *et al.* (1986) Treatment of multiple myeloma with recombinant alpha-interferon. *Blood*, **67**, 275–8.

Rai, K. R. *et al.* (1975) Clinical staging of chronic lymphocytic leukemia. *Blood*, **46**, 219–34.

Raich, P. C. *et al.* (1975) Acute granulocytic leukemia in Hodgkin's disease. *Am. J. Med. Sci.*, **269**, 237–41.

Ratain, J. J. *et al.* (1987) Durability of responses to interferon alfa-2b in advanced hairy cell leukemia. *Blood*, **69**, 872–7.

Ratain, M. J. *et al.* (1985) Treatment of hairy cell leukemia with recombinant alpha-2 interferon. *Blood*, **65**, 644–8.

Ravry, M. *et al.* (1972) Serious infection after splenectomy in the staging of Hodgkin's disease. *Ann. Intern. Med.*, **77**, 11–14.

Ray, G. R., Wolf, P. H. and Kaplan, H. S. (1973) Value of laboratory indicators in Hodgkin's disease: preliminary results. *Nat. Cancer Inst. Monogr.*, **36**, 315–23.

Redman, H. C. *et al.* (1977) Computed tomography as an adjunct in the staging of Hodgkin's disease and non-Hodgkin's lymphomas. *Radiology*, **124**, 381–5.

Risdall, R., Hoppe, R. T. and Warnke, R. (1979) Non-Hodgkin's lymphoma: a study of the evolution of the disease based upon 92 autopsied cases. *Cancer*, **44**, 529–42.

Robertson, D. A. F. *et al.* (1982) Suppressor cell activity, splenic function and HLA status in man. *J. Clin. Lab. Immunol.*, **9**, 133–8.

Rogers, J. S. II and Shah, S. (1980) Spontaneous splenic rupture in plasma cell leukemia. *Cancer*, **46**, 212–14.

Rosen, P. R. *et al.* (1982) Predicting splenic abnormality in Hodgkin disease using volume response to epinephrine administration. *Radiology*, **143**, 627–9.

Rosenberg, S. A. (1988) Exploratory laparotomy and splenectomy for Hodgkin's disease: a commentary. *J. Clin. Oncol.*, **6**, 574–5.

Rosenberg, S. A. and Kaplan, H. S. (1966) Evidence for an orderly progression in the spread of Hodgkin's disease. *Cancer Res.*, **26**, 1225–31.

Rosenberg, S. A. and Kaplan, H. S. (1970) Hodgkin's disease and other malignant lymphomas. *Calif. Med.*, **113**, 23–38.

Rosenberg, S. A., Ribas-Mundo, M. and Goffinet, D. R. (1978) Staging in adult non-Hodgkin's lymphomas. *Rec. Res. Cancer Res.*, **65**, 51–7.

Rosenberg, S. A. *et al.* (1961) Lymphosarcoma: a review of 1269 cases. *Medicine*, **40**, 31–84.

Rosenberg, S. A. *et al.* (1982) NCI-sponsored study of classification of non-Hodgkin's lymphomas: summary and description of a working formulation for clinical usage. *Cancer*, **49**, 2112–35.

Rosier, R. P. and Lefer, L. G. (1977) Spontaneous rupture of the spleen in hairy cell leukemia. Letter to the Editor. *Arch. Pathol. Lab. Med.*, **101**, 557.

Rosove, M. H. *et al.* (1980) Severe platelet dysfunction in hairy cell leukemia with improvement after splenectomy. *Blood*, **55**, 903–6.

Roth, M. S. and Foon, K. A. (1986) Alpha interferon in the treatment of hematologic malignancies. *Am. J. Med.*, **81**, 871–82.

Rowbotham, B. J., Brearley, R. L. and Collins, R. J. (1986) Non-tropical idiopathic splenomegaly and chronic T-cell lymphocytosis. *Pathology*, **18**, 187–9.

Rubin, A. D. *et al.* (1969) Chronic reticulolymphocytic leukemia. Reclassification of 'leukemic reticulo-endotheliosis' through functional characterization of the circulating mononuclear cells. *Am. J. Med.*, **47**, 149–62.

Ruco, L. P. *et al.* (1982) Natural killer activity in spleens and lymph nodes from patients with Hodgkin's disease. *Cancer Res.*, **42**, 2063–8.

Sacks, E. L. *et al.* (1978) Epithelioid granulomas associated with Hodgkin's disease. *Cancer*, **41**, 562–7.

Sagar, V. V., DelDuca, V., Jr and Mecklenburg, R. L. (1979) Spleen scan in histiocytic lymphoma: response to therapy. *Clin. Nucl. Med.*, **4**, 18–19.

Schaefer, H. E. *et al.* (1975) Zytochemischer Polymorphismus der sauren phosphatase bei Haarzell-Leukamie. *Blut*, **31**, 365–70.

Schechter, G. P. and Soehnlen, F. (1978) Monocyte-mediated inhibition of lymphocyte blastogenesis in Hodgkin's disease. *Blood*, **52**, 261–71.

Schiffer, C. A., Levi, J. A. and Wiernik, P. H. (1975) The significance of abnormal circulating cells in patients with Hodgkin's disease. *Br. J. Haematol.*, **31**, 177–83.

Schimpff, S. C. *et al.* (1975) Infections in 92 splenectomized patients with Hodgkin's disease. A clinical review. *Am. J. Med.*, **59**, 695–701.

Schmitt, G. T. *et al.* (1981) Rupture spontanée de rate au cours des leucémies a tricholeucocytes. Deux observations. *Nouv. Presse Med.*, **10**, 257.

Schrek, R. and Donnelly, W. J. (1966) Hairy cells in blood in lymphoreticular neoplastic disease and flagellated cells of normal lymph nodes. *Blood*, **27**, 199–211.

Schulof, R. S., Lacher, M. J. and Gupta, S. (1981) Abnormal phytohemagglutinin-induced T-cell proliferative responses in Hodgkin's disease. *Blood*, **57**, 607–13.

Schwartz, P. E. *et al.* (1982) Post-splenectomy sepsis and mortality in adults. *J. Am. Med. Assoc.*, **248**, 2279–83.

Scott, J. L. *et al.* (1971) Leukocyte labelling with chromium. II. Leukocyte kinetics in chronic myelocytic leukemia. *Blood*, **38**, 162–73.

Seabold, J. E. *et al.* (1976) Gallium citrate (Ga 67) scanning. *Arch. Intern. Med.*, **136**, 1370–4.

Seligmann, M., Preud' Homme, J. L. and Brouet, J. C. (1973) B and T cell markers in human proliferative blood diseases and primary immunodeficiencies, with special reference to membrane bound immunoglobulins. *Transplant. Rev.*, **16**, 85–113.

Seligmann, M. *et al.* (1968) Alpha chain disease: a new immunoglobulin abnormality. *Science*, **162**, 1396–7.

Senn, N. (1903) Case of spleno-medullary leukemia successfully treated by use of roentgen ray. *Med. Rec. New York*, **63**, 281.

Sharp, R. A. and MacWalter, R. S. (1983) A role for splenic irradiation in the treatment of hairy-cell leukaemia. *Acta Haematol.*, **70**, 59–62.

Sherman, R. (1980) Perspectives in management of trauma to the spleen. *J. Trauma*, **20**, 1–13.

Shimoyama, M., Abe, T. and Miyamoto, K. (1987) Chromosome aberrations and clinical features of adult T cell leukemia-lymphoma not associated with human T cell leukemia virus type I. *Blood*, **69**, 984–9.

Shimoyama, M. *et al.* (1983) Anti-ATLA (antibody to adult T-cell leukemia-lymphoma virus-associated antigen)-negative adult T-cell leukemia-lymphoma. *Jpn. J. Clin. Oncol.*, (Suppl. 2), **13**, 245–376.

Sibbit, W. L., Bankhurst, A. D. and Williams, R. C., Jr (1978) Studies of cell subpopulations mediating mitogen hyporesponsiveness in patients with Hodgkin's disease. *J. Clin. Invest.*, **61**, 55–63.

Siegal, F. P. (1976) Inhibition of T-cell rosette formation by Hodgkin-disease serum. Editorial. *N. Engl. J. Med.*, **295**, 1314–15.

Siler, J. *et al.* (1980) Increased echogenicity of the spleen in benign and malignant disease. *Am. J. Roentgenol.*, **134**, 1011–14.

Silverman, S. *et al.* (1972) Evaluation of the liver and spleen in Hodgkin's disease. II. The value of splenic scintigraphy. *Am. J. Med.*, **52**, 362–6.

Singer, D. B. (1973) Postsplenectomy sepsis. in *Perspectives in Pediatric Pathology* (eds. H. S. Rosenberg and R. P. Bolande), Year Book Medical Publishers, Chicago.

Singh, A. K., Bates, T. and Wetherley-Mein, G. (1986) A preliminary study of low-dose splenic irradiation for the treatment of chronic lymphocytic and prolymphocytic leukaemias. *Scand. J. Haematol.*, **37**, 50–8.

Skarin, A. T., Davey, F. R. and Moloney, W. C. (1971) Lymphosarcoma of the spleen. Results of diagnostic splenectomy in 11 patients. *Arch. Intern. Med.*, **127**, 259–65.

Smith, F. W. (1984) Prospects for tumour monitoring by nuclear magnetic resonance. *Reviews on Endocrine-Related Cancer*, **17**, 25–30.

Smithers, D. W. (1970) Spread of Hodgkin's disease. *Lancet*, i, 1262–7.

Smithers, D. W., Lillicrap, S. C. and Barnes, A. (1974) Patterns of lymph node involvement in relation to hypotheses about the modes of spread of Hodgkin's disease. *Cancer*, **34**, 1779–86.

Soederstroem, N. (1970) Cytologie der Milz in Punktaten. in *Der Milz* (eds. K. Lennert and D. Harms), Springer-Verlag, Berlin.

Soederstroem, N. (1979) Cytology of infradiaphragmatic organs. 9. Spleen. *Monogr. Clin. Cytol.*, **7**, 224–47.

Sokol, J. E. and Primikiros, N. (1961) The delayed skin test response in Hodgkin's disease and lymphosarcoma. *Cancer*, **14**, 597–607.

Solbiati, L. *et al.* (1983) Focal lesions in the spleen: sonographic patterns and guided biopsy. *Am. J. Roentgenol.*, **140**, 59–65.

Spencer, R. P. and Knowlton, A. H. (1975) Radiocolloid scans in evaluating splenic response to external radiation. *J. Nucl. Med.*, **16**, 123–6.

Spiegel, R. J. (1987) The alpha interferons: clinical overview. *Sem. Oncol.*, (Suppl 2), **14**, 1–12.

Spiers, A. S. D., Parekh, S. J. and Bishop, M. B. (1984) Hairy cell leukemia: induction of complete remission with pentostatin (2-deoxycoformycin). *J. Clin. Oncol.*, **2**, 1336–42.

Spiers, A. S. D. *et al.* (1985) Hairy cell leukemia (HCL): pentostatin (dcf, 2-deoxycoformycin) is effective both as initial treatment and after failure of splenectomy and alpha interferon. *Blood*, **66**, 208.

Spiro, S. *et al.* (1975) Follicular lymphoma, a survey of 75 cases with special reference to the syndrome resembling chronic lymphocytic cell leukaemia. *Br. J. Cancer*, (Suppl. 11), **31**, 60.

Spivak, J. L. and Perry, S. (1970) Lymphocyte kinetics in chronic lymphocytic leukaemia. *Br. J. Haematol.*, **18**, 511–22.

Stahel, R. A., Maurer, R. and Cavalli, F. (1982) Idiopathische Splenomegalie: Vorstufe eines malignen Lymphoms? Bericht ueber zwei Falle. *Schweiz. Med. Wochenschr.*, **112**, 725–30.

Stathopoulos, G. *et al.* (1977) The T and B lymphocyte content of lymph nodes and spleen in Hodgkin's disease. *Br. J. Exp. Pathol.*, **58**, 712–16.

Stein, R. S. *et al.* (1978) Anatomic substages of stage III Hodgkin's disease: implications for staging, therapy and experimental design. *Cancer*, **42**, 429–36.

Stein, R. S. *et al.* (1982) Anatomic substages of stage IIIA Hodgkin's disease: followup of a collaborative study. *Cancer Treat. Rep.*, **66**, 733–41.

Stephens, P. J. T. and Hudson, P. (1969) Spontaneous rupture of the spleen in plasma cell leukemia. *Can. Med. Assoc. J.*, **100**, 31–4.

Sterchi, J. M., Buss, D. H. and Beyer, F. C. (1984) The risk of improperly staging Hodgkin's disease with partial splenectomy. *Am. Surg.*, **50**, 20–2.

Sterchi, J. M. and Myers, R. T. (1980) Staging laparotomy in Hodgkin's disease. *Ann. Surg.*, **191**, 570–5.

Stewart, D. J. *et al.* (1979) The effectiveness of rubidazone in hairy cell leukemia (leukemic reticuloendotheliosis). *Blood*, **54**, 298–304.

Strauch, G. O. (1979) Accessory spleen in Hodgkin's disease. Letter to the Editor. *J. Am. Med. Assoc.*, **241**, 1792–3.

Straus, D. J., Filippa, D. A. and Lieberman, P. H. (1983) The non-Hodgkin's lymphomas. A retrospective clinical and pathologic analysis of 499 cases diagnosed between 1958 and 1969. *Cancer*, **51**, 101–9.

Strijk, S. P. *et al.* (1985) The spleen in Hodgkin disease: diagnostic value of CT. *Radiology*, **154**, 753–7.

Strum, S. B., Allen, L. W. and Rappaport, H. (1971) Vascular invasion in Hodgkin's disease: its relationship to involvement of the spleen and other extranodal sites. *Cancer*, **28**, 1329–34.

Strum, S. B., Park, J. K. and Rappaport, H. (1970) Observation of cells resembling Sternberg-Reed cells in conditions other than Hodgkin's disease. *Cancer*, **26**, 176–90.

Strumia, M. M., Strumia, P. V. and Bassert, D. (1966) Splenectomy in leukemia; hematologic and clinical effects on 34 patients and review of 299 published cases. *Cancer Res.*, **26**, 519–28.

Sugarbaker, E. D. and Craver, L. F. (1940) Lymphosarcoma. Study of 196 cases with biopsy. *J. Am. Med. Assoc.*, **115**, 17.

Sutcliffe, S. B. *et al.* (1978) Post-treatment laparotomy in the management of Hodgkin's disease. *Lancet*, ii, 57–9.

Sutcliffe, S. B. *et al.* (1982) Post-treatment laparotomy as a guide to management in patients with Hodgkin's disease. *Cancer Treat. Rep.*, **66**, 759–65.

Swerdlow, S. H. *et al.* (1984) Caribbean T-cell lymphoma/leukemia. *Cancer*, **54**, 687–96.

Takatsuki, K. *et al.* (1982) Adult T-cell leukemia: proposal as a new disease and cytogenic, phenotypic, and functional studies of leukemic cells. *Gann Monogr.*, **28**, 13–22.

Takatsuki, K. *et al.* (1985) Clinical diversity in adult T-cell leukemia lymphoma. *Cancer Res.* (Suppl.) **45**, 4644–5s.

Thompson, J. A. and Fefer, A. (1987) Interferon in the treatment of hairy cell leukemia. *Cancer*, (Suppl. 1), **59**, 605–9.

Thompson, J. A. *et al.* (1985) Recombinant alpha-2 interferon in the treatment of hairy cell leukemia. *Cancer Treat. Rep.*, **69**, 791–3.

Toge, T. *et al.* (1983) Concanavalin A-induced and spontaneous suppressor cell activities in peripheral blood lymphocytes and spleen cells from gastric cancer patients. *Cancer*, **52**, 1624–31.

Traetow, D., Fabri, P. J. and Carey, L. C. (1980) Changing indications for splenectomy. *Arch. Surg.*, **115**, 447–51.

Traub, A. *et al.* (1987) Splenic reticuloendothelial function after splenectomy, spleen repair, and spleen autotransplantation. *N. Engl. J. Med.*, **317**, 1559–64.

Trigg, M. E. (1979) Immune function of the spleen. *South Med. J.*, **72**, 593–9.

Tubiana, M. *et al.* (1981) Five-year results of the E.O.R.T.C. randomized study of splenectomy and spleen irradiation in clinical stages I and II of Hodgkin's disease. *Eur. J. Cancer*, **17**, 355–63.

Twomey, J. J. *et al.* (1975) Hodgkin's disease: an immunodepleting and immunosuppressive disorder. *J. Clin. Invest.*, **56**, 467–75.

Twomey, J. J. et al. (1980) Spectrum of immunodeficiencies with Hodgkin's disease. *J. Clin. Invest.*, **66**, 629–37.

Uchiyama, T. et al. (1977) Adult T-cell leukemia: clinical and hematologic features of 16 cases. *Blood*, **50**, 481–92.

Uchiyama, T. et al. (1978) Effect of adult T-cell leukemia cells on pokeweed mitogen-induced normal B-cell differentiation. *Clin. Immunol. Immunopathol.*, **10**, 24–34.

Uddstroemer, M. (1934) On the occurrence of lymphogranulomatosis (Sternberg) in Sweden, 1915–1931 and some considerations as to its relation to tuberculosis. *Acta Tuberc. Scand.* (Suppl. 1), 1–225.

Urba, W. J. and Longo, D. L. (1985) Clinical spectrum of human retroviral-induced diseases. *Cancer Res.* (Suppl.), **45**, 4637–43s.

van Leeuwen, F. E., Somers, R. and Hart, A. A. M. (1987) Splenectomy in Hodgkin's disease and second leukemias. *Lancet*, **ii**, 210–11.

Vanhaelen, C. P. J. and Fisher, R. I. (1981) Increased sensitivity of lymphocytes from patients with Hodgkin's disease to concanavalin A-induced suppressor cells. *J. Immunol.*, **127**, 1216–20.

Variakojis, D., Rosas-Uribe, A. and Rappaport, H. (1974) Mycosis fungoides: pathologic findings in staging laparotomies. *Cancer*, **33**, 1589–600.

Videbaek, A. A., Christensen, B. E. and Jonsson, V. (1982) *The Spleen in Health and Disease*. FADL, Yearbook Medical Publishers, Copenhagen and Chicago.

Vincent, P. C. (1977) Granulocyte kinetics in health and disease. *Clin. Haematol.*, **6**, 695–717.

von Fliedner, V. et al. (1980) Polymorphonuclear neutrophil function in malignant lymphomas and effects of splenectomy. *Cancer*, **45**, 469–75.

Wagener, D. J. T., Geestman, E. and Wessels, H. M. C. (1975) The influence of splenectomy on the in vitro lymphocyte response to phytohemagglutinin and pokeweed mitogen in Hodgkin's disease. *Cancer*, **36**, 194–8.

Wagener, D. J. T. et al. (1976) The influence of splenectomy on cellular immunologic parameters in Hodgkin's disease. *Cancer*, **37**, 2212–19.

Wagstaff, J. and Crowther, D. (1984) Human alpha-2 interferon (Schering Plough 30500) in the non-Hodgkin's lymphomas. (NHL): a report of 2 phase II studies. *Br. J. Cancer*, **50**, 244.

Wagstaff, J. et al. (1981) Human lymphocyte traffic assessed by indium-111 oxine labelling: clinical observations. *Clin. Exp. Immunol.*, **43**, 443–9.

Waldman, I. and Suissa, L. (1978) Lymphosarcoma in an ectopic pelvic spleen. *Clin. Nucl. Med.*, **3**, 417–19.

Wano, Y. et al. (1987) Interleukin 1 gene expression in adult T cell leukemia. *J. Clin. Invest.*, **80**, 911–16.

Wedelin, C. et al. (1981) Routine laboratory tests in relation to spleen size and tumour involvement in untreated Hodgkin's disease. *Acta Med. Scand.*, **209**, 309–13.

Weintraub, J. and Warnke, R. A. (1982) Lymphoma in cardiac allotransplant recipients. *Transplantation*, **33**, 347–51.

Weiss, S. H. et al. (1987) Emerging high rates of human T-cell lymphotropic virus type I (HTLV) and HIV infections among US drug abusers. *Proceedings of the Third International Conference on AIDS*, Washington, DC.

Weitzman, S. and Aisenberg, A. C. (1977) Fulminant sepsis after the successful treatment of Hodgkin's disease. *Am. J. Med.*, **62**, 47–50.

Weitzman, S. A. et al. (1977) Impaired humoral immunity in treated Hodgkin's disease. *N. Engl. J. Med.*, **297**, 245–8.

Westling, P. (1965) Studies of the prognosis in Hodgkin's disease. *Acta Radiol.*, (Suppl.), **245**, 5–125.

Wetherley-Mein, G. et al. (1952) Follicular lymphoma. *Q. J. Med.*, **21**, 327–51.

Whang-Peng, J. et al. (1979) Cytogenic abnormalities in patients with cutaneous T-cell lymphomas. *Cancer Treat. Rep.*, **63**, 575–80.

Winkelstein, J. A. and Lambert, G. H. (1975) Pneumococcal serum opsonizing activity in splenectomized children. *J. Pediatr.*, **87**, 430–3.

Wong-Staal, F. and Gallo, R. C. (1985) The family of human T-lymphotropic leukemia viruses: HTLV-1 as the cause of adult T cell leukemia and HTLV-III as the cause of acquired immunodeficiency syndrome. *Blood*, **65**, 253–63.

Worthy, T. S. (1981) Evaluation of diagnostic laparotomy and splenectomy in Hodgkin's disease. Report #12. *Clin. Radiol.*, **32**, 523–6.

Wright, D. H. (1970) Gross distribution and haematology. In *Burkitt's Lymphoma* (eds. D. P. Burkitt and D. H. Wright), E & S Livingstone, Edinburgh and London, pp. 64–81.

Yam, L. T. and Crosby, W. H. (1974) Early splenectomy in lymphoproliferative disorders. *Arch. Intern. Med.*, **133**, 270–4.

Yam, L. T. and Crosby, W. H. (1979) Spontaneous rupture of spleen in leukemic reticuloendotheliosis. *Am. J. Surg.*, **137**, 270–3.

Yam, L. T. and Li, C. Y. (1976) Histogenesis of splenic lesions in Hodgkin's disease. *Am. J. Clin. Pathol.*, **66**, 976–85.

Yam, L. T., Li, C. Y. and Finkel, H. E. (1972) Leukaemic reticuloendotheliosis. *Arch. Intern. Med.*, **130**, 248–56.

Yanes, B. *et al.* (1975) Impaired response to neoantigens in treated lymphoma patients. *Clin. Res.*, **23**, 1349.

Yeager, A. S. *et al.* (1981) Prevention of transfusion-acquired cytomegalovirus infections in newborn infants. *J. Pediatr.*, **98**, 281–7.

Young, R. C. *et al.* (1972) Delayed hypersensitivity in Hodgkin's disease. A study of 103 untreated patients. *Am. J. Med.*, **52**, 63–72.

Yu, A. *et al.* (1977) Concomitant presence of tumor-specific cytotoxic and inhibitor lymphocytes in patients with osteogenic sarcoma. *N. Engl. J. Med.*, **297**, 121.

Zarling, J. M., Berman, C. and Raich, P. C. (1980) Depressed cytotoxic T-cell responses in previously treated Hodgkin's and non-Hodgkin's lymphoma patients. *Cancer Immunol. Immunother.*, **7**, 243–9.

Ziegler, J. L. (1981) Burkitt's lymphoma. *N. Engl. J. Med.*, **305**, 735–45.

Ziegler, J. L., Beckstead, J. A. and Volberding, P. A. (1984) Non-Hodgkin's lymphoma in 90 homosexual men. *N. Engl. J. Med.*, **311**, 565–70.

Zucker-Franklin, D. (1974) Properties of the Sezary lymphoid cell: an ultrastructural analysis. *Mayo Clin. Proc.*, **49**, 567–74.

THE SPLEEN IN SICKLE CELL DISEASE 16

G. R. Serjeant

16.1 INTRODUCTION

The spleen is central to much of the early pathology in children with homozygous sickle cell (SS) disease, and abnormal splenic function secondary to the defective erythrocytes in SS disease is a major determinant of the morbidity and mortality of the disease in childhood.

Early observations in patients with sickle cell disease presented a confusing picture of splenomegaly in some patients and splenic atrophy in others. The sequence of splenic pathology in these patients was first recognized in detail by Diggs (1935) who noted that splenomegaly developed in young patients and then gradually disappeared with age as a result of a progressive splenic fibrosis.

The rate of progression of this process varies markedly between individuals with SS disease, and the basic pattern may be complicated by episodes of acute splenic enlargement ('acute splenic sequestration') or sustained enlargement, with or without hypersplenism. Furthermore, splenic immune function is frequently compromised early in life even in the presence of splenomegaly (functional asplenia), and this loss of splenic function predisposes to overwhelming infections, especially with encapsulated organisms such as the pneumococcus.*

16.2 THE PREVALENCE OF SPLENOMEGALY

Most patients with SS disease develop palpable splenomegaly early in life. The Jamaican cohort

*See also Chapters 11 and 12 (cd.)

study followed from birth all 308 children with SS disease detected among 100 000 consecutive newborns. Analysis of the incidence of splenomegaly revealed that the spleen had become palpable in 82% by the age of 6 months and in 93% by the age of one year. Since splenomegaly may be appearing in some patients while disappearing in others, its prevalence at any individual age is lower than the cumulative incidence. Palpable splenomegaly in surviving cohort children without splenectomy occurred in 35% at 6 months, 43% at one year, and in 10% at 10 years (Figure 16.1). These figures may be biased by the exclusion of 33 children who underwent splenectomy, and in whom splenomegaly might have been more likely to persist. With the assumption that splenomegaly would have persisted in all these patients, the maximum expected prevalence of splenomegaly is 48% at 2 years, 29% at 5 years, and 16% at 10 years.

This prevalence may be modified in different geographic areas by the frequency of other genetic factors (see later) and by environmental factors such as malaria. The higher levels of fetal hemoglobin (HbF) and the greater frequency of alpha-thalassemia in some Saudi and Indian populations with SS disease result in a greater prevalence of splenomegaly among these groups (Gelpi, 1970; Kar et al., 1986). The effect of malaria on the pattern of splenomegaly in SS disease is unclear although the reduction in spleen size with malaria chemoprophylaxis (Hendrickse, 1965) suggests that malaria may contribute to more frequent and more marked splenomegaly in SS disease.

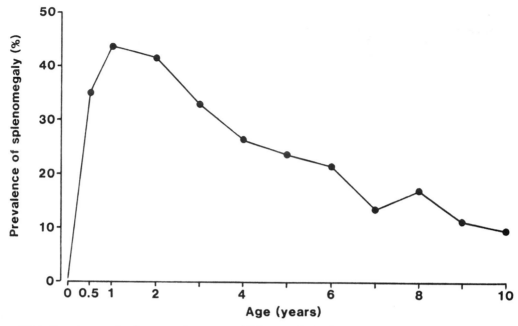

Figure 16.1 Prevalence of splenomegaly among children with SS disease in Jamaican cohort study.

The splenomegaly is usually modest in size, commonly measuring 1–2 cm from the costal margin, although a spleen measuring 4 cm or more occurred at some time in 118 of 308 cohort study children (38%). In 51 of these children the splenomegaly was transient and represented an episode of acute splenic sequestration (ASS); in the remaining 67 children, the splenomegaly persisted for more than one month. There are no hematological consequences to be recognized with the moderate splenomegaly characteristic of most patients with SS disease, although marked hematological changes may be associated with acute or chronic splenic enlargement.

16.3 THE DETERMINANTS OF SPLENOMEGALY

16.3.1 DEVELOPMENT OF SPLENOMEGALY

The splenomegaly typical of most children with SS disease in the first year of life probably results from their relatively rigid red cells, which have difficulty in negotiating the inter-endothelial slits in the basement membrane as these cells pass from the cordal tissue to the vascular sinus lumen. The elegant studies by Weiss and his colleagues (Weiss and Tavassoli, 1970; Weiss, 1983) have illustrated the extreme deformability needed by erythrocytes (Figure 16.2), and those containing intracellular HbS polymer cannot deform to the required extent. Sickled erythrocytes therefore obstruct passage through the reticular network and the inter-endothelial slits (de Boisfleury Chevance and Allard, 1982), resulting in passive splenic engorgement.

Indirect evidence for this process is available from the observation that fetal hemoglobin (HbF), which inhibits HbS polymer formation, is significantly correlated with the age at which splenomegaly develops (Stevens, Vaidya and Serjeant, 1981): patients with rapidly declining HbF levels tend to develop splenomegaly early, whereas those with high levels of HbF, and relatively less intravascular sickling, tend to develop splenomegaly late.

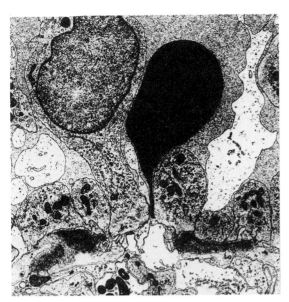 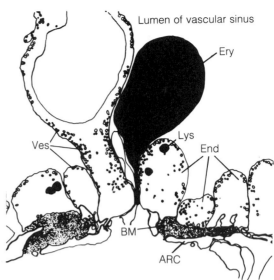

Figure 16.2 Red cell (Ery) traversing an interendothelial slit from the cordal tissue below to the vascular sinus above, demonstrating the extreme deformability required. BM, basement membrane; ARC, adventitial reticular cell; End, endothelium; Lys, lysosome; Ves, vesicles (From Weiss (1983) *Clin. Haematol.*, **12**, 384–5, with the permission of the author and Baillière Tindall Limited.)

16.3.2 DISAPPEARANCE OF SPLENOMEGALY

The gradual disappearance of splenomegaly, which is associated pathologically with progressive splenic fibrosis, is probably also a sequel of splenic microvascular obstruction. The early development of intravascular sickling would therefore be expected to lead to the early appearance of splenomegaly and to its early disappearance. Factors inhibiting sickling should therefore favor the persistence of splenomegaly, and this is supported by findings in patients with high levels of HbF or with alpha-thalassemia.

The presence of high levels of HbF at later ages is associated with persistence of splenomegaly (Serjeant, 1970) and there is a simple relationship between HbF level and the proportion of patients with splenomegaly at each age (Figure 16.3). In individuals, splenomegaly still tends to disappear with age but the process occurs at a later age in patients with higher HbF levels.

Alpha-thalassemia also influences persistence of splenomegaly. Heterozygous alpha[+] thalassemia, in which one of a pair of linked alpha globin genes is deleted, occurs in approximately 35% of populations of West African ancestry. The homozygous form which occurs in 3–4% affects the hematological expression of SS disease, lowering the mean cell hemoglobin concentration (MCHC) and inhibiting HbS polymerization. There is consequently a lower hemolytic rate, higher hemoglobin levels, amelioration of some clinical complications, and persistence of splenomegaly (Higgs *et al.*, 1982).

The association of genetic factors known to inhibit sickling with the persistence of splenomegaly, suggests that this clinical feature may be used as a tool in the search for other factors inhibiting intravascular sickling.

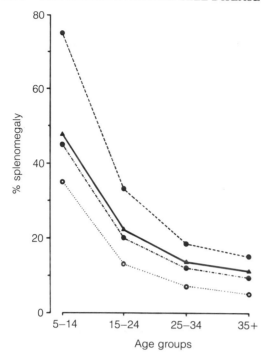

Figure 16.3 Prevalence of splenomegaly with relation to HbF level. Whole group (▲——▲), HbF < 4% (○······○), HbF 4–7.9% (●-·-·-●), HbF ≥ 8% (●-----●). (From Serjeant (1970) *Br. J. Haematol.*, **19**, 635–641 with the permission of Blackwell Scientific Publications Limited.)

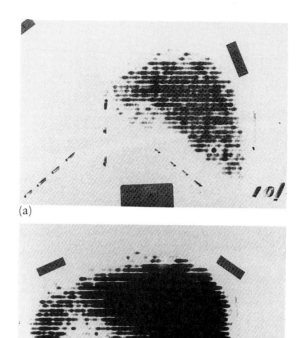

(a)

(b)

Figure 16.4 ^{99m}Tc-sulfur colloid scan (posterior view) in a 2-year-old child with SS disease and splenomegaly showing (a) hepatic uptake but absence of splenic uptake and (b) restoration of splenic uptake 6 days after transfusion. (From Pearson *et al.* (1970) *N. Engl. J. Med.*, **283**, 334–7 with the permission of the publishers.)

16.4 SPLENIC FUNCTION IN SS DISEASE

16.4.1 FUNCTIONAL ASPLENIA

The reduced red cell deformability of patients with SS disease compromises the processing functions of the spleen and influences not only the development of splenomegaly and later splenic atrophy but also produces other abnormalities of splenic function. These abnormalities develop early even while splenomegaly persists and have given rise to the concept of 'functional asplenia' (Pearson, Spencer and Cornelius, 1969). The ability of the spleen to take up ^{99m}Tc-sulfur colloid was abnormal in eight of nine children with SS disease and splenomegaly (Figure 16.4) but could be restored by transfusion in some young children

(Pearson *et al.*, 1970, 1979), suggesting that red cells diverted through intrasplenic shunts could once again traverse the interendothelial slits and be normally processed. At later ages this defect becomes irreversible.

16.4.2 PITTING FUNCTION

The early impairment in splenic function is also reflected in the loss of the normal 'pitting' function of the spleen and the proportion of pitted red cells rises early to levels characteristic of asplenic patients (Figure 16.5). (See also sections 11.2.2 and 11.3.2 (ed.)).

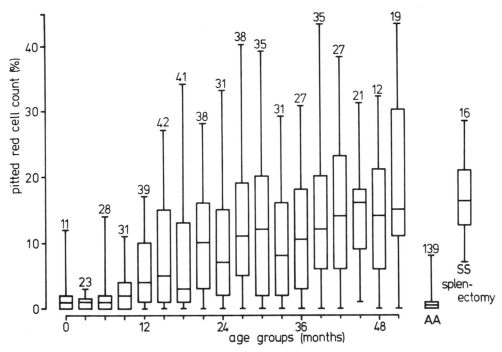

Figure 16.5 Pitted red cells (mean, quartiles, range) and age in children with SS disease, AA controls, and SS disease postsplenectomy. Figures above bars indicate numbers in each group. (From Rogers *et al.* (1982) *Arch. Dis. Child.*, 57, 338–42 with the permission of the publishers.)

16.4.3 OVERWHELMING INFECTIONS

The clinical consequence of this loss of processing and phagocytic function of the spleen is a susceptibility to overwhelming infections especially by encapsulated organisms such as the pneumococcus and *Haemophilus influenzae* b (see also Chapter 12). This susceptibility appears to be greatest in the first year of life and 80% of pneumococcal septicemias in the Jamaican cohort study were observed before the age of 2 years (John *et al.*, 1984). However, despite this early susceptibility, resistance to pneumococcal antigens is gradually acquired and pneumococcal septicemia is increasingly infrequent with advancing age.

16.4.4 PREDICTION OF INFECTIONS

Since the appearance of splenomgaly in SS disease is believed to signal the onset of splenic dysfunction, a relationship might be expected between early splenomegaly and the subsequent development of overwhelming septicemia. This hypothesis was tested by dividing children in the cohort study into three groups according to the age at the time of appearance of palpable splenomegaly: before 6 months, between 6 and 12 months, and after 12 months or not at all (Rogers, Vaidya and Serjeant, 1978). The frequency of subsequent overwhelming septicemias or meningitis in the three groups indicated a highly significant association with early splenomegaly (Table 16.1). These observations are clearly of practical importance since effective prophylactic programs may be concentrated in the highest risk group, which comprises only one-third of the entire SS population.

16.5 ACUTE SPLENIC SEQUESTRATION

Acute splenic sequestration (ASS) is a syndrome of sudden splenic enlargement associated with

Table 16.1 First severe infections by spleen group

Group	Age when spleen first palpable	No. of children	Observed infections	Expected infections[a]	Observed/expected
I	Up to 6 months	50	12	4.88	2.46
II	7–12 months	38	2	3.84	0.52
III	Over 12 months or not at all	47	0	5.27	0

[a]Expected number of first infections calculated from log-rank test (from Rogers *et al.*, 1978).

trapping of red cells, a decrease in hemoglobin in the peripheral blood and often reticulocytosis. There is a spectrum of severity which at its most severe, results in peripheral circulatory failure, shock, and death (Seeler and Shwaiki, 1972).

16.5.1 ETIOLOGY

The etiology is unknown. Non-specific symptoms and fever are common but there is no specific symptom-complex or associated bacteriology (Topley *et al.*, 1981) and this complication probably represents a non-specific response to increased intravascular sickling. There is no epidemiological evidence to support an infec-

tive etiology, although the behavior of the two sets of non-identical twins with SS disease in the cohort study was of interest. In the first set one twin developed ASS at 11 and the other at 19 months, before the spleen became impalpable in both at the age of 21 months. In the other pair of twins the first attacks of ASS occurred simultaneously at 366 days, and the third attacks were separated in time by only 3 days (Figure 16.6). A fourth attack occurred in twin II while awaiting splenectomy. The virtually simultaneous occurrences argue for an environmental factor which perhaps requires very close personal contact.

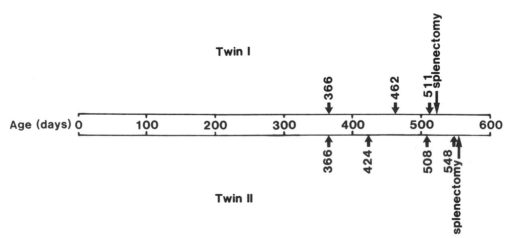

Figure 16.6 Pattern of attacks of ASS in one pair of twins in Jamaican cohort study.

16.5.2   RISK FACTORS

Patients prone to ASS have significantly lower HbF levels (Stevens, Vaidya and Serjeant, 1981; Emond et al., 1985) although no differences are apparent in the total hemoglobin, MCV, MCHC, or reticulocyte counts between patients with and without histories of ASS. Patients with homozygous alpha-thalassemia appear less likely to develop ASS (Emond et al., 1985) although this possibility was not statistically proved, perhaps because of the small numbers of patients in the study.

16.5.3   PREVALENCE

Estimates of the prevalence of ASS depend on the definition adopted for inclusion. Topley et al. (1981) argued for the recognition of minor episodes characterized by a fall in the Hb of at least 2 g/dl, since these may have prognostic significance identifying patients at risk for proceeding to severe or fatal attacks. However, since such mild attacks frequently pass unrecognized, accurate assessment of their prevalence is not possible. When analysis is confined to attacks which are clinically apparent either to the physician or the parent, the cumulative probability is 0.225 by 2 years, 0.265 by 3 years, and 0.297 by 5 years (Emond et al., 1985). Approximately 30% of Jamaican children with SS disease therefore experience episodes of ASS by the age of 5 years.

16.5.4   AGE OF ONSET

Fatal episodes of ASS have been reported to occur as early as 4 months of age (Walterspiel, Rutledge and Bartlett, 1984). The distribution of age at first attack among 89 affected children in the cohort study indicated the period of highest risk to be the second 6 months of life (Figure 16.7), and that 75% of first attacks (67 of 89) occurred before the age of 2 years. First attacks of ASS are rare after the age of 6 years although these occasionally occur in adolescents and may be seen in adults with the genotype sickle cell-hemoglobin C disease or sickle cell-beta°-thalassemia.

Attacks tend to be recurrent (Figure 16.8), 49% of patients at risk after the first attack proceeding to a second attack, and 21% of

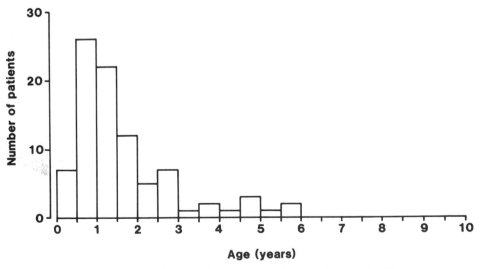

Figure 16.7 Age at first attack of ASS for 89 affected children in the cohort study. (From Emond et al. (1985) J. Pediatr., **107**, 201–6 with the permission of the publishers.)

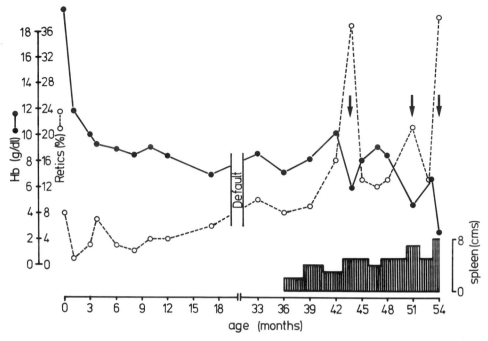

Figure 16.8 Recurrent pattern of ASS. Hemoglobin, reticulocyte count, and spleen size during three episodes of ASS (marked by arrows) in a child dying in the third attack. (From Topley *et al.* (1981) *Arch. Dis. Child.*, 56, 765–9 with the permission of the publishers.)

those at risk after the second attack proceeding to a third attack. There is also a tendency for attacks to recur at progressively shorter intervals (Emond *et al.*, 1985).

16.5.5   CLINICAL FEATURES

The clinical features of attacks are dominated by the anemia and associated clinical symptoms. In one study (Topley *et al.*, 1981) the mean hemoglobin level was 4.8 g/dl (range 0.8–7.3) with an average fall from steady-state values of 3.2 g/dl. The mean hemoglobin in fatal cases was 2.6 g/dl (range 0.8–4.8). Mean reticulocyte counts were elevated at 19% (range 4–43%); in particularly acute episodes, the reticulocyte count may not have had time to rise, but normoblasts are usually present in the peripheral blood. The average spleen size was 4 cm from the costal margin. Clinically the worst affected patients have signs of peripheral circulatory failure with tachycardia, tachyp-

noea and shock, and the time course may be precipitate with patients passing from apparently normal health to gross pallor and shock within as little as 6 hours.

Associated clinical features are common, and in 132 events of ASS in the Jamaican cohort study these included upper respiratory tract infection in 27 (20%), acute chest syndrome in 27 (20%), gastroenteritis in 7 (5%) and dactylitis in 7 (5%). In 25% of events there were no other clinical findings.

Bacteriological investigations do not suggest a common etiology. Review of 97 blood cultures in 132 Jamaican episodes indicated growth of *Streptococcus pneumoniae* in two, *Haemophilus influenzae* in two, *Klebsiella pneumoniae* in two and *Escherichia coli* in two. However, prophylactic penicillin did not reduce the prevalence of ASS, implying that penicillin-sensitive organisms are not a common cause of ASS.

16.5.6 TREATMENT

The treatment of ASS is both corrective and prophylactic. Treatment of the acute episode requires immediate transfusion and correction of any underlying pathology. Early detection and presentation to hospital in such episodes is vital if therapy is to be effective. The education of parents or guardians in the methods of diagnosis and the significance of ASS has had a profound impact on the outcome of this complication in Jamaica. Comparing the results of the 5 years before and after this education program (Table 16.2) reveals that although the apparent incidence of ASS has risen by two and a half times, representing parental detection of mild attacks not normally observed by doctors, the mortality rate has fallen by 90%.

Mortality associated with recurrent attacks may be prevented by prophylactic splenectomy, which in the Jamaican environment is usually performed after two attacks and has been similarly recommended in the United States (Seeler and Shwaiki, 1972). Occasionally with adverse social circumstances, splenectomy may be performed after the first attack, or if social circumstances are good, may be delayed until the third attack. Elective splenectomy has been well tolerated at this age in Jamaican patients (Emond et al., 1984) and effective prophylaxis may be achieved by parenteral penicillin (John et al., 1984). The alternative to splenectomy in the prophylaxis of recurrent attacks of ASS is a chronic transfusion program, which may have the desirable side effect of restoring or improving splenic function at this age (Pearson et al.,

1970). However, it is unclear how to monitor or when to stop such a transfusion program, and episodes of ASS may recur on cessation of transfusion even at an age when ASS is no longer expected (Rao and Pang, 1982). It is possible, therefore, that transfusion therapy delays but does not abolish the natural history of ASS.

16.6 HYPERSPLENISM

In some patients splenomegaly persists, causing a sustained pathological hemolysis accompanied by reactive erythropoietic expansion. A new equilibrium is reached at lower hemoglobin levels and higher reticulocyte counts than had characterized the patient previously. There is a spectrum of severity: the most severe cases present with a spleen measuring 10–15 cm below the costal margin, hemoglobin levels of 2–3 g/dl and reticulocyte counts of 40–50% (Figure 16.9). Estimates of mean red cell survival may be as short as 1–2 days and the erythropoietic expansion leads to skeletal changes with diploic widening, expansion of the zygoma and maxillary bones, and a generalized osteoporosis with cortical thinning.

16.6.1 RISK FACTORS

The risk factors for hypersplenism in SS disease in Jamaica appear to include high levels of HbF (unpublished observations) and homozygous alpha$^+$ thalassemia (Higgs et al., 1982). Approximately half the affected children with hypersplenism in the Jamaican cohort study developed this complication acutely with a clinical picture similar to an attack of ASS which did not resolve and was attended by increasing bone marrow compensation.

16.6.2 PREVALENCE

The frequency of hypersplenism is unclear, partly because there has not been a clear definition. In the Jamaican cohort study, children in whom splenectomy was considered clinically

Table 16.2 Incidence and case fatality rate for ASS before and after parental education program

	Preceding 5 years	Succeeding 5 years
Standardized incidence rates/100 pt years	4.6	11.3
Case fatality rate per 100 events	29.4	3.1

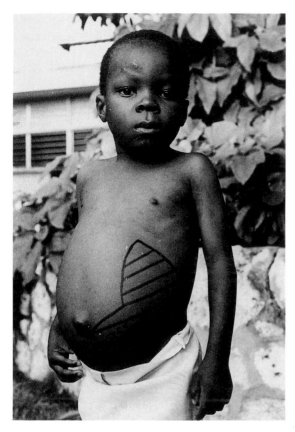

Figure 16.9 Hypersplenism in Jamaican child aged 5 years. The spleen measured 16 cm and weighed 460 g at splenectomy. At the time of photograph blood values included Hb 2.6 g/dl and reticulocytes 38%. (From Serjeant (1985) *Sickle Cell Disease*, with the permission of Oxford University Press.)

indicated for hypersplenism had in common a spleen size of at least 4 cm, a hemoglobin of less than 6.5 g/dl, a fall in hemoglobin of at least 2 g/dl from previous steady-state levels, and a platelet count below 260×10^9/l. Using this definition, hypersplenism occurred in 17 of 308 children (6%) in the cohort study. Comparable data elsewhere are unavailable, although there is a clinical impression that hypersplenism may be more common among Indian patients with SS disease in Orissa (Kar *et al.*, 1986).

16.6.3 AGE OF ONSET

Hypersplenism is essentially a pediatric complication, and is rare after the age of 15 years in Jamaican patients. In the cohort study, hypersplenism developed at a median age of 3.1 years with a range from 0.7 to 8.0 years.

16.6.4 CLINICAL FEATURES

The clinical features of hypersplenism result from the low hemoglobin, bone marrow expansion, and growth failure. The low hemoglobin necessitates a hyperdynamic circulation, maintained by a tachycardia and increased cardiac work. The increased erythropoietic activity is associated with increased requirements of hematinics and of amino acids and calories, which compete with the demands for normal growth. Growth failure is common and a marked growth spurt generally follows splenectomy (Emond *et al.*, 1988). Splenectomy is associated with reductions of 23–47% in protein turnover (Badaloo *et al.*, 1987). The post-splenectomy increase in height velocity was significantly related to the increase in hemoglobin (Figure 16.10) and impaired height velocity consistently occurred when the hematological changes persisted for more than 6 months.

16.6.5 OUTCOME

The outcome of untreated hypersplenism is unknown. Since hypersplenism is rarely the cause of death, and furthermore is rare in Jamaican adult patients, it must be assumed that spontaneous resolution generally occurs. Spontaneous resolution has been observed in mildly affected cases, but no data are available on prospectively observed severely affected cases (Emond *et al.*, 1989) since the natural course is usually interrupted by treatment. It is also unknown whether the low hemoglobin levels, bone changes secondary to erythropoietic expansion, or the growth failure have any permanent effects.

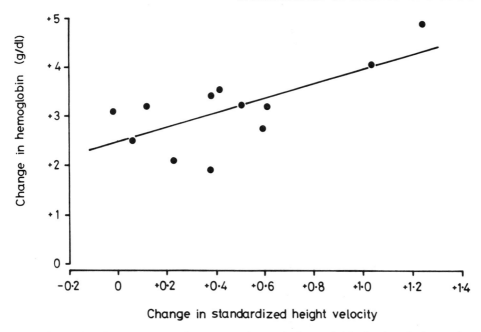

Figure 16.10 Relationship between postsplenectomy change in hemoglobin level and change in standard height velocity.

16.6.6 TREATMENT

Treatment of hypersplenism is based on removal of splenic tissue (either by splenectomy or splenic embolization) or alleviation of the hematological effects by chronic transfusion while awaiting the expected spontaneous splenic regression. Chronic transfusion avoids the surgical and anesthetic risks of operation, but may inhibit the tendency to spontaneous regression in SS disease by allowing hypersplenism to recur at the end of the transfusion program. The necessary duration of transfusion is unknown and there are also the customary problems of chronic transfusion programs which include iron overload, the risk of hepatitis, problems with venous access, transfusion reactions, and the increased destruction of transfused blood by hypersplenism. Splenic embolization (Politis *et al.*, 1987), advocated in the treatment of hypersplenism in beta-thalassemia, theoretically allows a controlled splenic ablation, leaving some residual functional splenic tissue. However, it is unclear whether any immune function persists in the hypersplenic spleen in SS disease and the procedure has been associated with marked pain and infection. Elective splenectomy is well tolerated, and has the advantage of rectifying the underlying pathology immediately; it has generally been used in Jamaica where conditions do not favor conservative management.

16.7 SIGNIFICANCE OF SPLENIC PATHOLOGY

The role of the spleen is central to much of the early morbidity and mortality in sickle cell disease. The first year of life carries the highest risk of death of any period in the life of a child with SS disease (Figure 16.11) and much of this early mortality is attributable either to acute splenic sequestration or pneumococcal septicemia (Thomas, Pattison and Serjeant, 1982). Hypersplenism adds significant morbidity through its effects on the blood picture and growth and development of the child.

Conversely the persistence of splenomegaly is

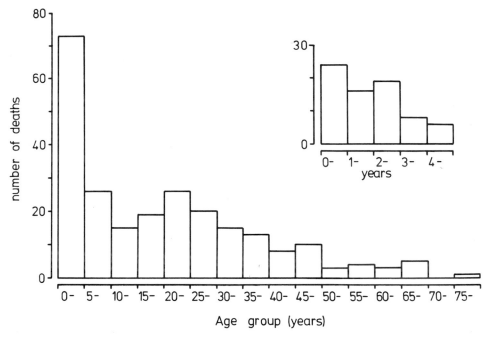

Figure 16.11 Distribution of age at death in Jamaican patients with SS disease. (From Thomas, Pattison and Serjeant (1982) *Br. Med. J.*, **285**, 633–5 with the permission of the publishers.)

frequently a manifestation of relatively mild disease, and reflects a splenic microvasculature that has not been destroyed by the vaso-occlusive processes of the disease. The behavior of the spleen in SS disease is, therefore, not only a cause of severe complications, but also a valuable indicator of the pathological processes active in this disease.

REFERENCES

Badaloo, A. V. *et al.* (1987) Whole-body protein turnover before and after splenectomy in children with homozygous sickle-cell disease. Abstract CCMRC Meeting, British Virgin Islands. *West Indian Med. J.*, **36**, 46–7.

de Boisfleury Chevance, A. and Allard, Ch. (1982) Scanning electron microscopy of the spleen in a case of sickle cell anemia. *Blood Cells*, **8**, 467–70.

Diggs, L. W. (1935) Siderofibrosis of the spleen in sickle cell anemia. *J. Am. Med. Assoc.*, **104**, 538–41.

Emond, A. M. *et al.* (1984) Role of splenectomy in homozygous sickle cell disease in childhood. *Lancet*, **i**, 88–90.

Emond, A. M. *et al.* (1985) Acute splenic sequestration in homozygous sickle cell disease; natural history and management. *J. Pediatr.*, **107**, 201–6.

Emond, A. M. *et al.* (1989) Persistent splenomegaly and hypersplenism in sickle cell disease. (In preparation).

Gelpi, A. P. (1970) Sickle cell disease in Saudi Arabs. *Acta Haematol.*, **43**, 89–99.

Hendrickse, R. G. (1965) The effect of malaria chemoprophylaxis on spleen size in sickle-cell anemia. in *Abnormal Haemoglobins in Africa* (ed. J. H. P. Jonxis). Blackwell Scientific Publications, Oxford, pp. 445–9.

Higgs, D. R. *et al.* (1982) The interaction of alpha-thalassemia and homozygous sickle-cell disease. *N. Engl. J. Med.*, **306**, 1441–6.

John, A. B. *et al.* (1984) Prevention of pneumococcal infection in children with homozygous sickle cell disease. *Br. Med. J.*, **288**, 1567–70.

Kar, B. C. *et al.* (1986) Sickle cell disease in Orissa State, India. *Lancet*, **ii**, 1198–201.

Pearson, H. A., Spencer, R. P. and Cornelius, A. E. (1969) Functional asplenia in sickle-cell anemia. *N. Engl. J. Med.*, **281**, 923–6.

Pearson, H. A. *et al.* (1970) Transfusion reversible asplenia in young children with sickle-cell anemia. *N. Engl. J. Med.*, **283**, 334–7.

Pearson, H. A. *et al.* (1979) Developmental aspects of splenic function in sickle cell disease. *Blood*, **53**, 358–65.

Politis, C. *et al.* (1987) Partial splenic embolisation for hypersplenism of thalassaemia major; five year follow up. *Br. Med. J.*, **294**, 665–7.

Rao, S. and Pang, E. (1982) Transfusion therapy for subacute splenic sequestration in sickle cell disease. *Blood*, **60**, Suppl: 48a.

Rogers, D. W., Vaidya, S. and Serjeant, G. R. (1978) Early splenomegaly in homozygous sickle-cell disease: an indicator of susceptibility to infection. *Lancet*, **ii**, 963–5.

Rogers, D. W., Serjeant, B. E. and Serjeant, G. R. (1982) Early rise in 'pitted' red cell count as a guide to susceptibility to infection in childhood sickle cell anaemia. *Arch. Dis. Child.*, **57**, 338–42.

Seeler, R. A. and Shwaiki, M. Z. (1972) Acute splenic sequestration crises (ASSC) in young children with sickle cell anemia. *Clin. Pediatr.*, **11**, 701–4.

Serjeant, G. R. (1970) Irreversibly sickled cells and splenomegaly in sickle-cell anaemia. *Br. J. Haematol.*, **19**, 635–41.

Serjeant, G. R. (1985) *Sickle Cell Disease*. Oxford University Press, Oxford.

Stevens, M. C. G., Vaidya, S. and Serjeant, G. R. (1981) Fetal hemoglobin and clinical severity of homozygous sickle cell disease in early childhood. *J. Pediatr.*, **98**, 37–41.

Thomas, A. N., Pattison, C. and Serjeant, G. R. (1982) Causes of death in sickle-cell disease in Jamaica. *Br. Med. J.*, **285**, 633–5.

Topley, J. M. *et al.* (1981) Acute splenic sequestration and hypersplenism in the first five years in homozygous sickle cell disease. *Arch. Dis. Child.*, **56**, 765–9.

Walterspiel, J. N., Rutledge, J. C. and Bartlett, B. L. (1984) Fatal acute splenic sequestration at 4 months of age. *Pediatrics*, **73**, 507–8.

Weiss, L. (1983) The red pulp of the spleen: structural basis of blood flow. *Clin. Haematol.*, **12**, 375–93.

Weiss, L. and Tavassoli, M. (1970) Anatomical hazards to the passage of erythrocytes through the spleen. *Semin. Hematol.*, **7**, 370–80.

IMAGING OF THE SPLEEN

Richard J. Rolfes, Pablo R. Ros and Abraham H. Dachman

17.1 INTRODUCTION

In the past, the spleen had been considered radiologically an 'orphan' abdominal organ, since the ability to image it by conventional technology was limited. Recent advances in imaging, including computed tomography (CT), ultrasonography (US) and magnetic resonance imaging (MRI) have created a new interest in the spleen, as part of the technical armamentarium of the growing subspecialty of radiology known as 'abdominal imaging'. It is the intent of this chapter to describe the role of imaging in the study of the spleen, and to present the radiographical manifestations of normal and pathological conditions using the multiple imaging modalities currently available.

17.1.1 THE PLAIN FILM

The simplest and most non-specific means of imaging the spleen is by plain film. The presence of perisplenic fat often makes visualization of the spleen possible on plain film, due to the difference in density between fat and adjacent splenic tissue. However, the ability to see the spleen on plain radiographs is variable, depending on such factors as body habitus and film technique. While the spleen is frequently seen more easily in an individual having an average or moderately increased amount of body fat than in an asthenic person, excessively increased body fat as in morbid obesity will usually obscure most intra-abdominal organs.

. Visualization of the spleen on plain films is generally unreliable and detection of splenic pathology by this modality is limited. Due to normal variations in the size, shape and location of the spleen, only moderate or massive splenomegaly can be appreciated. The spleen normally does not extend below the left costal margin; if it projects below this level splenomegaly can usually be diagnosed. Plain films are, however, useful in detecting calcifications within the spleen; these are frequently found in granulomatous disease, aneurysms of the splenic artery, healed abscesses and cysts.

17.1.2 NUCLEAR SCINTIGRAPHY

Since 1950, nuclear scintigraphy has been considered a conventional means of studying the spleen radiographically. Although CT and US have come to occupy much of the field of splenic imaging, the radionuclide scan still provides a sensitive and simple means for identifying structural and functional pathology. Splenic scintigraphy demonstrates the entire spleen in one image, whereas the newer modalities offer only a cross-sectional view. Perhaps the most frequent clinical indications for nuclear scintigraphy of the spleen are evaluation of space-occupying lesions, splenomegaly or suspected functional pathology. Other indications include the detection of congenital abnormalities, and the evaluation of splenic trauma, left upper quadrant pain and suspected asplenia.

[51]Chromium was used initially for splenic

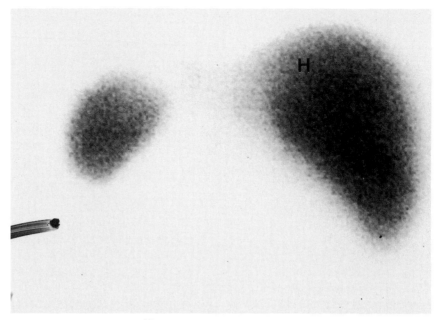

Figure 17.1 Normal liver-spleen scan (^{99m}Tc-sulfur colloid scintigraphy). On this posterior view, the spleen is located on the left. Note the homogeneous distribution of radionuclide activity in the spleen, which is slightly less than the hepatic activity (H). The spleen is best imaged from the posterior direction, since the spleen lies in the posterior abdomen. The spleen is not well visualized on anterior projections due to overlying stomach and bowel. (Image courtesy of W. Drane, MD.)

scintigraphy in the 1950s, but has been replaced by ^{99m}Technetium-sulfur colloid due to its optimal energy emission for imaging and its short 6-hour half-life which minimizes patient radiation exposure. ^{99m}Technetium-sulfur colloid is a suspension of sulfur colloid particles labeled with ^{99m}Technetium. The average particle diameter is 0.3–1.0 μm (Mettler, 1986). These particles are filtered out and trapped by the reticuloendothelial cells in the liver, spleen and bone marrow. Normally 80–90% of the particles injected are trapped by the liver and 5–10% by the spleen, with an insignificant amount trapped by the bone marrow, which is not normally visualized (Mettler, 1986).

^{99m}Technetium-sulfur colloid scintigraphy produces simultaneous imaging of both liver and spleen. Imaging of the spleen alone is possible using heat-damaged red blood cells labeled with ^{99m}Technetium, but is rarely necessary for clinical diagnosis (Mettler, 1986). In addition,

^{111}Indium platelet scanning can be performed to measure splenic blood flow and intrasplenic platelet transit time, a technique which may be useful in studying immune complex disease (Peters *et al.*, 1980, 1984).

The normal spleen scan demonstrates a homogenous distribution of radionuclide activity in the left upper quadrant which is equal to or less than the hepatic activity (Figure 17.1). A reversal of this distribution, with spleen activity greater than that of the liver, suggests hepatocellular disease or an intrinsic splenic abnormality (Figure 17.2). The following factors should be considered when observing a spleen scan: size, position, configuration, and amount and distribution of radionuclide uptake. In patients with congenital, post-surgical and acquired circulatory asplenia, a search for ectopic or accessory splenic tissue should be made.

Normal variations in size, shape and position

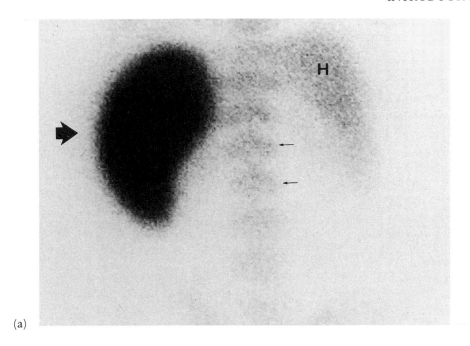

(a)

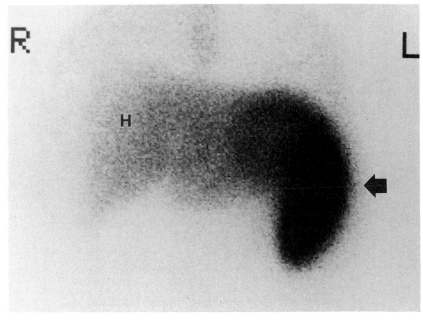

(b)

Figure 17.2 Liver–spleen scan in a patient with biopsy proven cirrhosis of the liver and ascites secondary to alcoholism. Posterior (a) and anterior (b) views. Note the intense radionuclide activity in an enlarged spleen (thick arrows), and the markedly reduced hepatic activity (H). This is an example of the reversal of the normal radionuclide distribution in the presence of hepatocellular disease, with marked shift of radionuclide to the enlarged spleen. Another manifestation of this hepatocellular disease is the abnormal activity present in the vertebral bodies (small arrows) which are not normally visualized. Again, note how the spleen is better visualized on the posterior view. (Images courtesy of W. Drane, MD.)

should be taken into consideration before describing an abnormality, as these normal variations may be demonstrable on nuclear scintigraphy. One such normal variant is the so-called 'upside down' spleen in which the hilum is identified as a concave defect superiorly, rather than in its usual location toward the inferior aspect of the spleen. Another is the presence of splenic lobulation, seen as small extensions of redundant, normally functioning spleen, usually at the anterior or inferior margin. This redundant tissue can cause a relative 'hot spot' when imaged in an overlapping fashion.

Other pitfalls in the interpretation of splenic radionuclide studies exist. A false focal defect in the spleen may be caused by barium retained in the colon from a previous barium study (Rao, Winebright and Dresser, 1979b). Significant enlargement of the left lobe of the liver may also create a false defect in the splenic contour. In addition, following surgical splenectomy, radionuclide uptake in the left lobe of the liver may mimic a normal or accessory spleen.

Single photon emission computed tomography (SPECT) is a form of nuclear scintigraphy which allows cross-sectional study of the spleen. SPECT imaging is useful in evaluating or detecting suspected space-occupying lesions.

17.1.3 ANGIOGRAPHY AND SPLENOPORTOGRAPHY

An extensive discussion of vascular imaging of the spleen can be found in Abrams (1983). On arteriography the splenic parenchymal phase, or 'blush', is seen as a region of homogeneous or slightly speckled contrast density (Figure 17.3b). The visualized density of perfused parenchyma depends on several factors, including contrast iodine content and volume injected, selectivity of the injection site and volume of the spleen. Large infarcts, hematomas, avascular or cystic masses and other non-perfused space-occupying lesions may sometimes be detected as defects in the parenchymal blush. The splenic vein can be visualized approximately 7 seconds after arterial injection,

during the venous phase. Immediate filling of the vein after arterial injection suggests arteriovenous shunting. Delayed filling raises the possibility of portal venous hypertension, whereas absent filling usually indicates splenic vein thrombosis or occlusion, or severe portal venous hypertension. In the presence of portal venous hypertension, gastric varices can frequently be identified. It is important to evaluate all phases of the arteriogram when performing splenic angiography.

Indications for splenoportography (venography of the splenic and portal veins) are limited and use of this procedure has diminished in recent years. In the past, splenoportography was performed by injecting contrast material into the splenic pulp by direct splenic puncture. However, adequate visualization of the splenoportal system can usually be obtained during the venous phase of selective splenic angiography, and this method now generally supplants direct splenic puncture when visualization of the splenic venous drainage is a primary concern. Percutaneous transhepatic splenoportography can also be performed. Since pancreatic veins in the body and tail contribute to splenic vein flow, this transhepatic approach is especially useful when obtaining blood samples in the splenic vein for localization of suspected small, active endocrine tumors of the pancreas.

17.1.4 ULTRASONOGRAPHY

A complete discussion of the technique of splenic ultrasound is outside the scope of this chapter. Adequate visualization of the spleen on ultrasonography is occasionally difficult due to the location of the spleen high in the left upper abdominal quadrant, since it is obscured by the adjacent ribs. In addition, air is a poor conductor of the beam, and the air-filled stomach and colon may further reduce sonographic access. While the spleen may be visualized for most purposes by scanning intercostally, these obstacles may create 'blind areas' within the spleen, especially in those portions adjacent to the dome of the left hemidiaphragm. Improved visualization, especially of the peridiaphragmatic

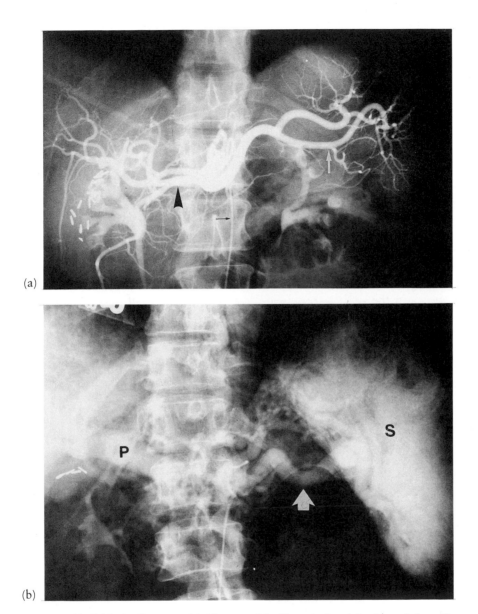

(a)

(b)

Figure 17.3 Normal splenic angiogram. (a) The arterial phase during injection of the celiac artery. The catheter (black arrow) has been positioned in the origin of the celiac artery via a femoral approach. The splenic (white arrow) and hepatic (arrowhead) arteries are well visualized. The splenic artery can normally be much more tortuous than this. Some renal excretion of contrast is seen bilaterally. (b) A relatively homogeneous parenchymal phase or 'blush'. This image was obtained in the late parenchymal phase, as early filling of the splenic vein (arrow) is noted. Portal vein (P).

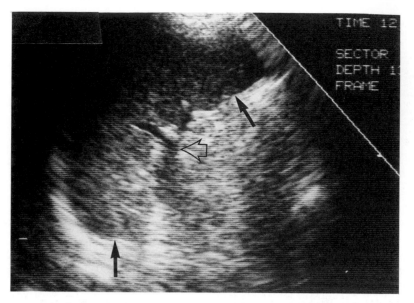

Figure 17.4 Normal spleen on ultrasound. Axial or transverse view demonstrates normal size and shape of the spleen (black arrows). Note the fine, homogeneous echo pattern of the parenchyma. Tubular, hypoechoic structures in the hilum of the spleen (open arrow) represent blood vessels.

portion of the spleen, can sometimes be obtained in the cooperative patient by using varying degrees of inspiration to move the non-visualized portions into view. For scanning in the supine position, it may be useful to have the stomach filled with fluid, which provides an excellent transmitter of ultrasound energy. Using a variety of these techniques the best images of the spleen are usually obtained with the patient in the left anterior oblique, left-side-up decubitus, or prone position. Both transverse and longitudinal (sagittal or coronal) views should be obtained.

On ultrasound, the parenchyma of the spleen produces a homogeneous pattern of echoes having a fine texture, with scattered echogenic foci representing blood vessels (Figure 17.4). The general pattern is similar to that of the liver, but the overall echogenicity is slightly greater. The size and shape of the spleen, its relationship to other organs and the position of the hilum should be defined during the examination. (See also section 15.2.4.)

17.1.5 COMPUTED TOMOGRAPHY

Computed tomography has revolutionized the examination of the spleen, as it has in evaluating other areas of the body. The spleen is usually well visualized on CT, unless technical artifacts or respiratory motion obscure the area (Federle, 1983). Beam-hardening is perhaps the most common technical artifact, and is seen with barium in the stomach or colon, or in the presence of multiple metallic surgical clips.

CT provides an excellent evaluation of the size, shape and position of the spleen, as well as identifying intrasplenic pathology. In addition, the relationship to adjacent organs is well demonstrated, particularly with respect to the pancreatic tail, diaphragm, left kidney and stomach. (See also section 15.2.5.)

By computed tomography obtained without intravenous contrast, the spleen appears homogeneous and of slightly lower density than the liver. The capsule and hilar vessels are often sharply delineated, due to the presence of peri-

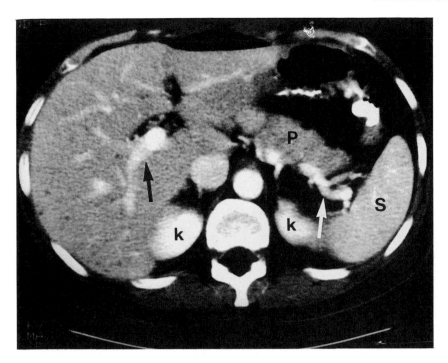

Figure 17.5 Normal spleen on contrast-enhanced computed tomography. Axial or transverse section through the mid-portion of the spleen (S) demonstrates relatively homogeneous contrast enhancement. The splenic hilar vessels are well visualized due to the presence of perisplenic fat (which appears black on this image). The branching vessel demonstrating marked contrast enhancement in the splenic hilum (white arrow) is the splenic artery. The splenic vein would be seen on a lower slice and would be much straighter in its course. Note the intense enhancement of the superior poles of the kidneys (k) and the branching portal vein (black arrow). The pancreas (P) is also well seen.

splenic fat. The splenic artery may appear curvilinear, and when tortuous, may be seen coursing in and out of the plane of section. The splenic vein usually pursues a straighter course and is of slightly greater diameter than the artery (Figure 17.5).

Use of intravenous contrast is generally indicated when looking for splenic pathology. Slow infusion of contrast yields a homogeneous increase in parenchymal density, which again, is slightly less than that of the liver. Rapid, or so-called 'dynamic', infusion of IV contrast may cause a heterogeneous blush initially, which is thought to be related to variable flow rates of contrast through the red pulp. However, a homogeneous splenic blush should be seen within two minutes after bolus injection (Glazer *et al.*, 1981), and persistent areas of heterogeneity beyond this point may be pathological.

The relative CT density of the liver and spleen is often useful in determining the presence of abnormalities. For example, when hepatic density is lower than that of the spleen, it may indicate fatty change of the liver. Lobulation of the spleen is a normal variant frequently appreciated on CT, and is usually more prominent inferiorly. An unusually prominent lobulation secondary to a deep fissure may give the appearance of a 'band' or 'waist' in the spleen (Wilson and Lieberman, 1983).

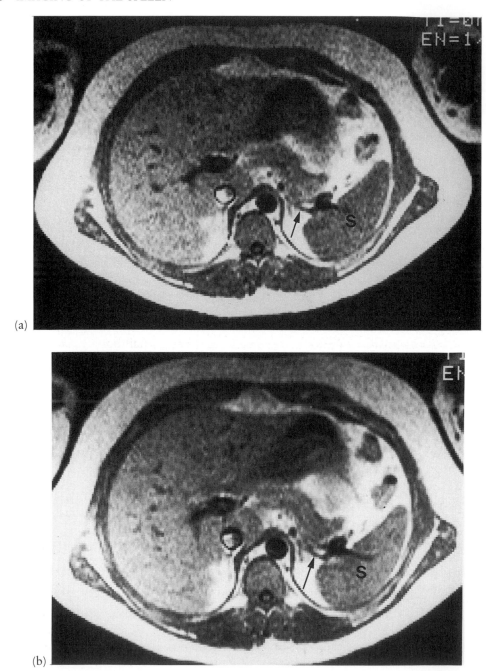

Figure 17.6 Normal spleen on MRI. Transverse sections of the upper abdomen in a normal individual. (a) and (b) were obtained at the same level using slightly different image-acquisition parameters, and (c) was obtained at a slightly more inferior level. The spleen is present at its normal location in the left upper posterior abdomen (S). Tissue of high intensity (white) surrounding the spleen represents fat. On (a) and (b), the tubular, curvilinear structure of low intensity (black) in the splenic hilum represents the splenic artery (black

17.1.6 MAGNETIC RESONANCE IMAGING

Magnetic resonance imaging (MRI) provides yet another means for evaluating the spleen, complementing but not replacing the other imaging modalities. MRI is thought to have superior soft tissue contrast resolution, while CT has superb spatial resolution. With continuing research into its clinical application, the full potential of MRI for solving clinical problems will be realized. The normal spleen is hypointense or isointense on T1-weighted images, compared with the liver, and is hyperintense on T2-weighted images. On MRI, fat is seen as areas of high-intensity (white), and fat in the splenic hilum and surrounding the spleen can thus be distinguished. Vessels, due to the blood flow within, are seen as low-intensity (black) tubular structures surrounded by high intensity fat. While the appearance of fat and vessels on MRI is relatively constant, the appearance of the splenic parenchyma may vary depending on the pulse sequences chosen for imaging (Figure 17.6). In addition, choice of appropriate pulse sequence depends on the particular clinical question to be answered and the type of pathology to be identified. These aspects of MRI are reserved for more comprehensive, technically oriented texts on the subject.

17.1.7 PERCUTANEOUS DRAINAGE AND BIOPSY AND SPLENIC EMBOLIZATION

There has traditionally been a reluctance to biopsy the spleen and to provide percutaneous drainage for splenic lesions; this has been related principally to the vascular structure of the spleen and the consequent risk of hemorrhage. However, there has been an increased interest in performing such procedures with the use of CT and ultrasound guidance. Percutaneous drainage of solitary splenic abscesses has been performed using small bore drainage catheters, without complications. This may be the proce-

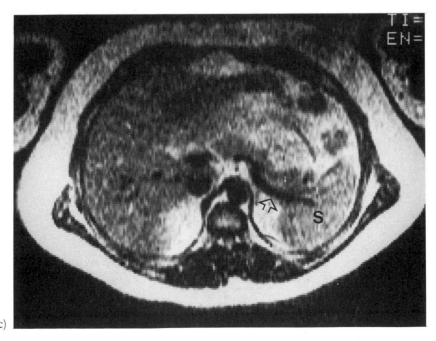

(c)

arrow). On (c), the low-intensity structure in the same location is of slightly larger caliber, and represents the splenic vein (open arrow). Note the differing intensity of the spleen in the same individual, depending on the image acquisition parameters utilized.

dure of choice when the abscess is very large, or when the patient is a poor surgical candidate and surgical splenectomy is not feasible. In addition, puncture of a splenic fluid collection makes the definitive diagnosis, identifies the infective organism and aids in planning therapy. Percutaneous needle aspiration of other splenic lesions for cytologic diagnosis has also been performed without complications using a 22 gauge needle, and this procedure can be useful in diagnosing lymphoma, metastasis and other malignancies involving the spleen. Such percutaneous drainage and biopsy procedures can aid materially in the clinical management of patients, and should be considered in appropriate circumstances.

Splenic artery embolization has been usefully employed in a variety of clinical situations: this consists of placing one of a variety of materials in an artery via a vascular catheter in order to induce thrombosis. Materials used for embolization include Gelfoam (small particles of a synthetic substance), detachable balloons, steel coils and Bucrylate (Goldman *et al.*, 1981). Embolization can be performed at the level of the small branch arteries, or in the main splenic artery. It can be used to stop bleeding in cases of trauma, without inducing hyposplenism with the risk of postsplenectomy infection. It can also be performed to produce a 'medical splenectomy', for example, to alleviate thrombocytopenia and anemia in hypersplenism, or to treat gastric varices secondary to splenic vein thrombosis or portal hypertension. Embolization in such cases reduces or eliminates the risk of surgery and reduces transfusion requirements. However, the complications of splenic embolization are not infrequent and include splenic and subphrenic abscess formation. (See also section 18.5.4.)

17.2 ANOMALIES AND CONGENITAL DISORDERS

17.2.1 WANDERING SPLEEN

'Wandering spleen' is the term usually applied to a spleen which is not located in the left upper quadrant of the abdomen. Supine and upright plain radiographs of the abdomen may demonstrate a mass in the left lower quadrant or mid-abdomen, which may correspond to a mass palpated clinically. There may be a marked difference in position of the mass on supine film when compared to the upright view, with bowel loops filling the left upper quadrant. Extrinsic compression of various intra-abdominal structures, especially the colon, may be detected by plain films or barium studies, and the splenic flexure of the colon may be interposed between the diaphragm and the spleen (Gordon *et al.*, 1977; Salomonowitz, Frick and Lund, 1984). In addition, the vascular pedicle of this spleen may cause a linear defect across the bowel in barium studies (Gordon *et al.*, 1977).

Nuclear scintigraphy using [99m]Technetium-sulfur colloid is a frequently performed study for diagnosing wandering spleen (McArdle,

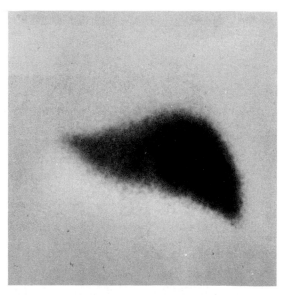

Figure 17.7 [99m]Technetium-sulfur colloid scan. This patient presented with acute abdominal pain. Posterior view of the abdomen demonstrates homogeneous radionuclide uptake in the liver. No splenic uptake was identified in the abdomen, indicating absence of vascular flow to the spleen consistent with torsion of the vascular pedicle and/or infarction. (The presence of a spleen in the left abdomen was confirmed by CT scan. See Figure 17.8.)

1980). Torsion can be diagnosed in the patient with acute abdominal pain, if there is absent or diminished radionuclide uptake at the site of a previously demonstrated wandering spleen (Rosenthall, Lisbona and Banerjee, 1974; Figure 17.7). Angiography also demonstrates the spleen definitively, and in anticipation of surgery can indicate the site of a vascular torsion and define abdominal vasculature. In the presence of chronic torsion or splenic vein compression, solitary gastric varices may be seen (Smulewicz and Clemett, 1975).

By ultrasound, an echogenic 'mass' is identified lying away from the left upper quadrant, with a peripheral indentation representing the splenic hilum. Decreased echogenicity of the spleen may be seen with infarction and necrosis secondary to torsion, and a complex mass may be seen with superimposed infection (Kelly, Chusid and Camitta, 1982). On CT, the spleen will be seen in an abnormal position, and a portion of the spleen or the entire organ may appear of low density in the presence of torsion with infarction (Toback, Steece and Kaye, 1984; Figure 17.8).

Overall, nuclear scintigraphy or ultrasound are probably the studies of choice for the diagnosis of a suspected wandering spleen. If there is no uptake of radionuclide on nuclear scan, as in torsion, ultrasound will identify the spleen. CT may be necessary if the spleen is obscured by bowel gas on ultrasound. If the diagnosis is still unclear, angiography may be indicated (Sheflin, Chung and Kretchmar, 1984).

17.2.2 ACCESSORY SPLEEN

'Accessory spleen' refers to a small body of splenic tissue of congenital origin, which is separate from the main body of the spleen and which may be ectopic in location. It is frequently discovered incidentally on radiological examination, particularly on CT. Accessory splenic tissue may be discovered by nuclear

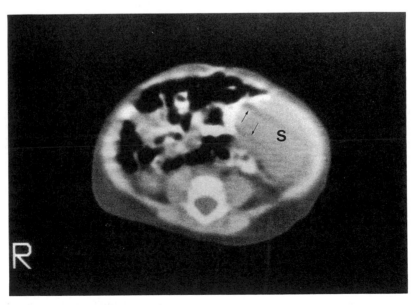

Figure 17.8 Wandering spleen on CT scan. Same case as Figure 17.7. Transverse section of the lower abdomen without IV contrast. Note absence of the liver or kidneys on this section, indicating that the spleen (S) lies much lower in the abdomen than normal. The spleen is somewhat 'plump', suggesting the presence of engorgement secondary to torsion of the vascular pedicle. No low density areas are identified within the spleen to suggest the presence of infarction. (The linear bands seen coursing through the spleen represent artifacts (arrows).)

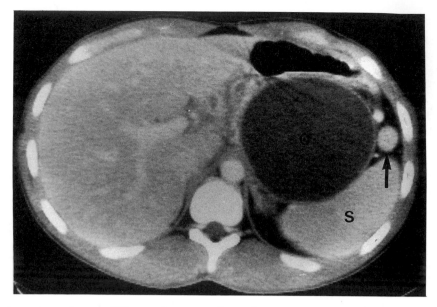

Figure 17.9 Accessory spleen on CT scan. Contrast-enhanced transverse section through the upper abdomen. A normal spleen (S) is seen in the usual position. A small focus of tissue measuring 2–3 cm in diameter is seen just anterior to the spleen (arrow), and was found to be an accessory spleen. A large, cystic structure (C) is seen just anterior to the spleen, which represents a manifestation of this patient's undifferentiated pancreatic carcinoma.

scintigraphy, ultrasound, CT or angiography, especially when hypertrophied following splenectomy (Figures 17.9–17.11). In subjects with intact spleens, accessory spleens are usually less than 2.5 cm in diameter as measured by CT and ultrasound (Beahrs and Stephens, 1980; Subramanyam, Balthazar and Horii, 1984). When hypertrophied following splenectomy, they may measure 3–5 cm in size. Differential diagnosis of an accessory spleen on CT and ultrasound depends on its location. Diagnosis can usually be made with confidence when the patient is asymptomatic and the tissue is located in the splenic hilus. However, location of the nodule of splenic tissue elsewhere in the left upper quadrant or abdomen may simulate a mass involving the pancreas, kidney, adrenal or other organ, and further diagnostic studies may be indicated to exclude the presence of a neoplasm. In such cases, nuclear scintigraphy using ^{99m}Technetium-sulfur colloid is diagnostic, demonstrating the presence of functioning splenic tissue in the area of concern. While the vascular supply was formerly demonstrated using arteriography (Clark, Korobkin and Palubinskas, 1972; Kaude, 1973), ultrasound appears to be capable of demonstrating the relationship of the accessory spleen to a splenic artery and vein in a large number of cases (Subramanyam, Balthazar and Horii, 1984).

17.2.3   SPLENIC–GONADAL FUSION

This is a rare congenital anomaly, usually found in males, which consists of ectopic splenic tissue in close association with the left gonad, sometimes with an abnormal connection between the left gonad and the spleen. The diagnosis is usually made postoperatively, following surgery for suspected gonadal neoplasm (Bearss, 1980; Ceccacci and Tosi, 1981). Ultrasound is frequently performed as an early study of a scrotal mass, and in the appropriate clinical setting, it is possible to suspect the diagnosis on

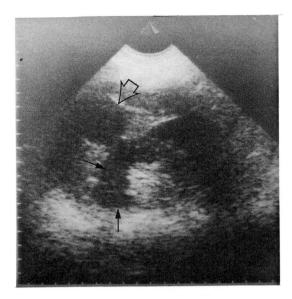

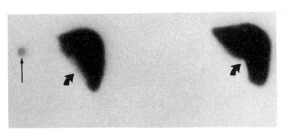

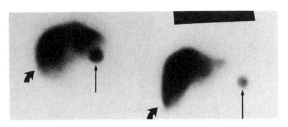

Figure 17.10 Accessory spleen on ultrasound. Scan of the left upper quadrant in a coronal plane demonstrates the presence of a normal left kidney (arrows). At the superolateral aspect of the left kidney, a spherical soft tissue mass of homogeneous echogenicity (open arrow) is seen. This structure demonstrates the same echo pattern as a normal spleen, and was found to represent an accessory spleen on 99mTechnetium-sulfur colloid scan. (See Figure 17.11.)

Figure 17.11 Accessory spleen on 99mTechnetium sulfur colloid scan. (Same case as Figure 17.10.) This patient has a past history of splenectomy. There is normal, homogeneous radionuclide uptake in the liver (curved arrows). A small focus of radionuclide uptake measuring several centimeters in diameter is seen in the left upper quadrant, representing an accessory spleen (straight arrows).

the basis of this study. The mass will probably have the scintigraphic characteristics of splenic tissue, such as accessory spleen, and 99mTechnetium-sulfur colloid scintigraphy may be diagnostic, demonstrating a focal area of uptake in close association with the left testicle (Mandell *et al.*, 1983; Guarin, Dimitrieva and Ashley, 1975).

17.2.4 ASPLENIA AND POLYSPLENIA SYNDROMES

In asplenia, or congenital absence of the spleen, there is usually a wide range of other congenital abnormalities, principally taking the form of situs ambiguous with bilateral right-sidedness. It occurs predominantly in males. Absence of the spleen only, as in vascular occlusion or

thrombosis, is thought to be an acquired abnormality which is usually found without other associated anomalies (Monie, 1982; Figure 17.12).

Radiographically, manifestations of the asplenia syndrome are as wide-ranging as the associated congenital abnormalities. Plain films of the chest and abdomen may demonstrate evidence of bilateral right-sidedness, with ultrasound and CT providing more definitive findings. Nuclear scintigraphy can be useful in demonstrating absence of the spleen, using 99mTechnetium-sulfur colloid, iminodiacetic agents (such as Disida) and tagged red blood cells (Freedom and Fellows, 1973; Rao *et al.*, 1982; Fitzer, 1976; Piepsz *et al.*, 1977; Figure 17.13). If the 99mTechnetium-sulfur colloid scan is equivocal for absence of the spleen, due

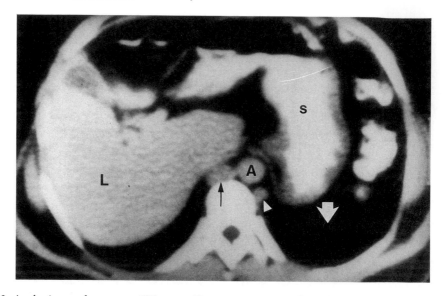

Figure 17.12 Asplenia syndrome on CT scan. Transverse section through the upper abdomen following administration of oral contrast. The spleen is absent from its normal location (white arrow). Scan of the remainder of abdomen and pelvis failed to demonstrate the presence of a spleen. Azygous continuation of the inferior vena cava (black arrow) is seen as an associated vascular anomaly. Stomach (S), liver (L), aorta (A), hemiazygous vein (white arrowhead).

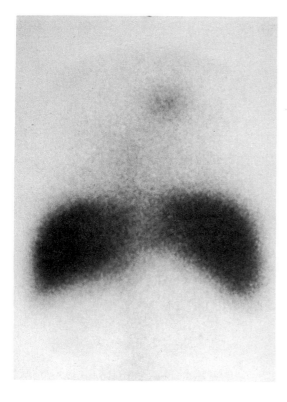

to the presence of bilaterally symmetrical hepatic tissue or a prominent left lobe, a hepatobiliary tract scan can be added to find the full extent of the liver. Angiography is useful for defining the cardiac anomalies and detecting absence of the splenic artery. The entire celiac axis may be absent, with the hepatic artery rising from the superior mesenteric artery (Rao et al., 1982).

In contrast to asplenia, polysplenia takes the form of multiple small masses of splenic tissue with features of bilateral left-sidedness and is seen predominantly in females. Like asplenia, polysplenia is associated with anomalies of other

Figure 17.13 Asplenia syndrome in a 27-month-old female with congenital heart disease. [99m]Technetium-sulfur colloid scan demonstrates the presence of homogeneous, bilaterally symmetrical radionuclide uptake in the upper abdomen. This radionuclide uptake is present in the liver, indicating the presence of bilateral right-sidedness and absence of the spleen.

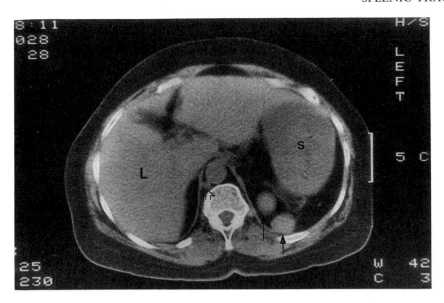

Figure 17.14. Polysplenia syndrome on CT scan. Transverse section of the upper abdomen obtained without intravenous contrast. Two small, round densities measuring approximately 2 cm in diameter are seen in the usual location of the spleen (arrows). No other splenic tissue was identified within the abdomen. These small soft tissue masses were found to represent splenic tissue in a patient with polysplenia. Again, note the enlarged caliber of the azygous vein (open arrow) in this patient with azygous continuation of the IVC as an associated anomaly. Stomach (S), Liver (L).

systems (Rose, Izukawa and Moes, 1975; Moller *et al.*, 1967; Rahimtoola, Marshall and Edwards, 1965; Van Mierop, Gessner and Schiebler, 1972). Radiographic findings are variable, depending on the congenital anomalies present. Again, radionuclide imaging and angiography can be used to demonstrate the multiple spleens in the upper quadrants, ranging in number from a few to as many as 16 (Peoples, Moller and Edwards, 1983). However, CT and ultrasound may be the best imaging methods for demonstrating the multiple features of this syndrome (Figure 17.14).

17.3 SPLENIC TRAUMA

The spleen is probably the most commonly injured organ in cases of blunt trauma to the abdomen (Stivelman, Glaubitz and Crampton, 1963). The main concern following trauma to the spleen is the possibility of splenic rupture, which is associated with a mortality of more than 75% if surgery is not performed promptly (Delany and Jason, 1981). Radiography has come to play an important role in the early diagnosis of splenic injury. With the realization of the important role of the spleen in preventing infection, it has become important to determine not only the presence of injury, but also the exact extent of the injury, to allow conservative surgical management when possible. While blunt abdominal trauma is the most common cause of splenic injury, iatrogenic injury is not uncommon, including injury during surgery, thoracentesis and left renal biopsy (Pachter, Hofstetter and Spencer, 1981; Rauch *et al.*, 1983).

17.3.1 PLAIN FILM

With intraparenchymal or subcapsular bleeding, plain radiographs may demonstrate evidence of splenic enlargement with medial displacement of the gastric air bubble and inferior displacement of the splenic flexure of the colon. Elevation of the left hemidiaphragm may also be seen. Significant splenic injury, such as laceration and rupture, is frequently associated with rib fracture and left pleural effusion (Figure 17.15). Hemoperitoneum due to splenic rupture may lead to an appearance of the abdomen simulating ascites, with diffusely increased density throughout. However, due to frequently poor visualization of the spleen even in normal patients, plain films can usually only be sugges-

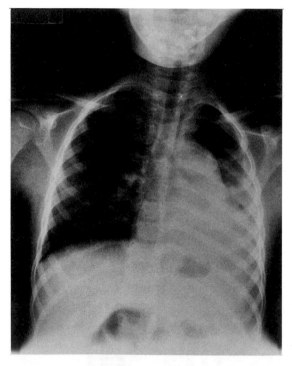

Figure 17.15 Plain film findings in the presence of splenic laceration. This patient suffered trauma to the left upper quadrant of the abdomen. The left costophrenic angle and left heart margin are obscured by a left pleural effusion. No rib fractures can be identified on this film. This patient was found to have a splenic laceration on follow-up studies.

tive of splenic trauma, and additional radiographic examination must be performed for definitive diagnosis. Evidence of previous splenic trauma may be detected on plain films in the form of calcification of old hematomas.

17.3.2 ULTRASOUND

Ultrasound and CT have come to assume much of the role of imaging in splenic trauma previously played by angiography and nuclear scintigraphy. Ultrasound can be very accurate in the diagnosis of splenic trauma, and may be very useful in situations in which a CT scanner is not immediately available. In addition, trauma involving other organs can be easily evaluated. Ultrasound can also be used to follow patients who are clinically stable and managed conservatively.

The appearance of a collection of blood on ultrasound, whether intracapsular or extracapsular, depends on the time of the examination relative to the time of injury. Immediately following trauma, a collection of blood is still liquid and may be easily differentiated from splenic tissue. However, after the blood clots, it may be very similar in echogenicity to the normal spleen for up to 48 hours or more. After several days, the blood collection begins to reliquefy and may again become more apparent. (Cooperberg, 1987).

In the presence of an intraparenchymal or subcapsular hematoma of the spleen without rupture of the capsule, the appearance on subacute examination is that of a focal inhomogeneous area within or at the periphery of the spleen (Figures 17.16 and 17.17). Subsequent scans may show clearing of this inhomogeneity, leading to the presence of a relatively anechoic, cystic structure representing the resolving hematoma (Lupien and Sauerbrei, 1984). These anechoic fluid collections may then decrease in size and disappear, or leave a small scar manifested as an echogenic line.

Rupture of the splenic capsule leads to intraperitoneal bleeding, which may be found as massive hemoperitoneum in the seriously injured

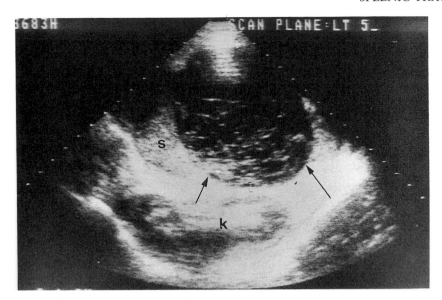

Figure 17.16 Splenic hematoma on ultrasound. Scan through the left upper quadrant in a coronal plane demonstrates a large area of mixed echogenicity measuring approximately 7 cm in diameter (arrows) at the inferior margin of the spleen (S). This region of mixed echogenicity represents a hematoma in the subacute stage of evolution. Irregular anechoic, hypoechoic and hyperechoic areas are seen within the hematoma, which has a well-defined margin. These anechoic areas will coalesce to form a relatively anechoic, cystic structure on follow-up scans. The left kidney (k) is also seen.

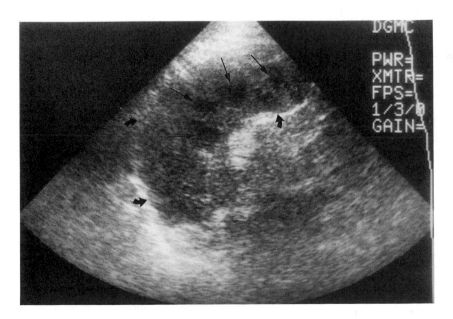

Figure 17.17 Splenic hematoma on ultrasound. View of the left upper quadrant in a coronal plane demonstrates the spleen to be relatively normal in size and contour (curved arrows). Intraparenchymal splenic hemorrhage in a subacute stage is seen as multiple hypoechoic areas (straight arrows). Again, these hypoechoic areas will become anechoic and may coalesce as the hemorrhage resolves.

patient, or as a more focal perisplenic hematoma. With a free hemoperitoneum, a fluid collection may be found distant from the spleen, in the left upper quadrant or elsewhere. While free intraperitoneal spread of blood is common, the blood occasionally becomes walled-off in the left upper quadrant and is seen as a large fluid collection or mass having irregular echogenicity. A smaller perisplenic hematoma may be seen as a focal area of inhomogeneous echogenicity adjacent to the spleen. Again, these fluid collections will undergo evolution, and may appear on subsequent scans as cystic structures adjacent to the spleen. A focal perisplenic hematoma can mimic a perisplenic abscess.

17.3.3 COMPUTED TOMOGRAPHY

CT has become established as an important means of evaluating splenic trauma in the stable patient, determining not only the presence of splenic injury but also its extent and the presence of injury in other organs. With the information obtained from CT, the surgeon can better decide between splenectomy and splenorrhaphy. A 96% accuracy for CT in diagnosing splenic trauma was observed by Jeffrey *et al.* (1981) in a prospective study: a normal CT virtually excludes significant splenic injury.

The severity of the injury determines whether radiological studies such as CT can be performed prior to surgery. With severe injury, where surgery seems necessary immediately, peritoneal lavage may be used to confirm hemoperitoneum prior to surgery. However, if there is time to perform CT, peritoneal lavage should be omitted or delayed; CT can identify a hemoperitoneum, as well as define other organ injury, and CT performed after peritoneal lavage may lead to uncertainty as to whether the intraperitoneal fluid is due to the trauma or the lavage.

As with ultrasound, the appearance of a hematoma on CT changes with time (Korobkin *et al.*, 1978; Moss *et al.*, 1979). Immediately

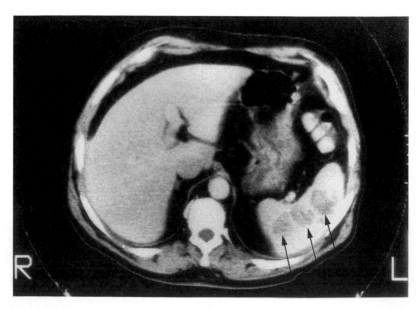

Figure 17.18 Splenic hematoma on CT. Transverse section through the upper abdomen obtained following administration of IV contrast. Several areas of low density are seen within the central portion of the spleen (arrows), representing intraparenchymal splenic hematomas. Note that these hematomas are relatively well-defined.

following injury, the hematoma is usually iso-dense with the spleen on non-contrast scan, and may only be detectable by causing abnormality of the splenic contour. Such hematomas become apparent on a contrast-enhanced scan as focal areas lacking contrast enhancement. With evolution of the hematoma, the blood components are broken down, leading to a decrease in hemoglobin content, and the hematoma becomes hypodense (Figure 17.18). It is clear that evaluation of acute splenic trauma requires intravenous contrast studies.

Subcapsular hematomas on contrast-enhanced CT are seen as peripheral areas of low density and may cause flattening of the splenic contour. Perisplenic hematomas are identified as low-density fluid collections surrounding the spleen. Splenic lacerations appear as low density bands with associated parenchymal defects, usually involving the lateral aspect of the spleen

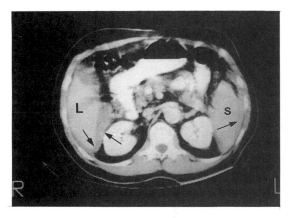

Figure 17.19 Free intraperitoneal blood associated with a fractured spleen. Transverse CT section obtained through the mid-abdomen following the administration of IV contrast. The spleen (S) and liver (L) are identified. Low density fluid is seen in a perisplenic location and in Morrison's pouch (arrows), representing free intraperitoneal blood. The splenic fracture cannot be identified on this image.

and having associated free intraperitoneal blood (Jeffrey *et al.*, 1981; Figure 17.19).

Anatomical variants of splenic anatomy may cause pitfalls in the evaluation of splenic trauma. For example, exaggerated splenic lobulation may form a 'cleft' or 'fissure' in the spleen and may be confused with laceration following trauma. However, an otherwise normal appearance of the spleen, with a thin linear configuration to the cleft and absence of intraperitoneal fluid, will usually lead to the correct diagnosis (Jeffrey *et al.*, 1981).

17.3.4   ANGIOGRAPHY

With the advent of CT and ultrasound, angiography has become less important to the diagnosis of splenic trauma. Angiography, however, continues to play an important role in identifying the exact sites of vascular injury and bleeding in the spleen. Splenectomy can be avoided in many instances by employing the various methods of angiographic occlusion of bleeding sites, including vasopressin infusion and therapeutic embolization using steel coils or Gelfoam particles. In this way, surgical morbidity can be avoided and functioning splenic tissue retained.

If angiography is performed following splenic injury, many signs of injury may be seen. Extravasation of contrast material is one of the more reliable signs of vascular laceration, especially if the extravasation is large. Extravasations may be intra- or extrasplenic, and are frequently ill-defined; however, they may be well-defined if associated with hematoma or pseudoaneurysm formation. Evidence of extravasation is usually seen early in the arterial phase of the angiogram. Other less common and less reliable signs of vascular injury include venous shunting (early venous filling). Multiple small arterial extravasations may produce mottling of the parenchymal phase. Amputated vessels due to spasm, transection, or thrombosis may be seen. Bowing or stretching of vessels around an avascular area is a reliable sign of hematoma. Linear or wedge-shaped defects in the parenchymal phase may be seen with splenic laceration and distal arterial occlusion, respectively (Delany and Jason, 1981). Displacement of the spleen from the chest wall by a lens-shaped peripheral avascular zone suggests the presence of subcapsular hematoma (Osborn *et al.*, 1973). Following penetrating injury, vascular occlusion and parenchymal defects predominate, rather than extravasation (Haertel and Ryder, 1979). In addition, angiography may reveal pseudoaneurysm formation or rupture, or formation of arteriovenous fistulae, as late complications of splenic trauma.

17.3.5 NUCLEAR MEDICINE

Like angiography, nuclear scintigraphy has also yielded to CT and ultrasound in the diagnosis of splenic trauma. Formerly, nuclear scintigraphy using ^{99m}Technetium-sulfur colloid was the procedure of choice in splenic trauma (Lutzker *et al.*, 1973), the signs of splenic trauma including linear, wedge-shaped and stellate intraparenchymal defects. Subcapsular hematoma may be seen as a concave defect along the splenic contour (Nesbesar, Rabinov and Potsaid, 1974). The fractured spleen may show a

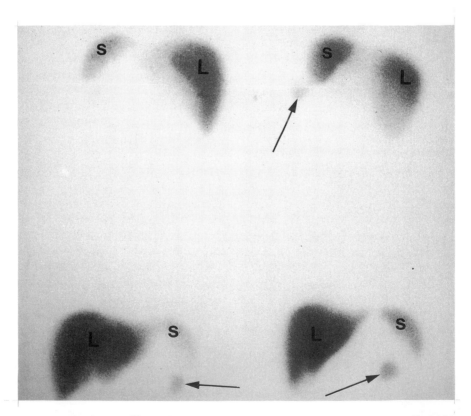

Figure 17.20 Fractured spleen on ^{99m}Technetium-sulfur colloid scan. This patient has suffered blunt trauma to the abdomen. Multiple views demonstrate homogeneous uptake of the radionuclide in the liver (L) and spleen (S). A small focus of uptake appears to be slightly displaced from the main body of the spleen (arrows), and was found at surgery to represent a small portion of splenic tissue which had been fractured away from the main body of the spleen.

linear defect, or a portion of splenic tissue may be displaced from the main body of the spleen (Figure 17.20).

With the recent improvement in instrumentation and availability of ultrasound and CT, reliance on these modalities for imaging in splenic trauma has increased. However, in rare instances, nuclear scintigraphy may still be useful, for example, in a patient with skin injury, which makes ultrasound difficult, and in whom contrast allergy and patient motion make the CT scan impractical.

17.3.6 SPLENOSIS

Splenosis is the result of autotransplantation of splenic tissue to ectopic sites following splenic rupture or penetrating injuries such as a gunshot wound. The nodules of splenic tissue may implant almost anywhere in the peritoneum, and may be found in the thorax following diaphragmatic penetration or tear (Dillion, Koster and Coy, 1977; Nielsen, 1981; Dalton, Strange and Downs, 1971). Patients having this condition are virtually all asymptomatic, with the splenosis frequently detected incidentally during radiological evaluation for an unrelated problem. For example, splenosis in the abdomen may be detected as multiple small masses on CT or as extrinsic masses on examination of the GI tract. In the thorax, CT or plain chest film may demonstrate the presence of a small, pleural-based soft tissue nodule. The nodules are usually multiple and small, ranging from several millimeters to several centimeters in size, and rarely larger than 3 cm (Nielsen, 1981). Differential diagnosis includes metastases in both the chest and abdomen, as well as endometriosis, hemangiomas and accessory spleens in the abdomen.

On CT scan, detection of multiple masses in the chest or abdomen demonstrating contrast-enhancement similar to splenic tissue may suggest the diagnosis. In patients with a known history of splenic trauma or surgery in which the diagnosis is suspected, confirmation can be obtained by radionuclide scan using either

[99m]Technetium-sulfur colloid or tagged, damaged red blood cells.

17.4 FOCAL DISEASE

17.4.1 CYSTS

Cystic lesions of the spleen have a varied etiology, and include the 'true' cyst containing an epithelial lining and believed to be congenital in origin, the 'false' cyst which is probably post-traumatic, and other less common lesions such as cystic neoplasms and parasitic cysts (McClure and Altemeier, 1942; Fowler, 1953). On radiographic examination, a large usually solitary splenic mass is identified in the left upper quadrant of the abdomen. While these are most commonly found in patients in the second or third decade (Sirinek and Evans, 1973), they may also be discovered in children (Griscom et al., 1977). Plain film may demonstrate evidence of a large left upper quadrant mass, with displacement of the gastric air bubble or elevation of the left hemidiaphragm (Figures 17.21 and 17.22). Curvilinear calcification may suggest the presence of a cystic structure, and has been found to occur in up to 25% of post-traumatic cysts (Denneen, 1942). It is less common in true cysts (Propper et al., 1979; Figure 17.23a).

On [99m]Technetium-sulfur colloid scintigraphy, a splenic cyst will be seen as a large photopenic zone representing the mass, often partially surrounded by a crescent of normal but compressed spleen (Figure 17.24). Barium study of the gastrointestinal tract may demonstrate dextrad displacement of the stomach, and possibly some inferior displacement of the splenic flexure of the colon. Such displacement of adjacent organs is common, as splenic cysts have been found in recent studies to average 10 cm in diameter (Garvin and King, 1981).

By CT a splenic cyst appears as a large, well-defined, non-enhancing, near-water density lesion having a smooth wall; however, there are few reports of the CT characteristics of these lesions (Davidson, Campbell and Hersh, 1980;

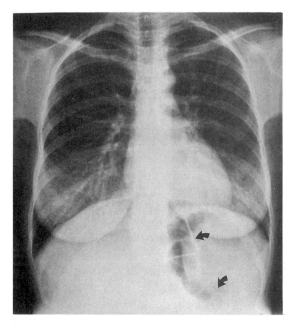

Figure 17.21 'True' cyst of the spleen on plain film. Chest X-ray demonstrates a left upper quadrant mass with displacement of the gastric bubble and air-filled splenic flexure to the midline (arrows). This mass corresponded to a 'true' cyst of the spleen.

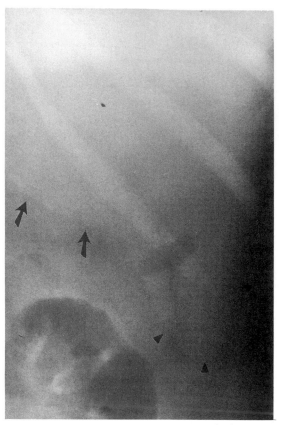

Figure 17.22 'True' cyst of the spleen on plain film. 'Tip of the spleen' sign. Localized view of the left upper quadrant demonstrates an enlarged spleen. The lower margin of the spleen suggests the presence of a large mass (arrows) as well as an intact inferior splenic tip (arrowheads). The identification of a normal appearing splenic tip suggests a discrete mass rather than splenomegaly. In splenomegaly the entire spleen is enlarged and a normal tip of the spleen cannot be identified. (Reproduced with permission from Dachman *et al.* (1986) *Am. J. Radiol.*, **147**, 537–42.)

Figure 17.23 'False' cyst of spleen by multiple imaging modalities. (a) Localized view of the left upper quadrant in a supine plain film of the abdomen demonstrates a curvilinear calcification (arrows). Calcification in a splenic cyst has a peripheral distribution. (b) Axial enhanced computed tomographic section in the same patient demonstrates a fluid density in the spleen corresponding to a 'false' or post-traumatic cyst (C). Observe the rim-like calcification (arrows) located in the periphery of the cyst and corresponding pathologically to calcification in the fibrous wall. These calcifications correspond to the findings seen in plain film (a). (c) Selective splenic artery injection during angiography demonstrates a large avascular zone in the spleen, corresponding to the plain film and CT findings. Note the stretching of the vessels around the cyst (arrows).

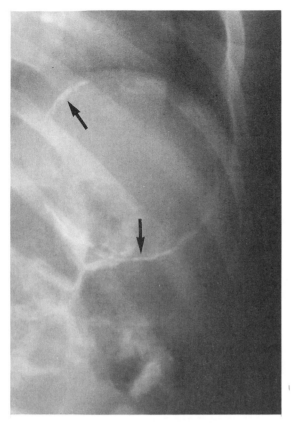

(a)

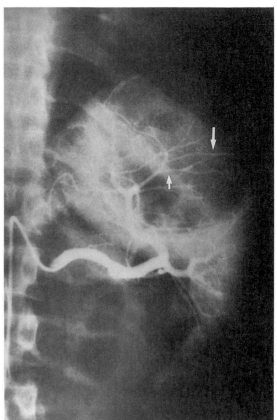

(c)

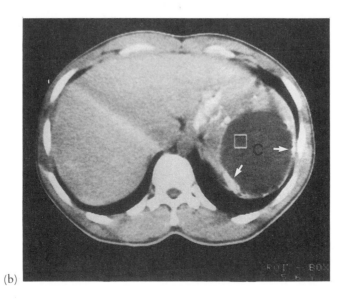

(b)

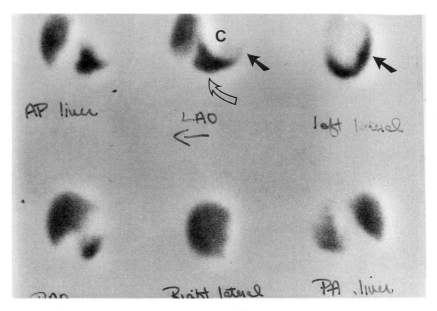

Figure 17.24 'True' cyst of the spleen on scintigraphy. [99m]Technetium-sulfur colloid scintigraphy demonstrates a large defect in the spleen (C), corresponding to the cyst, surrounded by a crescent of normal compressed splenic tissue (arrows). Note the normal tip of the spleen (open arrow), correlating with plain film findings demonstrated in Figure 17.22.

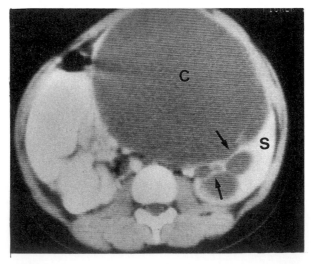

Figure 17.25 'True' cyst of the spleen on CT. There is a large fluid density (water) structure with smooth inner walls and homogeneous appearance (C). A small portion of normal appearing spleen with high density in this enhanced CT is noted (S). Note few trabeculations or septations (arrows). Septations are more commonly seen in 'true' cysts than in 'false' cysts. Observe how the cyst crosses the midline. This suggests the slow growing nature of 'true' cysts of the spleen and makes more aggressive lesions of the spleen (such as metastases, which may appear cystic) less likely.

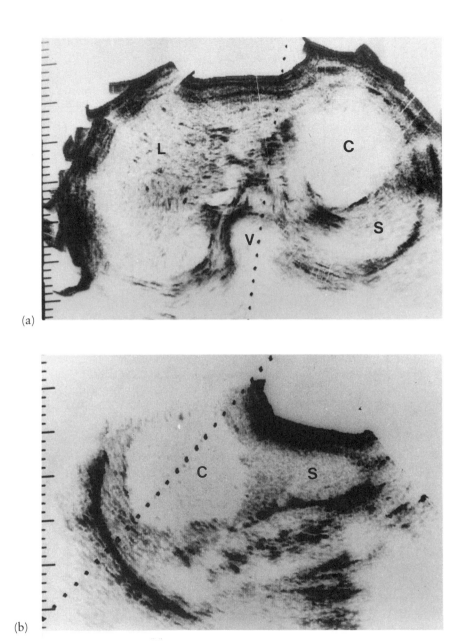

(a)

(b)

Figure 17.26 'True' cyst of the spleen on ultrasound. (a) Transverse view of the upper abdomen demonstrates a large anechoic area in the left upper quadrant (C). The liver (L), vertebral body (V) and the rest of the spleen (S) can also be identified. (b) In the same patient a longitudinal view again demonstrates an anechoic area in the upper portion of the spleen corresponding to a large 'true' cyst of the spleen (C). Note the tip of the normal spleen inferior to the cyst (S).

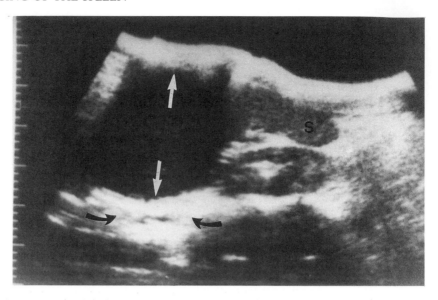

Figure 17.27 'True' cyst of the spleen on ultrasound. Note a large, well-defined anechoic area (white arrows) with smooth walls and increased echogenicity in its back wall (curved arrows). In addition, a normal tip of the spleen can be identified, suggesting splenic mass rather than splenomegaly (S).

Faer *et al.*, 1980; Shin and Ho, 1983; Piekarski, Federle and Moss, 1980; Figure 17.23b). It is usually found in a subcapsular location, but approximately one-third are located deep within the spleen. Although approximately 80% are solitary and unilocular, 20% are multiple or multilocular (Doolas *et al.*, 1978), and the septa may be visible on CT (Figure 17.25). The cyst walls are often trabeculated pathologically, and this trabeculation may also be seen (Dachman *et al.*, 1986). While the cyst may have the classic appearance on CT of a low (water) density structure, the presence of blood or other material within the cyst may give it a more complex appearance. The differential diagnosis on the basis of CT should include a large abscess or hematoma, cystic neoplasm or even echinococcal cyst if multiseptated. Pancreatic pseudocyst directly adjacent to, or (rarely) within, the spleen is also a possibility.

Ultrasound is also useful for identifying the splenic origin of the cyst, as well as in distinguishing cystic from solid or complex lesions (Wright and Williams, 1974). On ultrasound, a simple cyst is seen as a focal, usually well-defined area containing no echoes (anechoic). In addition, it demonstrates excellent transmission of the ultrasound waves to structures deep to the cyst, and increased echogenicity of the cyst wall furthest from the ultrasound transducer, or so-called 'back wall enhancement' (Figures 17.26a, b and 17.27). As on CT, trabeculation of the wall or septation may be seen, as well as wall calcification (Dachman *et al.*, 1986; Figure 17.28).

Angiography shows a large avascular zone with draping or stretching of vessels around the cyst (Figures 17.23c and 17.29). The splenic vessels are intrinsically normal in appearance, with no evidence of neovascularity in benign cysts (Bron and Hoffman, 1971; Shanser *et al.*, 1973). The parenchymal phase may demonstrate compression of the normal splenic tissue. However, CT and ultrasound usually make angiography unnecessary (Davidson, Campbell and Hersh, 1980).

While CT and ultrasound will usually provide the most revealing imaging studies, thin

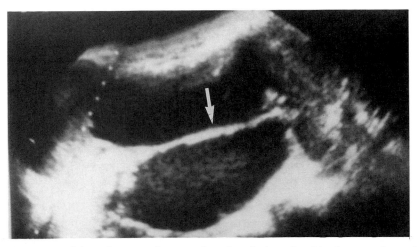

Figure 17.28 'True' cyst of the spleen on ultrasound: trabeculation. On this ultrasound a well-defined, thin septation or trabeculation is seen (white arrow).

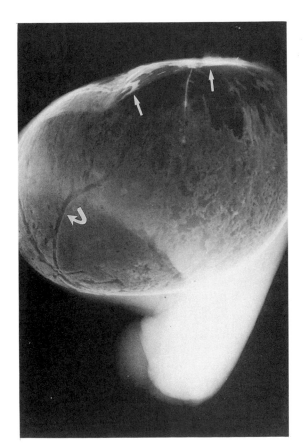

needle aspiration of cystic lesions in the spleen can be performed for diagnosis in equivocal cases, using a 22 gauge needle. However, caution should be used in selecting this procedure when there is the possibility of an echinococcal cyst. Frequently a clinical history of trauma will help differentiate a true cyst from a false cyst, but past trauma may not be reliably recalled by the patient.

17.4.2   SPLENIC ABSCESS

Before 1970, splenic abscess was largely diagnosed by clinical means, with available imaging modalities adding little to early diagnosis. Difficulty in diagnosis resulted in a high mortality. With subsequent widespread availability of

Figure 17.29 'False' cyst of the spleen on specimen radiograph. On this specimen radiograph several of the radiographic features of a splenic cyst can be noted. There is calcification in the periphery of the cyst (white arrows), commonly observed in 'false' cysts of the spleen. Note also stretching of vessels around the cyst (curved white arrow) as well as a tip of normal spleen inferiorly.

ultrasound and CT, the diagnosis of splenic abscess was made more confidently, and early enough to provide effective therapy and reduced mortality. While failure to diagnose this condition is frequently fatal, several studies indicate that early diagnosis and appropriate intervention increase the survival rate to greater than 93% (Lawhorne and Zuidema, 1976; Freund *et al.*, 1982).

Although splenic abscess is relatively uncommon overall, it is more frequent in the chronically debilitated or immunosuppressed, such as patients with malignancies, hematological disorders, endocarditis and diabetes. Commonly, hematogenous seeding from a distant site of infection creates multiple small abscesses throughout the spleen and other organs. Perhaps less common is a solitary splenic abscess seen with hematogenous seeding of a splenic hematoma or infarct, or rarely with inadvertent iatrogenic embolization of the spleen during angiography. Penetrating trauma may also cause a solitary septic lesion.

Plain film findings in splenic abscess are relatively non-specific, but such findings are present in the majority of patients with this condition. Standard frontal and lateral chest radiographs may demonstrate elevation of the left hemidiaphragm, left pleural effusion and left lower lobe infiltrates or atelectasis (Freund *et al.*, 1982; Pawar *et al.*, 1982). However, these findings can be seen in a number of other conditions including pancreatitis and subphrenic abscess. Occasionally, evidence of a left upper quadrant mass may be appreciated on a chest or abdominal film. Splenomegaly may also be evident, but this may be related to the underlying disorder rather than to the abscess itself. A focal adynamic ileus is frequently present in the left upper quadrant. The presence of gas or gas-fluid levels in the spleen is uncommon, but is more specific for the diagnosis if present (Figure 17.30). When splenic abscess is complicated by rupture, fistula formation or bowel obstruction, plain films may be altered accordingly.

Like plain films, contrast studies of the gastrointestinal tract usually demonstrate only indirect

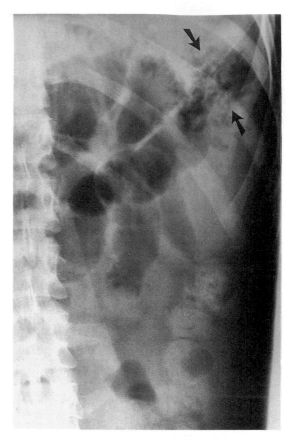

Figure 17.30 Splenic abscess on plain film. Localized view of the left upper quadrant in this supine film of the abdomen demonstrates extraluminal gas in the region of the spleen (arrows). Although extraluminal air in the left upper quadrant is not specific for splenic abscess, when present this diagnosis should be considered and CT of the upper abdomen should be performed to confirm the presence of a splenic abscess.

evidence of splenic abscess. The stomach or colon may be indented extrinsically or displaced. Focal edema, spasm or adynamic ileus of these structures may also be seen, due to the adjacent inflammatory process. Contrast studies of the gastrointestinal tract are principally required for the exclusion of disorders of the stomach or colon which might cause the left upper quadrant symptoms. When splenic abscess is suspected, CT or ultrasound provides

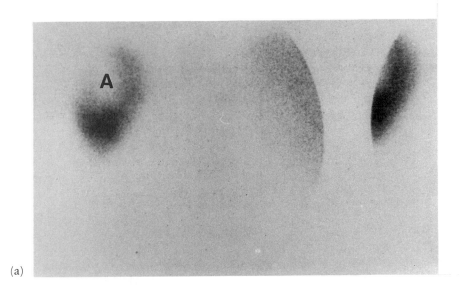

(a)

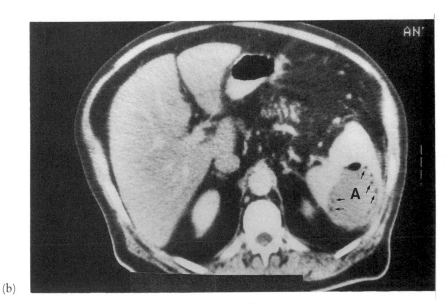

(b)

Figure 17.31 Splenic abscess on scintigraphy and CT. (a) ^{99m}Technetium-sulfur colloid scintigraphy demonstrates a focal defect within the spleen (A). This corresponded to a solitary splenic abscess. (b) CT of the same patient confirms the presence of a solitary lesion in the spleen. Note the presence of small bubbles of gas (arrows) in the periphery of a low density mass representing the abscess (A).

a much higher diagnostic yield and is more specific. Furthermore, prior gastrointestinal studies may compromise further evaluation by CT, particularly if barium is used. On ^{99m}Technetium-sulfur colloid scintigraphy, splenomegaly is a common but non-specific finding. If multiple abscesses are present, patchy, inhomogeneous splenic uptake of radionuclide may be seen. A solitary abscess produces a focal defect within the spleen (Figure 17.31a). In either case, there are multiple differential diagnostic possibilities, and clinical correlation with fever or sepsis aids in the diagnosis. As with any lesion studied by nuclear scintigraphy, lesions smaller than 2 cm in diameter may be missed unless SPECT imaging is utilized. In addition, splenic defects caused by the patient's underlying disease, such as myelofibrosis, or sickle cell disease with infarcts, may make scan interpretation difficult. However, other modalities are now preferred over nuclear scintigraphy in the diagnosis of this condition.

^{67}Gallium citrate has been used as an additional radionuclide for the detection of splenic abscess, often as a secondary study to increase the specificity of the diagnosis (Henkin, 1975). ^{67}Gallium will localize at the site of infection, permitting the detection of lesions which may be equivocal or inapparent in other studies. A focal defect in the spleen on ^{99m}Technetium-sulfur colloid scan caused by an abscess will be seen as a focal area of increased uptake on ^{67}gallium scan. However, an abscess will occasionally demonstrate no gallium uptake as, for example, with an infected infarct (Figure 17.32). Since gallium also localizes in a variety of tumors, distinction between tumor and abscess may at times be difficult.

Like other imaging modalities, angiography has come to have little role to play in the diagnosis of splenic abscess due to the widespread availability of CT and ultrasound. If angiography is performed, an avascular splenic mass associated with splenomegaly is the most common finding. The mass effect created by the abscess may stretch or displace splenic vessel

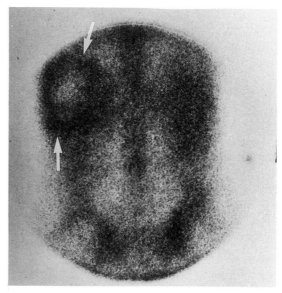

Figure 17.32 Splenic abscess on gallium scintigraphy. There is evidence of increased uptake in the left upper quadrant in this posterior view of the abdomen (white arrows). Note how the area of increased uptake has a central zone of decreased activity giving the impression of a 'crown' or 'doughnut'. This band of increased gallium uptake corresponds to the active zone of the abscess while the central area of liquefactive necrosis shows no activity.

branches. None of the abnormalities commonly seen with neoplastic lesions, such as neovascularity or vessel encasement, are seen. It may be impossible to distinguish an abscess from a wide variety of other avascular splenic lesions, such as cyst, infarct, metastasis or other hypovascular tumors (Jacobs *et al.*, 1974). In the event of splenic rupture secondary to a large abscess, extravasation of contrast material into the spleen or surrounding tissues may occur.

Ultrasound, together with CT, has become one of the principal imaging modalities in suspected splenic abscess. Early in its evolution, a splenic abscess may produce only subtle altera-

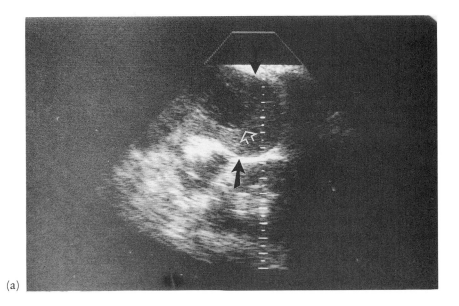

(a)

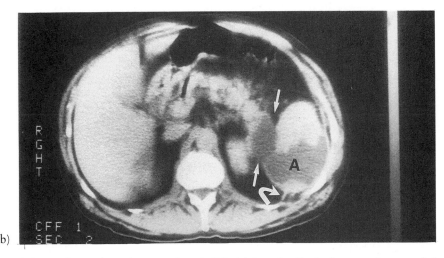

(b)

Figure 17.33 Splenic abscess on ultrasound and CT. (a) Longitudinal ultrasound scan of the left upper quadrant demonstrates a spleen (arrows) with an area of decreased echogenicity (white open arrow). Note the irregular internal wall of the abscess as well as the presence of scattered internal echoes corresponding to cellular debris and necrotic tissue. (b) In the same patient, enhanced computed tomography demonstrates an area of decreased density with irregular contours within the spleen (A). Note the extrasplenic extension of the abscess (arrows) into the hilus of the spleen and the region of the tail of the pancreas. Note also the thickening of the lateral conal fascia (curved arrow) suggesting perisplenic inflammation.

tions in the echogenicity of splenic tissue. In the presence of multiple small abscesses, ill-defined patchy areas of increased and decreased echogenicity may be seen diffusely throughout the spleen; these may coalesce and become more well-defined with time. With a solitary abscess, similar changes will be seen in a single area. Later in its development, a focal abscess will be seen as an irregular area of decreased echogenicity (Figure 17.33a). Septations and scattered internal echoes representing necrotic tissue, blood and other debris are often seen. Through-transmission is therefore less than that found with simple cyst (Pawar *et al.*, 1982; Ralls *et al.*, 1982). Distinguishing an abscess from a resolving hematoma may present difficulties.

The presence of multiple intrasplenic gas collections may compromise ultrasound examination of a splenic abscess, since gas appears intensely echogenic, and blocks through-transmission of the ultrasound beam. As mentioned previously, bowel gas in the left upper quadrant may also interfere with the examination, making CT scanning necessary (Moss *et al.*, 1980). In addition, very small lesions or lesions in the superior portion of the spleen may be missed.

Computed tomography is an excellent means of demonstrating splenic abscess, especially when ultrasound is equivocal or difficult due to presence of surrounding bowel gas. On CT, a splenic abscess is seen as an irregular area of low density which may be localized but which frequently replaces most of the normal splenic parenchyma (Figures 17.33b and 17.34). While gas is present in only a small number of splenic abscesses, it is easily seen on CT and may even be seen in the splenic or portal vein (Figure 17.31b). Evidence of inflammatory changes is frequently seen in tissues surrounding the abscess. While splenic abscesses are often poorly defined, use of IV contrast and appropriate CT imaging technique will frequently accentuate the subtle findings. Opacification of stomach and bowel with contrast is also crucial for

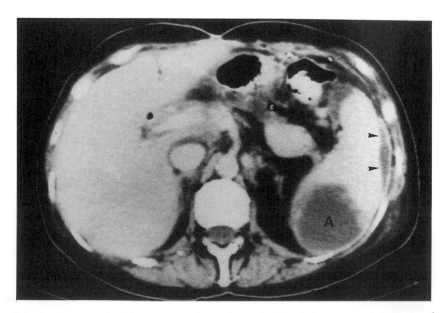

Figure 17.34 Splenic abscess on CT. Note on this enhanced CT of the upper abdomen a focal area of decreased density with irregular inner walls in the posterior portion of the spleen, corresponding to an abscess (A). Note in addition the subcapsular extension of the abscess (arrowheads). Perisplenic extension of an abscess is common and can be nicely detected by CT.

accurate diagnosis, as non-opacified bowel loops in a perisplenic location may lead to false-positive diagnoses or confusion in diagnosis.

CT has become the imaging modality of choice at many institutions for the diagnosis of abscess in any part of the body, and it provides a reliable method for follow-up. Whereas abscess of the spleen has been considered a surgical problem in the past, needle aspiration to confirm the diagnosis followed by percutaneous drainage using CT or ultrasound guidance, has been increasingly accepted and performed in recent years.

17.4.3 LYMPHOMA

Lymphomatous involvement of the spleen as a manifestation of systemic lymphoma is common, whereas primary splenic lymphoma is relatively uncommon. Lymphoma in the spleen characteristically involves the white pulp, frequently appearing as nodules (Burke, 1961). In advanced disease, the entire spleen may be replaced by tumor (Kim and Dorfman, 1974). Ahmann *et al.* (1966) described four categories of splenic lymphoma on gross pathology: (1) homogeneous enlargement without masses, (2) miliary masses, (3) 2–10 cm masses, and (4) a large solitary mass. However, it is important to realize that the spleen may be entirely normal in both cut section and size, with tumor cells seen only microscopically. (See also Chapter 15.)

The radiographic diagnosis of splenic lymphoma is often difficult due to the wide range of presentation, and the possibility of a normal appearance of the spleen despite the presence of tumor. No single imaging modality, including ultrasound (Carroll, 1982) and CT (Glazer *et al.*, 1981), has proved to be very accurate in diagnosis. However, there is interest in the possibility of more accurate radiological splenic evaluation, in order to avoid splenectomy and postsplenectomy infectious complications in patients with stage I and II clinical disease.

As a rule, splenomegaly is not a reliable sign of lymphomatous involvement. Although splenomegaly in most patients with non-Hodgkin's lymphoma indicates splenic involvement, up to one-third of patients with splenomegaly have no evidence of splenic lymphoma on histologic examination (Carroll, 1982). In addition, up to one-third of patients with lymphoma of any kind will have histologic involvement of the spleen in the absence of splenomegaly. Thus, radiographic demonstration of splenomegaly can only suggest or support a diagnosis of splenic involvement. Greater accuracy in the diagnosis of splenic lymphoma can be obtained with both CT and ultrasound by demonstrating adenopathy in the splenic hilum or focal splenic defects, in addition to splenomegaly (Carroll and Ta, 1980). Furthermore, demonstration of liver involvement indicates a high probability of splenic involvement, even if no splenic abnormalities can be identified radiographically (Carroll, 1982).

On ultrasound, lymphomatous involvement of the spleen is usually seen as single or multiple inhomogeneous, hypoechoic, nodular lesions of variable size (Carroll and Ta, 1980; Carroll, 1982). These lesions are often poorly defined. As described above, a single, large lesion involving most of the spleen or multiple smaller lesions may be seen (Figures 17.35 and 17.36). Lymphoma appearing as focal anechoic or hypoechoic defects can simulate an abscess (Castellino *et al.*, 1972; Cunningham, 1978; Bloom *et al.*, 1981) and may cause diagnostic difficulty in the individual with clinical features of abscess. Hyperechoic lesions have also been described (Carroll and Ta, 1980; Carroll, 1982). As described earlier, CT is susceptible to the same difficulties in identifying microscopic or diffuse splenic disease as ultrasound and other modalities. In diagnosing lymphoma at any site in the body, CT is least effective in identifying early disease, as microscopic infiltration may be seen in nodes of normal size or borderline enlargement. In more-advanced disease, the nodes may be unequivocally enlarged. In lymphomatous involvement of the spleen, contrast enhanced CT usually demonstrates inhomogeneous lesions of decreased density and variable size, either solitary or multiple (Figures

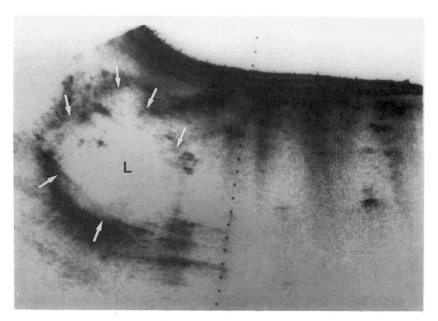

Figure 17.35 Splenic lymphoma on ultrasound. On this longitudinal, parasagittal scan of the left upper quadrant, an irregular, large area of decreased echogenicity can be seen (L) within the spleen. The mass is poorly defined (arrows) and markedly hypoechoic. There is no definite acoustic enhancement. The lack of acoustic enhancement suggests that the lesion is not cystic but solid. However, because of the marked hypoechogenicity of lymphoma, differentiation from cystic lesions such as abscess, cyst or necrotic metastases may be difficult.

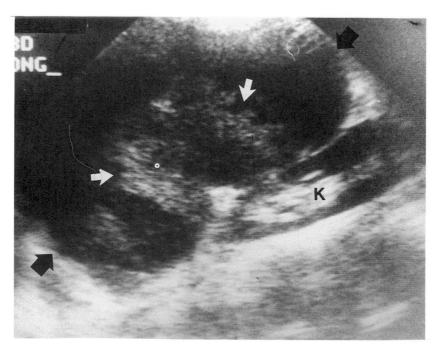

Figure 17.36 Splenic lymphoma on ultrasound. Lymphoma of the spleen can also appear with a hyperechoic pattern, as in this case. Note the markedly enlarged spleen (large arrows) with an irregular hyperechoic zone (white arrows) that corresponded to a mass of lymphoma. In addition, note how the left kidney is slightly compressed due to the splenomegaly (K).

17.37 and 17.38). As with ultrasound, the appearance can mimic an abscess, and the distinction may have to depend on clinical findings.

If the spleen is diffusely involved, some focal areas of low density may represent infarcts or hematomas. Some authors feel that abnormality of the spleen on CT is more likely to occur in non-Hodgkin's lymphoma (Koehler, 1983). CT using new contrast agents such as Ethiodol-oil-emulsion-13 (EOE-13) have demonstrated greater accuracy in the diagnosis of splenic lymphoma manifested as focal defects (Thomas *et al.*, 1982), and such agents may come to play a greater role in the future.

[99m]Technetium-sulfur colloid scintigraphy shows splenic lymphoma as solitary or multiple photopenic defects of variable size within the spleen (Figure 17.39). In certain clinical situations, nuclear scintigraphy using [67]gallium citrate is useful in demonstrating lymphomatous splenic involvement, since gallium may be taken up by lymphoma. Serial gallium imaging can be used to monitor the response to therapy and to detect recurrence. However, there are several major pitfalls to gallium imaging in lymphoma. Not all sites of involvement accumulate gallium, and lesions smaller than 1–2 cm in diameter may not be detected. In addition, many other neoplasms demonstrate gallium uptake, and activity in overlying colon and liver may present problems of interpretation. Therefore, this radionuclide study is probably most useful when correlated with other imaging studies and clinical findings.

17.4.4 HEMANGIOMA

Although rare, the hemangioma is the most common benign tumor of the spleen; it is usually asymptomatic and frequently presents as splenomegaly or as a mass in the left upper abdominal quadrant (Hushi, 1961; Ros *et al.*, 1987). However, it may be discovered incidentally at autopsy or radiologically during studies performed for other purposes. While usually solitary, it may be multiple, as in splenic hemangiomatosis.

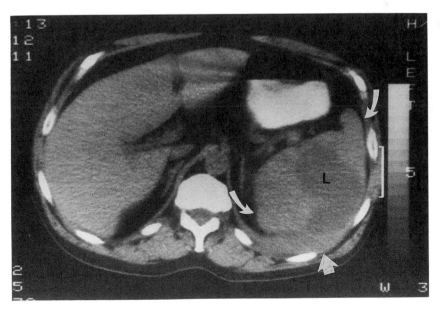

Figure 17.37 Splenic lymphoma on CT. In this CT section of the spleen there is an irregular area of decreased density (L) involving an enlarged spleen (curved arrows). Note how there is external splenic extension with thickening of the left hemidiaphragm (white arrow).

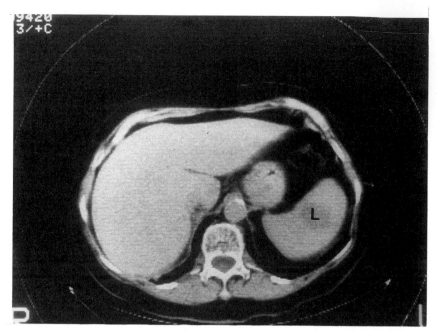

Figure 17.38 Splenic lymphoma on CT. In this enhanced CT of the abdomen a subtle area of decreased density is seen in a spleen of normal size (L). There is no extrasplenic involvement associated with this solitary deposit of lymphoma in the spleen.

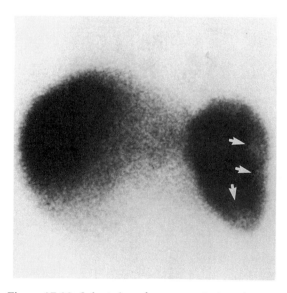

Figure 17.39 Splenic lymphoma on scintigraphy. On this [99m]Technetium-sulfur colloid scintigram, multiple defects are identified, primarily in the spleen (white arrows).

There are in fact relatively few reports in the literature of splenic hemangioma. When present, the radiographical appearance is similar to that of hemangiomas found elsewhere in the body. On plain radiographs, barium studies and excretory urography (IVP), a mass may be apparent in the left upper quadrant, which may displace adjacent organs. In cases in which an extensive hemangioma occupies most of the spleen, evidence of generalized splenomegaly may be seen. Calcification is occasionally present, and usually appears either peripherally in curvilinear form, or centrally and punctate (Ros et al., 1987).

[99m]Technetium-sulfur colloid scintigraphy shows the solitary splenic hemangioma as a single photopenic defect surrounded by a rim of normal splenic parenchymal uptake. Less commonly, multiple nodules of hemangioma will be present in the spleen, manifested on nuclear scintigraphy as multiple photopenic defects.

On sonography, two patterns have been iden-

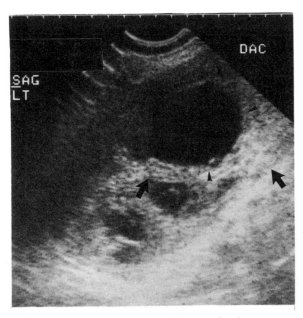

Figure 17.40 Hemangioma of the spleen on ultrasound. A longitudinal sonogram of the left upper quadrant shows a complex mass in the spleen. There are multiple, predominantly anechoic cystic areas (arrowheads), surrounded by echodense portions of solid hemangioma (arrows). This corresponds to a mixed solid tumor with cystic spaces; a pattern that can be observed in hemangioma of the spleen. The other pattern seen on CT scans and tomograms is that of a predominantly solid mass. (Reproduced with permission from Ros *et al.* (1987) *Radiology*, **162**, 73–7.)

tified. One is a predominantly echogenic mass corresponding to a solid hemangioma; the other is that of a complex echodense mass containing anechoic areas representing cystic chambers filled with fluid and debris (Figure 17.40).

Computed tomography also demonstrates two patterns. One is that of a homogeneous, well-margined solid mass that is either hypodense or isodense on non-enhanced studies in relation to the normal splenic parenchyma. The other pattern is that of a multicystic mass (Figure 17.41). The cystic areas demonstrate density similar to water, and lie within a mass which is isodense with normal spleen (Ros *et al.*, 1987). A single case report described peripheral enhancement with IV contrast, with delayed central enhancement, similar to the pattern observed in hepatic hemangioma (Paivansalo and Siniluoto, 1983).

The pattern of splenic hemangioma on angiography is variable and non-specific. Solid hemangiomas or cystic spaces may be seen as hypovascular areas, while hypervascularity, tumor vessels and pooling of contrast medium can also be seen (Figure 17.42). On magnetic resonance imaging, a round mass of homogeneous signal intensity is seen. The lesions demonstrate low signal intensity on T1-, and high signal intensity on T2-weighted images, similar in appearance to hepatic hemangioma (Ros *et al.*, 1987).

In summary, the radiographical appearance of splenic hemangioma ranges from a solid to a predominantly cystic tumor, and includes a variety of solid and cystic splenic masses in its differential diagnosis. The radiographical findings most suggestive of the diagnosis of splenic hemangioma are (1) a large, asymptomatic mass in the left upper abdominal quad-

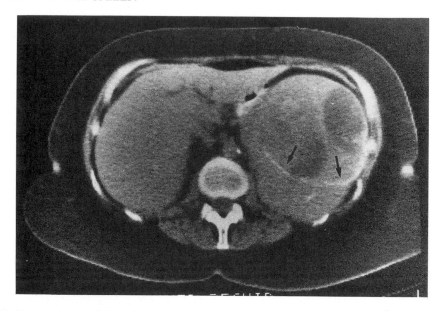

Figure 17.41 Hemangioma of the spleen on CT. Unenhanced CT scan of the upper abdomen demonstrates a faint rim of calcification (arrows) surrounding the posterior margin of an inhomogeneous splenic mass corresponding to a hemangioma. (Reproduced with permission from Ros *et al.* (1987) *Radiology*, **162**, 73–7.)

rant, (2) peripheral curvilinear or central punctate calcification in a left upper quadrant mass, and (3) a solid or combined solid and cystic intrasplenic mass seen on ultrasound or CT. The ability to diagnose this tumor radiographically is important, as needle biopsy is not indicated because of the location and vascular nature of the tumor, and unnecessary splenectomy may be avoided (Ros *et al.*, 1987).

17.4.5 ANGIOSARCOMA

Primary angiosarcoma of the spleen is a rare pathological entity, with less than 100 cases reported in the literature (Kishikawa *et al.*, 1977; Chen, Bolles and Gilbert, 1979; Garvin and King, 1981; Sordillo, Sordillo and Hajdu, 1981; Arbona *et al.*, 1982). While splenic angiosarcoma may be a primary lesion, it is frequently associated with hepatic lesions (Chen, Bolles and Gilbert, 1979; Locker *et al.*, 1979; Langhans, 1879) in which case the pri-

mary site cannot be definitely identified. Although many hepatic angiosarcomas are associated with toxic exposure (such as vinyl chloride or arsenic) or ionizing radiation (thorium), primary splenic angiosarcoma may not show such an association (Mahony, Jeffrey and Federle, 1982). Radiographical evaluation usually demonstrates no specific abnormality. Presentation frequently consists of abdominal pain, a left upper quadrant mass and anemia. [99m]Technetium-sulfur colloid scintigraphy performed on a patient with left upper quadrant symptoms may show an enlarged spleen containing single or multiple photopenic (cold) defects. Ultrasound and CT demonstrate nodules in the spleen of varying size, frequently involving the liver as well (Arbona *et al.*, 1982; Figure 17.43), but differentiation from other tumors cannot be made on the basis of these studies. Angiography will demonstrate the vascular nature of the lesion, with dilated arteries supplying vascular lakes (Chen, Bolles and Gilbert,

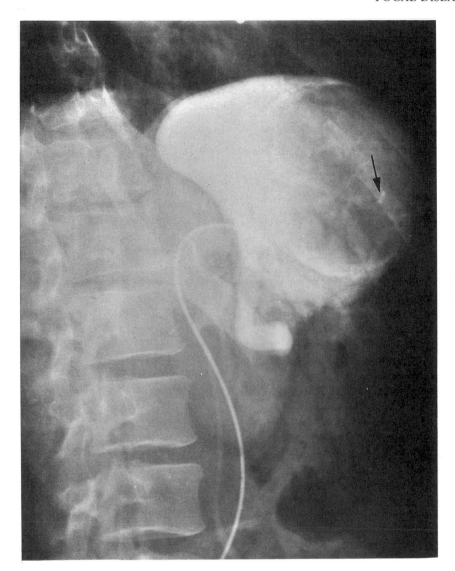

Figure 17.42 Hemangioma of the spleen on angiography. Selective splenic artery injection, oblique view, capillary phase. A well-delineated, large, hypovascular area is demonstrated within the spleen. Small areas of pooling of contrast can also be identified (arrow).

1979; Kishikawa *et al.*, 1977). Tumor vessels may or may not be present (Arbona *et al.*, 1982). The appearance is similar to angiosarcomas or hemangiomas elsewhere.

Splenic rupture is a major complication leading to hemoperitoneum which may be fatal. Discovery of hemoperitoneum in a patient with splenomegaly or splenic mass should lead to consideration of this diagnosis.

17.4.6 HAMARTOMA

Splenic hamartomas are usually solitary but may be multiple. White pulp or red pulp tissue,

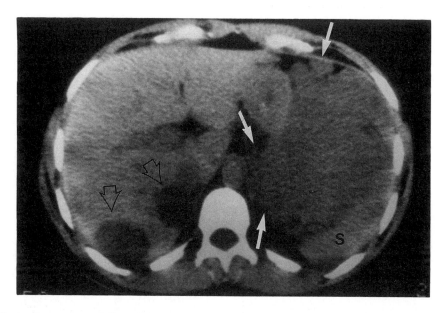

Figure 17.43 Angiosarcoma of the spleen on CT scan. On this enhanced CT of the upper abdomen, almost the entire spleen has been replaced by a large mass. This mass has irregular borders suggesting perisplenic infiltration (white arrows). Small peripheral areas of normal density spleen can be identified (S). Note multiple areas of decreased density in the liver representing angiosarcoma metastasis (open arrows).

or a mixture thereof, may predominate (Iozzo, Haas and Chard, 1980). As in many other splenic abnormalities, plain films are either normal or show some degree of splenomegaly. Calcifications found in splenic hamartomas have ranged from punctate to stellate in configuration (Langhans, 1879), and have been found to lie in the fibrotic portions of the lesions rather than within the vascular channels. There has been limited CT experience with this lesion, but the solid lesion may appear nearly isodense with the spleen on contrast-enhanced CT (Dachman *et al.*, 1986). Cystic hamartomas demonstrate both solid and cystic components on CT and ultrasound (Brinkley and Lee, 1981). However, it is again true that accurate differentiation of splenic hamartoma from other splenic masses cannot be made on the basis of these studies.

Likewise angiography is not diagnostic. Characteristically, however, splenic hamartoma is well-defined and usually has prominent tumor vessels. Aneurysmal dilatation, arter-iovenous shunting and vascular lakes have also been described, and are often similar to findings present in angiosarcoma (Wexler and Abrams, 1964; Teats, Seale and Allen, 1972; Komacki and Gombas, 1978; Kishikawa *et al.*, 1978).

17.4.7   SPLENIC LYMPHANGIOMATOSIS

Splenic lymphangiomatosis is a rare entity, with approximatly 90 cases reported in the literature (Pistoia and Markowitz, 1988). The lesion is characteristically diffuse, and involves almost the entire spleen, but solitary cystic lesions can be found (Asch, Cohen and Moore, 1974; Avigad *et al.*, 1976; Tuttle and Minielly, 1978). The lesion is composed of single or multiple cysts of varying sizes which are lined by endothelium and filled with proteinaceous fluid (Asch, Cohen and Moore, 1974; Pearl and Nassar, 1979), and therefore have a classic cystic appearance radiographically. Simultaneous involvement of other organ systems, includ-

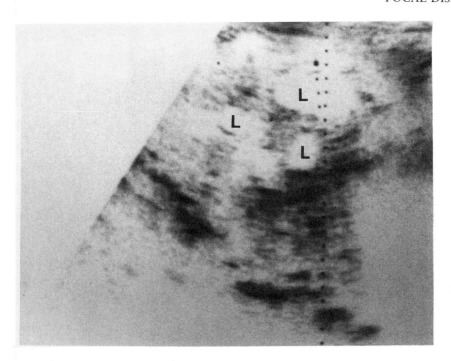

Figure 17.44 Lymphangioma of the spleen on ultrasound. Ultrasound of the left upper quadrant demonstrates multiple well-defined hypoechoic masses (L) corresponding to multiple cysts of variable size within the spleen. The normal contour of the spleen is altered due to the involvement by lymphangioma.

ing, skin, lungs, bones or other viscera ('angiomatosis') is occasionally present (Bill and Sumner, 1965). Curvilinear calcification in cyst walls has been described (Rao *et al.*, 1981).

Plain films may demonstrate splenomegaly, with mass effect on adjacent structures. On [99m]Technetium-sulfur colloid scintigraphy, single or multiple photopenic (cold) defects in the spleen are present (Dachman *et al.*, 1986; Novetsky and Epstein, 1982). On ultrasound, a single, well-defined cyst may be seen, which may be difficult to differentiate from other solitary cystic lesions. More commonly, in diffuse lymphangiomatosis, multiple well-defined hypoechoic masses (cysts) of various sizes will be seen throughout the spleen (Enzinger and Weiss, 1983; Figure 17.44). Septations or proteinaceous debris can sometimes be seen within these cystic masses as internal echoes (Rao *et al.*, 1981).

CT scanning may demonstrate an enlarged spleen containing single or multiple areas of low density. These lesions have a thin wall, are sharply marginated and do not enhance after administration of IV contrast material (Figure 17.45). Small, marginal, linear calcifications may be more easily detected than on plain film (Pistoia and Markowitz, 1988; Pyatt *et al.*, 1981).

Angiographically, numerous well-defined avascular lesions of various sizes are seen scattered throughout the spleen, creating a characteristic 'Swiss cheese' appearance, similar to that seen in renal polycystic disease (Avigad *et al.*, 1976; Tuttle and Minielly, 1978; Uflacker, 1979). The intrasplenic arteries are intrinsically normal and are stretched around these cystic masses. There is no neovascularity, arteriovenous shunting or venous pooling.

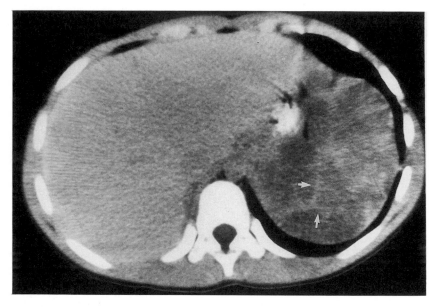

Figure 17.45 Lymphangioma of the spleen on CT scan. CT scan of the upper abdomen demonstrates an enlarged spleen with multiple areas of low density. Multiple small septations are identified (arrows).

17.4.8 METASTASES

Metastasis to the spleen is usually seen only late in the course of metastatic disease, and such patients generally have multi-organ involvement. However, solitary splenic metastases have been described without evidence of involvement of other organs (Federle and Moss, 1983). While most splenic metastases are of hematogenous origin, direct invasion from adjacent organs (including the stomach, left colon, left kidney and pancreas) and peritoneal seeding are also seen (Marymount and Gross, 1963).

Plain films are usually normal. However, diffuse metastases may create splenomegaly, which preserves the normal contour of the spleen. [99m]Technetium-sulfur colloid scintigraphy may show single or multiple photopenic (cold) defects within the spleen if macroscopic disease is present (Figure 17.46). Microscopic metastases may not be detected. Extensive splenic metastases may cause partial or complete non-visualization of the spleen, possibly by encasing or invading the splenic vessels, and in effect causing an 'autosplenectomy'.

On ultrasound, metastatic lesions in the spleen, as elsewhere, have a varied appearance. They can be homogeneously hypoechoic or echodense. In addition, lesions having mixed hypoechoic and echodense areas are seen, in the presence of solid masses having cystic or necrotic components (Figure 17.47).

By computed tomography, metastatic lesions usually have a lower density or are isodense relative to surrounding normal spleen, prior to IV contrast infusion. Following injection of IV contrast, the low-density lesions become accentuated against the enhancing normal splenic tissue (Figure 17.48). Frequently, isodense lesions on non-contrast CT are detected only after contrast injection, since the normal splenic tissue enhances to a greater degree than the metastatic disease (Piekarski, Federle and Moss, 1980). As on ultrasound, mixed density lesions having cystic or necrotic components are also seen. Frequently, metastatic lesions in the liver and other organs are also present. Evidence of

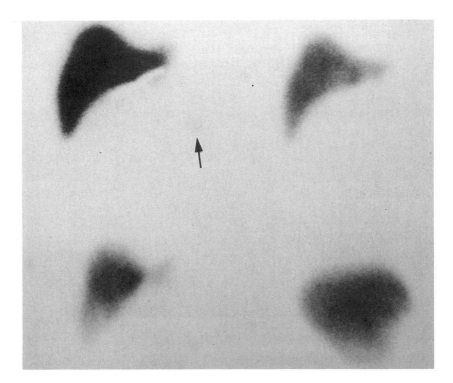

Figure 17.46 Metastases to the spleen on scintigraphy. ^{99m}Technetium-sulfur colloid scintigraphy shows almost no normal activity corresponding to the spleen in the left upper quadrant. A faint area of activity is identified (arrow) corresponding to a small portion of normal spleen that is not destroyed by necrotic metastasis. Non-visualization of the spleen secondary to metastasis essentially represents 'autosplenectomy', as in this case.

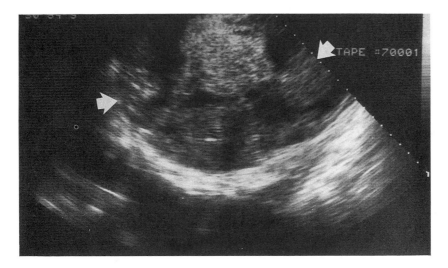

Figure 17.47 Metastases to the spleen on sonogram. This ultrasound of the left upper quadrant shows distortion of the normal architecture of the spleen. The spleen is essentially replaced by a large mass with complex echogenicity secondary to a large metastasis with central necrosis (white arrows).

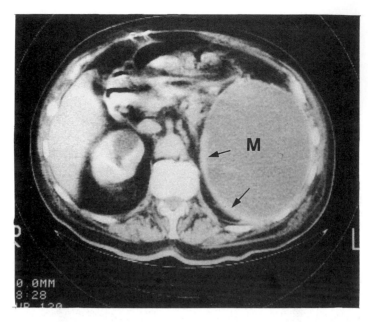

Figure 17.48 Metastasis to the spleen on CT. Enhanced CT scan of the upper abdomen demonstrates a large hypodense mass replacing the spleen (M). Note a thin rim of higher density (arrows) corresponding to a thin shell of residual spleen. The hypodense center corresponds to necrosis. Aggressive metastasis to the spleen may produce a cystic-appearing mass on imaging studies.

necrosis is usually seen in the larger metastases. CT-guided percutaneous needle biopsy can be performed on splenic lesions for definitive diagnosis.

17.5 DIFFUSE DISEASE

17.5.1 SPLENOMEGALY

Splenomegaly is probably the most common finding in the presence of diffuse splenic disease. While the differential diagnosis of splenomegaly is extensive, the degree of splenomegaly and associated findings may help in differentiating the various causes. However, many diseases causing splenomegaly without specific characteristics can be diagnosed only on the basis of clinical or laboratory data. Some of the causes of diffuse splenic disease will be discussed briefly here.

The myeloproliferative group of disorders, including certain leukemias and myelofibrosis, are often associated with massive splenomegaly. Such splenomegaly can be detected by almost any imaging modality (Figure 17.49). Diagnosis is made on the basis of hematological findings. Lymphoma was discussed previously under focal diseases (see section 17.4.3.) but may also present as diffuse splenic involvement.

Marked splenomegaly may be seen in cases of chronic passive congestion, which is commonly secondary to congestive heart failure or portal hypertension. The spleen is enlarged but uniform in texture. Dilatation of the splenic vein or associated varices may be identified by imaging studies.

In sarcoidosis, splenomegaly may be found even when relatively few lesions are present elsewhere (Figures 17.50 and 17.51): up to one-quarter of cases show hepatosplenomegaly

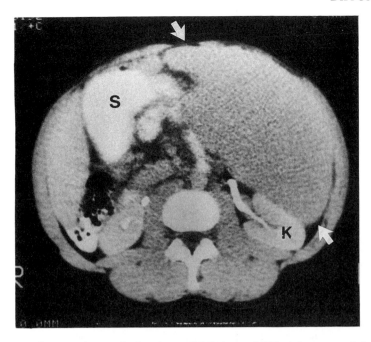

Figure 17.49 Splenomegaly secondary to leukemia on CT. Enhanced CT of the upper abdomen at the level of the left kidney demonstrates a markedly enlarged spleen (white arrows). This marked splenomegaly was due to chronic leukemia. Note that the spleen is homogeneous in density. There is compression of the left kidney posteriorly (K) and of the stomach (S) to the right of the midline.

(Longscope and Freiman, 1952). A pattern of multifocal defects on ^{99m}Technetium-sulfur colloid scan, apparently secondary to sarcoid granulomas, has been reported (Iko *et al.*, 1982).

Many storage diseases cause splenomegaly. Gaucher's disease is one of the more common lipid storage diseases, caused by accumulation of glucocerebroside in macrophages of the spleen, liver and bone marrow. Massive hepatosplenomegaly results, and is associated with characteristic skeletal lesions.

17.5.2   QUANTITATIVE MEASUREMENT OF SPLEEN SIZE AND VOLUME

As discussed above, splenomegaly is a non-specific finding caused by many different disorders of the spleen. Measurement of spleen volume is, in some instances, useful both in the initial assessment and the later follow-up of patients with splenomegaly. One of the earliest approaches to predicting spleen weight radiologically was devised by Whitley, Maynard and Rhyne (1966), in which a computer-based system was used to predict spleen weight from routine films of the abdomen. However, for routine use without the aid of a computer, plain films can only give an approximate estimate of spleen size, with only marked changes being detectable. More recently, with the use of newer imaging modalities, determination of spleen size has become increasingly accurate.

Nuclear scintigraphy has been used in the past for volume determination, and has achieved a reasonable degree of accuracy Mattson, 1982). In addition, SPECT imaging, previously applied to the liver for volume determination (Kan and Hopkins, 1979), may also be applied to the spleen.

Sonography has been used by many for

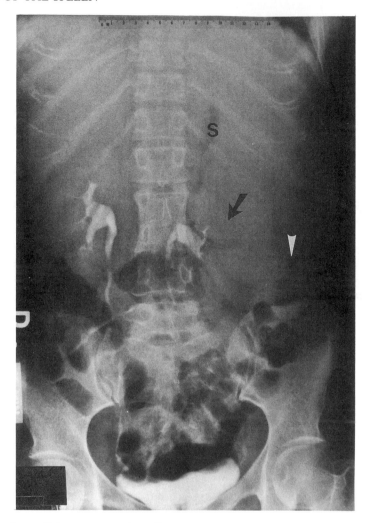

Figure 17.50 Sarcoidosis of the spleen on plain film. Supine view of the abdomen on an excretory urogram demonstrates displacement of the left kidney inferiorly and medially (arrow), due to a markedly enlarged spleen. Note also how the gastric air bubble (S) is displaced medially and the splenic flexure is displaced inferiorly (white arrowhead). A tip of normal spleen is not identified, indicating splenomegaly rather than a focal splenic mass.

volume determination, calculated by the summation of multiple, parallel, cross-sectional areas (Kardel *et al.*, 1971; Koga *et al.*, 1972; Rasmussen *et al.*, 1973). More recently, Pietri and Boscaini (1984) proposed sonographic calculation of a splenic volumetric index using measurements of the maximum breadth, thickness and height of the spleen. However, measurement of the spleen using sonography is ham-

pered by the inaccessibility of those portions of the spleen which are hidden by overlying bowel gas or ribs, and the difficulty of scanning under the left hemidiaphragm. In addition, the manual nature of sonography and its extreme operator dependency make reproducibility of measurements difficult (Breiman *et al.*, 1982).

The easiest and most accurate method of measuring spleen size is by computed tomog-

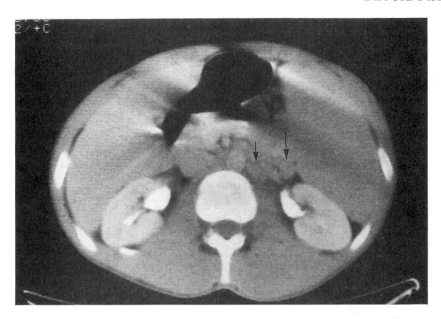

Figure 17.51 Sarcoidosis of the spleen on CT. Enhanced CT of the abdomen at the level of the renal hila demonstrates an enlarged spleen. Note the presence of periaortic and juxtacaval adenopathy (arrows), also secondary to sarcoidosis.

raphy, especially in view of its widespread availability and routine use. Several authors have described computer analysis of CT sections (Heymsfield *et al.*, 1979; Henderson *et al.*, 1981), using complex mathematical formulas. Breiman *et al.* (1982) simplified and refined this method, obtaining contiguous sections through the spleen at 2 cm intervals and calculating volume using a summation-of-areas technique. The area of the spleen on each CT section is calculated by tracing the spleen outline with a cursor and then using a computer program. The mean percentage error of volume measurements using this technique is about 3.6%. The advantages of the summation-of-areas technique using CT are: (1) the CT scans are completely automated, reproducible, and easily obtainable; (2) the boundaries of the spleen are easily recognized by CT; and (3) the method does not require the use of complex mathematical formulae.

While a relatively accurate determination of spleen size and volume can be obtained by CT,

in routine daily practice an experienced observer can judge spleen size and volume by simple study of the CT scans. Typically, the craniocaudal length of the normal spleen is less than 15 cm, and the inferior tip does not usually extend to the level of the tip of the right lobe of the liver. In addition, the anterior edge of the spleen does not usually extend anteriorly beyond the mid-axillary line (Federle, 1983). Splenomegaly can be strongly suspected if either of these boundaries is transgressed.

17.5.3   INFECTIONS

Infection involving the spleen may result simply in diffuse splenomegaly, as is found frequently in malaria, mononucleosis, leishmaniasis, trypanosomiasis (Chaga's disease), histoplasmosis, schistosomiasis, echinococcosis and congenital syphilis. Splenic infection may also take the form of multiple microabscesses or granulomas. Radiological manifestations of focal splenic abscess were discussed in section 17.4.2.

Infectious mononucleosis causes mild spleno-megaly in the second week of illness in 75% of patients, but marked splenomegaly may occasionally occur (Wintrobe *et al.*, 1981). Splenic rupture and hemoperitoneum are rare complications, and CT or ultrasound can be used to evaluate the spleen for suspected rupture.

In schistosomiasis, splenomegaly is produced secondary to the characteristic cirrhosis, which produces perisplenic vein fibrosis and splenic vein thrombosis (Wintrobe *et al.*, 1981). Thrombosis of the portal or splenic vein can be detected by ultrasound (Mousa *et al.*, 1967). A positive correlation has been demonstrated between portal venous pressure and splenic and portal vein measurements, and ultrasound can also be used to measure the portal and splenic veins in these patients to evaluate for portal hypertension (Abdel-Latif, Abdel-Wahab and El-Kady, 1981). Other findings on ultrasound in patients with schistosomiasis include periportal fibrosis, thickening of the gallbladder wall, echogenic hepatic nodules and hypertrophy of the left lobe of the liver with associated atrophy of the right lobe (Cerri, Alves and Magelhaes, 1984).

Splenic infection by echinococcus is usually associated with liver and/or lung involvement; this is the only parasite to produce splenic cysts. The cysts, solitary or multiple, may cause a focal mass effect or splenic enlargement which may be detected on plain films. These cysts may demonstrate peripheral, ring-like calcification, as is seen with other types of cysts (Soler-Bechara and Soscia, 1964). However, the presence of multiple cysts, the appearance of daughter cysts within a larger cyst, and similar calcified cystic structures in the liver or lung, help to differentiate echinococcal cysts from other forms. As with other types of cysts, photopenic defects are seen on ^{99m}Technetium-sulfur colloid scintigraphy. On ultrasound, solitary or multiple cysts are identified, sometimes with a 'cyst-within-a-cyst' pattern (Wurtele, Tondreau and Pollack, 1982). Extensive echoes may be seen within the cyst, representing internal debris or scolices (Schulman *et al.*, 1983). Similar findings are seen on CT.

Granulomatous disease of the spleen is most commonly secondary to tuberculosis and histoplasmosis, and is usually found with generalized disease. Mild to moderate splenomegaly may be present acutely, and calcified granulomas are frequently seen at a later stage. These calcifications are small and round in appearance, are frequently identified on plain film, and may be associated with similar calcifications in the lungs or liver. On ultrasound, the calcified granulomas are seen as small, bright echogenic foci with shadowing.

As discussed earlier, splenic abscess is usually a solitary focal lesion, but diffuse microabscesses may also be seen. The most common cause of microabscesses is *Candida albicans*, usually in immunocompromised patients, particularly in patients with leukemia on therapy (Bodey, 1966). On ^{99m}Technetium-sulfur colloid scintigraphy, hepatosplenomegaly is seen in association with diffuse, small defects in the spleen. These small defects represent microabscesses and show variably increased or decreased radionuclide uptake on gallium scan (Miller, Greenfield and Wald, 1982). Ultrasound may demonstrate a diffusely hypoechoic spleen, or multiple small hypoechoic or anechoic foci. The small hypoechoic lesions may contain an echogenic center ('target lesions'), which may represent fungus growing within the microabscess (Sumner *et al.*, 1983). Computed tomography demonstrates similar findings, with multiple small, low-density lesions in the spleen and/or liver, some having a target appearance which does not enhance with contrast media (Figure 17.52).

17.6 VASCULAR DISEASE

17.6.1 ARTERIOSCLEROSIS AND SPLENIC ARTERY ANEURYSM

As with many arteries affected by arteriosclerosis, involvement of the splenic artery leads to calcification of the wall and tortuosity. These changes principally affect the main splenic artery and its major divisions and tend to become more apparent with age (Abrams, 1983),

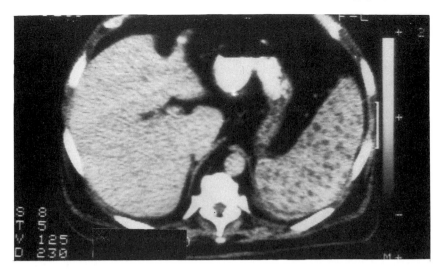

Figure 17.52 Candida microabscesses of the spleen on CT. CT of the upper abdomen demonstrates multiple small areas of decreased density throughout the spleen. These correspond to microabscesses due to *Candida albicans* in a patient immunocompromised by leukemia. The spleen is markedly enlarged.

although severe stenosis is unusual. Although aneurysms of visceral arteries are uncommon, the splenic artery is the most commonly affected (Cobos *et al.*, 1982). Splenic artery aneurysm is usually diagnosed by the presence of ring calcification in the left upper quadrant on plain film (Figure 17.53), CT or ultrasound. The aneurysms are cystic in appearance on ultrasound and demonstrate contrast enhancement on CT (Figure 17.54), that may be parti-

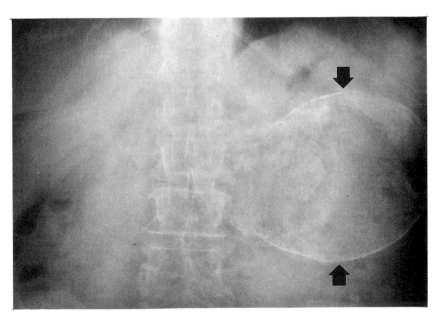

Figure 17.53 Splenic artery aneurysm on plain film. Localized view of the upper abdomen from a supine abdominal radiograph demonstrates a large ring-like calcification (arrows) characteristic of an aneurysm.

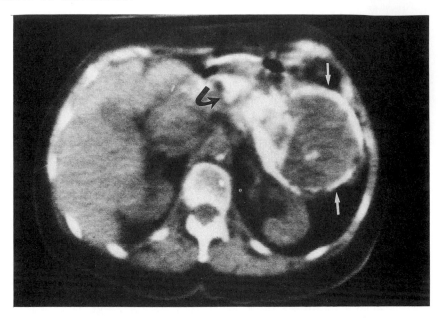

Figure 17.54 Aneurysm of the splenic artery on CT. Corresponding CT scan in the same patient as in Figure 17.53 demonstrates a mass in the left upper quadrant with a thick rim of calcification (white arrows) and a hypodense center. There is some oral contrast in the stomach (curved arrow).

ally due to blood clot. Due to the presence of flowing blood, a low-signal round mass is seen on MRI. Angiography is useful for demonstrating splenic artery aneurysms, as well as associated findings such as rupture or fistula formation. Trans-catheter embolization may be utilized for treatment of a bleeding aneurysm (Probst *et al.*, 1978). Pseudoaneurysms of the splenic artery may also be seen, especially following trauma or in association with chronic pancreatitis; the findings are similar to those of true aneurysms.

Most arteriovenous fistulas involving the splenic vessels are secondary to rupture of a splenic aneurysm, but they also occur as a result of penetrating (stab or gunshot) wounds. In the presence of splenic arteriovenous fistula, splenomegaly is often present with portal hypertension, esophageal varices and ascites (Donovan *et al.*, 1969; Van Way *et al.*, 1971). These findings may be detected by a variety of imaging studies: angiography with selective splenic artery injection yields the definitive diagnosis. Early

filling of the splenic vein is seen, often in association with the presence of a splenic artery aneurysm. In addition, the splenic vein may appear dilated secondary to increased pressure, and gastro-esophageal varices may be present. While surgery is usually regarded as the treatment of choice, transcatheter embolization of the involved splenic artery may be considered.

17.6.2 SPLENIC VEIN THROMBOSIS

The pathophysiology of splenic vein thrombosis includes compression, encasement and inflammation about the splenic vein. In most cases thrombosis is related to pancreatic carcinoma or chronic pancreatitis; however, the list of causes is long and includes trauma and large masses causing compression.

Radiographical findings may demonstrate evidence of the underlying cause of the splenic vein thrombosis; for example, pancreatic calcifications on plain films in a patient with chronic pancreatitis, or a large pancreatic mass seen on

CT. A primary finding is the presence of solitary gastric varices, which can be seen on contrast-enhanced CT scan, angiography or even barium study. Such varices are usually located in the region of the gastric fundus or cardia, but they may also occur in the body and antrum, especially along the greater curvature (Itzchak and Glickman, 1977). Splenomegaly may or may not be present.

Angiography demonstrates splenic vein thrombosis definitively following high dose injection of the celiac or splenic artery. Percutaneous transhepatic portography can also be used; percutaneous splenoportography is now only of historical interest (see section 17.1.3). Diagnostic findings on angiography include partial or complete non-opacification of the splenic vein with visualization of venous collaterals (varices).

Ultrasound has also been used to diagnose splenic vein thrombosis, and is being increasingly utilized for this purpose (Weinberger, Mitra and Yoeli, 1982; Jeanty *et al.*, 1982). On ultrasound, echogenic material may be seen occluding the splenic vein, which demonstrates no flow on Doppler ultrasound. CT scan can demonstrate non-patency of the splenic vein on dynamic contrast-enhanced scans, in association with gastric varices. CT and ultrasound are also useful in discovering the underlying cause of splenic vein thrombosis.

While the treatment of choice for gastrointestinal bleeding secondary to splenic vein thrombosis is surgical splenectomy (Little and Moosa, 1981; Salam, Warren and Tyras, 1973), transcatheter embolization of the splenic artery is an alternative form of treatment in poor risk patients.

17.6.3 SPLENIC INFARCTION

Splenic parenchymal arterial branches are end-arteries which do not intercommunicate (MacPherson, Richmond and Stuart, 1973). Therefore, occlusion of the splenic artery or its branches leads to infarction. Causes of splenic artery occlusion include sickle cell disease (thrombosis), embolic disease (for example, in mitral valve disease), atherosclerosis, arteritis, splenic artery aneurysm, splenic torsion and a mass lesion such as pancreatic carcinoma (Cohen, Mitty and Mendelson, 1984; Anderson and Kissane, 1977).

Findings on plain film may include splenomegaly, an elevated left hemidiaphragm and left pleural effusion, but these are infrequently seen (Balcar *et al.*, 1984). Despite the advent of newer imaging modalities, nuclear scintigraphy is probably still the best method of diagnosis of splenic infarction. On ^{99m}technetium-sulfur colloid scintigraphy, the area of infarction creates a defect which is classically periphery-based and wedge-shaped, with the apex of the defect directed toward the splenic hilum (Lin and Donati, 1981; Figure 17.55). However, the infarct may be irregular in shape or even multiple ('spotted spleen'), but these findings are less specific for infarction (Freeman and Tonkin, 1976). SPECT imaging is useful in equivocal cases, and may detect an infarct not seen on planar images.

Angiographically, occlusion of the splenic artery or one of its branches may be seen, with a peripheral, triangular defect in the splenic contour visualized in the parenchymal phase (Abrams, 1983). Sonographically, splenic infarct has been described as a sharply demarcated, hypoechoic area in an enlarged spleen (Yeh, Zacks and Jurado, 1981), correlating pathologically with edema and necrosis (Figure 17.56). A similar appearance has been described following transcatheter therapeutic embolization of the spleen (Weingarten *et al.*, 1984). However, echogenicity varies with the age of the infarct, which is hypoechoic acutely and becomes more echogenic with time.

As with ultrasound, the CT appearance of a splenic infarct depends on the period which has elapsed since the acute event. Balcar *et al.* (1984) demonstrated four phases of splenic infarction: hyperacute (day 1), acute (days 2–4), subacute (days 4–8) and chronic (2–4 weeks). In the hyperacute phase an area of decreased density (by comparison with the normal spleen)

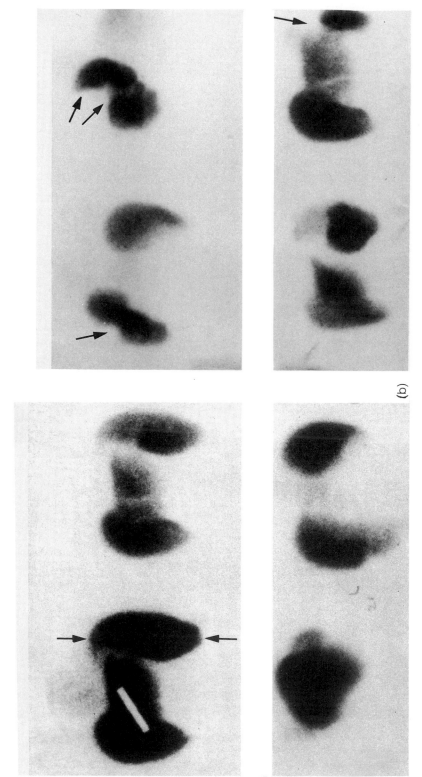

(b)

(a)

Figure 17.55 Splenic infarct on scintigraphy. (a) ^{99m}Technetium-sulfur colloid scintigraphy in this patient with polycythemia vera demonstrates a large spleen with increased uptake (arrows). (b) One month later, in the same patient, a large wedge-shaped defect can be identified in the spleen (arrows) in different projections. This defect represents an infarct, commonly seen in polycythemia vera. Splenic infarcts appear on scintigraphy as a defect, wedge-shaped and peripherally based, with the apex directed toward the splenic hilus.

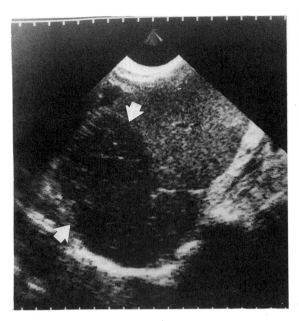

Figure 17.56 Splenic infarction on ultrasound. Ultrasound of the left upper quadrant, on a longitudinal parasagittal plane demonstrates in the same patient as in Figure 17.55 a large area of decreased echogenicity (white arrows). The spleen is enlarged, corresponding to the scintigraphic findings. This sharply demarcated, triangular-shaped hypoechoic area corresponds to the infarction seen on scintigraphy.

is usually seen on non-contrast scan, which shows a diffusely mottled pattern on contrast enhancement. However, a large, focal hyperdense lesion without contrast enhancement may also be seen hyperacutely. In the acute and subacute phases, focal, well-defined areas of low density are seen, which become progressively better demarcated, and which demonstrate no contrast enhancement. Again, infarcts may be wedge-shaped, irregular or multiple. Density of the infarcted area may return to normal in the chronic phase on both pre- and post-contrast scans. The infarct gradually decreases in size and may completely disappear. Frequently, however, a residual contour defect representing scarring is seen at the site of infarction.

17.6.4 SPLENORENAL SHUNT

Splenorenal shunts are seen in patients with chronic portal hypertension, and are most often secondary to cirrhosis: the definitive diagnosis is made angiographically. Transhepatic splenoportography demonstrates reverse flow in the splenic vein, with dilated collaterals communicating with the left renal vein and opacification of the inferior vena cava (Nunez *et al.*, 1978; Redman and Reuter, 1969). Enlarged perisplenic veins and left renal vein, and splenomegaly, are seen on CT and ultrasound. Postoperative patency of splenorenal shunts created surgically for treatment of portal hypertension may also be evaluated angiographically.

17.6.5 SPLENIC VASCULAR CHANGES IN PANCREATIC DISEASE

The pancreas is intimately associated with the splenic vessels along their entire course. A mass in the tail of the pancreas may cause displacement of these vessels without intrinsic damage to them. However, pancreatic carcinoma may cause encasement of the splenic artery, resulting in stenosis or complete occlusion. Occasionally, this encasement mimics atherosclerotic disease, in which case evaluation of the splenic vein can help differentiate benign from malignant disease. The splenic vein is normal in the presence of atherosclerosis, while involvement or obstruction of the splenic vein suggests pancreatic adenocarcinoma. Pancreatitis can also cause narrowing of splenic vessels due to fibrosis (Abrams, 1983), mimicking angiographically the findings seen in adenocarcinoma.

17.7 MISCELLANEOUS DISORDERS

17.7.1 SICKLE CELL DISEASE

Sickle cell disease has widespread manifestations, with frequent involvement of the spleen secondary to slow blood flow through this organ (see also Chapter 16). Sickled cells lodge in end-arteries, causing occlusion and infarction. Repetitive splenic infarction gradually causes autosplenectomy in homozygous subjects, resulting in complete loss of splenic function, usually by the age of 5. In heterozygous patients with sickle cell trait, there are fewer and less severe episodes of vaso-occlusion, and the spleen may be damaged without being functionally destroyed. Unlike the homozygous patient who has undergone vaso-occlusive autosplenectomy, continued function of the spleen in heterozygous patients provides the continuing potential for complications such as abscess formation and rupture. Due to their frequent episodes of 'crisis', with abdominal pain and other symptoms, sicklers often require medical care and concomitant imaging.

Splenomegaly may be seen at any age on plain film in the heterozygous population, but is usually seen only to about the age of 5 years in homozygous patients. An acute and marked increase in spleen size may indicate splenic sequestration crisis. In addition, splenic enlargement may be secondary to abscess or infarction. Likewise, non-specific perisplenic inflammatory changes may be detected, including left pleural effusion, an elevated left hemidiaphragm and left lower lobe atelectasis or infiltrates.

In older homozygous patients, the fibrotic, end-stage spleen following autosplenectomy may result in diffuse or patchy splenic calcification. These calcifications are most commonly diffuse and punctate or stippled, although larger, amorphous calcifications may also be seen. By the time these appear on plain film, splenic function has been greatly impaired or lost.

^{99m}Technetium-sulfur colloid scintigraphy may show multiple infarcts prior to autosplenectomy in the homozygous patient. In addition there is progressively decreasing uptake on serial scans secondary to declining splenic function. Following autosplenectomy, the spleen does not visualize on sulfur colloid scan. While radionuclide uptake may be impaired in heterozygous patients, at least partial splenic uptake persists into adult life, and frequently the uptake is normal. Such changes in the heterozygous population are usually proportional to the amount of abnormal hemoglobin. In the presence of splenic abscess, infarct or hemorrhage, focal photopenic defects may be seen. On radionuclide bone scanning, activity may accumulate in calcified areas of the spleen, and such accumulations may be seen prior to the appearance of calcification on plain film. This finding corresponds to microscopic deposits of calcium in splenic tissue.

By ultrasound, sickle cell-related splenomegaly is easily imaged, and permits the detection of infarction, abscess and other complications of the disease. (See previous sections for a full discussion of these conditions.) In the homozygous patient with a small, fibrotic, end-stage spleen, adequate visualization is often impossible due to the location of the spleen high up under the rib cage, and frequently the presence of diffuse calcification creates a major imaging pitfall for ultrasound. However, this is rarely of critical importance, since active splenic disease is unlikely following autosplenectomy.

CT is probably the most reliable means of imaging the spleen in the patient with sickle cell disease. Since these patients frequently present with abdominal pain, the entire abdomen can be imaged easily. The study is first performed without IV contrast to allow demonstration of splenic calcification and density, and is followed by the contrast-enhanced study. The spleen in sickle cell disease, even if normal or enlarged, is frequently of higher density than normal. This is thought to be secondary to the presence of diffuse and sometimes microscopic calcification, and also to increased iron deposition due to hemolysis and red cell transfusions. The CT manifestations of the complications of sickle cell disease have been described in previous sections of this chapter.

17.7.2 THE DENSE OR OPACIFIED SPLEEN

There are several causes of a radiographically dense spleen. Abnormal iron deposition in hemochromatosis causes increased density in the spleen, as well as in the liver, pancreas and other organs. This is evident on CT scan but very rarely seen on plain films (Mitnick *et al.*, 1981).

Increased density of the spleen due to the prior use of Thorotrast is also occasionally seen. Thorotrast, a solution containing thorium dioxide, was introduced in 1930 as a radiographic contrast agent, and was most commonly used for cerebral angiography. It was subsequently withdrawn due to the high radiation dose emitted during decay of thorium to lead, and due to its biological half-life of 400 years. Thorotrast particles are phagocytosed by reticuloendothelial cells and therefore the radiation dose is highest in the spleen, liver and bone marrow. Thorotrast causes the spleen to shrink in size and undergo fibrous replacement, sometimes resulting in functional asplenia (Burroughs *et al.*, 1982; Rao, Winebright and Dresser, 1979a). Thorotrast-induced splenic angiosarcoma has been described, but splenic neoplasms are rare following use of this contrast material (Levy *et al.*, 1986; Gardner and Ogilvie, 1959) when compared to the incidence of hepatic neoplasms such as angiosarcoma, hepatocellular carcinoma and cholangiocarcinoma.

On plain films and CT, the post-Thorotrast spleen is small and dense and contains diffusely scattered punctate opacities (Figure 17.57). Opacification of the liver, lymphatics and peripancreatic nodes may also be seen. If a splenic mass is present, a filling defect may be identified within the dense spleen (Levy *et al.*, 1986). Dense calcification of the spleen mimicking Thorotrast may be seen in diffuse splenic infarction, most commonly in sickle cell disease. However, in this case the pattern of splenic opacification is less dense and is limited to the spleen, and high density in the liver or perisplenic lymph nodes is lacking.

17.7.3 HYPOSPLENISM (FUNCTIONAL ASPLENIA)

Hyposplenism is the functional condition which follows autosplenectomy and other causes of

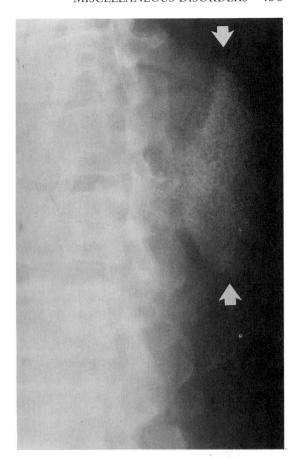

Figure 17.57 Thorotrast spleen on plain films. Oblique plain film of the left upper quadrant demonstrates a spleen with diffusely scattered punctate opacities (arrows). This fine, dense, well-delineated network pattern is typical of Thorotrast deposition (white arrows) in the reticuloendothelial system of the spleen.

splenic atrophy. Splenic atrophy, with a small or dense spleen, results from inflammatory bowel diseases, dermatitis herpetiformis, celiac disease, thyrotoxicosis and the post-Thorotrast spleen (see Chapter 11; Corozza and Gasbarrini, 1983; Eichner, 1979). Hyposplenism associated with a normal or enlarged spleen may be seen in sarcoidosis, amyloidosis, sickle-cell disease, and possibly with administration of high-dose corticosteroids (Eichner, 1979).

Nuclear scintigraphy using heat-damaged red

blood cells is the best procedure for confirming the presence of hyposplenism. The half-time for the blood clearance of heat-damaged ^{51}chromium labeled red blood cells is 10–16 minutes for normal subjects, and is increased to the range of 35 minutes to several hours in functionally asplenic patients.

17.8 SUMMARY

In this chapter we have attempted to demonstrate the imaging appearance of the normal spleen, as well as congenital anomalies, trauma, focal and diffuse diseases, vascular disorders and the miscellaneous processes involving the spleen.

A systematic approach reviewing the radiological findings by modality has been used, covering plain films, ultrasound, computed tomography, scintigraphy, angiography and magnetic resonance imaging.

Although a specific pathological diagnosis may be difficult to achieve, the information provided by imaging, coupled with the clinical and laboratory data, is capable in many instances of providing information affecting clinical management. Surgery, percutaneous intervention, medical therapy or simple observation can then be pursued, with greater assurance because of the radiological findings.

REFERENCES

Abdel-Latif, Z., Abdel-Wahab, F. and El-Kady, N. M. (1981) Evaluation of portal hypertension in cases of hepatosplenic schistosomiasis using ultrasound. *J. Clin. Ultrasound*, 9, 409–12.

Abrams, H. L. (1983) Splenic arteriography, in *Abrams Angiography: Vascular and Interventional Radiology* (ed. H. L. Abrams), Little Brown, Boston, MA, pp. 1531–73.

Ahmann, D. L. *et al.* (1966) Malignant lymphoma of the spleen. A review of 49 cases in which the diagnosis was made at splenectomy. *Cancer*, 19, 826–34.

Anderson, W. A. D. and Kissane, J. M. (eds) (1977) *Pathology*, 7th edn, C. V. Mosby, St Louis, MI, vol 2 pp. 1489–513.

Arbona, G. L. *et al.* (1982) Computed tomographic demonstration of angiosarcoma of the spleen. *South Med. J.*, 75, 348–50.

Asch, M. J., Cohen, A. H. and Moore, T. C. (1974) Hepatic and splenic lymphangiomatosis with skeletal involvement: report of a case and review of the literature. *Surgery*, 76, 334–9.

Avigad, S. *et al.* (1976) Lymphangiomatosis with splenic involvement. *J. Am. Med. Assoc.*, 236, 2315–17.

Balcar, I. *et al.* (1984) CT patterns of splenic infarction: a clinical and experimental study. *Radiology*, 151, 723–9.

Beahrs, J. R. and Stephens, D. H. (1980) Enlarged accessory spleens: CT appearance in postsplenectomy patients. *Am. J. Radiol.*, 135, 483–6.

Bearss, R. W. (1980) Splenic-gonadal fusion. *Urology*, 16, 277–9.

Bill, A. H. and Sumner, D. S. (1965) Unified concept of lymphangioma and cystic hygroma. *Surg. Gynecol. Obstet.*, 120, 79–86.

Bloom, R. A. *et al.* (1981) Acute Hodgkin's disease masquerading as splenic abscess. *J. Surg. Oncol.*, 17, 279–82.

Bodey, G. P. (1966) Fungal infections complicating acute leukemia. *J. Chronic Dis.*, 19, 667–87.

Breiman, R. S. *et al.* (1982) Volume determinations using CT. *Am. J. Radiol.*, 138, 329–33.

Brinkley, A. A. and Lee, J. K. T. (1981) Cystic hamartoma of the spleen: CT and sonographic findings. *J. Clin. Ultrasound*, 9, 136–8.

Bron, K. M. and Hoffman, W. J. (1971) Preoperative diagnosis of splenic cysts. *Arch. Surg.*, 102, 459–61.

Burke, J. S. (1961) Surgical pathology of the spleen: an approach to the differential diagnosis of splenic lymphomas and leukemias. *Am. J. Surg. Pathol.*, 5, 551–63.

Burroughs, A. K. *et al.* (1982) Absence of splenic uptake of radiocolloid due to thorotrast in a patient with thorotrast-induced cholangiocarcinoma. *Br. J. Radiol.*, 55, 598–600.

Carroll, B. A. (1982) Ultrasound of lymphoma. *Semin. Ultrasound*, 3, 114–22.

Carroll, B. A. and Ta, H. N. (1980) The ultrasonic appearance of extranodal abdominal lymphoma. *Radiology*, 135, 419–25.

Castellino, R. A. *et al.* (1972) Splenic arteriography in Hodgkin's disease: a roentgenographic-pathologic study of 33 consecutive untreated patients. *Am. J. Radiol.*, 114, 574–82.

Ceccacci, L. and Tosi, S. (1981) Splenic-gonadal fusion: case report and review of the literature. *J. Urol.*, 126, 558–9.

Cerri, G. G., Alves, V. A. F. and Magalhaes, A. (1984) Hepatosplenic schistosomiasis mansoni: Ultrasound manifestation. *Radiology*, **153**, 777–80.

Chen, K. T. K., Bolles, J. C. and Gilbert, E. F. (1979) Angiosarcoma of the spleen. *Arch. Pathol. Lab. Med.*, **103**, 122–4.

Clark, R. E., Korobkin, M. and Palubinskas, A. J. (1972) Angiography of accessory spleens. *Radiology*, **102**, 41–4.

Cobos, J. M. *et al.* (1982) Multiple calcified aneurysms of splenic artery, hypersplenism and concomitant cholelithiasis. *Jpn J. Surg.*, **12**, 448–52.

Cohen, B. A., Mitty, H. A. and Mendelson, D. S. (1984) Case report: computed tomography of splenic infarction. *J. Comp. Assist. Tomogr.*, **8**, 167–8.

Cooperberg, P. L. (1987) Ultrasonography of the spleen, in *Diagnostic Ultrasound, Text and Cases* (ed. D. A. Sarti), Year Book Medical Publishers, Chicago, IL, p. 312.

Corozza, G. R. and Gasbarrini, G. (1983) Defective splenic function and its relation to bowel disease. *Clin. Gastroenterol.*, **12**, 651–69.

Cunningham, J. J. (1978) Ultrasonic findings in isolated lymphoma of the spleen simulating splenic abscess. *J. Clin. Ultrasound*, **6**, 412–14.

Dachman, A. H. *et al.* (1986) Nonparasitic splenic cysts: a report of 52 cases with radiologic-pathologic correlation. *Am. J. Radiol.*, **147**, 537–42.

Dalton, M. L. Jr, Strange, W. H. and Downs, E. A. (1971) Intrathoracic splenosis: case report and review of the literature. *Am. Rev. Respir. Dis.*, **103**, 827–30.

Davidson, E. D., Campbell, W. G. and Hersh, T. (1980) Epidermoid splenic cyst occurring in an intrapancreatic accessory spleen. *Dig. Dis. Sci.*, **25**, 964–7.

Delany, H. M. and Jason, R. S. (1981) *Abdominal Trauma: Surgical and Radiological Diagnosis*, New York, Springer-Verlag.

Denneen, E. V. (1942) Hemorrhagic cyst of the spleen. *Ann. Surg.*, **116**, 103–8.

Dillion, M. L., Koster, J. K. and Coy, J. (1977) Intrathoracic splenosis. *South Med. J.*, **70**, 112.

Donovan, A. J. *et al.* (1969) Systemic-portal arteriovenous fistulas: pathologic and hemodynamic observations in two patients. *Surgery*, **66**, 474–82.

Doolas, A. *et al.* (1978) Splenic cysts. *J. Surg. Oncol.*, **10**, 369–87.

Eichner, E. R. (1979) Splenic function: normal, too much and too little. *Am. J. Med.*, **66**, 311–20.

Enzinger, F. M. and Weiss, S. W. (1983) *Soft Tissue Tumors*, C. V. Mosby, St Louis, MI, p. 485.

Faer, M. J. *et al.* (1980) RPC from AFIP. *Radiology*, **134**, 371–6.

Federle, M. P. (1983) Computed tomography of the spleen, in *Computed Tomography of the Body* (eds A. A. Moss, G. Gamsu and H. K. Genant), W. B. Saunders, Philadelphia, PA, p. 879.

Federle, M. and Moss, A. A. (1983) computer tomography of the spleen. *CRC Crit. Rev. Diagn. Imaging*, **19**, 1–16.

Fitzer, P. M. (1976) An approach to cardiac malposition and the heterotaxy syndrome using ^{99m}Tc-sulfur colloid imaging. *Am. J. Radiol.*, **127**, 1021–5.

Fowler, R. H. (1953) Collective review: nonparasitic benign cystic tumors of the spleen. *Int. Abstr. Surg.*, **96**, 209–27.

Freedom, R. M. and Fellows, K. E., Jr (1973) Radiographic visceral patterns in the asplenia syndrome. *Radiology*, **107**, 387–91.

Freeman, M. H. and Tonkin, A. K. (1976) Focal splenic effects. *Radiology*, **121**, 689–92.

Freund, R. *et al.* (1982) Splenic abscess: clinical symptoms and diagnostic possibilities. *Am. J. Gastroenterol.*, **77**, 35–8.

Gardner, D. C. and Ogilvie, R. F. (1959) The late results of injection of thorotrast: 2 cases of neoplastic disease following contrast angiography. *J. Pathol. Bacteriol.*, **78**, 133–44.

Garvin, D. E. and King, F. M. (1981) Cysts and nonlymphomatous tumors of the spleen. *Pathol. Ann.*, **16** (Part I), 61–80.

Glazer, G. M. *et al.* (1981) Dynamic CT of the normal spleen. *Am. J. Radiol.*, **137**, 343–6.

Goldman, M. L. *et al.* (1981) Intra-arterial tissue adhesive for medical splenectomy in humans. *Radiology*, **140**, 341–9.

Gordon, D. H. *et al.* (1977) Wandering spleen – the radiological and clinical spectrum. *Radiology*, **125**, 39–46.

Griscom, N. T. *et al.* (1977) Huge splenic cyst in a newborn: comparison with 10 cases in later childhood and adolescence. *Am. J. Radiol.*, **129**, 889–91.

Guarin, U., Dimitrieva, Z. and Ashley, S. (1975) Spleno-gonadal fusion: a rare congenital anomaly demonstrated by ^{99m}Tc-sulfur colloid imaging. *J. Nucl. Med.*, **16**, 922.

Haertel, M. and Ryder, D. (1979) Radiologic investigation of splenic trauma. *Cardiovasc. Radiol.*, **2**, 27–33.

Henderson, J. M. *et al.* (1981) Measurements of liver and spleen volume by CT. *Radiology*, **141**, 525–7.

Henkin, R. E. (1975) Selected topics in intraabdominal imaging *via* nuclear medicine techniques. *Radiol. Clin. North. Am.*, **17**, 39–54.

Heymsfield, S. B. *et al.* (1979) Accurate measurement of liver, kidney and spleen volume and mass by CT. *Ann. Intern. Med.*, **90**, 185–7.

Hushi, E. A. (1961) The clinical course of splenic hemangioma. *Arch. Surg.*, **83**, 681–5.

Iko, B. W. *et al.* (1982) Multifocal defects and splenomegaly in sarcoidosis: a new scintigraphic pattern. *J. Natl. Med. Assoc.*, **74**, 739–41.

Iozzo, R. V., Haas, J. E. R. and Chard, R. L. (1980) Symptomatic splenic hamartoma: a report of two cases and review of the literature. *Paediatrics*, **66**, 261–5.

Itzchak, Y. and Glickman, M. G. (1977) Splenic vein thrombosis in patients with a normal size spleen. *Invest. Radiol.*, **12**, 158–63.

Jacobs, R. P. *et al.* (1974) Angiography of splenic abscess. *Am. J. Radiol.*, **122**, 419–24.

Jeanty, P. *et al.* (1982) Case report: portal and splenic vein thrombosis: ultrasonic demonstration. *J. Belge Radiol.*, **65**, 45–7.

Jeffrey, R. B. *et al.* (1981) Computed tomography of splenic trauma. *Radiology*, **141**, 729–32.

Kan, M. K. and Hopkins, G. B. (1979) Measurement of liver volume by emission computed tomography. *J. Nucl. Med.*, **20**, 514–20.

Kardel, T., Halm, H. H., Rasmussen, S. N. *et al.* (1971) Ultrasonic determination of liver and spleen volumes. *Scand. J. Clin. Lab. Invest.*, **27**, 123–8.

Kaude, J. (1973) Accessory spleens as demonstrated by celiac angiography. *Radiology*, **13**, 53–6.

Kelly, K. J., Chusid, M. J. and Camitta, B. M. (1982) Splenic torsion in an infant associated with secondary disseminated Haemophilus influenzae infection. *Clin. Pediatr.*, **21**, 365–6.

Kim, H. and Dorfman F. R. (1974) Morphological studies of 84 untreated patients subjected to laparotomy for the staging of non-Hodgkin's lymphomas. *Cancer*, **33**, 557–647.

Kishikawa, T. *et al.* (1977) Hemangiosarcoma of the spleen with liver metastasis: angiographic manifestations. *Radiology*, **123**, 31–5.

Kishikawa, T. *et al.* (1978) Angiographic diagnosis of benign and malignant splenic tumors. *Am. J. Radiol.*, **130**, 339–44.

Koehler, R. E. (1983) Spleen, in *Computed Body Tomography* (eds J. K. Lee and S. R. J. Sagel), Raven Press, New York, NY, pp. 243–56.

Koga, T. M. *et al.* (1972) Ultrasonic tomography of the spleen. VII. Ultrasonic determination of the spleen volume from parallel sectional areas. *Med. Ultrason.*, **10**, 2–14.

Komacki, S. and Gombas, O. F. (1978) Angiographic demonstration of a calcified splenic hamartoma. *Radiology*, **121**, 77–8.

Korobkin, M. *et al.* (1978) Computed tomography of splenic subcapsular hematoma. *Radiology*, **129**, 441–5.

Langhans, T. (1879) Pulsating cavernous neoplasm of spleen with metastatic nodules to liver. *Virchows Arch. (Pathol. Anat.)*, **75**, 273–91.

Lawhorne, T. W. and Zuidema, G. D. (1976) Splenic abscess. *Surgery*, **79**, 686–9.

Levy, D. W. *et al.* (1986) Thorotrast-induced hepatosplenic neoplasia: CT identification. *Am. J. Radiol.*, **146**, 997–1004.

Lin, M. S. and Donati, R. M. (1981) Wedged appearance of splenic infarcts on scans. *Clin. Nucl. Med.*, **11**, 556.

Little, A. and Moosa, A. (1981) Gastrointestinal hemorrhage from left-sided portal hypertension. *Am. J. Surg.*, **141**, 153–8.

Locker, G. Y. *et al.* (1979) The clinical features of hepatic angiosarcoma: a report of four cases and a review of the English literature. *Medicine*, **58**, 48–64.

Longscope, W. T. and Freiman, D. G. (1952) Study of sarcoidosis. *Medicine*, **31**, 1.

Lupien, C. and Sauerbrei, E. E. (1984) Healing in the traumatized spleen: Sonographic investigation. *Radiology*, **151**, 181–5.

Lutzker, L. *et al.* (1973) The role of radionuclide imaging in spleen trauma. *Radiology*, **110**, 419–25.

Macpherson, A. I. S., Richmond, J. and Stuart, A. E. (1973) *The Spleen*, Charles C. Thomas, Springfield, IL, p. 101.

McArdle, C. (1980) Case of the winter season. Diagnosis: torsion of a wandering spleen. *Semin. Roentgenol.*, **15**, 7–8.

McClure, R. D. and Altemeier, W. A. (1942) Cysts of the spleen. *Ann. Surg.*, **116**, 98–102.

Mahony, B., Jeffrey, R. B. and Federle, M. P. (1982) Spontaneous rupture of hepatic and splenic angiosarcoma demonstrated by CT. *Am. J. Radiol.*, **138**, 965–6.

Marymount, J. H., Jr and Gross, S. (1963) Patterns of metastatic cancer in the spleen. *Am. J. Clin. Pathol.*, **40**, 58–66.

Mandcll, G. A. *et al.* (1983) A case of microgastria with splenic-gonadal fusion. *Pediatr. Radiol.*, **13**, 95–8.

Mattson, O. (1982) Scintigraphic spleen volume calculation. *Acta Radiol. Diag.*, **23**, 471–7.

Mettler, F. A. (1986) *Essentials of Nuclear Medicine Imaging*, Grune and Stratton, Orlando, Florida, p. 223.

Miller, J. H., Greenfield, L. D. and Wald, B. R. (1982) Candidiasis of the liver and spleen in childhood. *Radiology*, **142**, 375–80.

Mitnick, J. S. *et al.* (1981) CT in β-thalassemia: iron deposition in the liver, spleen and lymph nodes. *Am. J. Radiol.*, **136**, 1191–4.

Moller, J. H. *et al.* (1967) Congenital heart disease associated with polysplenia. A developmental complex of bilateral 'left-sidedness'. *Circulation*, **36**, 789–99.

Monie, I. W. (1982) The asplenia syndrome: an explanation for absence of the spleen. *Teratology*, **25**, 215–19.

Moss, A. A. *et al.* (1979) Computed tomography of splenic subcapsular hematomas: an experimental study in dogs. *Invest. Radiol.*, **1**, 60–4.

Moss, M. *et al.* (1980) CT demonstration of a splenic abscess not evident at surgery. *Am. J. Radiol.*, **135**, 159–60.

Mousa, A. H. *et al.* (1967) Hepatosplenic schistosomiasis, in *Bilharziasis* (ed. F. K. Mostofi), Springer-Verlag, New York, NY, p. 15.

Nesbesar, R. A., Rabinov, K. R. and Potsaid, M. S. (1974) Radionuclide imaging of the spleen and suspected splenic injury. *Radiology*, **110**, 609–14.

Nielsen, J. L. (1981) Splenosis on the right kidney and diaphragmatic surface following traumatic rupture of the spleen. *Acta Chir. Scand.*, **147**, 721–4.

Novetsky, G. S. and Epstein, A. J. (1982) Cystic lymphangiomatosis: an unusual cause of splenic scintigraphic defects. *Clin. Nucl. Med.*, **7**, 416–17.

Nunez, D., Jr *et al.* (1978) Portosystemic communication studied by transhepatic portography. *Radiology*, **127**, 75–9.

Osborn, D. J. *et al.* (1973) The role of angiography in abdominal nonrenal trauma. *Radiol. Clin. North Am.*, **11**, 579–92.

Pachter, H. L., Hofstetter, S. R. and Spencer, F. C. (1981) Evolving concepts in splenic surgery. Splenography versus splenectomy and post-splenectomy drainage: experience in 105 patients. *Ann. Surg.*, **194**, 262–7.

Paivansalo, M. and Siniluoto, T. (1983) Cavernous hemangioma of the spleen. *Fortschr. Rontgenstr.*, **142**, 228–30.

Pawar, S. *et al.* (1982) Sonography of splenic abscess. *Am. J. Radiol.*, **138**, 259–62.

Pearl, G. S. and Nassar, V. H. (1979) Cystic lymphangioma of the spleen. *South. Med. J.*, **72**, 667–9.

Peoples, W. M., Moller, J. H. and Edwards, J. E. (1983) Reviews: polysplenia, a review of 146 cases. *Pediatr. Cardiol.*, **4**, 129–37.

Peters, A. M. *et al.* (1980) Use of indium-111 labelled platelets to measure spleen function. *Br. J. Haematol.*, **46**, 587–93.

Peters, A. M. *et al.* (1984) Methods of measuring splenic blood flow and platelet transit time with ^{111}In-labelled platelets. *J. Nucl. Med.*, **25**, 86–90.

Piekarski, J., Federle, M. P. and Moss, A. A. (1980) Computed tomography of the spleen. *Radiology*, **135**, 683–9.

Piepsz, A. *et al.* (1977) A real clinical indication for selective spleen scintigraphy with ^{99m}Tc-labelled red blood cells. *Radiology*, **123**, 407–4.

Pietri, H. and Boscaini, M. (1984) Determination of a splenic volumetric index by ultrasound scanning. *J. Ultrasound Med.*, **3**, 319–23.

Pistoia, F. and Markowitz, S. K. (1988) Splenic lymphangiomatosis: CT diagnosis. *Am. J. Radiol.*, **150**, 121–2.

Probst, P. *et al.* (1978) Nonsurgical treatment of splenic artery aneurysms. *Radiology*, **128**, 619–23.

Propper, R. A. *et al.* (1979) Ultrasonography of hemorrhagic splenic cysts. *J. Clin. Ultrasound*, **7**, 18–20.

Pyatt, R. S. *et al.* (1981) CT diagnosis of splenic cystic lymphangiomatosis. *J. Comput. Assist. Tomogr.*, **5**, 446–8.

Rahimtoola, S. H., Marshall, H. J. and Edwards, J. E. (1965) Anomalous connection of pulmonary veins to right atrium associated with anomalous inferior vena cava, situs inversus and multiple spleens: developmental complex. *Mayo Clin. Proc.*, **40**, 609–13.

Ralls, P. W. *et al.* (1982) Sonography of pyogenic splenic abscess. *Am. J. Radiol.*, **138**, 523–5.

Rao, B. K., Winebright, J. W. and Dresser, T. P. (1979a) Functional asplenia after thorotrast administration. *Clin. Nucl. Med.*, **4**, 437–8.

Rao, B. K., Winebright, J. W. and Dresser, T. P. (1979b) Splenic artifact caused by barium in the colon. *Clin. Nucl. Med.*, **4**, 249.

Rao, B. K. *et al.* (1981) Cystic lymphangiomatosis of the spleen: a radiologic–pathologic correlation. *Radiology*, **141**, 781–2.

Rao, B. K. *et al.* (1982) Dual radiopharmaceutical imaging in congenital asplenia syndrome. *Radiology*, **145**, 805–10.

Rasmussen, S. N. *et al.* (1973) Spleen volume determination by ultrasonic scanning. *Scand. J. Haematol.*, **10**, 298–304.

Rauch, R. F. *et al.* (1983) CT detection of iatrogenic percutaneous splenic injury. *J. Comput. Assist. Tomogr.*, 7, 1018–21.

Redman, H. C. and Reuter, S. R. (1969) Angiographic demonstration of portocaval and other decompressive liver shunts. *Radiology*, 92, 790.

Ros, P. R. *et al.* (1987) Hemangioma of the spleen: radiologic–pathologic correlation in ten cases. *Radiology*, 162, 73–7.

Rose, V., Izukawa, T. and Moes, C. A. F. (1975) Syndromes of asplenia and polysplenia: a review of cardiac and non-cardiac malformations in 60 cases with special reference to diagnosis and prognosis. *Br. Heart J.*, 37, 840–52.

Rosenthall, L., Lisbona, R. and Banerjee, K. (1974) A nucleographic and radioangiographic study of a patient with torsion of the spleen. *Radiology*, 110, 427–8.

Salam, A., Warren, D. and Tyras, D. (1973) Splenic vein thrombosis: a diagnosable and curable form of portal hypertension. *Surgery*, 74, 961–72.

Salomonowitz, E., Frick, M. P. and Lund, G. (1984) Radiologic diagnosis of wandering spleen complicated by splenic nodules and infarction. *Gastrointest. Radiol.*, 9, 57–9.

Schulman, A. *et al.* (1983) Pseudosolid appearance of simple and echinococcal cysts in ultrasonography. *S. Afr. Med. J.*, 63, 905–6.

Shanser, J. D. *et al.* (1973) Angiographic evaluation of cystic lesions of the spleen. *Am. J. Radiol.*, 119, 166–74.

Sheflin, J. R., Chung, M. L. and Kretchmar, K. A. (1984) Torsion of the wandering spleen and distal pancreas. *Am. J. Radiol.*, 142, 100–1.

Shin, M. S. and Ho, K. (1983) Mesodermal cyst of the spleen: computed tomographic characteristics and pathogenetic considerations. *J. Comput. Tomogr.*, 7, 295–9.

Sirinek, K. R. and Evans, W. E. (1973) Nonparasitic splenic cysts: case report of epidermoid cyst with review of the literature. *Am. J. Surg.*, 126, 8–13.

Smulewicz, J. J. and Clemett, A. R. (1975) Torsion of the wandering spleen. *Dig. Dis.*, 20, 274–9.

Soler-Bechara, J. and Soscia, J. L. (1964) Calcified echinococcus (hydatid) cyst of the spleen. *J. Am. Med. Assoc.*, 187, 162.

Sordillo, E. M., Sordillo, P. P. and Hajdu, S. I. (1981) Primary hemangiosarcoma of the spleen: report of four cases. *Med. Pediatr. Oncol.*, 9, 314–24.

Stivelman, R. L., Glaubitz, J. P. and Crampton, R. S. (1963) Laceration of the spleen due to nonpenetrating trauma. One hundred cases. *Am. J. Surg.*, 106, 888–91.

Subramanyam, B. R., Balthazar, E. J. and Horii, S. C.

(1984) Sonography of the accessory spleen. *Am. J. Radiol.*, 143, 47–9.

Sumner, T. E. *et al.* (1983) Radiologic case of the month: hepatic and splenic candidiasis in acute leukemia. *Am. J. Dis. Child.*, 137, 1193–4.

Teats, C. D., Seale, D. L. and Allen, M. S. (1972) Hamartoma of the spleen. *Am. J. Radiol.*, 116, 419–22.

Thomas, J. L. *et al.* (1982) EOE-13 in detection of hepatosplenic lymphoma. *Radiology*, 145, 629–34.

Toback, A. C., Steece, D. M. and Kaye, M. D. (1984) Case report. Splenic torsion: an unusual cause of splenomegaly. *Dig. Dis. Sci.*, 29, 868–71.

Tuttle, R. J. and Minielly, J. A. (1978) Splenic cystic lymphangiomatosis. *Radiology*, 126, 47–8.

Uflacker, R. (1979) Cystic lymphangioma of the spleen. A cause of splenomegaly. *Br. J. Radiol.*, 52, 148–9.

Van Mierop, L. H. S., Gessner, J. H. and Schiebler, G. L. (1972) Asplenia and polysplenia syndromes. *Birth Defects*, 8, 36–44.

Van Way, C. W. *et al.* (1971) Arteriovenous fistula in the portal circulation. *Surgery*, 70, 876–90.

Weinberger, G., Mitra, S. K. and Yoeli, G. (1982) Case report: Ultrasound diagnosis of splenic vein thrombosis. *J. Clin. Ultrasound*, 10, 345–6.

Weingarten, M. J. *et al.* (1984) Sonography after splenic embolization: the wedge-shaped acute infarct. *Am. J. Radiol.*, 142, 957–9.

Wexler, L. and Abrams, H. L. (1964) Hamartoma of the spleen: angiographic observations. *Am. J. Radiol.*, 92, 1150–5.

Whitley, J. E., Maynard, C. D. and Rhyne, A. L. (1966) A computer approach to the prediction of spleen weight from routine films. *Radiology*, 86, 73–6.

Wilson, D. G. and Lieberman, L. M. (1983) Unusual splenic band appearance on liver–spleen scan. *Clin. Nucl. Med.*, 8, 270.

Wintrobe, M. M. *et al.* (1981) *Clinical Hematology*, 7th edn, Lea and Febiger, Philadelphia, PA, pp. 94–5; 1426–46.

Wright, F. W. and Williams, F. W. (1974) Large post-traumatic splenic cyst diagnosed by radiology, isotope scintigraphy and ultrasound. *Br. J. Radiol.*, 47, 454.

Wurtele, L. H., Tondreau, R. L. and Pollack, H. (1982) Ultrasonographic appearance of splenic echinococcal cyst. *Penn. Med.*, 85, 55–6.

Yeh, H-C., Zacks, J. and Jurado, R. A. (1981) Ultrasonography of splenic infarct. *Mt Sinai J. Med. NY*, 48, 446–8.

THE SURGERY OF THE SPLEEN 18

Carol E. H. Scott-Conner

18.1 INTRODUCTION

As recently as twenty years ago, splenectomy was routinely performed for even minor splenic injuries. Because of the fragile parenchyma, repair of lacerations was considered difficult at best, and likely to be followed by delayed bleeding. An increased awareness of the several important functions of the spleen has led surgeons to re-evaluate critically the indications for splenectomy and to develop techniques for splenic conservation. These surgical techniques, initially developed for use in trauma surgery, are being applied to an increasing number of situations in which elective splenectomy would previously have been the only option.

In this chapter, the most common indications for splenic surgery will be reviewed. Surgical options, including partial splenectomy, will be considered. The surgical anatomy and the techniques of partial and total splenectomy will be detailed, and measures to avoid or manage surgical complications will be discussed.

18.2 HEMATOLOGICAL INDICATIONS FOR SURGERY

Most elective splenic surgery is performed for diagnosis, palliation, or definitive management of hematological disorders. In most reported series, a majority of splenectomies are performed for treatment of cytopenias (Schwartz, Adams and Bauman, 1971; Traetow, Fabri and Carey, 1980; Ly and Albrechtsen, 1981; Musser *et al.*, 1984).

18.2.1 HEMOLYTIC ANEMIAS

Accelerated destruction of the circulating erythrocyte may occur as a result of increased clearance by the reticuloendothelial system or from intravascular hemolysis (see Chapter 13). Factors contributing to increased reticuloendothelial clearance include surface abnormalities of erythrocytes, such as membrane-bound IgG, or a physical abnormality of the erythrocyte which renders it unable to survive passage through the spleen. Intravascular hemolysis may be caused by trauma to the erythrocytes, exogenous toxins, or the fixation of complement to the erythrocytes with subsequent lysis. When the spleen is the major cause of abnormal erythrocyte destruction either by splenic destruction of red blood cells or by production of antibody or opsonizing factors, splenectomy may be indicated (NIH, 1977).

(a) General considerations

The hemolytic anemias may be conveniently divided into the congenital hemolytic anemias (including hereditary spherocytosis and the thalassemias) and the acquired hemolytic anemias (including autoimmune hemolytic anemia). In the congenital anemias, abnormalities of erythrocyte surface membrane or hemoglobin structure render the erythrocyte more vulnerable to destruction in the spleen. Splenectomy may significantly lengthen erythrocyte survival in these cases even though the underlying red cell defect remains unchanged. In contrast, the acquired anemias are generally immunologically mediated, the site of red cell destruction is frequently intravascular, and the response to splenectomy is variable.

(i) Prediction of the response to splenectomy

Accurate diagnosis of the cause and site of hemolysis is important. A family and ethnic history may be valuable in cases of hereditary spherocytosis or thalassemia, but is sometimes lacking. The direct antiglobulin (Coombs') test is usually negative in the congenital hemolytic anemias, which are more likely to respond to splenectomy than the acquired immune hemolytic anemias.

If the site of hemolysis is uncertain, a chromium (^{51}Cr) tagged red cell study may be helpful in determining whether or not the spleen is the site of significant erythrocyte destruction.

(ii) Treatment of associated biliary tract disease

The increased bilirubin load associated with chronic hemolysis leads to gallstone formation in a significant percentage of patients. The stones contain a black insoluble pigment composed of polymerized hemoglobin breakdown products (Bissel, 1986). In a representative series, concomitant cholecystectomy was performed in nine of 113 patients undergoing splenectomy for congenital or acquired hemolytic anemia (Coon, 1985c). The incidence varies with the duration and severity of hemolysis and is highest in adult patients with congenital hemolytic anemias. In adults with hereditary spherocytosis, the reported incidence of biliary tract disease averages 30%, although a 55% incidence was reported in one series (Lawrie and Ham, 1974). As part of the preoperative evaluation of patients with hemolytic anemia, ultrasound examination of the gallbladder should be performed. Careful assessment of the gallbladder at the time of laparotomy may disclose small stones not noted on ultrasound. Cholecystectomy and operative cholangiography, with common duct exploration if needed, may then be performed at the time of elective splenectomy.

In some patients, hemolysis is reduced but not eliminated by splenectomy. Such a result is particularly likely in autoimmune hemolytic anemias, or in some of the congenital anemias such as pyruvate kinase deficiency. In these cases pigment gallstones may occasionally form after splenectomy, even if the gallbladder appeared normal at the time of surgery. However, the possibility of subsequent gallstone formation does not justify removal of a gallbladder which appears normal at the time of splenectomy.

(b) Hereditary spherocytosis and related disorders

The hemolytic anemia resulting from hereditary spherocytosis is the type most commonly and predictably responsive to splenectomy. The incidence of hereditary spherocytosis is 1:4500 of the general population. Although in most cases an autosomal dominant pattern of inheritance can be demonstrated, approximately 20% of cases arise sporadically. The characteristic triad of anemia, splenomegaly and acholuric jaundice is initially mild and the illness may escape detection until adult life. The level of jaundice fluctuates, being less pronounced in early childhood. The degree of anemia varies from slight to moderate depending upon the balance between hemolysis and red cell production. A precarious state of compensation may be disrupted by systemic infection, resulting in jaundice and profound anemia.

An abnormality in red cell membrane structure, related to a deficiency of spectrin synthesis, causes the characteristic spheroidal shape of the erythrocytes and renders them either vulnerable to destruction in the spleen, or conditioning them to destruction elsewhere. Splenectomy corrects the anemia by allowing the abnormal erythrocytes to survive in the circulation. The differential diagnosis includes spherocytic hemolytic anemias associated with anti-erythrocyte antibodies, in which the direct antiglobulin (Coombs') test is positive. Spherocytes are also seen in patients with cirrhosis, chronic infections and occasionally in other hematologic disorders. The negative Coombs' test provides evidence that the diagnosis is hereditary spherocytosis, especially when a positive family history is obtained.

Most, but not all, patients with hereditary spherocytosis will require splenectomy. The surgery should be delayed at least until after the age of four, when the risk of postsplenectomy sepsis is decreased. Generally surgery can be postponed until early adulthood; however, it is unwise to defer surgery unduly as continued hemolysis will lead to gallstone formation. In the most severe form of hereditary spherocytosis, splenectomy may be required in infancy (Croom et al., 1986).

The spleen is generally slightly to moderately enlarged. Total splenectomy is the treatment of choice. Accessory spleens should be sought diligently since their subsequent enlargement can produce significant recurrence of hemolysis. The biliary tract should be assessed prior to surgery so that any associated biliary tract disease can be dealt with at the time of elective splenectomy. The postoperative course in these otherwise healthy patients is usually uncomplicated and the response to splenectomy is gratifying; erythrocyte survival is prolonged and the evidence for hemolysis subsides.

Hereditary elliptocytosis is a related disorder which is also transmitted as an autosomal dominant trait. The incidence is between 1:4000 and 1:5000. The usually mild degree of hemolysis does not require treatment in most patients. In approximately 10–15% of cases, significant hemolysis warrants splenectomy.

Other less-common congenital defects in erythrocyte membrane structure include hereditary pyropoikilocytosis and hereditary stomatocytosis. In hereditary pyropoikilocytosis, a spectrin structural abnormality causes red cells to assume bizarre shapes. *In vitro* thermal disruption occurs at 44–45°C, rather than the normal 49°C. Severe hemolysis is characteristic of the disorder; in contrast to hereditary spherocytosis, splenectomy only partially corrects the hemolytic tendency. In hereditary stomatocytosis, anemia is generally mild. The indications for splenectomy are similar to those for hereditary spherocytosis. Splenectomy decreases the rate of hemolysis but does not halt it completely.

(c) **Thalassemia**

The thalassemias constitute a group of congenital disorders characterized by a defect in synthesis of one or more subunits of hemoglobin. In general, the hemoglobin subunits are normal in structure but are produced at a greatly decreased rate.

The most common disorder is β-thalassemia. The gene frequency of this condition approaches 0.1 in southern Italy and some of the islands of the Mediterranean. It is also commonly encountered in regions of central Africa, Asia, the South Pacific and parts of India. Individuals who are homozygous are said to have β-thalassemia major (Cooley's anemia).

In β-thalassemia major, severe anemia is accompanied by hemolysis, iron overload, and active erythropoiesis. The hemolysis occurs in several locations, not just within the spleen, and is only partially improved by splenectomy. Affected individuals develop skeletal abnormalities from the increased mass of the highly erythropoietic marrow, cardiomegaly, often with congestive heart failure, and hepatosplenomegaly.

Although splenectomy may be of some benefit in decreasing transfusion requirements, it is accompanied by an inordinately high risk of septic complications, especially in childhood. Some of the earliest observations of overwhelming postsplenectomy sepsis were made in children who underwent splenectomy for Cooley's anemia (Smith et al., 1964). In an attempt to balance the potential benefits of splenectomy against the risks in this condition, both partial splenic embolization and partial splenectomy have been used. Politis et al. (1987) reported a five-year follow-up of six patients with thalassemia major who were treated with partial splenic embolization, and compared their clinical course to that of seven patients who underwent total splenectomy. Partial splenic embolization successfully reduced transfusion requirements, and no infectious complications were noted during the five-year follow-up. In contrast, two patients in the splenectomized group subsequently suffered recurrent infections.

(d)   Sickle cell disease

An abnormal hemoglobin (HBS) is synthesized in sickle cell disease. The tendency for this abnormal molecule to polymerize when deoxygenated causes the diverse clinical manifestations characteristic of the condition (see Chapter 16). Approximately 8% of black Americans have the heterozygous variant of the disorder ('sickle cell trait'). The incidence of the trait is substantially higher in certain regions of Africa, and exceeds 30% in Nigeria. In America, 0.15% of black children are homozygous for the disorder.

The erythrocytes of homozygous individuals tend to assume a rigid, sickled configuration when the Hbs is desaturated. In this configuration, the erythrocytes are vulnerable to destruction by the spleen and are also prone to lodge in the microvasculature of various organs. In the microcirculation a vicious cycle of microthrombosis, interruption of blood flow, local decrease in oxygen tension, and further sickling of more erythrocytes causes progressive infarction of the spleen and kidneys and produces the characteristic periodic vaso-occlusive crises. Between crises, anemia and hemolysis continue. The spleen is enlarged in the early stages in childhood, but later shrinks as sequential infarction occurs (Charache, 1975; Ballas *et al.*, 1982; see section 16.3).

Acute splenic sequestration crises, characterized by sudden enlargement of the spleen and worsening anemia, may occur. Thrombocytopenia and signs of hypovolaemia may be present. The pathogenesis is unclear; however, the syndrome resembles splenic vein occlusion in animal models. It is thought that transient splenic vein obstruction, possibly by sickled erythrocytes, may result in distension of the spleen and sequestration of a significant, and sometimes massive, amount of blood (Solanki, Kletter and Castro, 1986). Such crises are most common in patients under the age of six (Topley *et al.*, 1981). They are less common in adolescents and adults because progressive splenic infarction renders the spleen fibrotic and incapable of acute distension.

In heterozygous individuals splenic infarction is less likely to occur, and splenic sequestration crises have been reported in adolescents and adults with mixed sickle-cell syndromes, including sickle-cell hemoglobin C disease and sickle-cell thalassemia (Solanki, Kletter and Castro, 1986). The treatment is transfusion with normal red cells and hydration, and the crisis generally resolves with time. Rarely, splenectomy is indicated for the treatment of recurrent crises in adults, or in patients in whom transfusion is difficult because of erythrocyte alloantibodies.

Even before splenic atrophy develops, splenic function is diminished in homozygous individuals with hemoglobin S, and a hyposplenic state in which bacterial clearance is decreased can be detected (see Serjeant, Chapter 16). Splenectomy is rarely indicated in these individuals, since the spleen usually atrophies in time. Occasionally, splenic abscesses form within the parenchyma of an infarcted spleen, requiring drainage or splenectomy.

(e)   Other hemolytic anemias

Many forms of hereditary hemolytic anemia associated with erythrocyte enzyme deficiency have been identified. The two major forms of surgical importance are pyruvate kinase (PK) deficiency and glucose-6-phosphate dehydrogenase (G-6-PD) deficiency. Most patients with enzyme deficiencies maintain an adequate hemoglobin level and do not require splenectomy. The spleen is generally enlarged in PK deficiency, and splenectomy may be required in severe forms. In contrast, splenectomy is rarely indicated in G-6-PD deficiency (Ravindranath and Beutler, 1987).

Autoimmune hemolytic anemia is an acquired disorder which, in later life especially, tends to be secondary to other disorders. A positive direct antiglobulin (Coombs') test is characteristic, although in some cases the surface antibody is below the threshold of detection by this method. Collagen vascular diseases and lymphoproliferative disorders must especially be sought. Approximately 75% of patients will respond at least temporarily to corticosteroid therapy. Patients who do not respond after 6–8 weeks of steroids, or those in whom a contraindication to steroid use exists, may be referred for splenectomy. Careful evaluation to exclude other causes of hemolysis, particularly acute self-limited forms, is essential. Chromium-51 tagged erythrocyte sequestration studies may be helpful if carefully standardized. Schwartz *et al.* (1981) noted a greater probability of a good response to splenectomy in patients with splenomegaly, a positive direct antiglobulin test, the demonstrated presence of warm antibodies, and an absence of complement fixing antibodies and cold agglutinins. (See also Chapters 8 and 13.)

Hemolytic anemia may complicate the course of lymphoproliferative disorders, including chronic lymphatic leukemia and Hodgkin's disease. In some instances other cytopenias may be superimposed, and splenectomy may be required.

Paroxysmal nocturnal hemoglobinuria is an acquired erythrocyte membrane disorder in which red cells become inordinately sensitive to complement. The sensitivity to complement also involves neutrophils and platelets, and is thought to arise from a change in the pluripotent stem cell which gives rise to all three cell lines. Splenectomy is not recommended because of its limited therapeutic value and inordinately high operative risk.

18.2.2 DISORDERS ASSOCIATED WITH THROMBOCYTOPENIA

Recently one large series showed that 81% of elective splenectomies were performed for cytopenias, especially thrombocytopenia (Dotevall *et al.*, 1987). The most common disorder for which splenectomy is recommended is idiopathic thrombocytopenic purpura (Schwartz, Hoepp and Sachs, 1980).

(a) General considerations

The profound thrombocytopenia which is present in most of these patients renders bleeding complications more likely at the time of surgery. In addition, many have been on corticosteroid treatment preoperatively, necessitating perioperative steroid therapy and resulting in diminished wound healing.

(i) Preoperative evaluation

Accurate diagnosis is important. Response to previous therapy, as discussed in subsequent sections, is the most important predictor of response to splenectomy in ITP. Platelet sequestration studies with ^{51}Cr-tagged platelets are no longer recommended. Although a significant percentage of patients with thrombocytopenia undergo platelet destruction in liver as well as spleen, the majority respond favorably to splenectomy (Ries and Price, 1974; Schwartz, Hoepp and Sachs, 1980).

(ii) Measures to increase safety of operation in profoundly thrombocytopenic patients

An incision that does not require muscle transection is recommended, to minimize wound bleeding and hematoma formation. Initial control of the splenic artery in the lesser sac, as described in section 18.4.2(b), allows dissection to proceed under controlled conditions. After control of the splenic artery has been achieved, platelet transfusion may be used to raise the platelet count and decrease intraoperative oozing. If platelets are infused prior to control of the splenic artery, a significant number of them will be destroyed in the spleen. Because platelet counts start to rise rapidly after surgery, platelet transfusion may not be required.

Reperitonealization of raw surfaces after splenectomy and the use of topical hemostatic agents may help to control oozing from the splenic bed in profoundly thrombocytopenic patients.

(b) Idiopathic thrombocytopenic purpura

Idiopathic thrombocytopenic purpura is a hemorrhagic disorder characterized by a decreased platelet count, despite the presence of normal or increased megakaryocytes in the bone marrow. Definitive diagnosis depends upon ruling out other systemic illnesses capable of producing thrombocytopenia, and there must likewise be no history of ingestion of drugs known to produce thrombocytopenia. ITP is divided into two forms: acute and chronic.

Acute ITP is seen most commonly in children, following a viral illness or upper respiratory tract infection. Over 80% of affected individuals recover spontaneously within three to six months. In adults, approximately 10% of cases of ITP are of the self-limited acute form (Lacey and Penner, 1977).

Chronic ITP accounts for most adult cases. The typical patient is a female between the ages of 20 and 40 years. Bleeding, most commonly from the gingiva, vagina, gastrointestinal tract or urinary tract, is the presenting symptom. The platelet count is low, typically under 50 000/ mm^3. Bone marrow examination to confirm the presence of normal or increased numbers of megakaryocytes and to identify hematologic malignancy is required. Systemic lupus erythematosus should be sought by the antinuclear antibody test (ANA). Hepatitis, or infection with cytomegalovirus, Epstein–Barr virus, toxoplasmosis, and HTLV III virus should be investigated by appropriate serological tests. Treatment may not be necessary unless the platelet count is below 20 000/mm^3 or there is extensive bleeding.

Elevated levels of platelet-associated IgG have been found in this condition (see Chapter 13). The antibody-coated platelets are removed by the spleen and, to a lesser extent, by the liver. Platelet survival is markedly diminished, and platelet turnover increased. The survival of infused platelets is markedly decreased. Splenectomy is effective in ITP, not only because the spleen is the major site of platelet destruction, but also because it is commonly the site of production of antiplatelet antibodies.

Initial therapy of ITP consists of corticosteroid treatment for six weeks to two months. Patients who respond to corticosteroids are subsequently tapered off; a significant percentage will remain in remission. Patients who respond to steroids but relapse after steroid withdrawal are candidates for splenectomy, as are those patients who do not respond to steroid treatment. Emergency splenectomy may be necessary if serious bleeding complications, particularly intracranial hemorrhage, occur.

Of 216 patients who underwent splenectomy for ITP, Coon (1987) reported a satisfactory response, with platelet counts over 150 000/ mm^3 in 72%. This result is similar to those of other reported series. Patients who responded favorably to steroids were more likely to respond to splenectomy, but no other predictive factors could be identified. Patients who do not respond to splenectomy may require long-term treatment with immunosuppressive agents. Picozzi, Roeske and Creger (1980) studied 15 patients who were considered treatment failures after splenectomy for ITP. Patients who initially responded favorably to splenectomy and then relapsed were more likely to respond to immunosuppressive therapy than were those who did not respond to splenectomy. However, eight patients eventually achieved normal platelet counts after failing both splenectomy and immunosuppressive therapy, underscoring the unpredictable long-term natural history of the disorder.

Spleen size is usually close to normal in ITP. The mean splenic weight was 217 g in Schwartz' series (1980). Initial control of the splenic artery, as previously discussed, facilitates splenectomy by allowing platelet transfusion to be performed. Many patients do not require intra-operative platelet infusion: in a series of 120 patients who underwent splenectomy for ITP (Schwartz, Hoepp and Sachs,

1980), platelet transfusion was used intra-operatively or postoperatively in only nine patients.

(c) Systemic lupus erythematosus

Autoimmune thrombocytopenic purpura is the most common indication for splenectomy in systemic lupus erythematosus (SLE). Occasionally, autoimmune hemolytic anemia or hypersplenism due to portal hypertension occur and necessitate removal of the spleen. Thrombocytopenia occurs in approximately 20% of patients with SLE and is related to the presence of antiplatelet antibodies. Although the pathogenesis differs, patients with SLE respond to the same medical management as is used in ITP, and splenectomy is available when conservative treatment fails. In a representative series, Gruenberg, Van Slyck and Abraham (1986) reported that 1.9% of patients diagnosed with SLE required splenectomy during the study period. Of sixteen patients, twelve underwent splenectomy for thrombocytopenia. Eight had satisfactory results, the platelet counts being maintained at normal levels without the need for steroids, although these might be required for other manifestations of SLE. Splenectomy did not accelerate the development of other manifestations of SLE in this series.

The spleen is usually normal in size but may be enlarged. Five of 16 spleens in the Gruenberg series weighed more than 200 g. In a series reported by Homan and Dineen (1978), four of ten spleens removed for SLE showed the characteristic 'onion-skin lesions', with perivascular fibrosis surrounding central and penicilliary arteries. Only two of 16 patients in Gruenberg's series (1986) showed characteristic pathological changes of SLE, although when present, the histological characteristics provided important diagnostic confirmation of the disorder.

(d) Thrombotic thrombocytopenic purpura

Thrombotic thrombocytopenic purpura (TTP) has been regarded as an uncommon syndrome, but it is now being recognized with increasing frequency. The classical pentad is characterized by thrombocytopenic purpura, microangiopathic hemolytic anemia, fluctuating neurological abnormalities, renal disease and fever. The diverse manifestations are related to the formation of microthrombi within the capillaries and terminal arterioles of many organs. Platelet survival is decreased due to consumption of platelets in the thrombotic material within the microvasculature. The mortality rate without treatment is between 80 and 90%.

Prior to 1977, treatment with corticosteroids and splenectomy was used with a response rate averaging 50% (Hill and Cooper, 1968). The present treatment of choice is plasma exchange with the transfusion of fresh frozen plasma, which is believed to remove a platelet-aggregating agent. Antiplatelet drugs, dextran, and corticosteroids may be used in addition. Splenectomy is reserved for patients who fail to respond to plasma exchange. In one series (Schneider et al., 1985), eleven patients with TTP were treated initially with plasma exchange and infusion of fresh frozen plasma. Six patients who did not respond to plasma exchange underwent splenectomy and treatment with antiplatelet drugs, corticosteroids and dextran. All patients survived splenectomy and remained in remission during subsequent observation. Thompson and McCarthy (1983) detailed the clinical course of two patients who failed with plasma exchange and underwent splenectomy. Both went into remission and subsequently remained without evidence of TTP. Thus, although the preferred treatment of TTP is plasma exchange with plasma infusion, there is a subset of patients in whom splenectomy may be necessary to induce remission when this fails (Myers et al., 1980; Rowe et al., 1985; Liu, Linker and Shuman, 1986).

(e) Other disorders associated with thrombocytopenia

(i) Hematological malignancies

Thrombocytopenia may complicate the course of patients with malignant lymphoma, chronic lymphocytic leukemia, and myeloproliferative disorders, but this is rarely an indication for splenectomy in these circumstances (Lehman *et al.*, 1987). These situations are discussed further in section 18.2.3, and also in Chapters 14 and 15.

(ii) Chronic liver disease

Thrombocytopenia also occurs in the context of chronic liver disease and usually results from hypersplenism secondary to portal hypertension. Splenomegaly due to chronic splenic congestion leads to the splenic sequestration of platelets, leukocytes and erythrocytes, and may result in neutropenia and anemia as well as thrombocytopenia. Skootsky, Rosove and Langley (1986) reported two patients who underwent splenectomy for thrombocytopenia associated with chronic liver disease who had only minimally enlarged spleens (230 g and 375 g). They postulated that increased levels of platelet-associated IgG may be important in the pathogenesis of thrombocytopenia in chronic liver disease.

Soper and Rikkers (1982) described a series in which 36% of 76 patients with cirrhosis and portal hypertension had platelet counts under $100\,000/mm^3$, 41% had neutropenia, and 25% had both thrombocytopenia and neutropenia. The majority of patients with thrombocytopenia associated with chronic liver disease are asymptomatic and do not require treatment; however, when bleeding occurs, surgical intervention may be needed.

Although splenectomy has been used in the past as a means of treating symptomatic hypersplenism in this setting, it is rarely indicated (Crosby, 1987; El-Khishen *et al.*, 1985). Correction of the portal hypertension by portal–systemic shunting procedures alleviates the hypersplenism (Soper and Rikkers, 1982). Avoidance of splenectomy allows use of a selective distal splenorenal shunt, which will alleviate the hypersplenism (El-Khishen *et al.*, 1985).

(iii) Acquired immunodeficiency syndrome

Thrombocytopenic purpura occurs in association with the acquired immunodeficiency syndrome (AIDS) and AIDS-related complex. It has been termed immunodeficiency-associated thrombocytopenic purpura (Walsh *et al.*, 1985; Schneider *et al.*, 1987). It may be the presenting symptom in a patient previously undiagnosed as having AIDS or the AIDS-related complex. Splenomegaly was present clinically in 20% of patients in one series, and this is one characteristic in which the syndrome differs from ITP. Other findings include seropositivity to the HTLV-III virus, and depressed T-cell helper: suppressor ratios (Schneider *et al.*, 1987).

The condition shares many features with ITP, and treatment with corticosteroids and splenectomy has been patterned empirically after that used for ITP. Of 15 homosexual men treated by splenectomy for immunodeficiency-associated thrombocytopenic purpura, 14 initially responded favorably with an increase in platelet count to greater than $150\,000/mm^3$ (Schneider *et al.*, 1987). In nine of these patients, the clinical response was sustained; with additional therapy (corticosteroids and danazol) the response was sustained in an additional two patients. However, the precise role of splenectomy in the treatment of this disorder is still being clarified and the ultimate effect of losing the spleen in these patients is unknown. The initial data suggest, however, that the procedure can be accomplished without undue risk and with a significant percentage of patients achieving relief of thrombocytopenia.

18.2.3 MYELOPROLIFERATIVE AND LYMPHOPROLIFERATIVE DISORDERS

The indications for splenectomy and staging laparotomy in malignant hematological disorders will be considered in this section.

(a) Myeloid metaplasia

In myeloid metaplasia (MM) there is extra-medullary proliferation of hematopoietic stem cells (see Chapter 14). Enlargement of the spleen and liver result, and there is progressive replacement of the bone marrow by fibrous tissue (myelofibrosis). Primary myeloid metaplasia (Bowdler and Prankerd, 1961), also termed agnogenic myeloid metaplasia (Jackson, Parker and Lemon, 1940), arises *de novo*, in contrast to secondary myeloid metaplasia which occurs as a complication of other disorders. Splenectomy is selectively performed for hypersplenism or symptomatic splenomegaly. At one time, splenectomy was believed to be contraindicated because of an inordinately high postoperative mortality. Morbidity and mortality rates after splenectomy for MM remain higher than those following any other hematological disorder, with the exception of chronic myelogenous leukemia. In one series (Coon and Liepman, 1982), four of 34 patients died within 30 days of surgery. Complications occurred in an additional 12 patients. The mean survival in male patients surviving splenectomy was only 22 months; it was somewhat longer for female patients. Despite these discouraging statistics, splenectomy may be indicated for palliation of massive splenomegaly or excessive transfusion requirements. Compensatory hepatomegaly has been reported to occur after splenectomy, presumably in response to continued extramedullary hematopoiesis (Towell and Levine, 1987). Subtotal splenectomy has been used (Morgenstern, Kahn and Weinstein, 1966) to avoid postsplenectomy sepsis and also to preserve some of the hematopoietic function of the spleen. The role of subtotal splenectomy in the palliation of this disorder is at present unclear.

The spleen is commonly massively enlarged in MM, with spleen weights ranging from 400 to 6120 g in one series (Mulder, Steenberger and Haanen, 1977). Occasionally, the spleen is adherent to the abdominal parietes in the left upper quadrant due to previous radiation therapy or infarcts; in these cases initial control of the splenic artery and vein prior to mobilization of the spleen may be desirable (Coon and Liepman, 1982).

(b)   Chronic myelogenous leukemia

The first splenectomy for leukemia was performed in 1866; the patient died two hours after surgery from uncontrolled hemorrhage. Since that time, splenectomy has frequently been employed in the treatment of blast crisis. In a representative series (Coon, 1985a), eleven patients underwent splenectomy for chronic myelogenous leukemia (CML). Two of these splenectomies were performed as a prelude to bone marrow transplantation; other indications included severe thrombocytopenia, massive splenomegaly, splenic infarction, and impending splenic rupture. Three of eleven patients died during the immediate postoperative period. Similar results have been reported from other centers (Didolkar *et al.*, 1976; Ihde *et al.* (1976); McBride and Hester, 1977; Wolf, Silver and Coleman, 1978; Wilson *et al.*, 1985). Gomez *et al.* (1976) reported a case in which splenectomy in the terminal phase of CML resulted in removal of a clone of leukemic cells, resulting in a three-year remission before relapse.

In contrast to the high complication rate of splenectomy when performed late in the course of the disease, Rodigas *et al.* (1981) reported no mortality and only one serious complication among 20 patients undergoing splenectomy as part of a planned treatment protocol early in the course of CML. Early splenectomy prior to bone marrow grafting has been reported to result in more rapid hematological reconstitution (Goldman *et al.*, 1980). Thus, although the role of splenectomy in the treatment of CML is still not completely defined, there may be a place for this modality in the treatment of selected patients.

The spleen is usually enlarged, especially so when splenectomy is performed late in the disease. In the series described by Didolkar *et al.* (1976) the spleen weighed between 170 and 3650 g in patients splenectomized during the chronic phase, and between 270 and 6000 g in those who underwent operation during the blastic phase. In the series by Rodigas *et al.* (1981) of patients who underwent early splenectomy, splenic weights were considerably smaller, ranging from 60 to 800 g.

Histological examination of the spleen almost invariably reveals leukemic infiltration. In Didolkar's series (1976) only two of 46 spleens failed to reveal leukemic cells; in most cases, a diffuse pattern of leukemic involvement was noted. Extramedullary hematopoiesis, infarction, and fibrosis of the spleen may also be seen (see also Chapter 14).

(c)   Chronic lymphocytic leukemia

Chronic lymphocytic leukemia (CLL) is the most common chronic form of leukemia in the United States and Europe. The clinical course is frequently indolent, and the diagnosis is made on the basis of an incidental finding in an asymptomatic adult in 25%. The development of symptomatic splenomegaly, anemia or thrombocytopenia may necessitate treatment. Splenectomy is sometimes useful in treating cytopenias associated with late-stage, refractory CLL. In the past splenectomy was performed very late in the course of the disease, and the earlier series reported discouraging results. Recently, a reassessment of splenectomy (Delpero et al., 1987; Pegourie et al., 1987), sometimes combined with chemotherapy, has led some investigators to advocate splenectomy for splenomegaly with cytopenias associated with CLL. In Delpero's series (1987), 32 patients underwent splenectomy for CLL. Twenty-two of 23 patients with thrombocytopenia were improved, and an improvement was also noted in 15 of 19 patients who had anemia preoperatively. No consistent effect upon peripheral blood leukocyte counts was noted. Favorable response to splenectomy was noted in the majority of patients studied by Stein et al. (1987) and Pegourie et al. (1987). In Pegourie's series, the blood lymphocyte clone disappeared in four of 15 patients after splenectomy and discontinuous high-dose chlorambucil therapy.

The spleen is typically enlarged; splenic weight ranged from 1000 to 3572 g in a representative series (Stein et al., 1987). Generally

the histology reflects extensive involvement by leukemic cells.

(d)   Hairy cell leukemia*

Hairy cell leukemia is a rare lymphoproliferative disorder of adults, presenting with cytopenias and splenomegaly. Only 500 to 600 new cases are reported in the United States each year (Cheson and Martin, 1987). The cell of origin is generally a B-lymphocyte, but isolated instances of T-lymphocyte origin have been reported. Until recently, splenectomy has been virtually the only effective treatment and resulted in improvement in blood counts in virtually all patients (Golomb, 1987; Brochard et al., 1987). However, not all patients showed improvement in all hematological parameters, and almost half the patients subsequently required further treatment after a median interval of 8.3 months from splenectomy. Alpha-interferon and 2'-deoxycoformycin have been used as first-line treatment in clinical trials and initial results are encouraging (Cheson and Martin, 1987). In contrast to splenectomy, which is essentially a palliative treatment, these agents hold some promise for cure and long-term survival. Trials are presently under way to define the role of these agents alone and in combination, and to redefine the role of splenectomy.

Splenomegaly is generally moderate. The mean splenic weight in one series (Van Norman et al., 1986) was 1460 g with a range of 245–5012 g. The hairy cells show a highly characteristic pattern in the spleen on histological examination (Jansen and Hermans, 1981; Van Norman et al., 1986).

(e)   Hodgkin's disease and non-Hodgkin's lymphomas

The lymphomas are tumors of the lymphoid system. They are classically divided into Hodgkin's disease and the non-Hodgkin's lymphomas, and further subdivided by histological

---

*See also Chapter 15. (ed.)

type (see Chapter 15). Of 34 000 new cases of malignant lymphoma diagnosed in 1985, 40% were Hodgkin's disease and the remainder were non-Hodgkin's lymphomas. The diagnosis of Hodgkin's disease usually requires the presence of characteristic Sternberg–Reed cells, but these are not pathognomonic in themselves. Approximately 90% of cases of Hodgkin's disease arise in lymph nodes and there is frequently a pattern of contiguous spread to adjacent nodal groups or organs. The spleen is involved in approximately one-third of patients with Hodgkin's disease (Cohen *et al.*, 1977). The involved spleen is frequently normal in size, and the involvement may consist of nodules that are below the resolution of currently available imaging methods. Accurate determination of splenic involvement by non-invasive means is therefore difficult.

In contrast, the non-Hodgkin's lymphomas are a heterogeneous group of disorders. Accurate histological classification and staging are important for therapy and prognosis. Only 60% of non-Hodgkin's lymphomas arise in nodal tissue and the remainder arise in extranodal sites, including the gastrointestinal tract, lung and skin. Spread is generally non-contiguous in the non-Hodgkin's lymphomas, and many appear to be disseminated at the time of diagnosis (Williams and Golomb, 1986).

Splenectomy for lymphoma is most commonly performed as part of a staging laparotomy (discussed below). Occasionally, the diagnosis of lymphoma is initially made when splenectomy is performed for undiagnosed splenomegaly (Spier *et al.*, 1985). Hypersplenism with secondary cytopenias may be an indication for splenectomy in selected patients. These issues will be discussed individually.

(i) Staging laparotomy

Staging laparotomy was introduced at a time when radiotherapy to clinically involved areas was the initial treatment of Hodgkin's disease, and when non-invasive imaging methods were in an early stage of development. It is a diagnostic maneuver designed to determine precisely the extent of disease within the abdomen. It is currently performed only when clinical staging is uncertain or when a difference in stage will affect treatment (see Table 15.10, Chapter 15). Total splenectomy is performed for diagnostic purposes and also to avoid the subsequent need to irradiate the spleen. In the initial series of 65 carefully selected patients with Hodgkin's disease who underwent staging laparotomy, splenic involvement was incorrectly predicted preoperatively in almost half (Glatstein *et al.*, 1969). These patients had, however, been selected partially on the basis of difficulty in clinical staging. A recent review of the Stanford University Hospital experience (Taylor, Kaplan and Nelsen, 1985) shows remarkably similar results. The clinical stage was changed in 43.2% of 825 patients who underwent staging laparotomy. In 296 patients (36.1% of all cases), the stage was increased by findings at laparotomy. In 60 patients (7.3%), the stage was decreased. In this series, as in the earlier series, splenic involvement correctly predicted visceral involvement. There was only one postoperative death, and 37 patients (4.5%) sustained major complications.

The technique of staging laparotomy has been carefully developed to maximize diagnostic accuracy (Grieco and Cady, 1980). Preoperative evaluation usually includes CT scan of the abdomen. Bipedal lymphangiography has been found useful in outlining iliac and para-aortic nodes and to identify suspicious nodes for special attention at operation. Because of inability to evaluate mesenteric, splenic, and celiac nodes by this route, and because histological changes may be produced by the injected dye, this procedure is now used less frequently.

At operation, an incision which gives wide exposure and access to all quadrants of the abdomen is used, most commonly a midline or left paramedian. A general abdominal exploration is performed. Wedge and needle biopsies of both lobes of the liver are obtained. Splenectomy, with excision of splenic hilar nodes, is next performed. The spleen is submitted to immediate gross and histological examination. If Hodgkin's disease is confirmed within the spleen, then biopsy of intra-abdominal node groups may be curtailed. Abdominal node sampling should include the left para-aortic nodes, nodes from the small bowel mesentery, from the celiac axis, and the region of the inferior vena cava or iliac region. If suspicious nodes have been noted on preoperative lymphangiogram, then an X-ray may be obtained in the operating room to confirm that the node of interest has been excised. Clips are used to mark the splenic hilum, sites of node sampling, and any gross intra-abdominal disease. In females of reproductive age, oöphoropexy is performed to remove the ovaries from an anticipated radiation portal. Some pediatric surgeons perform incidental appendicectomy, generally by an inversion technique which does not involve opening the lumen of the appendix, at the time of staging laparotomy.

Because of the high incidence of postsplenectomy sepsis, particularly in children (Lanzkowsky et al., 1976; Brogadir et al., 1978; Hays et al., 1986), there has been an interest in the possibility of staging without total splenectomy (Lally et al., 1986). Laparoscopy has been used as a means of obtaining directed liver and splenic biopsies in selected patients with Hodgkin's disease (DeVita et al., 1971; Gasparini et al., 1976). It provides an attractive alternative to laparotomy in some patients because it can be performed under local anesthesia. Partial splenectomy has also been considered as an alternative to total splenectomy. Unfortunately, the pattern of splenic involvement in Hodgkin's disease is typically focal rather than diffuse. Nodules of variable size and distribution are typical. In a review of 112 spleens removed at staging laparotomy in which Hodgkin's disease was present, 13 spleens were identified in which the disease was limited to a few nodules in a localized distribution without visible subcapsular lesions (Dearth et al., 1978). These splenic lesions might well have been missed if splenic biopsy or partial splenectomy, rather than total splenectomy, had been employed for staging.

Both partial splenectomy and splenic biopsy are thus useful if positive and may be misleading if negative. Splenic irradiation is not a benign alternative to surgical splenectomy. Splenic atrophy, hyposplenism, and postsplenectomy sepsis have all been reported to occur (Dailey, Coleman and Kaplan, 1980).

Alternative techniques of non-operative and operative staging have been devised in an attempt to avoid total splenectomy with the corresponding risk of sepsis. However, staging laparotomy remains the most accurate method for determining the pathological stage of Hodgkin's disease and is indicated whenever the clinical stage is uncertain or when a change in clinical stage will alter treatment (Kaplan et al., 1973; Gamble, Fuller and Martin, 1975; Gill, Sauter and Morris, 1980; Irving, 1985; Mann, Hafez and Longo, 1986).

(ii)   Splenectomy for splenomegaly or hypersplenism

Cytopenias in patients with malignant lymphoma may arise from several causes; they are most commonly seen in patients with stage III and stage IV disease. Depression of the bone marrow by chemotherapy, infiltration by tumor cells, effects of radiation therapy, increased splenic pooling of blood, and hypersplenism may all be factors. Selection of patients who benefit from splenectomy is difficult. Tagged erythrocyte or platelet sequestration studies have been of limited value in predicting the response to splenectomy. Bone marrow involvement by lymphoma is not considered a contraindication to surgery, as many of these patients show a good response to splenectomy (Mitchell and Morris, 1985; Gill, Sauter and Morris, 1981). Splenectomy may allow resumption of chemotherapy, and thus contribute to remission. Removal of a bulky spleen relieves symptoms due to pressure and eliminates the risk of rupture with minor trauma.

Splenectomy was performed for cytopenias in 41 patients with malignant lymphoma (Gill, Sauter and Morris, 1981). All patients with

Hodgkin's disease had correction of their cytopenias, and 87% of those with non-Hodgkin's lymphoma had good results. There were no deaths. In this series, as in others, splenic irradiation did not prove to be a useful alternative to splenectomy.

18.2.4   HYPERSPLENISM

Hypersplenism is a syndrome in which there is enlargement of the spleen, deficits in one or more cell lines in the peripheral blood, evidence for adequate production of the deficient cells, and (in retrospect) correction of the condition by splenectomy (Bowdler, 1983; Coon, 1985b). It is divided into primary and secondary hypersplenism, and encompasses a wide range of disorders, many of which have already been discussed. Its presence usually implies abnormal sequestration or destruction of circulating blood cells in the spleen, but the mechanisms involved are diverse, and the term does not, in fact, refer to any specific process by which the cell deficit is generated. Mechanisms which may be involved include production of anti-erythrocyte, antigranulocyte, or antiplatelet antibodies, abnormal splenic hemodynamics, or maldistribution cytopenias and the effects of expanded blood volume (Eichner, 1979).

18.2.5   UNDIAGNOSED SPLENOMEGALY

The spleen may be palpable in as many as 3% of young adults on physical examination, and many enlarged spleens are not palpable or are difficult to palpate (see Chapter 10). Splenomegaly may be detected by palpation or by percussion of the area of splenic dullness, but radiographic techniques are important to confirm the diagnosis of splenic enlargement (Chapter 17). Radioisotope scan, CT scan, and ultrasound are all useful in delineating splenic size and to demonstrate lesions such as cysts and abscesses (Eichner and Whitfield, 1981).

Splenectomy is occasionally performed for diagnosis when a full diagnostic evaluation has otherwise failed to reveal the cause of spleno-megaly, particularly when signs of chronic illness are present. The terms primary splenic neutropenia or primary hypersplenism have been used to describe the combination of splenomegaly of unknown cause and neutropenia (Knudson et al., 1982).

Earlier series have emphasized a high incidence of lymphoma in patients with splenomegaly of unknown origin. In a review by Hermann, DeHaven and Hawk (1968), lymphoma was diagnosed in 31% of 52 patients who underwent splenectomy for the diagnosis of splenomegaly. Long and Aisenberg (1974) reported that lymphoma was found in 15 of 25 such patients. A more recent review of 28 patients failed to reveal any patient in whom the diagnosis of lymphoma was made at splenectomy; only one patient developed lymphoma in the postoperative period (Knudson et al., 1982). The cause of splenomegaly was determined at laparotomy in only seven of these 28 patients. Three patients were found to have cirrhosis, three were found to have undiagnosed splenic cysts (CT scanning was not available preoperatively), and one patient was found to have sarcoid of the spleen.

Preoperative evaluation of these patients demands close cooperation between surgeon and hematologist: the evaluation will generally require a blood count, bone marrow aspiration and biopsy, serum protein electrophoresis, erythrocyte sedimentation rate, and serological studies for collagen–vascular disorders. Liver function studies and additional tests such as percutaneous liver biopsy, angiography or upper gastrointestinal series, may be required to identify hepatic cirrhosis and portal hypertension. Cultures of blood, urine, sputum and bone marrow aspirates should be performed, and sometimes appropriate studies for viral and fungal infection. In the most recent series, one patient was subsequently diagnosed with the acquired immunodeficiency syndrome; hence, testing for antibodies to human immunodeficiency virus (HIV) may need to be included in the preoperative workup. CT of the abdomen may be necessary to diagnose splenic cyst or abscess which may present in this fashion (Knudson *et al.*, 1982; Coon, 1985b; Goonewardene *et al.*, 1979).

If a full evaluation has failed to reveal the cause of splenomegaly, laparotomy with splenectomy may be considered. Although a diagnosis may be made in a significant number of patients, delay in proceeding to laparotomy may still be justified, especially in young asymptomatic patients with a history of recent infection (Knudson *et al.*, 1982; Coon, 1985b).

18.2.6   OTHER CONDITIONS

Splenic surgery is occasionally required for the diagnosis or treatment of several other conditions, mostly associated with splenomegaly and hypersplenism; these will be discussed here.

In some parts of the world, tropical splenomegaly (usually secondary to infection with malaria, schistosomiasis, or leishmaniasis) may affect as many as 60% of the population. Symptomatic tropical splenomegaly with associated hypersplenism and cytopenias, may require splenic surgery (Cooper and Williamson, 1984).

(a)   Felty's syndrome

The characteristic triad of rheumatoid arthritis, splenomegaly, and neutropenia was described by Felty in 1924. Anemia and chronic leg ulcers may also be present. Felty's syndrome develops in approximately one of every 300 patients with rheumatoid arthritis. Splenectomy may be indicated for the relief of intractable neutropenia or chronic, non-healing leg ulcers; however, the response to splenectomy is variable and unpredictable, with an estimated 60–80% of patients having a favorable response (Coon, 1985d; Riley and Aldrete, 1975; O'Neill *et al.*, 1968; Barnes, Turnbull and Vernon-Roberts, 1971). In addition, there is substantial risk when splenectomy is performed during the course of an acute infectious episode. Three of nine patients died after splenectomy in one series, and only five had a rise in granulocyte count postoperatively (Ruderman, Miller and Pinals, 1968). It is therefore clear that patient selection is extremely important; however, the criteria which will select for both effectiveness and safety are not yet clearly defined.

Splenectomy is not felt to be indicated solely on the basis of the observed hematologic abnormalities in the absence of infectious complications. Severe neutropenia, with less than 500 cells/mm^3, has been used as an indication for operation in the past; however, in Coon's series (1985d) no correlation was found between the degree of neutropenia, the frequency or severity of infection, and response to splenectomy. Serious or refractory recurrent infections constitute an indication for splenectomy; under certain circumstances refractory cutaneous ulcers may also be an indication for surgery.

The pathogenesis of the neutropenia is incompletely understood at present. Increased levels of serum IgG which binds to neutrophils have been measured in patients with Felty's syndrome. The spleen is the site of destruction of IgG-coated granulocytes, and may be the site of production of serum granulocyte binding IgG as well. Blumfelder, Logue and Shimm (1981) measured serum granulocyte-binding IgG levels in 14 patients before and after splenectomy for Felty's syndrome, in an attempt to identify a subset of patients who might be expected to respond favorably to splenectomy. In this series, a partial or complete response to splenectomy was obtained in nine patients. They found that markedly elevated amounts of serum granulocyte-binding IgG preoperatively correlated with a favorable response to splenectomy. Mild or moderate elevation did not predict a response. The postoperative fall in serum granulocyte-binding antibody also correlated with the degree of response to splenectomy. A better understanding of the pathogenesis of the disorder is needed to identify more precisely those patients likely to respond favorably to splenectomy.

(b)   Gaucher's disease

Gaucher's disease is the commonest of the lysosomal storage diseases. It is an autosomal recessive disorder in which lysosomal β-

glucocerebrosidase is deficient and consequently the cerebroside β-glucosylceramide accumulates in reticuloendothelial cells of liver and spleen, and in the bones. Hypersplenism with pancytopenia, and progressive, eventually massive, enlargement of the spleen result. Several forms of the disorder have been identified, corresponding to several structural enzyme abnormalities.

Splenectomy has been used to alleviate the mechanical symptoms caused by the massively enlarged spleen and pancytopenia. However, postsplenectomy sepsis may result and acceleration of bone destruction has been reported. Whenever possible, splenectomy should be postponed until the second decade of life, in an attempt to minimize infectious and osteolytic complications (Ashkenazi, Zaizov and Matoth, 1986).

Partial splenectomy for Gaucher's disease was initially described by Govrin-Yehudain and Bar-Maor (1980) and has subsequently been employed at several centers (Rodgers, Tribble and Joob, 1987; Guzzetta et al., 1987). In one series (Rubin et al., 1986), partial splenectomy was attempted in 11 children with Gaucher's disease and was successfully performed in seven. Long-term follow up of these seven children showed improvement in hematological indices, with no episodes of postsplenectomy sepsis or clinical problems related to increased hepatic or bone accumulation of β-glucocerebroside. Partial splenic embolization has also been used in this disorder (Thanopoulos and Frimas, 1982).

(c) Wiskott–Aldrich syndrome

This is an X-linked hereditary immunodeficiency disorder characterized by the triad of eczema, hemorrhage, and recurrent infections. Profound thrombocytopenia is observed, with a characteristic decrease in mean platelet size. Some have suggested that this is due to the production of intrinsically abnormal platelets. Megakaryocytes are generally present in adequate numbers in the bone marrow of patients with Wiskott–Aldrich syndrome, however, and

platelet size and number increase after splenectomy. Corash, Shafer and Blaese (1985) studied 14 patients with Wiskott–Aldrich syndrome and reported increased levels of platelet-associated IgG in 13 of them. After splenectomy, levels of platelet-associated IgG fell to normal levels in these patients. Platelet size and number increased after splenectomy, suggesting that the spleen was involved in an immunologically mediated process.

(d) Schistosomiasis

Approximately 150 million persons worldwide are infected with *Schistosoma mansoni*. Splenomegaly and hypersplenism result from chronic infection and are frequently indications for splenectomy in endemic areas of the world. Partial splenectomy has been described for this disorder (Kamel and Dunn, 1982; Kamel et al., 1986). Fifty-one patients who underwent segmental splenectomy and 44 patients treated by total splenectomy for schistosomiasis were followed: the percentage of T-lymphocytes increased after segmental splenectomy, and there was also an increased T-helper:T-suppressor cell ratio after segmental splenectomy (Kamel et al., 1986). Only two patients required conversion from a partial to a total splenectomy for technical reasons, and no increase in size of the splenic remnant was noted during the subsequent two to four years. This is the largest series of elective partial splenectomies reported to date, and provides encouraging data in favor of the concept of partial splenectomy for hypersplenism.

18.3 OTHER CONDITIONS REQUIRING SPLENIC SURGERY

Surgery is occasionally required for a wide spectrum of other lesions of the spleen. The radiological aspects of these disorders are considered in Chapter 17.

18.3.1 SPLENIC CYST AND PSEUDOCYST

Splenic cysts present with symptoms of pressure, secondary infection, or rupture. They may be asymptomatic until much enlarged. Occasionally a calcified splenic cyst is noted radiographically in an otherwise asymptomatic individual.

The simplified classification proposed by Martin (1958) is still useful. He divided cystic masses of the spleen into two broad categories: true cysts with an epithelial lining, and false cysts or pseudocysts in which no epithelial lining can be identified. True cysts are further divided into parasitic and non-parasitic cysts, and the latter into congenital and neoplastic cysts.

Parasitic cysts are the most common on a world-wide basis: the majority of these are hydatid cysts. *Echinococcus granulosa* is the most commonly implicated species. This parasite is epidemic in regions of south central Europe, South America, Australia, and Alaska. Even in regions of high prevalence of echinococcal disease, splenic involvement is rare, occurring in 1.7–4% of all patients with hydatid disease (Al-Mohaya *et al.*, 1986). Infection of the spleen with *E. granulosa* results in the formation of a cyst which is typically unilocular, with a wall composed of several layers including an outer fibrous membrane. The fluid within the cyst is under pressure and contains infective scolices and daughter cysts. The cyst wall may become calcified; however, this is not sufficiently characteristic to distinguish a hydatid cyst from a cyst of non-parasitic origin. Ultrasound may show the characteristic appearance of the cyst containing daughter cysts and scolices. The diagnosis is best confirmed by hemagglutination inhibition and complement fixation tests. Splenectomy remains the treatment of choice. Care must be taken at laparotomy to avoid spillage of the cyst contents, not only to prevent infective material from seeding the peritoneal cavity, but also to avoid anaphylactic reactions. Because the cyst fluid is under pressure, dissection may be accomplished more safely if the cyst is first carefully aspirated and then 1% formalin solution or 3% NaCl solution instilled to kill the scolices. Mebendazole may be useful as an adjunctive treatment in inoperable cases, in patients with multiple cysts,

and those in whom spillage occurs at laparotomy.

The non-parasitic true cysts are less common. In young patients, epidermoid and dermoid cysts are encountered. Cystic lymphangiomas and true mesothelial cysts also occur. In the past, splenectomy was usually performed (Browne, 1963; Sirinek and Evans, 1973). Since these are generally benign lesions, partial splenectomy is a reasonable alternative and has been reported (Morgenstern and Shapiro, 1980). This is performed by mobilizing the spleen, identifying a plane external to the cyst, carefully enucleating it, and then obtaining hemostasis in the splenic remnant. By this method the cyst can be removed intact and a substantial amount of splenic parenchyma preserved. Partial splenectomy is not presently recommended for parasitic splenic cysts because of the danger of spillage of cyst contents.

Pseudocysts of the spleen are generally related to previous trauma. They are more common in women and tend to occur in young adults. The incidence of these cysts will probably increase as more patients with splenic trauma are treated with splenic conservation techniques or non-operatively. Partial splenectomy is recommended when surgery is required (Morgenstern and Shapiro, 1980).

Occasionally a pseudocyst of the tail of the pancreas will involve the spleen, and should be distinguished from a splenic cyst. A history of chronic pancreatitis, or the presence of characteristic pancreatic calcifications radiographically, indicate the possibility of the diagnosis. The serum amylase may be elevated, and the amylase content of the cyst fluid will also be elevated. Treatment of the underlying pancreatic ductal abnormality is critical; simple removal of the cyst and the spleen is likely to result in formation of a pancreatic fistula from the tail of the pancreas.

18.3.2 PRIMARY AND METASTATIC TUMORS INVOLVING THE SPLEEN

Both benign and malignant splenic neoplasms are distinctly uncommon. The most common benign neoplasm is the cavernous hemangioma. Small hemangiomas are asymptomatic and do not require surgery. Larger tumors may cause symptoms by pressure, hypersplenism, consumption coagulopathy, or spontaneous rupture. The treatment is splenectomy. The possibility of malignant degeneration to hemangiosarcoma has been discussed, but it is not clear whether or not this occurs. Lymphangiomas are less common and are frequently part of a generalized lymphangiomatosis. Hamartomas, lipomas, and fibromas also occur and are the least common benign tumors. Morgenstern *et al.* (1984) reported a series of hamartomas, many of which were multiple, and expressed the opinion that splenic hamartomas are more common than previously suspected. Because these lesions are frequently multiple, total splenectomy is generally required.

Primary malignant tumors of the spleen are extremely rare. Older series often include many patients with lymphoma and myeloproliferative disorders presenting with splenic involvement; at present these are usually excluded from the category of primary splenic neoplasms. The majority of the remaining malignant tumors are hemangiosarcomas (also called angiosarcomas and hemangioendothelialsarcomas). These lesions present with splenomegaly, microangiopathic hemolytic anemia, ascites, pleural effusion, and occasionally spontaneous rupture. The prognosis is poor. Etiological factors, such as thorium dioxide, vinyl chloride, or arsenic, are rarely identified when hemangiosarcoma occurs as a primary splenic tumor, in contrast to angiosarcomas in other locations (Das Gupta, Coombes and Brasfield, 1965; Chen, Bolles and Gilbert, 1979; Sordillo, Sordillo and Hajdu, 1981; Morgenstern, Rosenberg and Geller, 1985).

Although it is often stated that the spleen rarely harbours metastatic tumors, tumor cells are frequently found within the splenic sinuses at autopsy in cancer patients, and gross metastases were found within the spleens of 7% of patients with carcinoma at autopsy (Berge, 1974). The most common primary sites were breast, lung, skin and colon. Because metastatic disease to the spleen frequently coexists with widespread systemic metastases, splenectomy is rarely recommended. However, when spontaneous rupture occurs, or if splenomegaly is pronounced, resection of the spleen may be required. Klein *et al.* (1987) described four patients in whom isolated splenic metastases were identified. All four patients were treated by splenectomy and multi-modality treatment of their underlying malignancy. One patient survived for over twelve years, two survived for greater than two years, and the remaining patient lived for over one year after splenic resection for isolated metastatic disease. Thus it appears that isolated splenic metastases, although extremely rare, should be treated by resection and aggressive therapy directed at the underlying malignancy (Zamora and Halpern, 1987; Klein *et al.*, 1987).

18.3.3 SPLENIC ABSCESS

The spleen is rarely the site of intra-abdominal abscess formation. When an abscess forms within the parenchyma of the spleen, a predisposing factor such as an old splenic hematoma or splenic infarction from sickle cell disease or splenic embolization is frequently present. An increasing number of splenic abscesses are being reported in intravenous drug abusers, presumably in association with systemic bacteremia or bacterial endocarditis (Nallathambi *et al.*, 1987). Splenic abscess occasionally occurs when a splenic hematoma becomes infected; the incidence of this particular complication may rise as more splenic injuries are treated nonoperatively (Sands, Page and Brown, 1986).

Although the majority of abscesses are bacterial in origin, an increasing number of fungal abscesses are being reported. Approximately 75% of splenic abscesses are related to systemic bacteremia, 15% are secondary to trauma, and 10% occur as a result of direct extension from an adjacent abscess involving colon, stomach or other organ. In many patients, the diagnosis is difficult because the symptoms of weight loss and fever are non-specific. When left upper quadrant pain, diminished breath sounds, and tenderness in the left upper quadrant are present in a patient with systemic sepsis, the diagnosis of splenic abscess should be suspected (Simpson, 1980; Sarr and Zuidema, 1982). Ultrasound of the left upper quadrant is occasionally helpful (Benderly *et al.*, 1981); radioisotope scan or CT scan may be more useful. Even at laparotomy, the diagnosis may not be apparent (Chulay and Lankerani, 1976). Occasionally intraperitoneal or transdiaphragmatic rupture may occur, causing generalized peritonitis or empyema.

Formerly the most common organism was *Staphylococcus aureus*; however, Gram-negative organisms are becoming increasingly common. Salmonella has been a common organism in the past, and is returning to prevalence. Unusual organisms such as *Clostridium difficile* have been reported in the elderly (Studemeister, Beilke and Kirmani, 1987). The treatment of choice is splenectomy and intravenous antibiotic therapy directed at the causative organism. In the past, splenotomy (incision and drainage of the splenic parenchyma) was used as an alternative to splenectomy. This more limited procedure may still be useful in patients in whom intense inflammatory reaction in the left upper quadrant renders splenectomy difficult. A series of four patients treated by percutaneous aspiration was reported by Lerner and Spataro (1984). This treatment was successful in three of the four cases. The overall mortality rate has decreased from over 60% to 10%, and most deaths are related to the underlying cause of the sepsis.

Helton *et al.* (1986) reported a series of eight patients with fungal splenic abscesses and identified several etiological factors including cytotoxic chemotherapy, long-term corticosteroid administration, neutropenia, treatment with antibiotics for more than three weeks, and gastrointestinal colonization with *Candida albicans*. Five patients were treated with splenectomy and antifungal drugs, and three patients received antifungal drugs alone. Seven of the eight were cured of their splenic abscesses and five were long-term survivors. This disorder may come to be recognized with increasing frequency and should be considered in any patient at risk who develops fever, tenderness over the left upper quadrant, and a non-toxic appearance. CT and ultrasound can be used to confirm the diagnosis.

18.3.4 SPLENIC ARTERY ANEURYSM

With the solitary exception of the aorta, the splenic artery is the most common site of intra-abdominal aneurysmal disease. During the childbearing years, approximately twice as many women as men present with splenic artery aneurysms. After the menopause, the incidence in men equals that in women. Etiological factors include atherosclerosis and congenital defects in the arterial internal elastic membrane. Trauma, pancreatitis and arteritis can cause splenic artery aneurysms, and mycotic aneurysms of the splenic artery occur. Although most splenic artery aneurysms are small (1.5–3.5 cm in diameter), occasionally aneurysms measuring up to 15 cm have been recorded. Many aneurysms are asymptomatic and are identified when the characteristic calcification is noted on an abdominal film. However, a significant number present with intraperitoneal rupture or rupture into the gastrointestinal tract.

Generally, an aneurysm of any size in a symptomatic patient should be treated by excision, as should an aneurysm in a pregnant woman. Splenic artery aneurysms caused by pancreatitis or pancreatic pseudocysts should be treated, as the risk of rupture is high. Asymptomatic, non-pregnant patients may be observed if the aneurysm is small (<1 cm if non-calcified, or <3 cm if calcified) or if the risk of operation is high because of severe systemic disease. The preferred management is exposure of the aneurysm in the lesser sac, with total excision. Depending on the location of the aneurysm, ligation of the splenic artery, vascular reconstruction, or splenectomy may be required (Stanley and Fry, 1974; Trastek *et al.*, 1982).

18.3.5 SPLENIC VEIN THROMBOSIS

Because splenic vein thrombosis causes elevated pressure in the veins of the left upper quadrant, and results in gastric and esophageal varices, most patients with this condition present with gastrointestinal bleeding (Roder, 1984). The thrombosis is generally secondary to pancreatitis, trauma, infection or a pancreatic pseudocyst (Nishiyama *et al.*, 1986; Hofer, Ryan and Freeny, 1987). Splenectomy is the treatment of choice. Splenic artery ligation without splenectomy is not recommended, as continued gastrointestinal hemorrhage may occur (Glynn, 1986; Roder, 1984).

18.3.6 SPLENIC INFARCTION

Splenic infarction occurs in several situations: typical autoinfarction of the spleen is associated with sickle cell disease, systemic embolization, and as a surgical complication of partial splenic embolization and splenic artery ligation, performed in an attempt to preserve splenic function.

Autoinfarction of the spleen occurs with the progression of sickle cell anemia and does not require treatment unless secondary bacterial infection causes abscess formation (see Chapter 16).

Acute splenic infarction has been reported in association with systemic thromboembolism. The presentation is non-specific, with fever, left upper quadrant pain, and tachycardia. In a review of 96 cases of thromboembolic splenic infarction, O'Keefe *et al.* (1986) reported that although 44% of splenic infarcts had caused significant additional morbidity, only 10% had been suspected clinically. Atheromatous debris from the aorta, mural thrombus from the left ventricle, and vegetations on infected valves in bacterial endocarditis were the three most common sources. The diagnosis may be confirmed by CT scan.

Finally, splenic infarction can occur as a complication of partial splenic embolization or splenic artery ligation, which are discussed in subsequent sections.

Management of pain and treatment of the underlying cause, if systemic embolization is suspected, are the initial therapeutic approach. If secondary bacterial infection occurs or signs of sepsis develop, splenectomy may be required.

18.3.7 RUPTURE OF THE DISEASED SPLEEN AFTER MINOR TRAUMA

When the spleen ruptures after minor trauma, this is usually called spontaneous or pathological rupture. Most cases of pathological rupture have occurred in malaria, typhoid fever, infectious mononucleosis, pregnancy, or in patients with hematologic malignancies or coagulation abnormalities (Autry and Weitzner, 1975; Andrews *et al.*, 1980). The initial trauma may have been so slight as to have been forgotten. There is frequently a delayed presentation, characterized by diffuse or localized abdominal pain, left shoulder pain, and fatigue. Tachycardia, hypotension and tachypnea may be present, but a significant proportion of patients present with normal vital signs (Bauer, Haskins and Armitage, 1981). The diagnosis may be confirmed by ultrasound, CT scan, or diagnostic paracentesis. Splenectomy is usually required: most deaths have been related to delay in diagnosis and treatment (Brook and Newman, 1965; Hunter and Shoemaker, 1957). According to Bauer, Haskins and Armitage (1981), in rupture of the spleen associated with hematological malignancies, the single factor which correlated best with survival was appropriate surgical intervention.

18.3.8 ABDOMINAL TRAUMA

Although the spleen lies in a relatively protected position, high in the left upper quadrant and sheltered by the costal structures, it is frequently injured by both blunt and penetrating abdominal trauma.

Blunt trauma may cause a variety of injuries including transverse fracture along an intersegmental plane (especially in children), a stellate laceration, avulsion injuries from traction on the upper or lower pole, and subcapsular hematomas. Sometimes bleeding is initially slight and there is a variable latent period before the signs and symptoms of splenic rupture are clinically evident. This has given rise to the term 'delayed rupture'. It is generally felt that this is a misnomer, and that the rupture occurred at the time of the initial injury and was simply delayed in its presentation.

In contrast to the earlier belief that all splenic injuries require splenectomy, the current preferred management of many injuries is to utilize one of several techniques of splenorrhaphy, or splenic repair (Burrington, 1977; Benjamin *et al.*, 1978; Sherman, 1984; Seufert and Mitrou, 1985; Kidd *et al.*, 1987). These include suture of capsular lacerations, application of topical hemostatic agents, partial splenectomy, or wrapping the spleen with absorbable mesh. The commonly used techniques are described in section 18.4.4(c). Most require extensive mobilization of the spleen and meticulous, time-consuming control of bleeding. For patients who are hemodynamically unstable, or for those with extensive injuries elsewhere, splenectomy is still the procedure of choice, since it can be accomplished more rapidly, and frequently with less blood loss than splenic salvage (Mucha, Daly and Farnell, 1986).

Non-operative management of blunt abdominal trauma, despite suspected splenic injury, was introduced after the chance post-mortem observation of a child who had died in a motor vehicle accident, and in whom splenic injury had been suspected in the past (Douglas and Simpson, 1971). A well-healed, completely transected spleen was found, providing the first evidence that significant splenic injuries could heal spontaneously. Advantages of the non-operative approach include the avoidance of laparotomy and the possibility that further injury to spleen might occur during splenic mobilization, precluding splenic salvage. Against this must be balanced the potential disadvantages of possibly increased transfusion requirements, conversion of a simple laceration (which might easily be repaired at laparotomy) to a complex subcapsular hematoma which would necessitate splenectomy, and the possibility of overlooking injury to other organs such as bowel and kidney. The non-operative approach to blunt abdominal trauma has gradually been formalized, and is now the standard management of suspected splenic injuries in children. It is estimated from combined series that only 10% of children who are observed under a careful protocol will require laparotomy, and that splenic salvage will still be possible in 25% of those requiring surgical exploration (Luna and Dellinger, 1987).

Some have attempted to extend these results to the adult, in whom stellate lacerations, complex fractures, and fragmentation of the splenic parenchyma are more common, and which stand in contrast to the pattern of transverse fractures along intrasegmental planes seen in children. The importance of strict adherence to a protocol was emphasized by Mucha, Daly and Farnell (1986). Non-surgical management was unsuccessful in 19 of 70 patients in whom it was attempted. However, from this series and several other combined series, it appears that non-operative management may be successful in as many as 60% of carefully selected patients with isolated splenic injuries (Mucha, Daly and Farnell, 1986; Kidd *et al.*, 1987; Splenic Injury Study Group, 1987).

Penetrating abdominal trauma requires celiotomy; and the decision whether or not to attempt splenorrhaphy is made on the basis of hemodynamic stability, integrity of hilar vessels, and the severity of associated injuries. Injuries to adjacent organs such as stomach, pancreas, duodenum, colon, diaphragm and lung are common and must be carefully sought and dealt with.

Polyvalent pneumococcal vaccine and the selective use of antibiotic prophylaxis are recommended in patients who undergo splenectomy for trauma. Patients in whom non-operative management or splenorrhaphy has been utilized should avoid strenuous physical activity and contact sports for at least three months. They should have follow-up splenic imaging by CT or radioisotope scan one to two months after injury (Mucha, Daly and Farnell, 1986).

Post-traumatic cysts and splenic abscesses have been reported after the non-operative management of splenic injuries. These may require surgical excision, drainage, or splenectomy (Sands, Page and Brown, 1986).

18.4 SPECIFIC SURGICAL CONSIDERATIONS

In this section, the surgical anatomy of the spleen and the techniques of splenectomy and splenorrhaphy will be discussed.

18.4.1 THE SURGICAL ANATOMY OF THE SPLEEN

The spleen is tethered in position by several avascular peritoneal folds or ligaments. The phrenosplenic ligament attaches the spleen to the undersurface of the diaphragm. The splenocolic ligament attaches the inferior margin of the spleen to the splenic flexure of the colon. The splenorenal ligament tethers the spleen posteriorly to the abdominal wall and left kidney. These normally avascular structures may contain large venous collaterals in patients with portal hypertension. During surgery, traction on the stomach, esophagus, colon, or other intra-abdominal viscus may pull on the splenic capsule, and result in iatrogenic injury to the spleen (Cioffiro, Schein and Gliedman, 1976).

The normal adult spleen weighs between 100 and 175 g. The capsule varies from one to two millimeters in thickness and anchors the connective tissue trabeculae which traverse the organ and give it some structural rigidity. The spleen is a fragile, pulpy organ made up largely of vascular sinuses, and the capsule is the only part of the spleen which will reliably hold sutures.

The splenic artery, a branch of the celiac artery, courses along the upper margin of the pancreas in the lesser sac and then divides into several branches before entering the substance of the spleen. Each segmental artery supplies its own territory, and the vascular segments are divided by relatively avascular planes. The splenic vein passes posterior to the pancreas to enter the portal vein. Segmental venous drainage runs in parallel with the arterial distribution (Dawson, Molina and Scott-Conner, 1986). Hence the spleen can be divided into vascular segments separated by relatively avascular planes; this characteristic is important when partial splenectomy is performed. The number of identifiable segments varies. The larger segments are oriented in a roughly transverse plane and correspond with notches on the surface of the spleen; smaller segments are less predictable.

18.4.2 TECHNIQUE OF SPLENECTOMY

The technique of elective splenectomy will be described first. Splenic surgery for trauma will be discussed in section 18.4.4. Partial splenectomy is discussed with the surgery of trauma, although it may be utilized in the elective situation in some conditions.

(a) Choice of incision

A variety of incisions have been employed for splenic surgery. When the spleen is of normal size, a left subcostal incision provides the best access (Figure 18.1a). Extension of the incision vertically upwards in the midline may be used to provide additional exposure. As the spleen enlarges, it descends and the hilum is displaced medially. For massively enlarged spleens, a midline or left paramedian incision (Figure 18.1b) then provides better exposure. In children, a left subcostal incision made lateral to the rectus muscle, which is retracted rather than divided, may be used (Kiesewetter, 1975).

In the profoundly thrombocytopenic patient, it may be preferable not to divide the rectus muscle, and in this situation a midline or paramedian incision may also be preferred. Splenic surgery for trauma is best performed through a vertical midline incision, which gives excellent access to all quadrants of the abdomen.

(b) Preliminary ligation of splenic artery

When difficulty in dissection is anticipated, ligation of the splenic artery in the lesser sac should

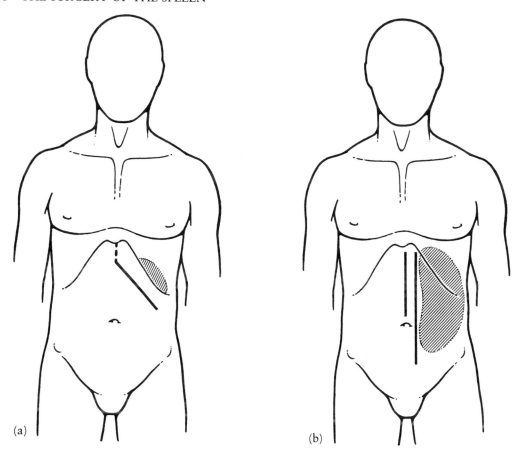

Figure 18.1 (a) When the spleen is normal in size, a left subcostal incision provides good exposure for splenic surgery. The incision may be extended upward in the midline, as indicated by the dotted line. This incision transects the abdominal muscles; persistent oozing or the development of a wound hematoma may occur in profoundly thrombocytopenic patients. For this reason, many surgeons prefer a midline or paramedian incision for those cases. (b) As the spleen enlarges, it descends and the hilar structures are displaced medially. A vertical midline or left paramedian incision gives good exposure and access to the hilum. These incisions may be preferred in profoundly thrombocytopenic patients, even when the spleen is small, because no muscle is transected.

be performed before the spleen is mobilized (Figure 18.2). This allows control of the major blood supply to the spleen, and the effective transfusion of platelets systemically if necessary, in profoundly thrombocytopenic patients.

(c)   Preoperative embolization of splenic artery

Preoperative transcatheter embolization of the splenic artery is sometimes used as a means of decreasing hemorrhage during elective splenectomy, and may be useful in patients who present extremely high operative risks. Successful preoperative splenic infarction may decrease splenic volume, increase the platelet count, and decrease intra-operative bleeding (Levy, Wasserman and Pitha, 1979). In most patients, however, this is not necessary. Total infarction of the spleen by transcatheter embolization has largely been abandoned as an alternative to splenectomy because of its high complication

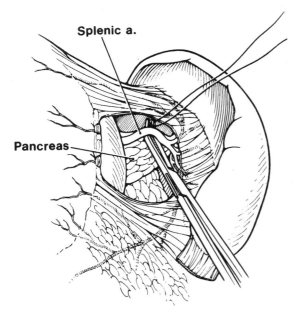

Figure 18.2 An opening is made in the lesser sac and the splenic artery encircled with a tape or ligature.

rate (Back *et al.*, 1987); however, partial splenic embolization shows promise as a technique of partial splenic ablation and will be discussed later.

(d) The technique of splenectomy

The patient is positioned supine on the operating table. Additional exposure may be obtained by placing a small roll under the left costal margin. The use of a framework which can anchor an 'upper hand' type of retractor may also facilitate exposure.

During the initial incision and subsequent steps, care is taken to effect meticulous hemostasis, since patients who undergo elective splenic surgery frequently have coagulation or immunological defects which may predispose to hematoma formation, or in whom poor wound healing can be anticipated. Placement of a nasogastric tube, unless contraindicated by extreme thrombocytopenia, facilitates operative exposure by decompressing the stomach.

The surgeon's hand is passed carefully up over the spleen to assess the size, consistency and mobility of the organ. A thorough intra-abdominal exploration is performed. In patients with hemolytic anemia, the gallbladder is carefully palpated. Accessory spleens are best sought at the beginning of the dissection, before blood stains the operative field, and again after mobilization of the spleen and tail of pancreas.

Preliminary ligation of the splenic artery may be performed by exposing the splenic artery in the lesser sac (Figure 18.2).

The spleen is mobilized by incising the lateral peritoneal attachments (Figure 18.3). The surgeon's left hand pulls the spleen medially and upwards. The dissection is performed in a plane deep to the tail of the pancreas and splenic vessels, which are mobilized gently out of the retroperitoneum. Further mobilization is limited by the gastrosplenic and splenocolic ligaments. The splenocolic ligament is generally avascular; occasionally a few small vessels may require ligature (Figure 18.4). The lower pole of the spleen is further freed by division of several branches of the gastroepiploic vessels (Figure 18.5).

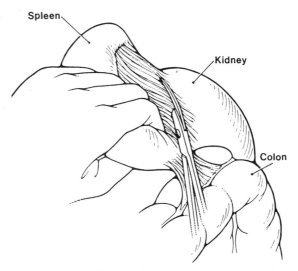

Figure 18.3 In the initial stage of splenectomy, the spleen is mobilized by incising the lateral peritoneal attachments to abdominal wall, diaphragm and left kidney.

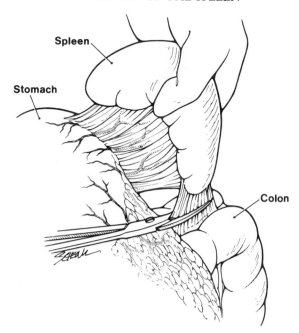

Figure 18.4 The splenocolic ligament is divided.

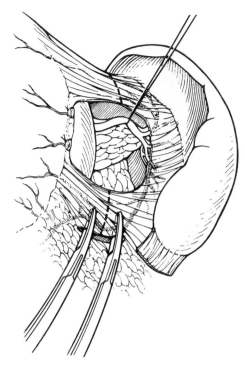

Figure 18.5 Branches of the left gastroepiploic artery and vein are serially clamped and tied. Similarly the short gastric vessels which connect the stomach to the spleen are ligated and divided.

The upper pole of the spleen is mobilized by dividing several short gastric vessels. These are carefully ligated (Figure 18.5). Care must be taken not to include a small portion of the wall of the stomach in the ligature, which may otherwise induce necrosis and gastric fistula formation.

The spleen is now attached only by the hilum and tail of the pancreas. The dissection of the splenic artery and vein should be performed with care to avoid damage to the tail of the pancreas, which extends for a variable extent into the hilum of the spleen. In many cases, serial ligation of several branches of the splenic artery and vein is preferable to ligation of the main arterial and venous trunk, because of the proximity to the pancreas. This dissection is most conveniently performed from the underside of the spleen, accessible now because of careful mobilization of spleen and pancreas (Figure 18.6). The artery should be ligated before the vein, to avoid sequestration of a significant volume of blood within the spleen.

Ligation of the splenic vein at the juncture with the inferior mesenteric vein has been recommended as a means of decreasing the probability of portal vein thrombosis after splenectomy, and may be advisable when massive splenomegaly, with a correspondingly large splenic vein, is encountered (Broe, Conley and Cameron, 1981).

(e) **Avoidance and management of hemorrhage**

Blood loss may be decreased significantly by preliminary control of the splenic artery in the lesser sac (Figure 18.2). Preoperative embolization of the splenic artery is an alternative, but is rarely necessary. If the spleen is torn during mobilization or dissection, it is best to control bleeding by direct pressure and continue mobil-

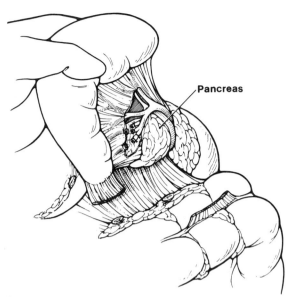

Pancreas

Figure 18.6 Careful dissection and ligation of the splenic vessels in the hilum, with identification and preservation of the tail of the pancreas, is often easier from the underside. Adequate mobilization of the spleen and tail of pancreas facilitates this maneuver.

ization. An atraumatic vascular clamp can be placed across the hilar vessels if necessary, for temporary control while dissection progresses. The major vascular trunks should be suture ligated; a double clamp technique may be advisable. Occasionally, the splenic vein is so large that oversewing the stump with a running vascular suture is safer than simple ligature or suture ligature.

The short gastric vessels can be the source of troublesome bleeding which is more easily controlled after the spleen has been removed. If there is any question that a ligature or suture ligature may have encroached on part of the wall of the stomach, the area in question should be imbricated with interrupted Lembert sutures to avoid the development of a gastric fistula.

The splenic bed is carefully checked for hemostasis. Bleeding from raw peritoneal and diaphragmatic surfaces may be controlled by packing, topical hemostatic agents, or by reperitonealizing the raw area with a running suture.

If there is any question of the adequacy of hemostasis, or injury to the tail of the pancreas, a drain should be placed. The closed-suction form of drain is preferred.

(f)   The search for accessory spleens

When accessory spleens are carefully sought at autopsy, they are found in about 10% of the general population (Halpert and Gyorkey, 1959). The most common location is within the splenic hilum, along the course of the splenic artery, or within the tail of the pancreas. Other common locations include the omentum, the gastrosplenic and splenocolic ligaments, and the mesentery of the small bowel. Occasionally an accessory spleen is found in a presacral, pelvic, or paratesticular location (Wick and Rife, 1981). The accessory spleen is generally involved by the same pathological process as the primary spleen (Curtis and Movitz, 1946; Halpert and Gyorkey, 1959).

When total splenectomy is performed for disorders such as hereditary spherocytosis, hereditary elliptocytosis, or idiopathic thrombocytopenic purpura, a careful search should be made and any accessory spleens present should also be removed. After splenectomy, an accessory spleen may enlarge and cause a recurrence of the symptoms for which the original surgery was performed (Appel and Bart, 1976; Seufert and Mitrou, 1985). Howell–Jolly bodies normally appear within the erythrocytes after splenectomy; when these are absent, an accessory spleen should be suspected. The combination of CT scan and radionuclide scan provides satisfactory diagnostic accuracy in identifying the location of the accessory spleen (Joshi *et al.*, 1980). The treatment of choice is surgical removal, if an accessory spleen causes recurrence of a hematological disorder.

(g)   Decision to drain or not to drain the splenic bed

Routine drainage of the splenic bed has largely been abandoned because of several studies which have demonstrated an increase in post-operative complications, particularly subphrenic abscess formation, when drains are used (Cohn, 1965; Olsen and Beaudoin, 1969). In most of these studies, prolonged drainage of the splenic bed with passive drains such as the Penrose drain was utilized. A recent study of the results of routine closed suction drainage in 282 patients undergoing splenectomy reported a subphrenic abscess rate of only 0.71% (Ugochukwu and Irving, 1985). In this study, drains were removed between the third and fifth postoperative day. Many surgeons utilize selective drainage, employing closed-suction drains when there are associated injuries in the setting of abdominal trauma, or if there is a possibility of incomplete hemostasis, or of injury to the tail of the pancreas.

18.4.3 SPLENIC ENLARGEMENT: EFFECT UPON SURGERY

As the spleen enlarges, the hilum is displaced medially and the spleen moves downward. In some ways, this facilitates dissection, but adhesions between the spleen and the diaphragm may be more troublesome and vascular (Goldstone, 1978). In one series of 49 patients who underwent removal of massively enlarged spleens, perisplenitis with dense adhesions was encountered in more than half (Wobbes, Van der Sluis and Lubbers, 1984). Although the mortality rate was not increased in those patients with massive splenomegaly, the complication rate was twice that of patients with smaller spleens. The most frequent operative complication was postoperative hemorrhage, which was generally related to thrombocytopenia or to perisplenitis.

18.4.4 SPLENIC TRAUMA

(a) Non-operative management of splenic trauma

Non-operative management of splenic trauma is the preferred approach in children, and may be applicable in some carefully selected adults. Mucha, Daly and Farnell (1986) listed three selection criteria for the non-operative management of patients with blunt splenic trauma. These included: hemodynamic stability, absence of peritoneal signs, and a maximum transfusion requirement of 2 units of blood for the splenic injury. They also emphasized the importance of using modern imaging techniques (double contrast CT scan) to exclude other intra-abdominal injuries. Careful serial observation and the capacity for prompt decision to proceed to laparotomy are critical to successful non-operative management. The precise role for this modality in the management of adults with blunt abdominal trauma is still being investigated, and many authorities continue to prefer laparotomy if splenic injury is suspected in an adult.

(b) Laparotomy for splenic trauma

Laparotomy for trauma is performed through a long midline incision which provides excellent access to all quadrants of the abdomen. A rapid and thorough abdominal assessment is performed. The presence of blood and clots within the left upper quadrant confirms the probability of splenic injury. All blood and clots should be evacuated and the abdomen packed in quadrants. Any continuing hemorrhage is dealt with first. If the patient's condition is stable and splenic salvage is to be attempted, the spleen is first carefully mobilized as described previously. This mobilization must be performed with extreme care to avoid further injury which might preclude successful splenorrhaphy. Occasionally, an isolated capsular avulsion injury of the lower pole of the spleen can be treated without full mobilization of the spleen. The decision to perform splenectomy, rather than splenorrhaphy, is based upon the hemodynamic stability of the patient, the severity of associated injuries, the age of the patient, and the severity of the splenic injury. If no blood or hematoma are found in the left upper quadrant, the spleen should not be mobilized, to avoid iatrogenic injury. Splenectomy for trauma is performed in a fashion similar to that described for elective splenectomy. Preliminary ligation of the splenic artery is generally not performed.

(c) Splenic conservation techniques

Careful, atraumatic mobilization of the spleen is performed. Division of the short gastrics and the splenocolic ligament may be required for adequate exposure. Temporary control of the splenic hilum by application of an atraumatic vascular clamp may be used to diminish blood loss while repair is being performed.

Minor capsular avulsion injuries may be managed by the application of topical hemostatic agents and pressure.

A simple capsular tear or laceration may be debrided and sutured with interrupted sutures (Figure 18.7a, b). Pledgets may be required to avoid the problem of sutures tearing through the delicate splenic capsule (Figure 18.7c). Viable omentum, with an intact vascular pedicle, may be used to buttress the repair (Figure 18.7d). Many surgeons prefer the use of a fine monofilament suture on a vascular needle for these repairs, to avoid injury from a large needle. Others prefer the use of chromic catgut on a gastrointestinal needle, which is less likely to cut through the delicate capsule. In any event, a fine suture on a small taper point needle should be used and care should be taken to avoid lacerating the capsule as the sutures are placed and tied.

When a stellate laceration of one pole of the spleen or damage to one of the hilar vessels has occurred, partial splenectomy may be necessary (Figure 18.8a). The segmental artery and vein supplying the involved pole are ligated and the spleen is allowed to demarcate (Figure 18.8b). The segment will become dusky and a line of demarcation will develop. The capsule is divided and the splenic parenchyma opened by a finger fracture technique. Occasional small vessels will be encountered and should be ligated or clipped with fine hemostatic clips. Hemostasis is again checked, and the capsule is sutured to

provide some additional compression and hemostasis (Figure 18.8c). Omentum may be used to wrap the splenic remnant.

A badly damaged spleen with intact hilar vessels may be salvaged by wrapping it with absorbable synthetic mesh (Figure 18.9). The mesh may be applied with several concentric pursestring sutures placed at the splenic hilum. Alternatively, a hole may be cut for the hilum, and the spleen wrapped and the mesh sutured around the front and towards the diaphragmatic surface of the spleen. It is critical that the mesh be sutured in such a manner as to apply firm but gentle compression of the splenic parenchyma without encroaching upon the vascular supply.

Splenic artery ligation is occasionally performed to control hemorrhage and allow splenic salvage. Some have stated that splenic artery ligation is safe and does not result in splenic infarction (Dalton and West, 1965). Recent experimental work demonstrating the importance of an intact splenic artery in bacterial clearance by the spleen raises the possibility that the spleen, even if viable, may no longer be an efficient bacterial filter after splenic artery ligation (Horton *et al.*, 1982; Scher, Wroczynski and Scott-Conner, 1985).

18.5 ALTERNATIVES TO TOTAL SPLENECTOMY

Total splenectomy remains the treatment of choice for patients with hemolytic anemias (with the possible exception of β-thalassemia major where partial splenectomy may be preferred), immune thrombocytopenias, and severely injured patients who are hemodynamically unstable and have sustained significant splenic injury. In patients undergoing elective splenectomy for hematological disorders, accessory spleens should be carefully sought and removed to avoid recurrent symptoms. In contrast, when splenectomy is required because of trauma, accessory spleens are preserved with the intent that they may provide some protection against the sequelae of hyposplenism (see Chapter 11).

The main alternatives to total splenectomy

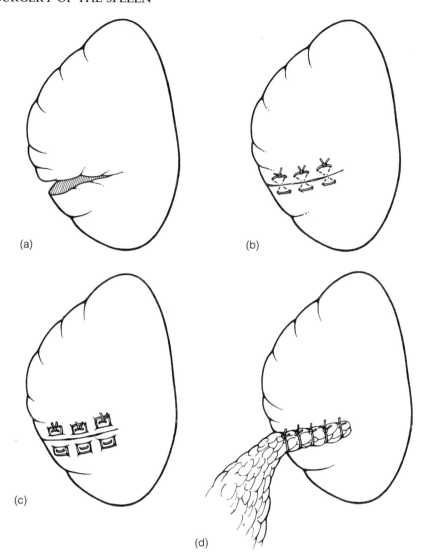

(a)

(b)

(c)

(d)

Figure 18.7 (a) A laceration of the spleen which may be managed by simple repair. (b) The laceration may be closed with interrupted sutures placed through the capsule. (c) Pledgets may be necessary to avoid the tendency of sutures to cut through the delicate capsule. (d) A buttress of viable omentum, with intact arterial and venous blood supply, may be used to reinforce the repair.

Figure 18.8 (a) A complex, stellate fracture of the lower pole of the spleen is typical of the sort of injury for which partial splenectomy is a good form of management. Partial splenectomy may also be utilized when a benign cyst or tumor occupies part of the spleen; or for preservation of some splenic function in selected disorders (such as schistosomiasis or thalassemia major). (b) The hilar artery and vein supplying the involved segment are ligated and the pole is allowed to demarcate. Resection is accomplished along the line of demarcation. Occasional intrasplenic branches of vessels may require ligation or control by fine hemostatic clips. (c) Sutures are placed to compress the raw surface. These may be placed over pledgets, if desired.

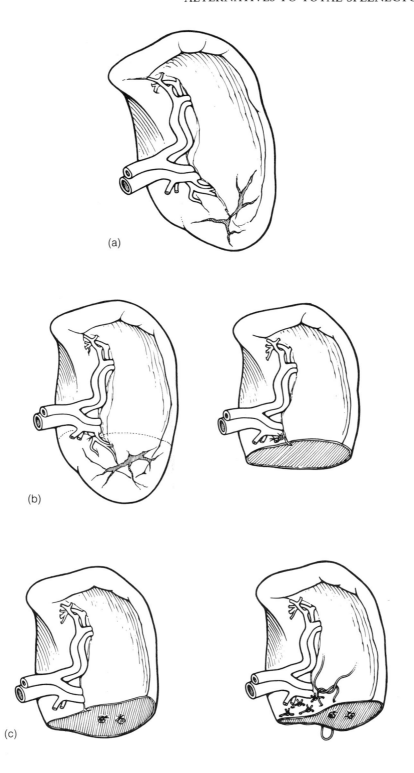

(a)

(b)

(c)

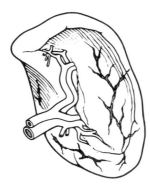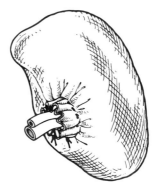

Figure 18.9 When the spleen has been severely damaged, but the hilar vessels are intact, a synthetic absorbable mesh wrap may be used to provide hemostasis by gentle compression. Several pursestring sutures are placed to assure that the mesh provides adequate compression.

are splenic biopsy, which may be performed under laparoscopic guidance, partial splenectomy, and partial splenic embolization. Techniques of splenic preservation during trauma surgery have been discussed in section 18.4.4.

18.5.1 LAPAROSCOPIC BIOPSY

Laparoscopic biopsy has been used mainly to determine splenic involvement in Hodgkin's disease; it has been shown to be a safe technique. However, because of the non-uniform involvement of the spleen, it is generally not regarded as a satisfactory alternative to full staging laparotomy with splenectomy.

18.5.2 PARTIAL SPLENECTOMY

Partial splenectomy is being used in an increasing number of situations to preserve some splenic function (Cooney et al., 1979). The technique of elective partial splenectomy is essentially the same as that described for trauma (Figure 18.8). When partial splenectomy is performed for Gaucher's disease, myeloid metaplasia, schistosomiasis or for some similar indication, the resection is generally planned so that the remaining splenic remnant is about the size of a normal spleen. This generally means ligating several segmental ves-

sels and carefully preserving the final segment. In contrast, partial splenectomy for a cyst or benign tumor is planned according to the location of the lesion. In all other respects, the partial resection is performed in the same manner as that performed for trauma.

18.5.3 SPLENOSIS

The occasional observation of generalized studding of omental and peritoneal surfaces in patients who undergo laparotomy years after unrecognized splenic injury, led to the speculation that such 'born-again spleens' might protect against subsequent sepsis (Fleming, Dickson and Harrison, 1976; Pabst and Kamran, 1986; Kusminsky et al., 1982). The spleen is minced and slices no thicker than 1 cm are placed on the greater omentum, which is then folded over to contain the splenic remnants. The location of these remnants may be marked by fine hemostatic clips. Such splenic autotransplants have been demonstrated to remain viable, and to achieve a blood supply from the omentum. Subsequent radionuclide scanning will frequently demonstrate uptake of radionuclide within the splenic fragments (Pearson et al., 1978; Livingston, Levine and Sirinek, 1983). However, several studies have failed to demonstrate normal bacterial clearance in experimental animals in the absence of a significant fragment of the spleen which is supplied by the splenic artery. The fragment may need to be as much as one-third of normal splenic size (Moore *et al.*, 1983; Scher, Wroczynski and Scott-Conner, 1985). In addition, overwhelming postsplenectomy sepsis has been documented in a patient found to have approximately 25 g of viable splenic tissue in splenosis of the omentum and mesentery (Holmes *et al.*, 1981). Thus, although splenic autotransplantation is feasible and may be performed with minimal difficulty, it is not clear that such autotransplants provide protection against overwhelming postsplenectomy sepsis. Many surgeons continue to place such autotransplants when splenectomy for trauma is unavoidable; however, these patients should probably also receive polyvalent pneumococcal vaccine and be considered for antibiotic prophylaxis as if they were asplenic.

18.5.4   PARTIAL SPLENIC EMBOLIZATION

Partial transcatheter embolization has been used in patients in whom partial ablation of splenic function is desired and in whom both surgery and the asplenic state carry considerable risk (Maddison, 1973; Chuang and Reuter, 1975; Spigos *et al.*, 1979; Yoshioka *et al.*, 1985). Mozes *et al.* (1984) conducted a prospective randomized study comparing partial splenic embolization with total splenectomy in patients requiring splenic ablation prior to renal transplantation. Partial splenic embolization resulted in a mean reduction in splenic mass of 65%. A significant number of patients experienced regeneration of the spleen after partial splenic embolization, and repeated procedures were performed in 11 patients. The immediate complication rate was similar in patients who underwent partial splenic embolization and splenectomy. Both groups subsequently underwent renal transplantation with similar results. Witte *et al.* (1982) confirmed the importance of occluding the intrasplenic, rather than the extrasplenic, vasculature. The use of large coils to occlude the main splenic artery has generally been associated with a high failure rate. In a series of 136 patients undergoing partial splenic embolization, fever, pain, atelectasis, leukocytosis, hyperamylasemia, and pleural effusion were commonly seen (Jonasson, Spigos and Mozes, 1985). More serious complications were infrequent however; two patients developed pancreatitis, two developed pancreatic pseudocysts, and two developed splenic abscesses. Partial splenic embolization shows promise as a relatively safe and effective technique for partial splenic ablation in selected patients. However, the risks and relatively high failure rate associated with partial and total splenic embolization in children were recently emphasized (Back *et al.*, 1987) and the precise role of these techniques in the management of splenic disorders remains to be defined.

18.6   COMPLICATIONS OF SPLENECTOMY

Careful preoperative preparation and meticulous operative technique have significantly decreased the complication rate associated with elective splenectomy. Improvements in postoperative care have also benefitted these patients.

18.6.1   IMMEDIATE COMPLICATIONS

Atelectasis is the most common complication of splenic surgery, occurring in 69 of 310 patients in a representative series (Hodam, 1970). This is higher than the expected rate following abdominal operations in general: the increased incidence of atelectasis and other pulmonary complications after elective splenectomy is related to the upper abdominal incision, and extensive dissection in the left upper quadrant. Careful preoperative pulmonary preparation, with instruction in deep breathing and coughing, as well as meticulous postoperative pulmonary care, can minimize this complication. Pleural effusion is less frequent, occurring in 10% of most series (Ellison and Fabri, 1983).

Pleural effusion was more common when prolonged drainage of the splenic bed with passive drains was employed; this is one reason that such drainage has been abandoned. It also occurs when mesh is used to wrap the spleen for splenic repair, and is apparently a reaction to the mesh in this setting. Pneumonia is generally reported to occur in approximately 10% of patients. Atelectasis, pleural effusion and pneumonia are more common in patients experiencing blunt trauma, where associated chest wall trauma and rib fractures cause diminished respiratory effort. The presence of such pulmonary complications after the third postoperative day should alert the surgeon to the possibility of a left subphrenic abscess (Ellison and Fabri, 1983).

(a)   Hemorrhage

Postoperative bleeding is most common when splenectomy is performed for hypersplenism, particularly when thrombocytopenia is present. Left shoulder pain from diaphragmatic irritation, hemodynamic instability, and the appearance of blood in drains (if these have been placed) suggest that bleeding is occurring. Prompt reoperation with evacuation of clot, irrigation of the left upper quadrant, and re-establishment of hemostasis is advisable. Most postoperative bleeding comes from raw peritoneal and diaphragmatic surfaces. Frequently no specific bleeding source is found at reoperation, but bleeding from the hilar vessels, short gastrics, or pancreatic surface may also occur (Ellison and Fabri, 1983).

(b)   Injury to the tail of the pancreas; pancreatic fistula

Pancreatic injuries are reported to occur in 1–3% of splenectomies in large series, and are believed to be related to injury during ligation of the splenic artery and vein. Ugochukwu and Irving (1985) measured serum and drain fluid amylase in ten patients who underwent elective splenectomy. Pancreatic injury was suspected in only one patient; however, all ten patients had an elevated level of amylase in the drain fluid in the early postoperative period. Pancreatic fistula results when the amount of drainage remains elevated and when a drainage tract becomes established. If there is no path to the skin, a collection of amylase-rich fluid in the left upper quadrant may predispose to subphrenic abscess formation, or may present as a pseudocyst of the tail of the pancreas. Occasionally, hemorrhagic pancreatitis occurs after splenectomy.

Careful dissection in the splenic hilum, and placement of closed suction drains when pancreatic injury is suspected, should minimize the occurrence of these complications.

(c)   Injury to the greater curvature of the stomach; gastric fistula

Gastrocutaneous fistula is a rare complication of splenectomy. Harrison, Glanges and Sparkman (1977) reviewed 14 previously reported cases and added four additional ones. They identified several factors as contributing to the development of this complication. Trauma to the greater curvature of the stomach by instruments or by ligatures placed when the short gastric vessels are controlled is probably the most important preventable cause of gastric fistula. This is most likely to occur at the extreme upper pole of the spleen, where the distance between the splenic capsule and the stomach may be relatively short and exposure difficult. The rich anastomotic blood supply of the stomach usually prevents ischemia when these vessels are ligated. Occasionally, previous gastric surgery or atherosclerosis may contribute to ischemia in the region of the greater curvature. Although this is not thought to be severe enough to result in fistula formation, it may prevent healing of otherwise minor serosal injuries. Gastric injury may result in a subphrenic abscess which can be confirmed by performing an upper gastrointestinal series with water-soluble contrast medium (Ellison and Fabri, 1983). Adequate drainage, antibiotic treatment of related infection, and prolonged nutritional support are necessary.

The complication can be prevented by careful surgical technique and by imbricating the greater curvature with interrupted Lembert sutures when injury is suspected. Postoperative gastric decompression with a nasogastric tube until peristalsis returns is also recommended (Harrison, Glanges and Sparkman, 1977).

(d) Subphrenic abscess

The incidence of subphrenic abscess is variable; it is more common when adjacent organs have been injured, either by trauma or iatrogenic injury, and is consistently more common when the splenic bed is drained. Cohn (1965) reported that subphrenic abscess occurred in 18.5% of patients in whom the splenic bed was drained; by contrast there were no abscesses in those patients in whom drainage was not employed. More recent studies using closed suction drainage demonstrate much lower rates of subphrenic abscess formation (Ugochukwu and Irving, 1985). However, there may be an element of selection bias in the association of abscess and drainage; many surgeons employ drainage when there is concern over the adequacy of hemostasis or injury to the tail of the pancreas, and do not drain routine uncomplicated splenectomies. Consequently, there may be a predisposition to local infection in those patients for whom drainage is deemed appropriate.

Pleural effusion, shoulder pain, singultus, and fever may be signs of a subphrenic abscess. The diagnosis can be confirmed by CT scan, and percutaneous CT-directed drainage may be performed. Adequate drainage and treatment with appropriate antibiotics are necessary. Surgical drainage may be required if adequate drainage cannot be accomplished under CT guidance.

18.6.2 DELAYED COMPLICATIONS

Late complications of splenectomy include overwhelming postsplenectomy sepsis and an increased tendency to develop thromboembolic and ischemic complications (see Chapters 11 and 12). Failure of the original operation due to undetected accessory spleens may also develop late in the postoperative period.

(a) Thrombocytosis and thrombotic complications

The platelet count will commonly rise by 30–100% after splenectomy, reaching a maximum 7–20 days after surgery (Balz and Minton, 1975). Thrombocytosis developed in 239 of 318 patients who underwent splenectomy; none of these patients had a myeloproliferative disorder (Boxer, Braun and Ellman, 1978). In 72 patients, platelet counts over $1\,000\,000/$ mm^3 were encountered. Ten patients developed a thromboembolic complication; however, no correlation with postoperative platelet count, preoperative diagnosis, or medication could be established in this series.

An impression of increased risk persists for splenectomy for myeloid metaplasia or congestive splenomegaly, especially when postoperative platelet counts are high (Gordon et al., 1978; Salter and Sherlock, 1957; Bowdler, 1982; Malmaeus et al., 1986). Broe, Conley and Cameron (1981) studied 28 patients who underwent splenectomy for myeloid metaplasia and identified thromboembolic complications in nine. The postoperative platelet count did not predict the occurrence of thrombosis. The incidence of thromboembolic disease reported in this series is considerably higher than the incidence reported when splenectomy is performed for other hematological indications. Antithrombin III deficiency may cause thrombosis in the postsplenectomy state even when platelet counts are normal (Peters et al., 1977).

Mesenteric infarction secondary to portal vein occlusion is a particularly lethal complication (Bull, Zikria and Ferrer, 1965). It has been reported most commonly in patients who underwent splenectomy for myeloid metaplasia and other myeloproliferative disorders. With massive splenomegaly, splenic vein enlargement occurs: it has been postulated that thrombus forms in the cul-de-sac which remains when the splenic vein is ligated near the hilum of the spleen. Clot then propagates into the portal vein. Ligation of the splenic vein close to the junction with the inferior mesenteric vein may diminish the incidence of this complication by eliminating this cul-de-sac (Broe, Conley and Cameron, 1981).

Postoperative thrombosis and thromboembolic complications are also found in patients treated for hemolytic anemia who remain anemic after splenectomy (Balz and Minton, 1975). The mechanism of this relationship, if in fact it is valid, continues to be conjectural.

Finally, whole blood viscosity increases significantly after splenectomy, partly due to the increase in platelets, but also due to a decrease in erythrocyte deformability and an increase in circulating protein aggregates normally removed by the spleen (Robertson, Simpson and Losowsky, 1981).

Treatment of postsplenectomy thrombocytosis remains controversial. Many recommend the use of acetylsalicylic acid and dipyridamole or low-dose heparin, and initiate such therapy when the platelet count exceeds 800 000–1 000 000/mm^3 (Hansen, Christensen and Jonsson, 1979). Chemotherapy with agents such as phenylalanine mustard has been used to treat symptomatic postsplenectomy thrombocytosis in patients with myeloproliferative disorders.

Thromboembolic complications remain one of the hazards of splenectomy. Mesenteric venous thrombosis should be considered when a patient develops abdominal pain or ileus after splenectomy. Surgery is required once thrombosis has occurred.

(b) Infectious complications: overwhelming sepsis (OPSI)

Early experimental work demonstrated an increased susceptibility to infection in splenectomized rats (Morris and Bullock, 1919), but it was not until King and Shumacker (1952) described an association between splenectomy in infancy and the subsequent occurrence of lethal sepsis that the syndrome of overwhelming postsplenectomy infection (OPSI) was recognized. Later reports confirmed the association and defined the nature of the syndrome more clearly (Smith et al., 1964; Eraklis et al., 1967; Diamond, 1969; Hays et al., 1986). OPSI was originally described as a fulminant, acute illness, frequently progressing to death within 36 hours of first symptoms (see also Chapter 12). The organisms most commonly implicated have been Streptococcus pneumoniae, meningococcus, and Hemophilus influenzae. Review of large numbers of splenectomized children by the Surgical Section of the American Academy of Pediatrics confirmed the existence of the syndrome, and showed a tendency for OPSI to occur more frequently when splenectomy was performed early in life. It also appeared to be more frequent in children with certain disorders, and initially it was thought that children splenectomized for trauma rarely developed OPSI (Hays et al., 1986).

Subsequently, OPSI was recognized in adults (Chaikof and McCabe, 1985). The incidence of various infections including OPSI is now recognized to be increased in previously splenectomized individuals of all ages, especially in those with underlying diseases which affect immune competence (Mower, Hawkins and Nelson, 1986; Dickerman, 1981; Green et al., 1986; O'Neal and McDonald, 1981; Willis, Deitch and McDonald, 1986).

Current recommendations include the administration of polyvalent pneumococcal vaccine, which should be given preoperatively when elective splenectomy is anticipated, and the selective use of prophylactic antibiotics. The value of vaccines against Haemophilus influenzae and other organisms is less clear. All patients who have undergone splenectomy should be warned of their increased susceptibility to infection, should be instructed to seek medical attention when signs of infection or systemic illness develop and should carry a warning card or device which indicates their asplenic state. Such patients should be followed indefinitely, as the risk does not appear to diminish with time.

(c) Undetected accessory spleens: recurrence of symptoms

Although accessory spleens have been documented at autopsy in 10–31% of cases, the incidence may be higher in patients with hematological disorders (Verheyden *et al.*, 1978). Accessory splenic tissue will generally enlarge after splenectomy and may cause a recurrence of symptoms if overlooked at the initial laparotomy.

The presence of Howell–Jolly bodies in erythrocytes after splenectomy is a good indicator that complete splenectomy has been performed. If Howell–Jolly bodies do not appear after splenectomy, or if they disappear months or years after splenectomy, then a return of splenic function due to retained splenic tissue may have occurred. Recurrent hemolytic anemia 25 years after splenectomy has been reported to have been caused by two accessory spleens (Bart and Appel, 1978). The larger of these weighed 225 g. In the more typical situation, the splenic residua are smaller (Verheyden *et al.*, 1978; Talarico *et al.*, 1987).

The diagnosis can be confirmed and the location of the accessory spleen determined by preoperative radioisotope and CT scan. Removal of the accessory splenic tissue is the treatment of choice (Wallace, Fromm and Thomas, 1982; Seufert and Mitrou, 1985).

18.6.3 COMPLICATIONS RELATED TO SPECIFIC DISORDERS

Because of the underlying immunodeficiency disorder, there is an increased incidence of septic complications when splenectomy is performed in the Wiskott–Aldrich syndrome. Until recently, splenectomy was felt to be contraindicated because of the high incidence of delayed postoperative deaths from sepsis. As with other postsplenectomy infections, the principal

organisms responsible for major septic complications are *Streptococcus pneumoniae* and *Hemophilus influenzae*. Active immunization with pneumococcal or *H. influenzae* vaccines does not protect these patients because they are unable to produce antibodies to polysaccharide antigens (Lum, 1980). Long-term prophylactic antibiotic treatment, directed against these two organisms, should be given indefinitely to these post-splenectomy patients. A recent review of 16 patients who underwent splenectomy for Wiskott–Aldrich syndrome documented fatal bacterial sepsis in five of seven patients who did not receive prophylactic antibiotics, in contrast to one death from sepsis in nine patients who did (Lum *et al.*, 1980). The single death in the antibiotic-treated group occurred two weeks after antibiotics were discontinued. Lum *et al.* (1980) emphasized the need for continuing prophylactic antibiotics and stated that inability to follow an antibiotic regimen should be regarded as a contraindication to splenectomy.

18.7 THE INFLUENCE OF PATIENT AGE ON SURGICAL DECISIONS

Deckinga and Printen (1977) reviewed a ten-year experience of elective splenectomy in patients over the age of 55 years. During the study period, 55 such patients, comprising 27% of all elective splenectomies, underwent elective splenectomy with five deaths. The complication rate was similar to that reported in larger series spanning all age groups. The response to splenectomy was comparable to that reported for younger patients with similar preoperative diagnoses.

18.8 SUMMARY

Increasing recognition of the unique and significant functions of the spleen has stimulated interest in the development of therapeutic alternatives to total splenectomy. Techniques for partial splenic resection and splenic salvage, initially developed for the management of splenic trauma, are being applied to an increasing number of conditions in which reduction, rather than total ablation, of splenic tissue is desired. The precise role of these techniques in the treatment of hematological conditions requiring splenic surgery is still being defined. In patients requiring total splenectomy, careful preoperative evaluation, meticulous surgical technique and postoperative care can minimize complications and operative mortality. Furthermore, awareness of the longer-term hazards of the hyposplenic state will stimulate a continued search for improved methods of management, and greater attention to the possible complications of those for whom total splenectomy cannot be avoided.

ACKNOWLEDGEMENT

The assistance of Michael P. Schenk, who skillfully rendered the illustrations, is gratefully acknowledged.

REFERENCES

Al-Mohaya, S. *et al.* (1986) Hydatid cyst of the spleen. *Am. J. Trop. Med. Hyg.*, **35**, 995–9.

Andrews, D. F. *et al.* (1980) Pathologic rupture of the spleen in non-Hodgkin's lymphoma. *Arch. Intern. Med.*, **140**, 119–20.

Appel, M. F. and Bart, J. B. (1976) The surgical and hematologic significance of accessory spleens. *Surg. Gynecol. Obstet.*, **143**, 191–2.

Ashkenazi, A., Zaizov, R. and Matoth, Y. (1986) Effect of splenectomy on destructive bone changes in children with chronic (Type I) Gaucher disease. *Eur. J. Pediatr.*, **145**, 138–41.

Autry, J. R. and Weitzner, S. (1975) Hemangiosarcoma of the spleen with spontaneous rupture. *Cancer*, **35**, 534–9.

Back, L. M. *et al.* (1987) Hazards of splenic embolization. *Clin. Pediatr.*, **26**, 292–5.

Ballas, S. K. *et al.* (1982) Clinical, hematological, and biochemical features of HbSC disease. *Am. J. Hematol.*, **13**, 37–51.

Balz, J. and Minton, P. (1975) Mesenteric thrombosis following splenectomy. *Ann. Surg.*, **181**, 126–8.

Barnes, C. G., Turnbull, A. L. and Vernon-Roberts, B. (1971) Felty's syndrome: a clinical and pathological survey of 21 patients and their response to treatment. *Ann. Rheum. Dis.*, **30**, 359–74.

Bart, J. B. and Appel, M. F. (1978) Recurrent hemolytic anemia secondary to accessory spleens. *South. Med. J.*, **71**, 608–9.

Bauer, T. W., Haskins, G. E. and Armitage, J. O. (1981) Splenic rupture in patients with hematologic malignancies. *Cancer*, **48**, 2729–33.

Benderly, A. *et al.* (1981) Splenic abscess in infancy: diagnosis by ultrasound. *Helv. Pediatr. Acta*, **36**, 175–8.

Benjamin, J. T. *et al.* (1978) Alternatives to total splenectomy: two case reports. *J. Pediatr. Surg.*, **13**, 137–8.

Berge, T. (1974) Splenic metastases: frequencies and patterns. *Acta Pathol. Microbiol. Scand.*, (A) **82**, 499–506.

Bissel, D. M. (1986) Heme catabolism and bilirubin formation. in *Bile Pigments and Jaundice: Molecular, Metabolic and Medical Aspects* (ed. J. D. Ostrow), Marcel Dekker, New York, pp. 133–56.

Blumfelder, T. M., Logue, G. L. and Shimm, D. S. (1981) Felty's syndrome: effect of splenectomy upon granulocyte count and granulocyte associated IgG. *Ann. Intern. Med.*, **94**, 623–8.

Bowdler, A. J. (1982) The spleen in disorders of the blood. in *Blood and its Disorders* (eds R. M. Hardisty and D. J. Weatherall), 2nd edn, Blackwell Scientific, London and Boston, Chapter 20.

Bowdler, A. J. (1983) Splenomegaly and hypersplenism. *Clin. Haematol.*, **12**, 467–88.

Bowdler, A. J. and Prankerd, T. A. J. (1961) Primary myeloid metaplasia. *Br. Med. J.*, i, 1352–8.

Boxer, M. A., Braun, J. and Ellman, L. (1978) Thromboembolic risk of postsplenectomy thrombocytosis. *Arch. Surg.*, **113**, 808–9.

Brochard, M. *et al.* (1987) Splenectomy performed upon thirty-seven patients with hairy cell leukemia. *Surg. Gynecol. Obstet.*, **165**, 305–8.

Broe, P. J., Conley, C. L. and Cameron, J. L. (1981) Thrombosis of the portal vein following splenectomy for myeloid metaplasia. *Surg. Gynecol. Obstet.*, **152**, 488–92.

Brogadir, S. *et al.* (1978) Morbidity of staging laparotomy in Hodgkin's disease. *Am. J. Med.*, **64**, 429–33.

Brook, J. and Newman, P. E. (1965) Spontaneous rupture of the spleen in hemophilia. *Arch. Intern. Med.*, **115**, 595–7.

Browne, M. K. (1963) Epidermoid cyst of the spleen. *Br. J. Surg.*, **50**, 838–41.

Bull, S. M., Zikria, B. A. and Ferrer, J. M. (1965) Mesenteric thrombosis following splenectomy: report of two cases. *Ann. Surg.*, **162**, 938–40.

Burrington, J. D. (1977) Surgical repair of a ruptured spleen in children: report of eight cases. *Arch. Surg.*, **112**, 417–19.

Chaikof, E. L. and McCabe, C. J. (1985) Fatal over-whelming postsplenectomy infection. *Am. J. Surg.*, **149**, 534–9.

Charache, S. (1975) The treatment of sickle cell anemia. *Arch. Intern. Med.*, **133**, 698–705.

Chen, K. T. K., Bolles, J. C. and Gilbert, E. F. (1979) Angiosarcoma of the spleen: a report of two cases and review of the literature. *Arch. Pathol. Lab. Med.*, **103**, 122–4.

Cheson, B. D. and Martin, A. (1987) Clinical trials in hairy cell leukemia. Current status and future directions. *Ann. Intern. Med.*, **106**, 871–8.

Chuang, V. P. and Reuter, S. R. (1975) Experimental diminution of splenic function by selective emboli-zation of the splenic artery. *Surg. Gynecol. Ob-stet.*, **140**, 715–20.

Chulay, J. C. and Lankerani, M. A. (1976) Splenic abscesses: report of ten cases and review of the literature. *Am. J. Med.*, **62**, 512–22.

Cioffiro, W., Schein, C. J. and Gliedman, M. L. (1976) Splenic injury during abdominal surgery. *Arch. Surg.*, **111**, 167–71.

Cohen, I. T. *et al.* (1977) Staging laparotomy for Hodgkin's disease in children. *Arch. Surg.*, **112**, 948–51.

Cohn, L. H. (1965) Local infections after splenec-tomy: relationship of drainage. *Arch. Surg.*, **90**, 230–2.

Coon, W. W. (1985a) The limited role of splenec-tomy in patients with leukemia. *Surg. Gynecol. Obstet.*, **160**, 291–4.

Coon, W. W. (1985b) Splenectomy for splenomegaly and secondary hypersplenism. *World J. Surg.*, **9**, 437–43.

Coon, W. W. (1985c) Splenectomy in the treatment of hemolytic anemia. *Arch. Surg.*, **120**, 625–8.

Coon, W. W. (1985d) Felty's syndrome: when is splenectomy indicated? *Am. J. Surg.*, **149**, 272–5.

Coon, W. W. (1987) Splenectomy for idiopathic thrombocytopenic purpura. *Surg. Gynecol. Obstet.*, **164**, 225–9.

Coon, W. W. and Liepman, M. K. (1982) Splenec-tomy for agnogenic myeloid metaplasia. *Surg. Gynecol. Obstet.*, **154**, 561–3.

Cooney, D. R. *et al.* (1979) Relative merits of partial splenectomy, splenic reimplantation, and immuni-zation in preventing postsplenectomy infection. *Surgery*, **86**, 561–9.

Cooper, M. J. and Williamson, R. C. N. (1984) Splenectomy: indications, hazards and alterna-tives. *Br. J. Surg.*, **71**, 173–80.

Corash, L., Shafer, B. and Blaese, R. M. (1985) Platelet-associated immunoglobulin, platelet size, and the effect of splenectomy in the Wiskott–Aldrich syndrome. *Blood*, **65**, 1439–43.

Croom, R. D. *et al.* (1986) Hereditary spherocytosis. Recent experience and current concepts of pathophysiology. *Ann. Surg.*, **203**, 34–9.

Crosby, W. H. (1987) Splenectomy for thrombocyto-penia in chronic liver disease. *Arch. Intern. Med.*, **147**, 195–7.

Curtis, G. M. and Movitz, D. (1946) The surgical significance of the accessory spleen. *Ann. Surg.*, **123**, 276–98.

Dailey, M. O., Coleman, C. N. and Kaplan, H. S. (1980) Radiation-induced splenic atrophy in patients with Hodgkin's disease and non-Hodgkin's lymphomas. *N. Engl. J. Med.*, **302**, 215–17.

Dalton, M. L. and West, R. L. (1965) Fate of the dearterialized spleen. *Arch. Surg.*, **91**, 541–4.

Dameshek, H. F. and Ellis, L. D. (1975) Hematologic indications for splenectomy. *Surg. Clin. North Am.*, **55**, 253–75.

Danforth, D. N. and Thorbjarnarson, B. (1976) Inci-dental splenectomy: a review of the literature and the New York Hospital experience. *Ann. Surg.*, **183**, 124–9.

Das Gupta, T., Coombes, B. and Brasfield, R. D. (1965) Primary malignant neoplasms of the spleen. *Surg. Gynecol. Obstet.*, **120**, 947–60.

Dawson, D. L., Molina, M. E. and Scott-Conner, C. E. H. (1986) Venous segmentation of the human spleen: a corrosion cast study. *Am. Surg.*, **52**, 253–6.

Dearth, J. C. *et al.* (1978) Partial splenectomy for staging Hodgkin's disease: risk of false negative results. *N. Engl. J. Med.*, **299**, 345–6.

Deckinga, B. G. and Printen, K. J. (1977) Elective splenectomy in the elderly patient. *Am. Surg.*, **43**, 195–9.

Delpero, J. R. *et al.* (1987) The value of splenectomy in chronic lymphocytic leukemia. *Cancer*, **59**, 340–5.

DeVita, V. T. *et al.* (1971) Peritoneoscopy in the staging of Hodgkin's disease. *Cancer Res.*, **31**, 1746–50.

Diamond, L. K. (1969) Splenectomy in childhood and the hazard of overwhelming infection. *Pediat-rics*, **43**, 886–9.

Dickerman, J. D. (1981) Traumatic asplenia in adults: a defined hazard? *Arch. Surg.*, **116**, 361–3.

Didolkar, M. S. *et al.* (1976) Evaluation of splenec-tomy in chronic myelogenous leukemia. *Surg. Gynecol. Obstet.*, **142**, 689–92.

Dotevall, A. *et al.* (1987) A retrospective analysis of a consecutive series of patients splenectomized for various haematologic disorders. *Acta Haematol. (Basel)*, **77**, 38–44.

Douglas, G. L. and Simpson, J. S. (1971) The conservative management of splenic trauma. *J. Pediatr. Surg.*, 6, 565–70.

Eichner, E. R. (1979) Splenic function: normal, too much, and too little. *Am. J. Med.*, 66, 311–20.

Eichner, E. R. and Whitfield, C. L. (1981) Splenomegaly: an algorithmic approach to diagnosis. *J. Am. Med. Assoc.*, 246, 2858–61.

El-Khishen, M. A. *et al.* (1985) Splenectomy is contraindicated for thrombocytopenia secondary to portal hypertension. *Surg. Gynecol. Obstet.*, 160, 234–8.

Ellison, E. C. and Fabri, P. J. (1983) Complications of splenectomy: etiology, prevention and management. *Surg. Clin. North Am.*, 63, 1313–30.

Eraklis, A. J. *et al.* (1967) Hazard of overwhelming infection after splenectomy in childhood. *N. Engl. J. Med.*, 276, 1225–9.

Fleming, C. R., Dickson, E. R. and Harrison, E. G. (1976) Splenosis: autotransplantation of splenic tissue. *Am. J. Med.*, 61, 414–19.

Gamble, J. F., Fuller, L. M. and Martin, R. G. (1975) Influence of staging celiotomy in localized presentations of Hodgkin's disease. *Cancer*, 35, 817–25.

Gasparini, M. *et al.* (1976) Laparoscopy in staging and restaging childhood neoplasia. *Proc. Am. Soc. Clin. Oncol.*, 17, 257.

Gill, P. G., Sauter, R. G. and Morris, P. G. (1980) Results of surgical staging in Hodgkin's disease. *Br. J. Surg.*, 67, 478–81.

Gill, P. G., Sauter, R. G. and Morris, P. G. (1981) Splenectomy for hypersplenism in malignant lymphomas. *Br. J. Surg.*, 68, 29–33.

Glatstein, E. *et al.* (1969) The value of laparotomy and splenectomy in the staging of Hodgkin's disease. *Cancer*, 24, 709–18.

Glynn, M. J. (1986) Isolated splenic vein thrombosis. *Arch. Surg.*, 121, 723–5.

Goldman, J. M. *et al.* (1980) Haematological reconstitution after autografting for chronic granulocytic leukemia in transformation: the influence of previous splenectomy. *Br. J. Haematol.*, 45, 223–31.

Goldstone, J. (1978) Splenectomy for massive splenomegaly. *Am. J. Surg.*, 135, 385–8.

Golomb, H. M. (1987) The treatment of hairy cell leukemia. *Blood*, 69, 979–83.

Gomez, G., Hossfeld, D. K. and Sokal, J. E. (1975) Removal of abnormal clone of leukemic cells by splenectomy. *Br. Med. J.*, 2, 421–3.

Gomez, G. A. *et al.* (1976) Splenectomy for palliation of chronic myelocytic leukemia. *Am. J. Med.*, 61, 14–22.

Goonewardene, A. *et al.* (1979) Splenectomy for undiagnosed splenomegaly. *Br. J. Surg.*, 66, 62–5.

Gordon, D. H. *et al.* (1978) Postsplenectomy thrombocytosis: its association with mesenteric, portal, and/or renal vein thrombosis in patients with myeloproliferative disorders. *Arch. Surg.*, 113, 713–15.

Govrin-Yehudain, J. and Bar-Maor, J. A. (1980) Partial splenectomy in Gaucher's disease. *Isr. J. Med. Sci.*, 16, 665–8.

Greco, R. S. and Alvarez, F. E. (1981) Intraportal and intrahepatic splenic autotransplantation. *Surgery*, 90, 535–40.

Green, J. B. *et al.* (1986) Late septic complications in adults after splenectomy for trauma: a prospective analysis in 144 patients. *J. Trauma*, 26, 999–1004.

Grieco, M. B. and Cady, B. (1980) Staging laparotomy in Hodgkin's disease. *Surg. Clin. N. Amer.*, 60, 369–379.

Gruenberg, J. C., Van Slyck, E. J. and Abraham, J. P. (1986) Splenectomy in systemic lupus erythematosus. *Am. Surg.*, 52, 366–70.

Guzzetta, P. C. *et al.* (1987) Operative technique and results of subtotal splenectomy for Gaucher disease. *Surg. Gynecol. Obstet.*, 164, 359–62.

Halpert, B. and Gyorkey, F. (1959) Lesions observed in accessory spleens of 311 patients. *Am. J. Clin. Pathol.*, 32, 165–8.

Hansen, M. S., Christensen, B. E. and Jonsson, V. (1979) The effect of acetylsalicylic acid and dipyridamole on thromboembolic complications in splenectomised patients with myelofibrosis. *Scand. J. Haematol.*, 23, 177–81.

Harrison, B. F., Glanges, E. and Sparkman, R. S. (1977) Gastric fistula following splenectomy: its cause and prevention. *Ann. Surg.*, 185, 210–13.

Hays, D. M. *et al.* (1986) Postsplenectomy sepsis and other complications after staging laparotomy for Hodgkin's disease in childhood. *J. Pediatr. Surg.*, 21, 628–32.

Helton, W. S. *et al.* (1986) The diagnosis and treatment of splenic fungal abscesses in the immunesuppressed patient. *Arch. Surg.*, 121, 580–6.

Hermann, R. E., DeHaven, K. E. and Hawk, W. A. (1968) Splenectomy for the diagnosis of splenomegaly. *Ann. Surg.*, 168, 896–900.

Heyman, M. R. and Walsh, T. J. (1987) Autoimmune neutropenia and Hodgkin's disease. *Cancer*, 59, 1903–5.

Hill, J. B. and Cooper, W. M. (1968) Thrombotic thrombocytopenic purpura: treatment with corticosteroids and splenectomy. *Arch. Intern. Med.*, 122, 353–6.

Hobbs, J. R. *et al.* (1987) Beneficial effect of pretransplant splenectomy on displacement bone marrow transplantation for Gaucher's syndrome. *Lancet*, **ii**, 1111–15.

Hodam, B. P. (1970) The risk of splenectomy. A review of 310 cases. *Am. J. Surg.*, **119**, 709–13.

Hofer, B. O., Ryan, J. A. and Freeny, P. C. (1987) Surgical significance of vascular changes in chronic pancreatitis. *Surg. Gynecol. Obstet.*, **164**, 499–505.

Holmes, F. F. *et al.* (1981) Fulminant meningococcemia after splenectomy. *J. Am. Med. Assoc.*, **246**, 1119–20.

Homan, W. P. and Dineen, P. (1978) The role of splenectomy in the treatment of thrombocytopenic purpura due to systemic lupus erythematosus. *Ann. Surg.*, **187**, 52–6.

Horton, J. *et al.* (1982) The importance of splenic blood flow in clearing pneumococcal organisms. *Ann. Surg..*, **195**, 172–6.

Hunter, R. M. and Shoemaker, W. C. (1957) Rupture of the spleen in pregnancy: a review of the subject and a case report. *Am. J. Obstet. Gynecol.*, **73**, 1326–32.

Ihde, D. C. *et al.* (1976) Splenectomy in the chronic phase of chronic myelogenous leukemia. *Ann. Intern. Med.*, **84**, 17–21.

Irving, M. (1985) Hodgkin's disease: is staging laparotomy necessary? *Br. J. Surg.*, **72**, 589–90.

Jackson, H., Parker, F. and Lemon, N. M. (1940) Agnogenic myeloid metaplasia of the spleen. *N. Engl. J. Med.*, **222**, 985–91.

Jansen, J. and Hermans, J. (1981) Splenectomy in hairy cell leukemia: a retrospective multicenter analysis. *Cancer*, **47**, 2066–76.

Jonasson, O., Spigos, D. G. and Mozes, M. F. (1985) Partial splenic embolisation: experience in 136 patients. *World J. Surg.*, **9**, 461–7.

Joshi, S. N. *et al.* (1980) Complementary use of computerized tomography and technetium scanning in the diagnosis of accessory spleen. *Dig. Dis. Sci.*, **25**, 888–92.

Kamel, R. and Dunn, M. A. (1982) Segmental splenectomy in schistosomiasis. *Br. J. Surg.*, **69**, 311–13.

Kamel, R. *et al.* (1986) Clinical and immunological results of segmental splenectomy in schistosomiasis. *Br. J. Surg.*, **73**, 544–7.

Kaplan, H. S. *et al.* (1973) Staging laparotomy and splenectomy in Hodgkin's disease: analysis of indications and patterns of involvement in 285 consecutive unselected patients. *Nat. Cancer Inst. Monogr.*, **36**, 291–301.

Kidd, W. T. *et al.* (1987) The management of blunt splenic trauma. *J. Trauma*, **27**, 977–9.

Kiesewetter, W. B. (1975) Pediatric splenectomy: indications, technique, complications and mortality. *Surg. Clin. North Am.*, **55**, 449–560.

King, H. and Shumacker, H. B. (1952) Splenic studies: I. Susceptibility to infection after splenectomy performed in infancy. *Ann. Surg.*, **136**, 239–42.

Klein, B. *et al.* (1987) Splenomegaly and solitary spleen metastasis in solid tumors. *Cancer*, **60**, 100–2.

Knudson, P. *et al.* (1982) Splenomegaly without an apparent cause. *Surg. Gynecol. Obstet.*, **155**, 705–8.

Kusminsky, R. E. *et al.* (1982) An omental implantation technique for salvage of the spleen. *Surg. Gynecol. Obstet.*, **155**, 407–9.

Lacey, V. Y. and Penner, J. A. (1977) Management of idiopathic thrombocytopenic purpura in the adult. *Semin. Thromb. Hemost.*, **3**, 160–74.

Lally, K. P. *et al.* (1986) A comparison of staging methods for Hodgkin's disease in children. *Arch. Surg.*, **121**, 1125–7.

Lanzkowsky, P. *et al.* (1976) Staging laparotomy and splenectomy: treatment and complications of Hodgkin's disease in children. *Am. J. Hematol.*, **1**, 393–404.

Lawrie, G. M. and Ham, J. M. (1974) The surgical treatment of hereditary spherocytosis. *Surg. Gynecol. Obstet.*, **139**, 208–10.

Lehman, H. A. *et al.* (1987) Complement-mediated autoimmune thrombocytopenia. Monoclonal IgM antiplatelet antibody associated with lymphoreticular malignant disease. *N. Engl. J. Med.*, **316**, 194–8.

Lerner, R. M. and Spataro, R. F. (1984) Splenic abscess: percutaneous drainage. *Radiology*, **153**, 643–5.

Levy, J. M., Wasserman, P. and Pitha, N. (1979) Presplenectomy transcatheter occlusion of the splenic artery. *Arch. Surg.*, **114**, 198–9.

Liu, E. T., Linker, C. A. and Shuman, M. A. (1986) Management of treatment failures in thrombotic thrombocytopenic purpura. *Am. J. Hematol.*, **23**, 347–61.

Livingston, C. D., Levine, B. A. and Sirinek, K. R. (1983) Improved survival rate for intraperitoneal autotransplantation of the spleen after pneumococcal pneumonia. *Surg. Gynecol. Obstet.*, **156**, 761–6.

Long, J. C. and Aisenberg, A. A. (1974) Malignant lymphoma diagnosed at splenectomy and idiopathic splenomegaly. *Cancer*, **33**, 1054–61.

Lum, L. G. *et al.* (1980) Splenectomy in the management of the thrombocytopenia of the Wiskott-Aldrich syndrome. *N. Engl. J. Med.*, **302**, 892–6.

Luna, G. K. and Dellinger, E. P. (1987) Nonoperative observation treatment for splenic injuries: a safe therapeutic option? *Am. J. Surg.*, **153**, 462–8.

Ly, B. and Albrechtsen, D. (1981) Therapeutic splenectomy in hematologic disorders. *Acta Med. Scand.*, **209**, 21–9.

Maddison, F. E. (1973) Embolic therapy of hypersplenism. *Invest. Radiol.*, **8**, 280–1.

Malmaeus, J. *et al.* (1986) Early postoperative course following elective splenectomy in haematological diseases: a high complication rate in patients with myeloproliferative disorders. *Br. J. Surg.*, **73**, 720–3.

Mann, J. L., Hafez, G. R. and Longo, W. L. (1986) Role of the spleen in the transdiaphragmatic spread of Hodgkin's disease. *Am. J. Med.*, **81**, 959–61.

Martin, J. W. (1958) Congenital splenic cysts. *Am. J. Surg.*, **96**, 302–8.

McBride, C. M. and Hester, P. J. (1977) Chronic myelogenous leukemia: management of splenectomy in a high-risk population. *Cancer*, **39**, 653–8.

Mitchell, A. and Morris, P. J. (1985) Splenectomy for malignant lymphomas. *World J. Surg.*, **9**, 444–8.

Moore, G. E. *et al.* (1983) Failure of splenic implants to protect against fatal postsplenectomy infection. *Am. J. Surg.*, **146**, 413–14.

Morgenstern, K., Kahn, F. H. and Weinstein, I. M. (1966) Subtotal splenectomy in myelofibrosis. *Surgery*, **60**, 336–9.

Morgenstern, L., Rosenberg, J. and Geller, S. A. (1985) Tumors of the spleen. *World J. Surg.*, **9**, 468–76.

Morgenstern, L. and Shapiro, S. J. (1980) Partial splenectomy for nonparasitic splenic cysts. *Am. J. Surg.*, **139**, 278–81.

Morgenstern, L. *et al.* (1984) Hamartomas of the spleen. *Arch. Surg.*, **119**, 1291–3.

Morris, D. H. and Bullock, F. D. (1919) The importance of the spleen in resistance to infection. *Ann. Surg.*, **70**, 513–21.

Mower, W. R., Hawkins, J. A. and Nelson, E. W. (1986) Postsplenectomy infection in patients with chronic leukemia. *Am. J. Surg.*, **152**, 583–6.

Mozes, M. F. *et al.* (1984) Partial splenic embolization an alternative to splenectomy – results of a prospective randomized study. *Surgery*, **96**, 694–702.

Mucha, P., Daly, R. C. and Farnell, M. B. (1986) Selective management of blunt splenic trauma. *J. Trauma*, **26**, 970–9.

Mulder, H., Steenberger, J. and Haanen, C. (1977) Clinical course and survival after elective splenectomy in 19 patients with primary myelofibrosis. *Br. J. Haematol.*, **35**, 419–27.

Musser, G. *et al.* (1984) Splenectomy for hematologic disease: the UCLA experience with 306 patients. *Ann. Surg.*, **200**, 40–5.

Myers, T. J. *et al.* (1980) Thrombotic thrombocytopenic purpura: combined treatment with plasmapheresis and antiplatelet agents. *Ann. Intern. Med.*, **92**, 149–55.

Nallathambi, M. N. *et al.* (1987) Pyogenic splenic abscess in intravenous drug addiction. *Am. Surg.*, **53**, 342–6.

NIH Conference (1977) Pathophysiology of immune hemolytic anemia. *Ann. Intern. Med.*, **87**, 210–22.

Nishiyama, T. *et al.* (1986) Splenic vein thrombosis as a consequence of chronic pancreatitis: a study of three cases. *Am. J. Gastroenterol.*, **81**, 1193–8.

O'Keefe, J. H. *et al.* (1986) Thromboembolic splenic infarction. *Mayo Clin. Proc.*, **61**, 967–72.

Olsen, W. R. and Beaudoin, D. E. (1969) Wound drainage after splenectomy: indications and complications. *Am. J. Surg.*, **117**, 615–20.

O'Neal, B. J. and McDonald, J. C. (1981) The risk of sepsis in the asplenic adult. *Ann. Surg.*, **194**, 775–8.

O'Neill, J. A. *et al.* (1968) The role of splenectomy in Felty's syndrome. *Ann. Surg.*, **167**, 81–4.

Pabst, R. and Kamran, D. (1986) Autotransplantation of splenic tissue. *J. Pediatr. Surg.*, **21**, 120–4.

Pearson, H. A. *et al.* (1978) The born-again spleen: return of splenic function after splenectomy for trauma. *N. Engl. J. Med.*, **298**, 1389–92.

Pegourie, B. *et al.* (1987) Splenectomy during chronic lymphocytic leukemia. *Cancer*, **59**, 1626–30.

Peters, T. G. *et al.* (1977) Antithrombin III deficiency causing postsplenectomy mesenteric venous thrombosis coincident with thrombocytopenia. *Ann. Surg.*, **185**, 229–31.

Picozzi, V. J., Roeske, W. R. and Creger, W. P. (1980) Fate of therapy failures in acute idiopathic thrombocytopenic purpura. *Am. J. Med.*, **69**, 690–4.

Politis, C. *et al.* (1987) Partial splenic embolisation for hypersplenism of thalassaemia major: five year follow up. *Br. Med. J.*, **294**, 665–7.

Ravindranath, Y. and Beutler, E. (1987) Two new variants of glucose-6-phosphate dehydrogenase associated with hereditary non-spherocytic hemolytic anemia. *Am. J. Hematol.*, **24**, 357–63.

Ries, C. A. and Price, D. C. (1974) ^{51}Cr platelet kinetics in thrombocytopenia. *Ann. Intern. Med.*, **80**, 702–7.

Riley, S. M. and Aldrete, J. S. (1975) The role of

splenectomy in Felty's syndrome. *Am. J. Surg.*, **130**, 51–2.

Robertson, D. A. F., Simpson, F. G. and Losowsky, M. S. (1981) Blood viscosity after splenectomy. *Br. Med. J.*, **283**, 573–5.

Roder, O. C. (1984) Splenic vein thrombosis with bleeding gastro-oesophageal varices. Reports of two splenectomised cases and review of the literature. *Acta Chir. Scand.*, **150**, 265–8.

Rodgers, B. M., Tribble, C. and Joob, A. (1987) Partial splenectomy for Gaucher's disease. *Ann. Surg.*, **205**, 693–9.

Rodigas, P. *et al.* (1981) Early splenectomy in chronic myelogenous leukemia: surgical aspects. *Am. Surg.*, **47**, 219–23.

Rowe, J. M. *et al.* (1985) Thrombotic thrombocytopenic purpura recovery after splenectomy associated with persistence of abnormally large von Willebrand factor multimers. *Am. J. Hematol.*, **20**, 161–8.

Rubin, M. *et al.* (1986) Partial splenectomy in Gaucher's disease. *J. Pediatr. Surg.*, **21**, 125–8.

Ruderman, M., Miller, L. M. and Pinals, R. S. (1968) Clinical and serologic observations on 27 patients with Felty's syndrome. *Arthritis Rheum.*, **11**, 377–84.

Salter, P. P. and Sherlock, E. C. (1957) Splenectomy, thrombocytosis and venous thrombosis. *Ann. Surg.*, **23**, 549–54.

Sands, M., Page, D. and Brown, R. B. (1986) Splenic abscess after nonoperative management of splenic rupture. *J. Pediatr. Surg.*, **21**, 900–1.

Sarr, M. G. and Zuidema, G. D. (1982) Splenic abscess: presentation, diagnosis, and treatment. *Surgery*, **92**, 480–5.

Scher, K. S., Wroczynski, A. F. and Scott-Conner, C. E. H. (1985) Intraperitoneal splenic implants do not alter clearance of pneumococcal bacteremia. *Am. Surg.*, **51**, 269–71.

Schneider, P. A. *et al.* (1985) The role of splenectomy in the multimodality treatment of thrombotic thrombocytopenic purpura. *Ann. Surg.*, **202**, 318–322.

Schneider, P. A. *et al.* (1987) Immunodeficiency-associated thrombocytopenic purpura (IDTP). *Arch. Surg.*, **122**, 1175–8.

Schwartz, S. I., Adams, J. T. and Bauman, A. W. (1971) Splenectomy for hematologic disorders. *Curr. Prob. Surg.*, **8**, 1–57.

Schwartz, S. I., Hoepp, L. M. and Sachs, S. (1980) Splenectomy for thrombocytopenia. *Surgery*, **88**, 497–506.

Schwartz, S. I. *et al.* (1981) Splenectomy for hematologic disease. *Surg. clin. North Am.*, **61**, 117–25.

Schwartz, S. I. (1985) Splenectomy for thrombocytopenia. *World J. Surg.*, **9**, 419–21.

Seufert, R. and Mitrou, P. (1985) *The Surgery of the Spleen* (H. A. Reber, translator). Theime, New York.

Sherman, R. (1984) Management of trauma to the spleen. in *Advances in Surgery*, Volume 17 (ed. G. T. Shires), Yearbook Medical Publishers, Chicago. pp. 37–71.

Simpson, J. N. L. (1980) Solitary abscess of the spleen. *Br. J. Surg.*, **67**, 106–10.

Sirinek, K. R. and Evans, W. E. (1973) Nonparasitic splenic cysts: case report of epidermoid cyst with review of the literature. *Am. J. Surg.*, **126**, 8–13.

Skootsky, S. A., Rosove, M. H. and Langley, M. B. (1986) Immune thrombocytopenia and response to splenectomy in chronic liver disease. *Arch. Intern. Med.*, **146**, 555–7.

Smith, C. H. *et al.* (1964) Postsplenectomy infection in Cooley's anemia. *Ann. NY Acad. Sci.*, **119**, 748–57.

Solanki, D. L., Kletter, G. G. and Castro, O. (1986) Acute splenic sequestration crises in adults with sickle cell disease. *Am. J. Med.*, **80**, 985–90.

Soper, N. J. and Rikkers, L. F. (1982) Effect of operations for variceal hemorrhage on hypersplenism. *Am. J. Surg.*, **144**, 700–3.

Sordillo, E. M., Sordillo, P. P. and Hajdu, S. I. (1981) Primary hemangiosarcoma of the spleen: report of four cases. *Med. Pediatr. Oncol.*, **9**, 319–24.

Spier, C. M. *et al.* (1985) Malignant lymphoma with primary presentation in the spleen. *Arch. Pathol. Lab. Med.*, **109**, 1076–80.

Spigos, D. G. *et al.* (1979) Partial splenic embolization in the treatment of hypersplenism. *Am. J. Roentgenol.*, **132**, 777–82.

Splenic Injury Study Group (1987) Splenic injury: a prospective multicentre study on non-operative and operative treatment. *Br. J. Surg.*, **74**, 310–13.

Stanley, J. C. and Fry, W. J. (1974) Pathogenesis and clinical significance of splenic artery aneurysms. *Surgery*, **76**, 898–909.

Stein, R. S. *et al.* (1987) Splenectomy for end-stage chronic lymphocytic leukemia. *Cancer*, **59**, 1815–18.

Studemeister, A. E., Beilke, M. A. and Kirmani, N. (1987) Splenic abscess due to *Clostridium difficile* and *Pseudomonas paucimobilis*. *Am. J. Gastroenterol.*, **82**, 389–90.

Talarico, L. *et al.* (1987) Late postsplenectomy recurrence of thrombotic thrombocytopenic purpura responding to removal of accessory spleen. *Am. J. Med.*, **82**, 845–8.

Taylor, M. A., Kaplan, H. S. and Nelsen, T. S. (1985)

Staging laparotomy with splenectomy for Hodgkin's disease: the Stanford experience. *World J. Surg.*, 9, 449–60.

Thanopoulos, B. D. and Frimas, C. A. (1982) Partial splenic embolisation in the management of hypersplenism secondary to Gaucher disease. *J. Pediatr.*, 101, 740–3.

Thompson, H. W. and McCarthy, L. J. (1983) Thrombotic thrombocytopenic purpura: potential benefit of splenectomy after plasma exchange. *Arch. Intern. Med.*, 143, 2117–19.

Topley, J. M. *et al.* (1981) Acute splenic sequestration and hypersplenism in the first five years in homozygous sickle cell disease. *Arch. Dis. Child.*, 56, 765–9.

Towell, B. L. and Levine, S. P. (1987) Massive hepatomegaly following splenectomy for myeloid metaplasia. *Am. J. Med.*, 82, 371–5.

Traetow, W. D., Fabri, P. J. and Carey, L. C. (1980) Changing indications for splenectomy: 30 years' experience. *Arch. Surg.*, 115, 447–51.

Trastek, V. F. *et al.* (1982) Splenic artery aneurysms. *Surgery*, 91, 694–9.

Ugochukwu, A. I. and Irving, M. (1985) Intraperitoneal low-pressure suction drainage following splenectomy. *Br. J. Surg.*, 72, 247–8.

Van Norman, A. S. *et al.* (1986) Splenectomy for hairy cell leukemia: a clinical review of 63 patients. *Cancer*, 57, 644–8.

Verheyden, C. N. *et al.* (1978) Accessory splenectomy in the management of recurrent idiopathic thrombocytopenic purpura. *Mayo Clin. Proc.*, 53, 442–6.

Wallace, D., Fromm, D. and Thomas, D. (1982) Accessory splenectomy for idiopathic thrombocytopenic purpura. *Surgery*, 91, 134–6.

Walsh, C. *et al.* (1985) Thrombocytopenia in homosexual patients: prognosis, response to therapy, and prevalence of antibody to the retrovirus associated with the acquired immunodeficiency syndrome. *Ann. Intern. Med.*, 103, 542–5.

Weiden, P. L. and Blaese, R. M. (1972) Hereditary thrombocytopenia: relation to Wiskott–Aldrich syndrome with special reference to splenectomy. *J. Pediatr.*, 80, 226–34.

Wheeler, W. E. and Hardy, J. D. (1986) Splenectomy: acute infectious complications. *South. Med. J.*, 79s, 64.

Wick, M. R. and Rife, C. C. (1981) Paratesticular accessory spleen. *Mayo Clin. Proc.*, 56, 455–6.

Williams, S. F. and Golomb, H. M. (1986) Perspective on staging approaches in the malignant lymphomas. *Surg. Gynecol. Obstet.*, 163, 193–201.

Willis, B. K., Deitch, E. A. and McDonald, J. C. (1986) The influence of trauma to the spleen on postoperative complications and mortality. *J. Trauma*, 26, 1073–6.

Wilson, R. E. *et al.* (1985) Splenectomy for myeloproliferative disorders. *World J. Surg.*, 9, 431–6.

Witte, C. L. *et al.* (1982) Ischaemia and partial resection for control of splenic hyperfunction. *Br. J. Surg.*, 69, 531–5.

Wobbes, T., Van der Sluis, R. F. and Lubbers, E.-J. C. (1984) Removal of the massive spleen: a surgical risk? *Am. J. Surg.*, 147, 800–2.

Wolf, D. J., Silver, R. T. and Coleman, M. (1978) Splenectomy in chronic myeloid leukemia. *Ann. Intern. Med.*, 89, 684–9.

Yoshioka, H. *et al.* (1985) Splenic embolization for hypersplenism using steel coils. *Am. J. Radiol.*, 144, 1269–74.

Zamora, J. U. and Halpern, N. B. (1987) Splenectomy for metastatic neoplasms. *South. Med. J.*, 80, 80S.

INDEX